INTERNATIONAL ENCYCLOPEDIA OF PHARMACOLOGY AND THERAPEUTICS

Sponsored by the International Union of Pharmacology (IUPHAR)

(Chairman: B. UVNÄS, Stockholm)

Executive Editor: G. PETERS, Lausanne

Section 78

RADIONUCLIDES IN PHARMACOLOGY

Section Editor

Y. COHEN

Gif-sur-Yvette

VOLUME I

INTERNATIONAL ENCYCLOPEDIA OF
PHARMACOLOGY AND THERAPEUTICS

Radionuclides in Pharmacology

VOLUME I

CONTRIBUTORS

L-E. APPELGREN

L. BUGNARD

J. R. CATCH

Y. COHEN

J. GLENN

L. HAMMARSTROM

J. INGRAND

J. F. LAMB

R. E. MCCAMAN

E. RICCI

J. S. ROBERTSON

U. ROSA

H. H. ROSS

J. C. STOCLET

S. ULLBERG

M. M. WINBURY

PERGAMON PRESS

OXFORD · NEW YORK · TORONTO
SYDNEY · BRAUNSCHWEIG

Pergamon Press Ltd., Headington Hill Hall, Oxford

Pergamon Press Inc., Maxwell House, Fairview Park, Elmsford,
New York 10523

Pergamon of Canada Ltd., 207 Queen's Quay West, Toronto 1

Pergamon Press (Aust.) Pty. Ltd., 19a Boundary Street,
Rushcutters Bay, N.S.W. 2011, Australia

Vieweg & Sohn GmbH, Burgplatz 1, Braunschweig

First edition 1971

Library of Congress Catalog Card No. 77-133090

Printed in Great Britain by A. Wheaton & Co., Exeter

08 016152 9

CONTENTS

CONTENTS OF VOLUME II

LIST OF CONTRIBUTORS

APPELGREN, LARS-ERIK, Department of Pharmacology, Royal Veterinary College, Stockholm, Sweden.

BUGNARD, LOUIS, Head of the Department of Biophysics, C.H.U. St. Antoine, University of Paris, Paris, France.

CATCH, J. R., The Radiochemical Centre, Amersham, Buckinghamshire, England.

COHEN, YVES, Departement des Radioéléments, Centre d'Études Nucleaires de Saclay, B.P. No. 2, 91-Gif-sur-Yvette, France.

GLENN, HOWARD J., Specialist, Radiopharmaceutical Medicine, Abbott Laboratories, North Chicago, Illinois, U.S.A.

HAMMARSTROM, LARS, Department of Pharmacology, Royal Veterinary College, Stockholm, Sweden.

INGRAND, J., Laboratoire de Physique Medicale, Faculte de Medecine-Cochin, Rue Faubourg St Jacques, Paris 14ᵉ, France.

LAMB, J. F., Department of Physiology, University of St. Andrews, Fife, Scotland.

MCCAMAN, R. E., Section of Cellular Microchemistry, Division of Neurosciences, City of Hope Medical Center, Duarte, California, U.S.A.

RICCI, ENZO, Analytical Chemistry Division, Oak Ridge National Laboratory, Oak Ridge, Tennessee, U.S.A.

ROBERTSON, JAMES S., Medical Physics Division, Medical Research Center, Brookhaven National Laboratory, Upton, New York, U.S.A.

ROSA, U., S.O.R.I.N., Saluggia, Italy.

ROSS, H. H., Analytical Chemistry Division, Oak Ridge National Laboratory, Oak Ridge, Tennessee, U.S.A.

STOCLET, J. C., Pharmacodynamics Laboratory, Faculty of Pharmacy, University of Strasbourg, Strasbourg, France.

ULLBERG, SVEN, Department of Pharmacology, Royal Veterinary College, Stockholm, Sweden.

WINBURY, MARTIN M., Department of Pharmacology, Warner-Lambert Research Institute, Morris Plains, New Jersey, U.S.A.

ix

PREFACE

THE reader may be surprised that an entire section has been devoted to "Radionuclides in Pharmacology", since it deals with a particular experimental method rather than with a class of drugs, as in the case of other sections. Thus the use of radioisotopes has created a category which interconnects physics, chemistry, and biology, and which has a humanitarian objective: the development of new drugs. The isotopists are specially trained; and, in the case of pharmacologists, they have followed a course of instruction in mathematics, physics, and advanced nuclear chemistry. The laboratory of the radiopharmacologist resembles that of the radiochemist more than it does the classical pharmacological laboratory. The possible health hazard makes it necessary to take special precautions while handling the radioactive substances used, which are classified as very toxic, toxic, or weakly toxic. These are concepts familiar in a nuclear research center, but less so in a pharmacology department.

Radiopharmacology has evolved its own individual character determined by such contingencies, methods of thinking, and techniques as have spontaneously occurred.

When, in the autumn of 1965, Professor Peters asked me to act as editor for this section, I hesitated before the size of the task, the diversity of subjects to cover, and the difficulty of bringing such a venture to a successful conclusion.

On this day in December 1968, when I write the final pages of the section, I am able to measure the distance traveled, the obstacles overcome, and the fatigue left behind. On reflection, I owe the successful completion of the work to the fact that I have personally met all but two of the authors, and that I discussed their plans with them, both at the beginning and on a number of occasions during the writing of their contributions. This direct contact, both at the beginning and during the course of the work, has been very fruitful, and has prevented misunderstandings, unnecessary repetition, and lack of unity. However, the "pilgrim's staff", or rather the "jet liner" which is necessary for such an undertaking, requires a continental and intercontinental mobility comparable to that of the commuter.

The authors whom I approached are eminent specialists in the subjects they covered: often having contributed already to the preparation of international scientific works, they were already familiar with teamwork. In general, the invitations to take part in this work met with favorable responses. The rare refusals were due to work on a book already in preparation and were accompanied by suggestions for alternative authors. The one abandonment during the work is to be deplored.

Happily no difficulty arose, but the effort demanded a constant determination to succeed in spite of the delays, the multiplicity of languages of the original manuscripts, and the need to place in a homogenous form all the paragraphs and chapters.

Because of the abundance of the material, the reader is presented with two volumes. In the first volume he will be able to enter the fields of physics and nuclear chemistry presented in a form which can be assimilated by the student or the non-specialist scientist. He will become familiar with modern mathematical methods which will allow him to understand the theories of compartments.

In the second volume he will find the pharmacological application presented in a form more specialized and more specific to the subject of the work. It is suggested that he start with the first chapters, but frequent cross-references from one chapter to another will make the reading of the two volumes independent. The clinician will come across the moral and ethical problems arising from the use of radioisotopes in man. The pharmacologist will be introduced to the problems of health physics.

The bibliography at the end of each chapter brings together a considerable number of references. These references, which include the complete title of the works quoted, are a mine of information never previously achieved in a work of this type. Carefully prepared, they have been frequently checked: however, their large number has made it impossible to check each one individually, and thus a guarantee of complete freedom from error cannot be given.

The illustrations are usually original and often come from well-known centers of nuclear research.

Before concluding this preface I should like to thank the individual authors for their enthusiastic and efficient collaboration, for their patience, and for the firmness of their intention.

I would like to express my gratitude to Professor Louis Bugnard, Director of Health Biology, who encouraged me in this project, who followed its development, and who has kindly written the Foreword.

I would also like respectfully to thank M. Henri Piatier, Directeur des

Materiaux et Combustibles Nucléaires, and M. Charlie Fisher, Chef du Département des Radioéléments, who authorized this undertaking.

This work would not have been possible without the collaboration of the staff of the laboratories of the Faculty of Pharmacy of the University of Paris and of the Center for Nuclear Studies at Saclay, and without the efficient help of Mrs. Rose-Marie Rolland of the Secretariat: to each and all I present my sincere thanks.

I hope my children will excuse the Sundays and the not less numerous evenings when I could not be with them.

To my wife, valuable and devoted collaborator, I dedicate my contribution to this work.

Finally, may I, as a Frenchman, hope that this work may rapidly become accessible to French-speaking pharmacologists, physicians and scientists.

Saclay YVES COHEN

FOREWORD

Professsor Louis Bugnard, M.D..

Head of the Department of Biophysics,
C.H.U. Saint Antoine, University of Paris

RADIATIONS emitted by naturally occurring radioactive substances (generally radium) and by X-rays have been used in diagnosis and therapy since the beginning of the century and have been an important factor in the advancement of medicine. The rapid progress in nuclear physics since 1930 has placed at the disposal of the biological and medical sciences new means of understanding the elementary processes of life and of benefiting man. They have aroused the interest of research workers, and have led to particularly desirable and useful collaboration between workers throughout the world, specialists in the most diverse branches of science—physicists, chemists, biophysicists, physiologists, pharmacologists, and physicians.

There are numerous works dealing with the use of radioactive elements in biology, particularly their use in the treatment of certain conditions, notably cancer. There are also numerous books dealing with the use of radioisotopes by the clinician. Their use as tracers, recognized by F. Joliot and R. Courrier, was the starting point of a very fruitful method of studying function. For these functional studies the radioelement chosen will depend, firstly, on its chemical properties, which will determine its distribution in the body; and, secondly, on its physical properties, which will determine its radioactive half-life and the type of radiation emitted. The number of radioisotopes at present available is very large, there being one for almost every known element. They are usually used in laboratory studies and in animal experiments. However, a fairly large proportion may be used for studies in man, and some have been available in pharmaceutical form for a number of years. In the early days they were available in oral or parenteral form, and were packaged in small bottles or containers like those used for other drugs such as penicillin. However, pharmaceutical companies have since set up special radioisotope departments whose aim is the development of new usable nuclides.

The work of those university laboratories dealing with radioactivity, and the realization by the pharmaceutical industry of the importance and value of radioactive elements, has led to the development of a new discipline with its own special features.

This explains the emergence on an international scale of this, the first work dealing with the utilization of radioisotopes in pharmacology. These articles are prepared with a didactic object: they are not merely the proceedings of a symposium. This section of the *International Encyclopedia of Pharmacology and Therapeutics* is intended for the pharmacologist who is not a specialist in the use of radioisotopes; and, beginning with the fundamentals of nuclear physics and chemistry, it leads to an understanding of its final conclusions, and the means of attaining them, as well as an understanding of interesting developments in various sections of pharmacology. Thus in this new field of nuclear medicine there exists a nuclear pharmacology and a nuclear therapy.

Professor Y. Cohen, the editor of this section, with whom I have had frequent contact since the beginning of his project, conceived a work divided into sections dealing with those areas where radiopharmacology (to use the current term) has already created interest.

After summarizing the basic physical and chemical principles and the methods available to detect ionizing radiations, the methods of preparing labeled molecules which are to be used as tracers in pharmacological studies are explained. In order to use tracers correctly, the pharmacologist must be aware of their stability and the strength of the binding of the radioisotope to the molecule carrying it. Using this knowledge he can, by measuring the emitted radiation and by studying the pathway and distribution of an element or molecule in the body, draw valid biological and pharmacological conclusions.

This is followed by a discussion of methods adapted from biochemistry and histology which are in general use. One comes across these methods both in metabolic studies and in therapeutic investigations, and it was therefore difficult to categorize them.

Special care has been taken with the kinetic aspects. Tracer elements are especially valuable in the study of this particular characteristic of living matter. The importance attributed to this problem is indicated by the choice of collaborators—mathematicians, physiologists, and pharmacologists. The kinetics of molecules and atoms is of fundamental importance to the understanding of the mechanism of action of drugs. The movement of ions and their distribution in the cellular medium, as well as changes in the properties of membranes that limit the movement of ions, are important to the understanding of the type and mechanism of pharmacological action that can occur. Special problems, such as drug metabolism, the permeability of the blood–brain barrier, cutaneous permeability, and the passage of drugs across the placenta, are treated separately. This selection has been determined by the quality of the results already obtained and the projects currently being developed.

Chemotherapy and the study of the metabolism of drugs has already derived considerable benefit from the use of radioactive tracers. More can still be expected. Two important sections have been devoted to the results already obtained. These interesting results cannot but persuade pharmacologists to use further the techniques described.

The last two chapters of this survey deal with the human aspects. The use of radioisotopes in man can incur both somatic and genetic risks which need major attention. This risk has already been studied on an international scale with particular reference to the distribution of weak doses of radiation which cause trouble especially when radioisotopes are used in radioactivation analysis. As long as one takes account of the correct choice of substance administered, the quantity of radioactivity introduced, and the speed of elimination, then the advantages to pharmacology already gained from the use of radioactive elements—advantages which must increase in the future—justify their use.

One cannot deny the value of using isotopes in diagnosis and for specific therapeutic purposes, nor the use of tracer elements in healthy man, to study the metabolism or the duration of action of a drug that has previously been studied only *in vitro* and in experimental animals. Nevertheless, one cannot allow the use of radioisotopes in clinical pharmacology without close control and severe limitations.

The clinical pharmacologist using radioisotopes must display a competence beyond criticism. A considerable amount of work has already been done on the technical aspects of studying the distribution of tracer elements in the body by means of scintillation counters and scintillation scanning methods. These techniques permit a considerable reduction in the dose of radiation received by the subject—for example, in a study of the absorption, distribution, and elimination of a labeled drug in relation to its therapeutic effect. Of course, the reduction in radiation dose applies not only to the subject but also to the scientific and medical staff involved.

The risks involved in exposure to ionizing radiations are outlined in a separate chapter which includes a thorough discussion of basic organization in any laboratory dealing with radioactive elements. The author has special experience in this field, which forms a sound basis for the facts discussed and makes them especially interesting.

The two volumes which form Section 78 of the *International Encyclopedia* finish, as previously mentioned, with an example based on everyday experience. The authors who have collaborated in the formation of the section have all had the privilege of living with the science which they are explaining. Their discussion is based on their own experience. They are members of that scientific élite created after the explosive birth of nuclear physics some 35 years ago, and they are unquestionably an international team. The team is united by friendships formed during international meetings and deepened by subsequent collaborations, and illustrate the splendid results of the efforts of numerous international bodies: the International Atomic Energy Agency (I.A.E.A.); the World Health Organization (W.H.O.); and the United Nations Economic Social and Cultural Organization (U.N.E.S.C.O.). The results of their present work and the promise of the future are certain to open new fields for research involving the use of radioactive elements in biology, pharmacology, and medicine, fields that are far from being fully explored. The tool provided by the use of radioactive tracers is a powerful and very effective one. As the diversity of authors of this section indicates, this requires the collaboration of research workers of widely differing disciplines whose theoretical and practical knowledge is very wide. They have accepted with enthusiasm the teamwork and discipline that this requires, with security given prime importance.

This instructive work should encourage the regular meeting of groups of workers interested in the problems of radiopharmacology; and it should stimulate creative efforts in a field concerned entirely with the wellbeing of man. The dynamic nature of this new science will, as I predicted in 1953, increase. The progress already achieved is very surprising, and it is likely that aspects different from those known at present will soon appear. Certainly it will retain the active and productive youthfulness which is at present its distinctive feature.

Subsection I

RADIOISOTOPIC METHODOLOGY
AND RADIOACTIVE TRACERS

International Encyclopedia of Pharmacology and Therapeutics
Section 78: Radionuclides in Pharmacology, vol. 1

Section Editor YVES COHEN

ERRATA

p. 440, line 23,   *for* C(ml/g min) per   *read* C(ml/g per min)

p. 499, Fig. caption, line 5,   *for* $(Z = C_1 e^{-k_i t})$ *read* $(Z = C_1 e^{-k_1 t})$

line 7,   *for* $(y - z = C_1 e^{-k_2 t})$ *read* $(y - z = C_2 e^{-k_2 t})$

line 8,   *for* $(y = C_2 e^{-k_2 t} + C_2 e^{-k_1 t})$ *read* $(y = C_1 e^{-k_1 t} + C_2 e^{-k_2 t})$

p. 529, under Iodine 131, last column,   *insert arrow to read*: $^{130}\text{Te}(n,\gamma)\ ^{131}\text{Te} \xrightarrow[25m]{\beta}\ ^{131}\text{I}$

$$\text{U}(n,f)\ ^{131}\text{Te} \nearrow$$

CHAPTER 1

THE PLACE OF RADIONUCLIDES
IN PHARMACOLOGY

Y. Cohen

Center for Nuclear Studies, Saclay, and University of Paris

1. SUMMARY OF THE MAJOR STEPS IN THE
DEVELOPMENT OF RADIOPHARMACOLOGY

THE progress of science has both a continuous and a discontinuous aspect. Its continuous aspect is the individual effort of innumerable scientists working in many laboratories who build a springboard from which a small number of scientists are able to make science leap from one orbit to another: the discontinuous aspect consists of that leap, which results in the creation of new means of research, of a new scientific philosophy, and often of a new doctrine and a new discipline.

The discovery of artificial radioactivity by Irène Curie and Frédéric Joliot (1934) is an example of such a discontinuity rich in potential energy, in original theories, and in new facts.

The extent of the impact produced by this discovery are incompletely appreciated even to this day. The repercussions on the progress of pharmacology have led the Editorial Board of the *International Encyclopedia of Pharmacology and Therapeutics* to devote an entire section to the presentation of the results and the hypotheses produced by these new scientific methods. It is thus that "radiopharmacology" is born with its own character and its own theories and methods.

Some two decades elapsed between the discovery of M. and Mme Joliot Curie and the first use by a pharmacologist of a radioactively labeled drug. Then in 1948 Geiling and his colleagues, working not far from the site of the first nuclear reactor in the world, synthetized by biological means digitoxin labeled with carbon-14.

At the same time Roth and his colleagues (1948) studied the metabolism in the mouse of nicotinic acid and nicotinamide labeled with

3

carbon-14. In this case the compounds were prepared by chemical synthesis (Murray *et al.*, 1947). Already the two major methods for the preparation of labeled drugs were outlined: chemical synthesis and biosynthesis.

Shortly afterwards the metabolism of a drug both in man (Okita *et al.*, 1955b) and in experimental animals had been studied, and the scientific methods, widely used at the present time, were already created.

The basic principles for the study of drug metabolism thus erected included:

   (i) detection of the labeled molecule in the blood, the urine, and the feces;

  (ii) determination of the radioactivity in these materials;

 (iii) identification of the molecule carrying the radioactivity ("radio-phore"), and measurement of its concentration;

 (iv) quantitative determination of the radioactivity in the tissues of the animal;

  (v) establishment of a model of the distribution in the organism.

Pharmacologists have taken up these principles and applied them to a large number of drugs. The techniques of analysis have obviously improved both by simplification and by increased precision. Present-day counting equipment, such as liquid scintillation, and multichannel analysis, increase the experimental data, and provide every experiment with a rich harvest of results. Completely automated equipment provides the data in a form immediately usable by the experimenter.

Another approach was started by the work of Niepce de Saint Victor (1867), Henri Becquerel (1896), and Lacassagne (1924), and this led to autoradiography—that is to say, the detection of radioactivity by its effect on a photographic plate. Autoradiography was rapidly taken up by biologists (Boyd, 1955), but was used by pharmacologists only after the work of Ullberg (1954), who developed whole-body autoradiography to study the distribution of ^{35}S-penicillin in the mouse. Whole-body autoradiography gives an immediate picture of the distribution of a radionuclide* in the body. The next step is the application of autoradiography to the study of the distribution of a drug within the cell—that is, autoradiography with the electron microscope (Rogers, 1967).

Finally, the combination of tracer methods with techniques of electronic calculation will, it is hoped, lead to a better knowledge of the distri-

---

  * In this chapter the terms radioelement, radionuclide, and radioisotope are taken as being synonymous.

bution and fate of pharmacological substances in the living organism. Garrett (1960) has used an analog computer, while Nodine (1964) has worked with a digital computer.

The development of the peaceful applications of nuclear energy in biology, and particularly in pharmacology, has been marked by a number of international conferences. Among these were the three United Nations conferences at Geneva (1955, 1958, and 1964); the Unesco conference in Paris (1957); the symposium at the University of Chicago (1964); and the meeting of the University of Geneva (1967).

Until 1945, artificial radioisotopes could only be obtained from large cyclotrons or by use of the weak neutron sources available in some laboratories. Only a few workers had access to radioisotopes, and then only in small quantities.

Since the discovery of the fission of uranium, numerous atomic reactors have made available to pharmacologists dozens of radioisotopes. These may be valuable to the pharmacologists by virtue of the energy of the radiation, their radioactive half-life, or by the possibility of introducing them in a biological molecule, physiological transmitter, vitamin, hormone, etc.

The first deliveries of radioisotopes were made by the Oak-Ridge National Laboratory of the United States Atomic Energy Commission, by the Atomic Energy Research Establishment at Harwell, by the Radiochemical Centre of Amersham in England, and by the Center for Nuclear Studies at Saclay, of the French Atomic Energy Commission. At the present time radioisotopes and labeled molecules are provided by numerous national nuclear centers as well as private companies. The names and addresses of suppliers of radioisotopes and labeled molecules are listed in the *Isotope Index 1967* (Sommerville, 1967).

Pharmaceutical companies now have the necessary equipment so that all new drugs worthy of therapeutic interest are labeled, their metabolism studied, and the kinetics of their distribution throughout the body calculated. These studies have given rise to a new branch of pharmacology, the so-called "pharmacokinetics", which deals with compartmental analysis.

In addition, the mechanism of action at the biochemical level of new therapeutic agents may be elucidated by the use of labeled molecules which are incorporated in normal physiological cycles. Thus some drugs may be shown to disturb a particular stage of the cycle, to displace this or that metabolite, to inhibit the uptake of a chemical mediator of neuronal activity, or to increase the rate of passage of such ions as sodium or potassium across cell membranes.

This use of radioisotopes as tracers of physiological activity leads to iso-topic studies in diagnosis. Those tracers, so called "radiopharmaceuticals" have led to a new class of drugs, which includes the nuclides used in radio-therapy. Radioisotopes are thus of increasing importance to the pharma-cologist both as a method of study and as a new class of medicinal agent.

The survey presented in this section reflects this importance, and there are covered, in a number of subsections, the fundamental chemical and physical aspects which are essential to an understanding of nuclear pheno-mena by the pharmacologist. In addition there are articles dealing with the systematic study of compartmental analysis at the local and cellular level; the study of physiological barriers, including the blood–brain barrier; the placental barrier and the cutaneous barrier; the study of the metabolism of drugs; and the use of radionuclides in chemotherapy, in therapeutics, and in diagnosis in man.

The inherent danger associated with radioactive substances is discussed, both from the ethical aspect and from the point of view of the risk to personnel (research workers, physicians, and patients) who come into contact with them.

2. CONCEPT OF NONDISCRIMINATION AND CHARACTERISTICS OF RADIONUCLIDES

A concept that is fundamental to the use of radioisotopes in biological research, in pharmacology, in diagnosis, and in therapeutics, is that the chemical behavior of a radioisotope is identical to that of the correspond-ing stable isotope: living organisms cannot, in the course of metabolism, distinguish between a radioisotope and the corresponding stable atom.

Nevertheless, stable and radioactive isotopes may be individually detected in tracer quantities by virtue of their different atomic weight or by the radiation they emit. In the case of radioactive elements, quantitative measurements may be made which take account of the loss of radioactivity with time (radioactive decay). This decay time is a characteristic of the radioisotope, as is the type of radiation emitted (α particles, β particles, or γ radiation). The ratio between the quantity of radioactive substance and the weight of the same element constitutes the specific radioactivity which is distributed throughout a living organism after the introduction of a radioactive tracer substance within a metabolite of that particular organ-ism. This distribution of specific radioactivity gradually decreases, indicat-ing that the radioactive tracer is becoming more and more diluted with stable isotopes of the same element already present within the living organism. The specific radioactivity must not be confused with the concentration of radioactivity. The latter is expressed as the amount of radioactivity in a given volume of solution containing the radioelement. A radionuclide may be present with another radioisotope of the same element, in which case the radioactive purity or radionuclidic purity will be affected, as will also be the case if the radionuclide is present with a radioisotope of another element. As an example of the former, one may cite the presence of iodine-131 in a solution of iodine-132; and of the latter, the presence of molybdenum-99 in solutions of technetium-99m.

The research worker should thus be aware of the energy of the radiation emitted by the isotope in which he is interested. He must verify that the chemical species carrying the radioactivity does not alter, neither by displacement of the radioactive atom within the molecule concerned, nor by partial degradation of the molecule itself (polymerization, hydrolysis, etc.). Such alterations are not infrequent with molecules labeled with iodine-131. Thus thyroxine-^{131}I or tetra-iodo-thyronine will yield triiodothyronine-^{131}I and an ^{131}I ion. When this occurs, one says that the radiochemical purity of the thyroxine is reduced. This degradation is due to radiation emitted by the radionuclide carried by the labeled molecule (Cohen *et al.*, 1968). Provided the elementary precautions cited below are taken, complex problems involving a series of many metabolic reactions may be elucidated by the use of radioactive tracers both *in vitro* and *in vivo*. This is particularly true since the introduction of the radioisotope in no way affects the equilibrium conditions provided one uses material of high specific radioactivity. Specific radioactivity (or specific activity) is expressed in Curies or fractions of Curies per mole or fraction of a mole. It may also be expressed in Curies or fractions of Curies per gram or fraction of a gram. With modern methods of detecting and measuring radioactivity, a nano-Curie of radioactivity may readily be detected; and so, if the specific activity of a sample of, say, noradrenaline is of the order of 10 Curies per millimole, picogram quantities of this chemical mediator may be estimated in tissue samples, after the introduction of a few micrograms of the radioactive material into the organism or reaction mixture.

The synthesis of a labeled molecule of high specific activity is far from easy. Firstly, the atom of the molecular structure to be labeled must be carefully selected in such a manner that the binding of the labeled atom with the remainder of the molecule is strong. This labeled atom will become a constituent of the molecule (e.g. replacement of stable ^{12}C by the radioactive ^{14}C), or a supplement grafted onto the molecule (e.g. ^{131}I attached to antipyrine gives iodo-^{131}I-antipyrine, which has been used as a tracer for antipyrine). Not all the atoms found in organic molecules can be replaced by a radioisotope; for instance, there are no readily usable radio-isotopes of nitrogen or oxygen. The radioisotope ^{13}N has a radioactive half-life of 9.96 min, while the radioisotope ^{15}O has a half-life of 124 sec. These short radioactive half-lives make them unsuitable for organic synthesis. In certain positions in the molecule hydrogen 3 can be exchanged readily for hydrogen 1 present in tissue water. In contrast one can obtain specific and useful information by varying the position of a labeled atom within the molecule. Thus some amino acids may be labeled on the ali-phatic chain, on the nuclear ring (if there is one), or on the carboxylic acid carbon. These variable linkages are of interest, as each can take part in different experiments. For example, histidine labeled with ^{14}C in the carboxyl group will be acted on by histidine decarboxylase, and will give off labeled carbon dioxide. Histidine labeled on the imidazoline ring, however, will yield histamine, imidazole 2-^{14}C. Whether one uses the histidine labeled on the carboxyl group or on the imidazole ring will depend on the metabolism of which part one is interested. In fact, for histidine there are a number of tracers:

(a) L-histidine carboxyl-^{14}C.
     D-histidine carboxyl-^{14}C.
     DL-histidine carboxyl-^{14}C.
(b) L-histidine, imidazole 2-^{14}C.
     DL-histidine, imidazole 2-^{14}C.
(c) DL-histidine, alpha ^{14}C.
(d) L-histidine uniformally labeled with ^{14}C.
(e) DL-Histidine, 2–5 ^{3}H.
(f) L-histidine tritiated in the side chain.
(g) DL-histidine uniformally tritiated.
     L-histidine uniformally tritiated.

The choice of the particular tracer will depend on the study contemplated.

One may ask whether the transmutation of the radioisotope produces any disturbance of the biological system. Thus iodine-131 becomes xenon-131; iodine-125 becomes tellurium-125; and phosphorus-32 becomes sulphur-32 (Table 1). The transmutation of the same element can give rise to two different elements with different biological properties. Little is known of the biological effects of such transmutations (see A.I.E.A. panel, 1968); in contrast, the isotopic effect has been quite thoroughly studied.

TABLE 1. TRANSMUTATION OF RADIONUCLIDES USED IN PHARMACOLOGY

Parent			Daughter		
Atomic number	Symbol	Mass number	Atomic number	Symbol	Mass number
1	H	3	2	He	3
6	C	14	7	N	14
15	P	32	16	S	32
16	S	35	17	Cl	35
24	Cr	51	23	V	51
26	Fe	55	25	Mn	55
26	Fe	59	27	Co	59
27	Co	57	26	Fe	57
27	Co	58	26	Fe	58
27	Co	60	28	Ni	60
29	Cu	64	{28	Ni	64
			{30	Zn	64
29	Cu	67	30	Zn	67
34	Se	75	33	As	75
35	Br	82	36	Kr	82
43	Tcᵐ	99	43	Tc	99
53	I	125	52	Te	125
53	I	131	54	Xe	131

3. ISOTOPIC EFFECT

The isotopic effect is readily accepted if it is remembered that the mass of tritium is three times that of the stable hydrogen isotope. The molecular steric hindrance will be different in the case of the molecule labeled with tritium, and the reaction processes of a triton will not necessarily be those of a proton. It follows that, although the effects are usually negligible, the isotopic effect may affect the results of a tracer experiment by a factor of two or more. The possible importance of the isotopic effect will depend on the particular biological phenomenon being studied. The equilibrium constants, distribution coefficients, diffusion constants, and vibrational frequencies, will all be affected. The isotopic effect will have its greatest effect in reactions involving the transfer of the isotopic atom itself from the reacting molecule to an acceptor. Thus in the case of an enzymatic reaction, the radioisotope, even if it does not react itself, may affect a reaction if it is near to the reacting atoms of the molecule.

In the case of tritium the isotopic effect may be quite large because of the large difference between the atomic masses of the radioactive and stable isotopes. For other radioisotopes the problem is correspondingly less marked as, in the case of carbon-14 for example, the atomic mass is 14/12th that of the stable isotope. In the case of iodine-131, the ratio is 131/127.

The strength of a carbon–hydrogen bond is greater than that of the carbon–tritium bond. The same is true for nitrogen–hydrogen in relation to the nitrogen–tritium bond. In contrast, the carbon-14–carbon-12 bond is stronger than the carbon-12–carbon-12 bond. The isotopic effect may occur not only from one molecule to another (intermolecular isotopic effect), but also within the molecule itself (intramolecular isotopic effect). The intramolecular isotopic effect will either strengthen or weaken the molecular structure, and will modify the reactivity.

Nevertheless, differences between the pharmacological properties of a labeled and unlabeled substance have never been detected, which leads one to believe that the isotopic effect, if it does occur at all in a manner that might alter results, does not do so frequently. It should be borne in mind when considering enzymatic reactions, but it should not be considered as a major limitation of the use of radioisotopes in pharmacology.

4. KINETIC STUDIES

One of the most important contributions from radiotracer studies was the proof that biological structures in living organisms are not in a static state but in a state of continuous change. A static concept was replaced by a dynamic one. In all metabolic reactions, the large and complex molecules, and their break-down products (fatty acids, amino acids, nucleic acids, carbohydrates), come both from absorption via the digestive tract and from the constituents of body cells. There is a continuous exchange between substances in the circulation and the cell. Living matter is thus in a dynamic state. In these equilibrium conditions, anabolism and catabolism compensate each other in such a manner that the total quantity of living substance remains constant. In a steady state there is continuous exchange, passive or active, which can be demonstrated only by the use of radioactive tracers.

What is true for living matter is also true for drugs. The linkage between drug and living tissue is not permanent. The molecules of a pharmacological substance combine with the receptor in a more or less stable fashion. Subsequently one molecule of the drug will dissociate from the receptor and another molecule will take its place.

The study of the mechanism of action of drugs has greatly benefited from the use of radioactive tracers. Thus it is not possible, by classical chemical and biological methods, to trace a compound within the organism; to localize the structures with which it combines; to enumerate the metabolic products to which it gives rise; or to determine the reactions of the metabolic products themselves.

In all areas of pharmacology the use of radioactive tracers sheds new light on the mechanism of biological action of drugs. Radioactive methods have demonstrated the importance of the organs of biotransformation such as the liver and kidney, in the distribution of drugs in the body. After their passage across the epithelium of the intestinal mucosa, the great majority of drugs are taken up by one or other of these organs. Drug molecules follow a cycle consisting of: effector organ to the blood; from the blood to the liver; from the liver to the intestine; and again the effector organ in the blood. In each cycle a fraction of the drug will be lost by metabolism and excretion.

We now have a much better understanding of the biotransformation of drugs than we had 20 years ago. At one time it was thought that the breakdown of drugs in the body was similar to the destructive analytic procedures then used. A better understanding of enzymology, and of the individualization of *n* metabolites originating from *one* drug, has corrected the erroneous ideas concerning the hypothetical opening or closing of rings. It is also claimed that some metabolites are more active than the parent drug. This has led to the suggestion that dimethyl or sulphoxyde derivatives could be substituted and used as drugs in place of the original parent molecule. One can envisage that the production of each new drug would be accompanied by the preparation of a card setting out all the metabolites produced both in man and in animals. It would thus be possible to predict any increase in toxicity or risk of over-dosage.

The biological half-life of a drug in the circulation, like the urinary half-life, provides a standard which makes it possible (by measuring changes in these physiological constants) to measure enzyme induction or delay in excretion due to a defect in the renal filtration mechanism. It is essential to distinguish between the drug itself and one or more of its metabolites. The nature of the latter may be quite different at the beginning of drug administration and after a period of drug treatment. Pharmacokinetics is only just beginning to be studied, and it is useful in the study of the fat depots, which play the role of "expansion tanks", thus allowing some degree of regularity in the distribution of drugs to the tissues and effector sites. A general scheme can be drawn up of the distribution of a drug in the body which takes account of these variables (Fig. 1). There is the absorption of the drug at the site of administration, the distribution in the tissues, the metabolism, and the excretion. The interaction of the drug at the effector site gives rise to the pharmacological action in the organism. The blood is the central compartment from which all the distributions are made. These may be in a single direction or they may be reversible. The speed of passage from one compartment to another is denoted by the letter λ, by the number of the compartment to which the transfer is taking place, and by the number of the compartment from which the change is occurring: thus λ_{31} represents the rate of transfer of a drug from the blood (compartment 1) to tissue depots (compartment 3), fatty depots, or the aqueous phase. This rate of transfer is often large. λ_{13} is the rate of transfer of the

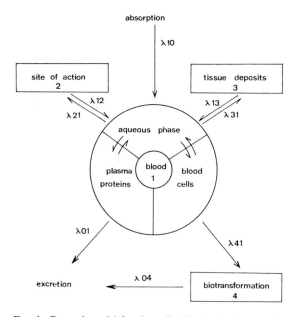

Fig. 1. General model for drug distribution in the organism.

drug from tissue depots (compartment 3) to the blood (compartment 1). This rate is usually less than that of the reverse process. The blood is not a homogenous tissue. There is an aqueous phase, plasma proteins on which a drug may become attached, and blood corpuscles which often are carriers of the drug. Such a schema applies only to the drug itself, and not to the metabolites. The latter must be considered separately and subtracted from the cycle of distribution of the parent. For this reason only the transfer of the drug from the blood to the organs of biotransformation (compartment 4) are indicated. This process takes place with a rate λ_{41}. Often the metabolic products pass again into the circulation, but they are no longer the drug itself. Biotransformation results in an abolition of or a decrease (or in contrast an increase) in the biological activity and to an alteration in the coefficient of hydrolipid solubility. Nevertheless, the presence of a metabolite can result in an alteration of the distribution of the drug by means of a feedback mechanism. A more complex schema has to be envisaged for each particular case. λ_{10} can be determined only for oral, rectal, subcutaneous, or intravenous administration. In the case of intravenous administration, λ_{10} is the speed of injection. In practice, λ_{10} will depend on the nature of the vessels into which the injection is being made, i.e. a peripheral vein such as the saphenous, or a vein near to the heart such as the external jugular.

It often happens that tolerance develops after prolonged administration of a drug. This will be indicated by a change in the rate of distribution of the drug in the tissues. λ_{13} will decrease because of an increased retention in the tissues. λ_{41} will increase because of increase in the amount of biotransformation. λ_{01} and λ_{04} will increase because of increased urinary excretion. In the case of a decrease in renal filtration, there will be a decrease in the values of λ_{01} and of λ_{04}.

There are now numerous substances that have been studied by radioactive tracer methods. Table 2 sets out a list of labeled drugs together with the relevant literature reference. We have listed only the first paper dealing with the particular labeled drug or that which we consider to be the most important. This list is not exhaustive, but merely indicative of the papers published. The reader should consult the specialized chapters of this section, or the general review articles listed in the bibliography. We have drawn up a list of endogenous substances present in the body and which have an important function in pharmacology. Table 3 lists the possible labels, thus underlining the flexibility of the radiotracer method.

5. STATIC STUDIES

Distribution studies have led to the rather disappointing conclusion that radioactively labeled drugs are, in general, concentrated in the sites of loss, and only small quantities gather in the sites of action. In the light of present studies it would seem that the distribution of a drug is determined by the physico-chemical properties of the molecule, while the particular pharmacological action depends on the nature and sensitivity of the receptor cell. Why does a cell of cardiac muscle respond more rapidly to a given concentration of digitalis than does a cell of skeletal muscle? One cannot yet give a satisfactory answer to such a question, although one knows the effect

TABLE 2. LIST OF LABELED DRUGS

Name	Label	References
Acetylsalicylic acid	^{14}C	Smith *et al.* (1956)
Acriflavine	^{3}H	Murray and Williams (1958)
Adrenochrome semi-carbazone	^{14}C	Sohler *et al.* (1967)
Amphetamine	^{14}C	Young and Gordon (1962)
Atropine	^{3}H	Gabourel and Gosselin (1958)
Barbital	^{14}C	Ebert (1962)
Bemegride	^{14}C	Nicholls (1960)
Bethanidine	^{14}C	Doyle and Morley (1965)
Bretylium	^{14}C	Boura *et al.* (1960)
Chloramphenicol	^{3}H	Felsenfeld and Carter (1961)
Chlormerodrine	^{197}Hg	
	^{203}Hg	
Chloroquine	^{14}C	Cohen *et al.* (1963)
Chlorothiazide	^{14}C	Bretell *et al.* (1960)
Chlorpromazine	^{14}C	Murray and Williams (1958)
Chlorpromazine	^{35}S	Cassano *et al.* (1965)
Chlortalidone	^{14}C	Beisenherz *et al.* (1966)
Cotinine	^{3}H	Bowman *et al.* (1964)
Decamethonium	^{14}C	Broen Christensen (1966)
Dextran sulphate	^{14}C	Weigel and Walton (1959)
Dextran	^{3}H	Hanngren *et al.* (1959)
Dicoumarol	^{14}C	Wosilait (1968)
Digitoxine	^{14}C	Geiling *et al.* (1948)
Dihydroxyphtalazine	^{14}C	McIsaac (1964)
Dihydromorphine	^{3}H	Van Praag and Simon (1966)
Diisopropylfluorophosphate	^{32}P	Ramachandran (1967)
Dimethyltubocurarine	^{3}H	Nedergaard and Taylor (1966)
Diphenylhydantoine	^{14}C	Noach *et al.* (1958)
Ephedrine	^{14}C	Bralet *et al.* (1968)
Ethanol	^{14}C	Scherrer *et al.* (1963)
Griseofulvine	^{14}C	Symchowicz and Wong (1966)
Hemicholinium	^{14}C	Domer and Schueller (1960)
Hydrochlorothiazide	^{3}H	Sheppard *et al.* (1960)
Indomethacin	^{14}C	Hucker *et al.* (1966)
Isocarboxazid	^{14}C	Schwartz (1960)
Isoniazid	^{14}C	Bonet-Maury *et al.* (1954)
Meprobamate	^{3}H	Walkenstein and Knebel (1958)
Mescaline	^{14}C	Neff *et al.* (1964)
Metformine	^{14}C	Cohen and Costerousse (1961)
Methaqualone	^{14}C	Cohen *et al.* (1962)
Methocarbamol	^{14}C	Campbell *et al.* (1961)
Morphine	^{14}C	Mulé (1965)
Morphine	^{3}H	Misra *et al.* (1961)
Nalorphine	^{3}H	Hug and Woods (1963)
N-benzyl-β-chloropropionamide	^{14}C	Quevauviller and Garcet (1956)
Neostigmine	^{14}C	Roberts *et al.* (1965)
Nicotine	^{14}C	Appelgren *et al.* (1962)
Norepinephrine	^{14}C	Reivich and Glowinski (1967)
Orphenadrine	^{3}H	Prins and Hespe (1968)

TABLE 2—*cont.*

Name	Label	References
Oxolinic acid	^{14}C	Di Carlo *et al.* (1968)
Para amino salicylic acid	^3H	Rydberg and Hanngren (1958)
Penicillin	^{35}S	Ullberg (1954)
Penicillin	^3H	Giovanozzi *et al.* (1960)
Pentaerythritol-tetranitate	^{14}C	Di Carlo *et al.* (1967)
Pentamidine	^{14}C	Pichat *et al.* (1956), Launoy *et al.* (1960)
Perhydrosqualene	^3H	Wepierre *et al.* (1968)
Perphenazine	^{35}S	Symchowicz *et al.* (1962a and b)
Persantin	^{14}C	Litwack *et al.* (1964)
Phenformin	^{14}C	Wick *et al.* (1960)
Phenobarbital	^{14}C	Glasson *et al.* (1959)
Pristinamycine	^3H	Benazet and Bourat (1965)
Psicofuranine	^3H	Garrett *et al.* (1960)
Pyribenzamine	^{14}C	Weinman and Geisman (1959)
Pyridostigmine	^{14}C	Husain *et al.* (1968)
Reserpine	^3H	Maggiolo and Haley (1964)
Stilboestrol	^{14}C	Fischer *et al.* (1966)
Succinyldicholine	^{14}C	Neubert *et al.* (1960)
Tetrabenazine	^3H	Stumpf *et al.* (1961)
Tetracycline	^3H	Takesue *et al.* (1960)
Tetracycline	^{131}I	Eskelson *et al.* (1963)
Tetramethylammonium	^{14}C	Smetana *et al.* (1964)
Thalidomide	^{14}C	Koransky and Ullberg (1964)
Tolbutamide	^{14}C	Tagg *et al.* (1967)
Toxiferin	^{14}C	Waser (1963)
Triamcinolone	^3H	Florini (1960)
Urethane	^{14}C	Cohen *et al.* (1967)

of digitalis-like drugs on ionic movements. With labeled drugs one is able to localize the point of attachment of a drug within the cell. If the receptor cell is also the effector cell, the drug–receptor link will produce a pharmacological response. This has been illustrated by the work of Waser (1963) on the site of localization of curare-like drugs and the structure of the motor end-plate. Nevertheless, the major quantity of the curarizing agent is found outside the motor end-plate in the sites of loss. It would appear that there should be a relation between the chemical structure of a drug and its affinity for certain tissues or cellular structures. Thus the relationship between chemical structure and pharmacological action should be refered to as: chemical structure–cellular affinity–pharmacological action. The relationship between chemical structure and cellular affinity is independent of the relationship between cellular affinity and pharmacological

R.I.P.—B

TABLE 3. LABELED BIOLOGICAL SUBSTANCES USED IN PHARMACOLOGICAL
RESEARCH

Labeled with carbon-14
  Acetylcholine labeled in position 1 of the acetyl group
  Adenosine labeled in position 8
  Adenosine monophosphate (same label)
  Epinephrine labeled in position 7
  Glucose uniformly labeled
  Glucose labeled in position 2
  Glucose labeled in position 6
  Histamine labeled in position 2 of the imidazole ring
  5 hydroxytryptamine (serotonin) labeled in position 2
  Methionine labeled in position 1 or 2
  Norepinephrine labeled in position 7
  Oestradiol labeled in position 4
  Progesterone labeled in position 4
  Saccharose uniformly labeled
  Thiamine labeled in position 2 of the thiazol ring
  Urea
  Vasopressine-2 phenyl uniformly labeled-8 lysine
  Vitamine D_3 labeled in position 4
Labeled with tritium
  Cortisol in position 1 and 2
  Dopamine
  Epinephrine in position 7
  Histamine uniformly labeled
  5 hydroxytryptamine (serotonin)
  Norepinephrine in position 7
  Progesterone labeled in position 16
  Prostaglandin E_1 (Holmes and Horton, 1968)
Labeled with iodine-131 *or* -125
  Fibrinogen
  Human serum albumin
  Insulin
  Thyroxine
Labeled with phosphorus-32
  Adenosine monophosphate
  Adenosine triphosphate
Labeled with sulfur-35
  Cystein
  Glutathione
  Thiamine
Labeled with selenium-75
  Methionine
Labeled with cobalt-57, -58, *or* -60
  Cyanocobalamin
Labeled with chromium-51
  Human serum albumin
  Pepsin

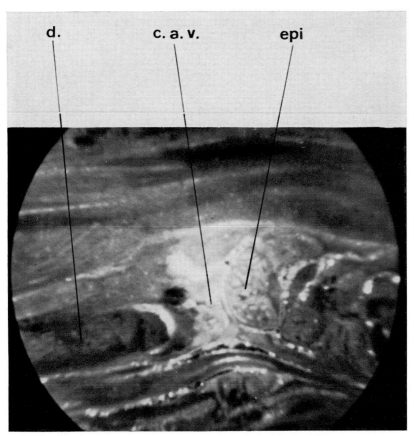

FIG. 2. Photograph in polarized light of rat phalangic joint. Section of normal joint (magnification × 6.6). c.a.v., articular cavity. epi, bony epiphysis. d, bony diaphysis.

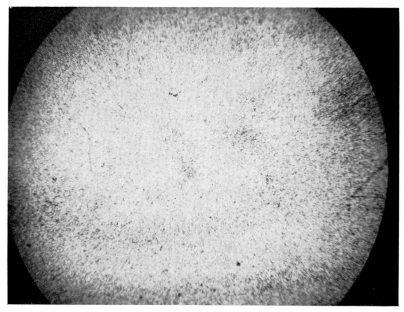

FIG. 3. Autoradiograph of the same joint, showing absence of fixation of ^{14}C-chloroquine.

action. Labeled molecules have provided the proof of a cellular affinity that does not result in a pharmacological action. The notion of a pharmacological receptor, which has been so fruitful, remains to be proved, and for a large number of drugs the concept has not passed the stage of hypothesis. Studies with labeled molecules will, little by little, afford the direct experimental proof which is still wanting.

On the other hand, one must distinguish between the effect on healthy tissue and on diseased tissue (Quevauviller, 1967). The chemical composition of the receptor on a diseased organ might be different from that of a healthy organ. Cohen *et al.* (1963) and Lacapere (1964) have shown that in the normal rat chloroquine labeled with ^{14}C is distributed in the pituitary, the adrenal medulla, the thymus, spleen, adrenal cortex, liver, salivary glands, and bone marrow. As is indicated in Figs. 2 and 3, there was no distribution of radioactivity in the joints. Figure 2 is a photograph, taken with a polarizing microscope, of the phalangic joint of an anterior limb. Figure 3 is an autoradiograph of the same section. There is no preferential concentration of radioactivity.

In the rat, in which an arthritic syndrome is produced by the injection of Freund's adjuvant into the skin of the neck, there develops some 3 weeks later an arthritis of the anterior and posterior limbs and of the tail. This phenomenon was first described by Pearson (1956).

The administration of ^{14}C-chloroquine to such rats results in a distribution in the pituitary, adrenal medulla, thymus, spleen, adrenal cortex, liver, salivary glands, bone marrow, and in the arthritic joints. Figure 4 shows a photograph, taken with a polarizing microscope, of a phalangic joint which is arthritic, and in which the synovial sack has hypertrophied and has passed the articular capsule. Figure 5 is an autoradiograph of the section shown in Fig. 4. It will be seen that the radioactivity is distributed in the periphery of the hypertrophied synovial pouch and in the bone of the joint. This observation is of interest in two respects:

(i) the arthritic response is produced at some distance from the arthrogenic substance;

(ii) the arthritis modifies the chemical properties of the structure of the joint. This alteration is demonstrated by the fact that the chloroquine, which is not concentrated in the joint of the normal rat, is concentrated in the joint of the arthritic rat.

What are the biological constituents which combine with the chloroquine molecule? The hypothesis has been put forward that the chondroitin–sulfuric acid groups could react with chloroquine, which is basic. This hypothesis must still be proved, but this example illustrates to what extent the concept of a pharmacological receptor needs to be investigated, since the receptors in a healthy organ are possibly different from those in a diseased organ. Chloroquine is claimed to have anti-arthritic properties. These claims are chiefly based on clinical observations, and little evidence has come from experimental pharmacology. Should one deny that chloroquine has any therapeutic activity in arthritis, or must one accept that the pharmacological methods are unsufficient for this particular problem? In such a case the theories and techniques of radioactive tracers may be very helpful. The distribution of ^{14}C-chloroquine in man and the monkey has been studied by McChesney *et al.* (1966, 1967). These workers found high concentrations in the choroid retina, the adrenals, the liver, and the pituitary of the rhesus monkey 4 days after drug administration.

6. NEW TRENDS: RADIOIMMUNO ASSAYS

Pharmacological methods for the detection of circulating levels of proteic hormones during hormone therapy used to be insufficiently sensitive. However, the study of the levels of proteic hormones in the circulation has been made possible by the method described by Berson *et al.* (1956), originally for insulin. This method allows the determination of levels of hormone of the order of a picogram per milliliter. The principle of the method is as follows: labeled insulin combines in plasma with specific anti-insulin antibodies. This combination is competitively inhibited by un-labeled hormone.

Thus the concentration of hormone present in an unknown solution may be determined by comparing the inhibition observed in the unknown solution in comparison with a series of standard solutions of the hormone. Figure 6, taken from the work of Yalow and Berson (1956a) may help in the understanding of this method of estimation. The reaction between insulin and anti-insulin antibodies is an equilibrium reaction which follows the law of mass action. The sensitivity of the method depends on the quality of the antibody used and the specific activity of the labeled insulin. The specificity of the reaction depends on the purity of the antigen and of the existence of and the degree of energy of the cross-linkage reaction. This method which is now widely used in clinical biology afforded the proof of the existence of hormonal antigenicity. Previously this concept was disputed.

Determinations by immuno-tracer methods have been extended to other

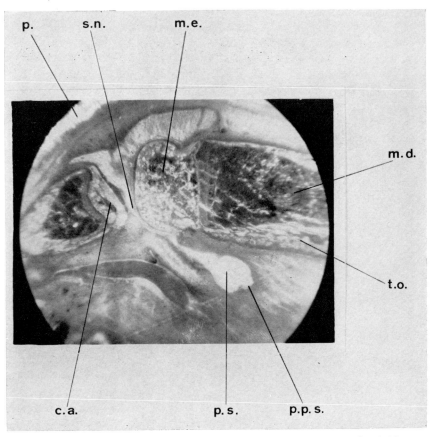

FIG. 4. Photograph in polarized light of rat phalangic joint. Section of arthritic joint (magnification ×6.6) p., skin. s.n., normal synovium. c.a., articular cartilage. m.e., epiphyseal bone marrow. p.p.s., periphery of synovial pouch. p.s., synovial pouch. t.o., bony tissue. m.d., diaphyseal bone marrow.

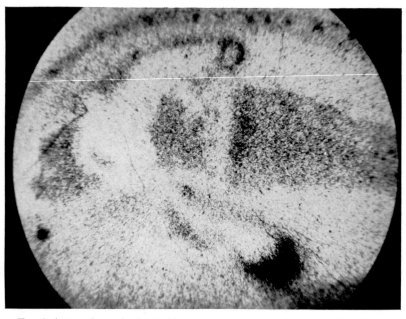

FIG. 5. Autoradiograph of arthritic articulation showing fixation of ^{14}C-chloroquine in the periphery of the extruded synovial pouch, in the epiphyseal bone marrow, and the diaphyseal bone marrow.

proteic hormones, including the growth hormone (Glick *et al.*, 1963) and the follicle-stimulating hormone (Rosselin and Dolais, 1968).

Yalow and Berson (1966b) emphasize two essential factors arising from their studies which they have enunciated in the form of theorems:

$$\text{Free hormone } ^{131}\text{I} + \text{hormone antibody} \rightleftharpoons \text{antibody-bound hormone } ^{131}\text{I}$$

$$+$$

unlabeled hormone
(in known standards
or in body fluids)

$$\updownarrow$$

antibody-bound unlabeled hormone

FIG. 6. Competitive reaction of labeled and unlabeled hormone with antibody. (From Yalow and Berson, 1966b.)

"THEOREM I. A labeled protein is a valid tracer for its parent unlabeled protein in a particular system *S* if and only if, the labeled and unlabeled proteins exhibit identical behaviour in *S*, similarities or dissimilarities of behaviour in all other systems being irrelevant.

"THEOREM II. A labeled protein may be used other than as a tracer for the parent unlabeled protein, in which case identity of behaviour of labeled and unlabeled proteins may be irrelevant to the validity of application of the labeled protein."

These techniques have been developed primarily in clinical biochemistry, and have as yet been little used in pharmacology. Nevertheless, it was necessary to mention them in this volume of the *Encyclopedia* since we feel that in future they will become widely used in pharmacology.

7. THE PHARMACODYNAMICS OF RADIOPHARMACEUTICALS

Thus far we have considered a radioactive element or a labeled molecule as a tracer rather than as a drug in its own right. However, when the tracer is administered to man it becomes, according to the pharmacopeias, a medicinal substance. This also applies if the radioisotope is administered to man for a therapeutic purpose. At the present time, therefore, the pharmacologist must consider the radioisotope as a medicament, and must study its pharmacological properties as in the case of any drug. This is becoming particularly true in the sense that the suppliers of radioisotopes for medical purposes must make a submission to the appropriate authority (e.g. the Ministry of Health) for permission to market the product. The procedure necessary for obtaining such authorization is the same as for other drugs.

It therefore follows that, in addition to clinical and physico-chemical studies, the normal pharmacological and toxicological (acute toxicity and chronic toxicity) studies must be carried out.

Radiopharmaceutical substances may be classified into five groups:

(1)   Irradiated substances that are used immediately.
(2)   Irradiated substances subsequently made in solution.
(3)   Radioisotopes prepared by chemical separation.
(4)   Radioisotopes used in the form of labeled organic molecules.
(5)   Radioisotopes in colloidal form.

The nature of the radiopharmaceutical preparations can itself vary. These may be:

(i) Isotope generators in elution columns (Fig. 7).
(ii) Solutions for oral administration.
(iii) Solutions for parenteral administration.

Elution columns are a source of solutions of radioisotopes with short half-lives: iodine-132, technetium-99m, indium-113m, barium-137, etc. The solutions for oral administration may be aqueous, aqueous–alcoholic, or oily. They contain the labeled molecule, inorganic or organic, and are used for the preparation of the oral dosage in the form of a "radiocapsule". This consists of a gelatin capsule filled with an inert powder on which the radio-active solution is poured.

The solutions for parenteral administration contain the labeled organic or inorganic molecule. They are sterile, pyrogen-free, isotonic, and buffered. In this group are labeled molecules of biological origin such as iodinated human serum albumin or radioactive colloids, etc. The solutions for parenteral administration may be presented in "one-shot syringes" (or disposable syringes) which deliver the appropriate single dose.

What is the role of the pharmacologist in respect of these radiopharmaceutical agents?

The pharmacologist must ensure that the radioactive molecule in solution is not toxic neither in the short nor long term. He should study the distribution of the labeled molecule in the body of an experimental animal (mouse, rat, rabbit, dog). He should determine the biological half-life in the circu-

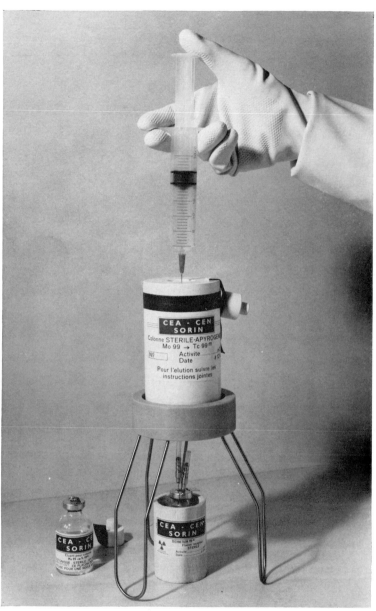

FIG. 7. Isotopic generator (Photograph from French Atomic Energy Commission, Center of Nuclear Studies, Saclay.)

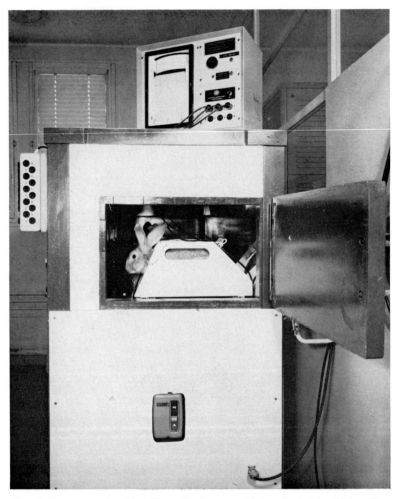
FIG. 8. Pyrogen test in rabbit. The radiopharmaceutical under test has high radio-activity and can be handled only behind shielding especially constructed for the test. (Photograph from French Atomic Energy Commission, Center for Nuclear Studies, Saclay.)

lation as well as the rate of urinary and fecal excretion. He should determine the target organ in which the radioactive molecule is preferentially concentrated. He should study the affinity of the blood cells for the radioactive molecule.

He should ensure that the administration of the radiopharmaceutical agents does not modify the principal physiological functions of the body since this is not the intention. Thus he should verify that arterial pressure, heart rate, body temperature, and so on remain normal (Fig. 8). He should determine the break-down products of the labeled molecule.

At the beginning of the use of radioisotopes in medicine, such studies were usually carried out on an empirical basis. At present, however, there is a tendency for systematic studies of this type to be carried out with all new radiopharmaceuticals which are developed.

A number of reviews are available concerning radiopharmaceutical agents (Cohen, 1961, 1962; Briner, 1963; Cohen *et al.*, 1964; Kristensen, 1966; Cohen, 1966; Tubis, 1967; Gopal and Iya, 1967). Two chapters of this section will deal in detail with this question, but it seemed appropriate to give here a synopsis of this rather special pharmacology.

8. CONCLUSIONS

We have attempted in this introductory chapter to present a point of view which, although personal, we consider to be objective of the importance of the use of radioactive substances in pharmacology as well as an indication of the use of radiopharmaceuticals in clinical biology. Their use in therapeutics has been steadily developing, but concerns only the destructive properties of the radiation. In functional studies, however, the diversity of the investigations is remarkable.

Radioisotopes have undeniably provided pharmacology with a new methodology for the study of mechanism of action of drugs and have made possible studies of metabolism.

However, their use has some limitations, and cannot replace the good old smoked drum which is so useful for recording muscular contractions. Nevertheless, the smoked drum is of no use in analyzing variations in the metabolic cycle of lipids for instance. Here only the labeled molecule comes to the assistance of the pharmacologist. As the pharmacology of the mechanism of drug action becomes more and more biochemical or molecular, so radioisotopes will be used to greater and greater extent in the pharmacological laboratory.

In 1957 I wrote: "Should we applaud the discoveries made possible by the use of radioisotopes, or should we regret the sometimes important errors which result from their uncritical use?" In 1968 the doubt has lifted. We must applaud.

REFERENCES

(A) BOOKS, REVIEWS AND MONOGRAPHS

Peaceful Uses of Atomic Energy (1956) Proceedings of the International Conference in Geneva, August 1955. United Nations, Geneva. Vol. 10. *Radioactive Isotopes and Nuclear Radiations in Medicine.* Vol. 12, *Radioactive Isotopes and Ionizing Radiation in Agriculture, Physiology and Biochemistry.*

Peaceful Uses of Atomic Energy (1958) Proceedings of the Second United Nations International Conference on the Peaceful Uses of Atomic Energy, September 1958. United Nations, Geneva. Vol. 24, *Isotopes in Biochemistry and Physiology*, Part 1. Vol. 25, *Isotopes in Biochemistry and Physiology*, Part 2. Vol. 26, *Isotopes in Medicine.*

Peaceful Uses of Atomic Energy (1965) Proceedings of the Third International Conference on the Peaceful Uses of Atomic Energy, August–September 1964, Geneva. United Nations, New York, U.S.A. Vol. 15, *Special Aspects of Nuclear Energy and Isotope Applications.*

INTERNATIONAL ATOMIC ENERGY AGENCY (1962) *Tritium in the Physical and Biological Sciences*, Vol. 2. Vienna.

INTERNATIONAL ATOMIC ENERGY AGENCY (1968) *Biological Effects of Transmutation and Decay of Incorporated Radioisotopes*, Panel Proceedings Series. Vienna.

ANDREWS, G. A., KNISELEY, R. M., and WAGNER, H. N. (eds.). (1966) *Radioactive Pharmaceuticals.* U.S. Atomic Energy Commission, Division of Technical Information, Oak Ridge, Tenn. U.S.A.

BOYD, G. A. (1955) *Autoradiography in Biology and Medicine.* Academic Press, New York, U.S.A.

BUGNARD, L. (1953) Les utilisations des isotopes comme indicateurs; applications à la pharmacologie. *Actual. Pharmacol.*, **6**:51–69.

COHEN, Y. (1957) L'emploi des isotopes en pharmacologie. Rapport à la séance solennelle de la Société de Thérapeutique et de pharmacodynamie. *Thérapie*, **12**:708–36.

COHEN, Y. (1961) Bases experimentales de l'emploi des colloides radioactifs en thérapeutique. *Produits Pharm.*, **16**:159–68.

COHEN, Y. (1962a) Les possibilités des applications des isotopes dans les études pharmacologiques. *Minerva Nucleare*, **6**:1–8.

COHEN, Y. (1962b) Une nouvelle classe de médicaments. Les isotopes radioactifs. *Produits Pharm.*, **17**:3–21.

COHEN, Y. (1963) Problèmes de pharmacodynamie générale abordés à l'aide de radioéléments. *Actual. Pharmacol.* **15**:45–98.

COHEN, Y. (1968) Transport function of blood. Pharmacological studies using radioisotopes. *J. Nucl. Biol. Med.*, **12**:26–34.

DUGGAN, D. E. and TITUS, E. O. (1961) The use of radioactive isotopes for pharmacological research, in *Künstliche radioaktive Isotope in physiologie, Diagnostik und Therapie*, Vol. II, (Schwiegk, H. and Turba, F. eds.). Springer Verlag, Berlin, pp. 433–48.

EXTERMANN, R. C. (1958) *Radioisotopes in Scientific Research.* Proceedings of the International Conference held in Paris in September 1957 under the Auspices of the United Nations Educational Scientific and Cultural Organisation, Vol. III, *Research with Radioisotopes in Human and Animal Biology and Medicine.* Pergamon Press, London, England.

GEILING, E. M. K. (1957) The value of radioactive isotopes in pharmacological research. *J. Amer. Geriatric Soc.,* **5**:202–13.

GOPAL, N. G. S. and IYA, V. K. (1967) Quality control of radiopharmaceuticals. *J. Scient. Industr. Res.,* **26**:153–8.

KAMEN, M. D. (1957) *Radioactive Tracers in Biology.* Academic Press Inc., New York, U.S.A.

KRISTENSEN, K. (1966) Radiopharmaceuticals, *Acta Radiol., Suppl.,* **254**:131–4.

MURRAY III, A. and WILLIAMS, D. L. (1958) Part I, *Compounds of Isotopic Carbon.* Part II, *Organic Compounds Labeled with Isotopes of the Halogens, Hydrogen, Nitrogen, Oxygen, Phosphorus, Sulfur.* Interscience Publ., New York, U.S.A.

ROGERS, A. W. (1967) *Techniques of Autoradiography.* Elsevier, Amsterdam.

ROSSELIN, G. and DOLAIS, J. (1968) Applications de la méthode radioimmunologique au dosage de l'insuline humaine et au dosage de l'hormone folliculostimulante humaine (H.F. S.H.), *Ann. Biol. Clin.,* **26**:763–91.

ROTH, L. J. (ed.). (1965) *Isotopes in Experimental Pharmacology.* The University of Chicago Press, Chicago, Ill., U.S.A.

SIRCHIS, J. (ed.). (1968) *Methods of Preparing and Storing Labelled Compounds.* European Atomic Energy Community—Euratom, Brussels.

SMITH, P. K., MANDEL, H. G. and DAVISON, C. (1956) Metabolism of radioisotope labeled drugs, in *Peaceful Uses of Atomic Energy,* Vol. XII. United Nations, Geneva, pp. 519–25.

SOMMERVILLE, J. L. (ed.), (1967) *The Isotope Index 1967.* Scientific Equipment Co., Indianapolis, U.S.A.

ULLBERG, S. (1958) Autoradiographic studies on the distribution of labelled drugs in the body, Proceedings of the Second United Nations International Conference on Peaceful Uses of Atomic Energy, Geneva, **24**:248–54.

WANG, C. H. and WILLIS, D. L. (1965) *Radiotracer Methodology in Biological Science.* Prentice-Hall, Englewood Cliffs, N.J., U.S.A.

WASER, P. G. and GLASSON, B. (eds.), (1969) *Radioactive Isotopes in Pharmacology.* John Wiley, London, England.

WOLF, W. and TUBIS, M. (1967) Radiopharmaceuticals, *J. Pharm. Sci.,* **56**:1–17.

(B) ORIGINAL PAPERS

APPELGREN, L. E., HANSSON, E. and SCHMITERLOW, C. G. (1962) The accumulation and metabolism of C^{14} labelled nicotine in the brain of mice and cats. *Acta Physiol. Scand.,* **56**:249–57.

BECQUEREL, H. (1896) Sur les radiations émises par phosphorescence. *C. R. Acad. Sci.,* **122**:420–1.

BEISENHERZ, G., KOSS, F. W., KLATT, L., and BINDER, B. (1966) Distribution of radio-activity in the tissues and excretory products of rats and rabbits following admini-stration of C^{14} hygroton. *Arch. Int. Pharmacodyn.,* **161**:76–93.

BENAZET, F. and BOURAT, G. (1965) Étude autoradiographique de la répartition du constituant I—A de la pristinamycine (7. 293 R.P.) chez la Souris. *C. R. Acad. Sci.,* **260**:2622–5.

BERSON, S. A., YALOW, R. S., BAUMAN, A., ROTHSCHILD, M. A. and NEWERLY, K. (1956) ^{131}I insulin metabolism in human subjects: Demonstration of insulin binding globulin in the circulation of insulin treated subjects. *J. Clin. Invest.*, **35**:170–80.

BONET-MAURY, P., DEYSINE, A. and PATTI, F. (1954) Enregistrement continu sur la souris vivante de la concentration sanguine en ^{14}C. *C. R. Soc. Biol.*, **148**:798–801.

BOURA, A. L. A., COPP, F. C., DUNCOMBE, W. G., GREEN, A. F. and McCOUBREY, A. (1960) The selective accumulation of bretylium in sympathetic ganglia and their post ganglionic nerves. *Brit. J. Pharmacol.*, **15**:265–70.

BOWEN, H. J. M. (1960) Biological fractionation of isotopes. *Intn. J. Appl. Rad. Isotopes* **7**:261–72.

BOWMAN, E. R., HANSSON, E., TURNBULL, L. B., McKENNIS, H. and SCHMITERLOW, C. G. (1964) Disposition and fate of (−)cotinine H^3 in the mouse. *J. Pharmacol. Exp. Therap.*, **143**:301–8

BRALET, J., COHEN, Y. and VALETTE, G. (1968) Métabolisme et distribution tissulaire de la *DL* ephedrine ^{14}C. *Biochem. Pharmacol.*, **17**:2319–31.

BRETELL, H. R., AIKAWA, J. K. and GORDON, G. S. (1960) Studies with chlorothiazide tagged with radioactive carbon (^{14}C) in human beings. *Arch. Int. Med.*, **106**:57–63.

BRINER, W. H. (1963) The preparation of radioactive chemicals for clinical use. *Amer. J. Hosp. Pharm.*, **20**:553–61.

BROEN, CHRISTENSEN, C. (1966) Rate and mechanism of the renal excretion of ^{14}C decamethonium by rabbits. *Acta Pharmacol. Toxicol.*, **24**:139–47.

CAMPBELL, A. D., COLES, F. K., EUBANK, L. L. and HUF, E. G. (1961) Distribution and metabolism of methocarbamol. *J. Pharmacol. Exp. Therap.*, **131**:18–26.

CARLSSON, A. and WALDECK, B. (1966) Release of ^{3}H metaraminol by different mechanisms. *Acta Physiol. Scand.*, **67**:471–80.

CASSANO, G. B., SJOSTRAND, S. E. and HANSSON, E. (1965) Distribution of ^{35}S-chlorpromazine in cat brain. *Arch. Int. Pharmacodyn.*, **156**:48–57.

COHEN, Y. (1969) Application des modèles à l'étude de mécanismes pharmacodynamiques, in *Radioactive Isotopes in Pharmacology*. Waser, P. G. and Glasson, B. (eds.). John Wiley, London, England, pp. 391–408.

COHEN, Y., BLANCHARD-PELLETIER, O. and BONFILS, S. (1966) Le marquage de la pepsine par le chlorure de chrome ^{51}Cr. Choix des conditions techniques et des contrôles. *C. R. Soc. Biol.*, **160**:2272–7.

COHEN, Y. and COSTEROUSSE, O. (1961) Étude autoradiographique chez la Souris d'un antidiabétique oral le *NN* diméthyl biguanide marqué au carbone 14. *Thérapie*, **16**:109–20.

COHEN, Y., BRALET, J. and FRAPART, P. (1968) Pureté radiochimique et conservation de la thyroxine marquée à l'iode 125 ou à l'iode 131, in *Methods of Preparing and Storing Labeled Compounds*, Proceedings of the Second International Conference on Methods of Preparing and Storing Labeled Compounds, held in Brussels, November 28–December 3, 1966. European Atomic Energy Community, Euratom, Brussels, pp. 1003–7.

COHEN, Y., COSTEROUSSE, O. and CHIVOT, J. J. (1964) Pharmacodynamie des colloides radioactifs. *Minerva Nucleare*, **8**:357–66.

COHEN, Y., FONT DE PICARD, Y. and BOISSIER, J. R. (1962) Étude de la distribution chez la Souris d'un hypnotique marqué au carbone 14, la méthyl 2-orthotolyl 3, quinazolone 4. *Arch. Int. Pharmacodyn.*, **137**:271–82.

COHEN, Y., LACAPERE, J. and VIAL, M.-C. (1963) Distribution de la ^{14}C chloroquine chez le Rat normal et arthritique. *Biochem. Pharmacol.*, *Suppl.*, **12**:174–5.

COHEN, Y., WEPIERRE, J. and LINDENBAUM, A. (1967) Relations entre les phases de l'anesthésie à l'uréthane ^{14}C et son accumulation dans le systeme nerveux central. *Biochem. Pharmacol.*, **16**:175–83.

CURIE, I. and JOLIOT, F. (1934) Un nouveau type de radioactivité. *C. R. Acad. Sci.*, **198**: 254–6.

DE SAINT VICTOR, N. (1867) Sur une nouvelle action de la lumière. *C. R. Acad. Sci.*, **65**: 505–7.

DI CARLO, F. J., CREW, M. C., COUTINHO, C. B., HAYNES, L. J. and SKLOW, N. J. (1967) The absorption and biotransformation of pentaerythritol tetranitrate 1,2 ^{14}C by rats. *Biochem. Pharmacol.*, **16**: 309–16.

DI CARLO, F. J., CREW, M. C., MELGAR, M. D., ROEMER, S., RINGEL, S. M., HAYNES, L. J. and WILSON, M. (1968) Oxolinic acid metabolism by man. *Arch. Int. Pharmacodyn.*, **174**: 413–27.

DOMER, F. R. and SCHUELLER, F. W. (1960) Synthesis and metabolic studies of ^{14}C labeled hemicholinium number three. *J. Amer. Pharm. Ass.*, Sci. Ed., **49**: 553–6.

DOYLE, A. E. and MORLEY, A. (1965) Studies on the absorption and excretion of ^{14}C bethanidine in man. *Brit. J. Pharmacol.* **24**: 701–4.

EBERT, A. G. (1962) Barbital C^{14} distribution and metabolism in tolerant and non tolerant rats. *Dissert. Abstr.*, **23**: 651–2.

EIDINOFF, M. L. (1963) Tritium in biochemical studies, in *Advances in Tracer Methodology*, Vol. I, Rothschild, S. (ed.). Plenum Press, New York, U.S.A., pp. 222–6.

ESKELSON, C. D., DUNN, A. L., OGBORN, R. E. and MCLEAY, J. F. (1963) Distribution of some radioiodinated tetracyclines in animals. *J. Nucl. Med.* **4**: 382–92.

FELSENFELD, H. and CARTER, C. E. (1961) Tritium labelled chloramphenicol in *E. Coli*. *J. Pharmacol. Exp. Therap.*, **132**: 1–5.

FISCHER, L. J., MILLBURN, P., SMITH, R. L., and WILLIAMS, R. T. (1966) The fate of (^{14}C) stilboestrol in the rat. *Biochem. J.*, **100**: 69P.

FLORINI, J. R. (1960) Isolation and characterisation of a tritium exchange labeled synthetic corticosteroid. *J. Biol. Chem.*, **235**: 367–70.

GABOUREL, J. D. and GOSSELIN, R. E. (1958) The mechanism of atropine detoxication in mice and rats. *Arch. Int. Pharmacodyn.*, **115**: 416–32.

GARRETT, E. R., THOMAS, R. C., WALLACH, D. P. and ALWAY, C. D. (1960) Psicofuranine: Kinetics and mechanisms *in vivo* with the application of the analog computer. *J. Pharmacol. Exp. Therap.*, **130**: 106–18.

GEILING, E. M. K., KELSEY, F. E., MCINTOSH, B. J. and GANZ, A. (1948) Biosynthesis of radioactive drugs using carbon 14. *Science*, **108**: 558–9.

GIOVANNOZZI-SERMANNI, G. and POSSAGNO, E. (1960) Preparation of tritium labeled antibiotics. *Energ. Nucl.*, **7**: 797–800.

GLASSON, B., LERCH, P. and VIRET, J. P. (1959) Étude du phénobarbital marqué dans l'organisme du rat. *Helv. Physiol. Pharmacol. Acta*, **17**: 146–52.

GLICK, S. M., ROTH, J., YALOW, R. S. and BERSON, S. A. (1963) Immunoassay of human growth hormone in plasma. *Nature, Lond.*, **199**: 784.

HANNGREN, Å., HANSSON, E., ULLBERG, S. and ÅBERG, B. (1959) Fate of injected dextran labelled with tritium in mice. *Nature, Lond.*, **184**: 373–4.

HOLMES, S. W. and HORTON, E. W. (1968) The distribution of tritium-labelled prostaglandin E_i injected in amounts sufficient to produce central nervous effects in cats and chicks. *Brit. J. Pharmacol.*, **34**: 32–37.

HUCKER, H. B., ZACCHEI, A. G., COX, S. V., BRODIE, D. A. and CANTWELL, N. H. R. (1966) Studies on the absorption, distribution, and excretion of indomethacin in various species. *J. Pharmacol. Exp. Therap.*, **153**: 237–49.

HUG, C. C. and WOODS, L. A. (1963) Tritium labeled nalorphine: Its C.N.S. distribution and biological fate in dogs. *J. Pharmacol. Exp. Therap.*, **142**: 248–56.

HUSAIN, M. A., ROBERTS, J. B., THOMAS, B. H. and WILSON, A. (1968) The excretion and metabolism of oral ^{14}C-pyridostigmine in the rat. *Brit. J. Pharmacol.*, **34**:445–50.

ISBELL, H. S., FRUSH, H. S. and SNIEGOSKI, L. T. (1962) Utilization of tritium and carbon-14 in studies of isotope effects, in *Tritium in the Physical and Biological Sciences*, Vol. 2. International Atomic Energy Agency, Vienna, pp. 93–101.

KORANSKY, W. and ULLBERG, S. (1964) Autoradiographic investigations of ^{14}C labelled thalidomide and glutethimide in pregnant mice. *Proc. Soc. Exp. Biol. Med.*, **116**: 512–16.

LACAPERE, J. (1964) Notes sur la polyarthrite chronique rhumatoide expérimentale du rat. *Presse Med.*, **72**:1549–54.

LACASSAGNE, A. and LATTES, J. S. (1924) Methode auto-histo-radiographique pour la détection dans les organes du polonium injecté. *C. R. Acad. Sci.*, **178**:488–90.

LAUNOY, L., GUILLOT, M., and JONCHERE, H. (1950) Étude du stockage et de l'élimination de la pentamidine chez la Souris et le Rat blanc. *Ann. Pharm. Fr.*, **18**:273–84, 424–39.

LITWACK, G., BERGER, N., TRYFIATES, G. P. and PRESSMAN, B. C. (1964) Subcellular distribution in surviving rat heart slices of Persantin-2,6 ^{14}C and its fixation to isolated subcellular particles. *Biochem. Pharmacol.*, **13**:609–14.

MAGGIOLO, C. and HALEY, T. J. (1964) Brain concentration of reserpine H^3 and its metabolites in the mouse. *Proc. Soc. Exp. Biol. Med.*, **115**:149–51.

McAFEE, J. G. and WAGNER, H. N. (1960) Visualization of renal parenchyma by scintiscanning with Hg 203 Neohydrin. *Radiology*, **75**:820–1.

McCHESNEY, E. W., CONWAY, W. D., BANKS, W. F., ROGERS, J. E. and SHEKOSKY, J. M. (1966) Studies of the metabolism of some compounds of the 4-amino-7-chloroquinoline series. *J. Pharmacol.*, **151**:482–90.

McCHESNEY, E. W., SHEKOSKY, J. M. and HERNANDEZ, P. H. (1967) Metabolism of chloroquine 3-^{14}C in the rhesus monkey. *Biochem. Pharmacol.*, **16**:2444–7.

McISAAC, W. M. (1964) The metabolic fate of I-4 dihydroxyphtalazine I-^{14}C. *Biochem. Pharmacol.*, **13**:1113–18.

MISRA, A. L., MULÉ, S. J. and WOODS, L. A. (1961) *In vivo* formation of normorphine in the rat as a metabolite of tritium nuclear labelled morphine. *Nature, Lond.*, **190**:82–3.

MULÉ, S. J. (1965) Distribution of N-C^{14} methyl labeled morphine. III : Effect of nalorphine in the central nervous system and other tissues of tolerant dogs. *J. Pharmacol. Exp. Therap.*, **148**:393–8.

MURRAY, A., FOREMAN, W. W. and LANGHAM, W. (1947) The halogen–metal interconversion reaction and its application to the synthesis of nicotinic acid labeled with isotopic carbon. *Science*, **106**:277.

NEDERGAARD, O. A. and TAYLOR, D. B. (1966) The uptake by skeletal muscle of tritium labeled decamethonium and dimethyltubocurarine. *Experientia*, **22**:521–2.

NEFF, N., ROSSI, G. V., CHASE, G. D. and RABINOWITZ, J. L. (1964) Distribution and metabolism of mescaline C^{14} in the cat brain. *J. Pharmacol. Exp. Therap.*, **144**:1–7.

NEUBERT, D., SCHAEFER, J. and BELITZ, H. D. (1960) Ausscheidung von ^{14}C Succinyl bis Cholin und seiner Spaltprodukte succinyl Monocholin und Cholin im Urin der Ratte. *Arch. (Naunyn-Schmiedeberg's) Exper. Pathol. Pharmakol.*, **239**:492–6.

NICHOLLS, P. J. (1960) Metabolism of bemegride labelled with carbon 14. *Nature, Lond.*, **185**:927.

NOACH, E. L., WOODBURY, D. M. and GOODMAN, L. S. (1958) Studies on the absorption, distribution, fate and excretion of 4-^{14}C labelled diphenylhydantoin. *J. Pharmacol. Exp. Therap.*, **122**:301–14.

NODINE, J. H., PLATT, J. M., CARRANZA, J., DYKYJ, R. and MAPP, Y. (1964) Digital computer analysis of human isotopic drug kinetics. *Int. J. Appl. Rad. Isotopes*, **15**:263–8.

OKITA, G. T., TALSO, P. J., CURRY, J. H., SMITH, F. D., and GEILING, E. M. K. (1955a) Blood level studies of C^{14} digitoxin in human subjects with cardiac failure. *J. Pharmacol. Exp. Therap.* **113**:376–82.

OKITA, G. T., TALSO, P. J., CURRY, J. H., SMITH, F. D. and GEILING, E. M. K. (1955b) Metabolic fate of radioactive digitoxin in human subjects. *J. Pharmacol. Exp. Therap.*, **115**:371–9.

PEARSON, C. M. (1956) Development of arthritis, periarthritis and periostis in rats given adjuvants. *Proc. Soc. Exp. Biol. Med.*, **91**:95–101.

PICHAT, L., BARET, C. and AUDINOT, M. (1954) Synthèse de l'hydrazide de l'acide isonicotinique (isoniazide, Rimifon) marqué au carbone 14 dans le noyau pyridine. *Bull. Soc. Chim. Fr.*, **21**:88–92.

PICHAT, L., BARET, C. and AUDINOT, M. (1956) Synthèses du dibromo 1,5-pentane (^{14}C-1) du *p*-hydroxy benzonitrile (cyano ^{14}C) et leur emploi pour la préparation de bis(*p*-amidino phenoxy)-1,5-pentane (Lomidine, pentamidine, 2512 R.P.). *Bull. Soc. Chim. Fr.*, pp. 151–6.

PRINS, H. and HESPE, W. (1968) Autoradiographic study of the distribution of radio-activity in mice after oral administration of tritium labelled orphenadrine hydro-chloride. *Arch. Int. Pharmacodyn.* **171**:47–57.

QUEVAUVILLER, A. (1967) Activité des médicaments en fonction de l'état pathologique experimental. *Actual. Pharmacol.*, **20**:133–67.

QUEVAUVILLER, A. and GARCET, S. (1956) Répartition d'un anti épileptique dans les differents tissus. Étude avec le *N* benzyl C^{14}-β chloropropionamide chez la Souris. *C. R. Soc. Biol.*, **150**:1148–50.

RABINOWITZ, J. L., SALL, T., BIERLY, J. N. and OLEKSYSHYN, O. (1956) Carbon isotope effects in enzyme systems. I: Biochemical studies with urease. *Arch. Biochem. Biophys.*, **63**:437–45.

RAMACHADRAN, B. V. (1967) Distribution of DF ^{32}P in mouse organs. III: Incorporation in the brain tissue. *Biochem. Pharmacol.*, **16**, 1381–3.

REIVICH, M. and GLOWINSKI, J. (1967) An autoradiographic study of the distribution of ^{14}C norepinephrine in the brain of the rat. *Brain*, **90**(3):633–46.

ROBERTS, J. B., THOMAS, B. H. and WILSON, A. (1968) Metabolism of neostigmine *in vitro*. *Biochem. Pharmacol.*, **17**, 9–12.

ROTH, L. J., LEIFER, E., HOGNESS, J. R. and LANGHAM, W. H. (1948) Studies on the metabolism of radioactive nicotinic acid and nicotinamide in mice. *J. Biol. Chem.*, **176**:249–57.

RYDBERG, J. and HANNGREN, Å. (1958) Radiation induced tritium labelling of *p*-amino-salicylic acid (PAS). *Acta Chem. Scand.*, **12**:332–9.

SCHERRER-ETIENNE, M. and POSTERNAK, J. M. (1963) Pénétration et répartition de l'éthanol et du pentobarbital dans le cerveau du chat. Etude autoradiographique. *Schweiz. Med. Wschr.*, **93**:1016–20.

SCHWARTZ, M. A. (1960) The metabolism of isocarboxazid (marplan) in the rat. *J. Pharmacol. Exp. Therap.*, **130**:157–65.

SHEPPARD, H., MOWLES, T. F., BOWEN, N., RENZI, A. A., and PLUMMER, A. J. (1960) Distribution and fate of hydrochlorothiazide ^{3}H. *Toxicol. Appl. Pharmacol.*, **2**, 188–94.

SIRI, W. and EVERS, J. (1962) Tritium exchange in biological systems, in *Tritium in the Physical and Biological Sciences*, Vol. 2. International Atomic Energy Agency, Vienna.

SMETANA, A. F., HABERMAN, J. and CASTORINA, T. C. (1964) The preparation of C^{14} labeled tetramethylammonium bromide. *Int. J. Appl. Rad. Isotopes*, **15**:345–50.

SODEE, D. B., RENNER, R. R., and DI STEFANO, B. (1965) Photoscanning localization of tumor, utilizing chlormerodrin Mercury 197. *Radiology*, **84**:873–6.

SOHLER, A., NOVAL, J. J., PELLERIN, P. and ADAMS, W. C. (1967) Metabolism of adrenochrom semi-carbazone in the rat. *Biochem. Pharmacol.*, **16**:17–24.

STUMPF, W., GRAUL, E. H. and HUNDESHAGEN, H. (1961) Experimentelle Untersuchungen zur Pharmakologie des mit ^3H markierten Tetrabenazins. *Arzneimittel-Forsch.*, **2**:47–9.

SYMCHOWICZ, S. and WONG, K. K. (1966) Metabolism of griseofulvin ^{14}C: Studies *in vivo*. *Biochem. Pharmacol.*, **15**:1595–1600.

SYMCHOWICZ, S., PECKHAM, W. D., EISLER, M. and PERLMAN, P. L. (1962a) The distribution and excretion of radioactivity after administration of ^{35}S labeled perphenazin (trilafon). *Biochem. Pharmacol.*, **2**:417–22.

SYMCHOWICZ, S., PECKHAM, W. D., KORDUBA, C. A., and PERLMAN, P. L. (1962b) The metabolism of ^{35}S labeled perphenazine (trilafon). *Biochem. Pharmacol.*, **2**:499–501.

TAGG, J., YASUDA, D. M., TANABE, M. and MITOMA, C. (1967) Metabolic studies of tolbutamide in the rat. *Biochem. Pharmacol.*, **16**:143–53.

TAKESUE, E. I., TONELLI, G., ALFANO, L. and BUYSKE, D. A. (1960) A radiometric assay of tritiated tetracycline in serum and plasma of laboratory animals. *Int. J. Appl. Rad. Isotopes.*, **8**:52–9.

ULLBERG, S. (1954) Studies on the distribution and fate of ^{35}S labelled benzylpenicillin in the body. *Acta Radiol.* Supplement **118**, pages 1–110.

VAN PRAAG, D. and SIMON, E. J. (1966) Studies on the intracellular distribution and tissue binding of dihydromorphine-7,8-H^3 in the rat. *Proc. Soc. Exp. Biol. Med.*, **122**:6–11.

WALKENSTEIN, S. S. and KNEBEL, C. M. (1958) The excretion and distribution of meprobamate and its metabolites. *J. Pharmacol. Exp. Therap*, **122**:80A.

WASER, P. G. (1963). Les recepteurs cholinergiques. *Actual. Pharmacol.*, **16**:169–93.

WEIGEL, H. and WALTON, K. (1959) Synthesis of dextran sulphate labelled with carbon 14 and tracer experiments in the rat. *Nature, Lond.*, **183**:981–2.

WEINMAN, E. O. and GEISSMAN, T. A. (1959) The distribution, excretion and metabolism of ^{14}C labeled tripelennamine (pyribenzamine) by guinea pigs. *J. Pharmacol. Exp. Therap.*, **125**:1–13.

WEPIERRE, J., COHEN, Y., and VALETTE, G. (1968) Percutaneous absorption and removal by the body fluids of ^{14}C ethyl alcohol, ^3H perhydro-squalene and ^{14}C *p*-cymene. *Eur. J. Pharmacol.*, **3**:47–51.

WICK, A. N., STEWART, C. J. and SERIF, G. S. (1960) Tissue distribution of ^{14}C labelled betaphenetylbiguanide. *Diabetes*, **9**:163–5.

WOSILAIT, W. D. (1968) The accumulation and distribution of dicoumarol in rat liver slices. *Biochem. Pharmacol.*, **17**:429–37.

YALOW, R. S. and BERSON, S. A. (1966a) Preparation of high specific activity iodine 131 labeled hormones: Use in radioimmunoassay of hormones in plasma, in *Radioactive Pharmaceuticals*, Andrews, G. A., Kniseley, R. M. and Wagner, H. N. (eds.). U.S. Atomic Energy Commission Division of Technical Information, Oak Ridge, Tenn., U.S.A., pp. 265–80.

YALOW, R. S. and BERSON, S. A. (1966b) Basic principles in the use of labeled peptide hormones with particular reference to radioimmunoassay, in *Labelled Proteins in Tracer Studies*. Donato, L., Milhaud, G. and Sirchis, J. (eds.). Euratom, Brussels, pp. 209–21.

YOUNG, R. L. and GORDON, M. W. (1962) The disposition of (^{14}C) amphetamine in rat brain. *J. Neurochem.*, **9**:161–7.

CHAPTER 2

ELEMENTARY PHYSICS OF RADIOACTIVATION AND RADIOISOTOPES

Enzo Ricci

Analytical Chemistry Division, Oak Ridge National Laboratory,* Oak Ridge, Tennessee

1. NUCLEAR PROPERTIES

1.1 THE ATOM AND ITS NUCLEUS

Structure. Classic experiments performed by Ernest Rutherford at the beginning of this century led to the conclusion that elements consist of atoms, each having a very small, heavy, positively charged center called the *nucleus*, which is surrounded by light, negative particles called *electrons* (Choppin, 1964; Friedlander *et al.*, 1964; Harvey, 1962; 1965; Weidner and Sells, 1960). A good model for the composition of the nucleus was obtained after James Chadwick (1932) demonstrated the existence of the *neutron*, a particle with no electric charge. The nucleus is formed by a group of neutrons and *protons* bound together by "nuclear forces" whose origin is still unknown. Protons bear one positive elementary charge, and have approximately the same mass as neutrons, as shown in Table 1 (Friedlander *et al.*, 1964); both particles are generically called *nucleons*. The number of protons in the nucleus of an atom is called the *atomic number*, (Z) of that particular nucleus or atom. The number of nucleons in the nucleus is called the *mass number* (A), and the number of neutrons, *neutron number* (N); clearly $A = Z + N$. Each of the electrons which surround the nucleus carries one negative elementary charge; thus a neutral atom should have Z electrons. Atoms and nuclei are represented by the symbol $_Z^A E$, where E is the corresponding chemical symbol. Some examples of light atoms are given in Table 2.

---

* Operated by the Union Carbide Corporation for the U.S. Atomic Energy Commission.

TABLE 1. SOME USEFUL PHYSICAL CONSTANTS AND CONVERSION FACTORS

Quantity	Symbol	Value
Velocity of light	c	2.997925×10^8 m/sec[a]
Elementary charge	e	1.60210×10^{-19}C[a]
Electron mass	m_e	9.1091×10^{-31} kg
		$(5.48597 \times 10^{-4}$ amu)
Proton mass	m_p	1.67252×10^{-27} kg
Neutron mass	m_n	1.67482×10^{-27} kg
Alpha particle mass	m_α	6.64426×10^{-27} kg
Mega electron-volt	MeV	1.60210×10^{-13} joule
		$(3.8291 \times 10^{-14}$ calories)
Atomic mass unit	amu	1.66044×10^{-27} kg
		(931.478 MeV)
Avogadro's number	N_0	6.02252×10^{-23} atoms/mol

[a] The MKS system of units is used throughout this chapter. These expressions mean, respectively, $c = 299,792,500$ m/sec, and $e = (1.60210/10^{19})$ coulomb.

TABLE 2. NOMENCLATURE FOR A FEW LIGHT ATOMS

Name	Symbol $_Z^A$E	Z	A	N	No. of electrons	Nucleus (symbol)
hydrogen-1 (or hydrogen)	$_1^1$H	1	1	0	1	proton (p)
hydrogen-2 (or deuterium)	$_1^2$H	1	2	1	1	deuteron (d)
hydrogen-3 (or tritium)	$_1^3$H	1	3	2	1	triton (t)
helium-3	$_2^3$He	2	3	1	2	helion-3 (^{3}He)
helium-4	$_2^4$He	2	4	2	2	alpha particle (α)
lithium-6	$_3^6$Li	3	6	3	3	
lithium-7	$_3^7$Li	3	7	4	3	
beryllium-9	$_4^9$Be	4	9	5	4	

Atoms or nuclei which have the same Z but different A are called *isotopes*. For example, the natural chemical *element* lithium is formed by a mixture of two of the isotopes mentioned in Table 2, $_3^6$Li (7.42%) and $_3^7$Li (92.58%) (Goldman, 1965; Strominger *et al.*, 1958; Sullivan, 1958); elemental hydrogen is also formed by two isotopes, hydrogen $_1^1$H (99.985%) and deuterium $_1^2$H (0.015%). All these are *stable* isotopes, but, for example, tritium $_1^3$H is unstable because it is radioactive; it is therefore a *radioisotope* of hydrogen. Some natural elements are formed by only one stable isotope (100%, abundance), e.g. beryllium $^9_4$Be, aluminum $^{27}_{13}$Al, cobalt $^{59}_{27}$Co, arsenic $^{75}_{33}$As, iodine $^{127}_{53}$I, gold $^{197}_{79}$Au, bismuth $^{209}_{83}$Bi, etc.; however, many radioisotopes of these elements can be produced artificially.

   If two nuclei differ only in internal energy, i.e. they have the same values for Z and A, they are called *isomers*. For example $^{60m}_{27}$Co (the m meaning metastable or unstable) and $^{60}_{27}$Co (Goldman, 1965; Strominger *et al.*, 1958;

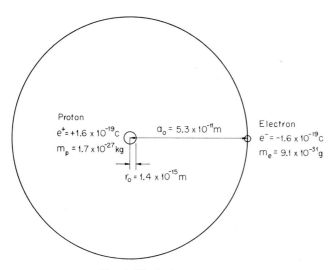

FIG. 1. The hydrogen atom.

Sullivan, 1958). In general, the isomer which is in a higher energy state ($^{60m}_{27}$Co) has a tendency to release its excess energy in the form of electromagnetic radiation (gamma-rays), and transform itself into its lower-energy isomer. This process is called *isomeric transition*. We have seen that the word isotope is used to refer both to one individual atom or nucleus and to a great number of identical ones. Analogously, another word, *nuclide*, refers both to one nucleus and to a great number of them having the same numbers Z and A and the same energy state; naturally, if the nuclide is unstable it will be called *radionuclide*.

   Chemical elements can be characterized either by their chemical symbol or by their atomic number; it is thus somewhat repetitious to use both, and the value of Z is frequently omitted. For example, lithium-6 may be referred to as ^6Li, instead of ^6_3Li, etc. Nuclei of some of the atoms of Table 2 have individual names because they play a very important role in nuclear physics research. These nuclei are listed in the last column, and they are known as *charged particles*; they are commonly used as projectiles to induce nuclear reactions in adequate targets, as will be shown in Section 1.3.

Dimensions. Approximate values for atomic and nuclear dimensions are given in Fig. 1, which represents a hydrogen atom. Exact values of these dimensions can be found in Table 1. We may immediately observe that the *mass* of the electron is negligible with respect to that of the proton:

$$\frac{m_p}{m_e} = \frac{1.67 \times 10^{-27} \text{ Kg}}{9.11 \times 10^{-31} \text{ Kg}} = 1833.$$

The *size* of the hydrogen atom is about twice the radius, a_0, of the electron orbit, i.e. about 10^{-10}m, or 0.0001 μ. The nucleus is much smaller still; its diameter, $2r_0$, is about 40,000 times smaller than the size of the atom:

$$\frac{2a_0}{2r_0} = \frac{5.3 \times 10^{-11} \text{ m}}{1.4 \times 10^{-15} \text{ m}} = 3.8 \times 10^4 = 38000.$$

If the proton had a radius of 10 cm, as has a basketball, the diameter of the atom would be of about 8 km, the size of a town.

Experimental measurements show that, in general, the *volume* V of a nucleus is directly proportional to its mass number A. Thus, assuming spherical shape,

$$V = \frac{4}{3} \pi r^3 = kA, \, k = \text{proportionality constant.}$$

Thus
$$r = \sqrt{\left(\frac{3kA}{4\pi}\right)} = r_0 \sqrt[3]{A} = r_0 A^{1/3}, \tag{1}$$

where $r_0 = \sqrt{(3k/4\pi)} = 1.4 \times 10^{-15}$ m = proton radius (Fig. 1), because for the proton $A = 1$ and $r = r_0$. Let us now calculate the volume of a ^{4}He nucleus (an α particle):

$$V_\alpha = \frac{4}{3} \pi r_\alpha^3 = \frac{4}{3} \pi r_0^3 A_\alpha, \quad \text{by Eq. (1)}$$

$$V_\alpha = \frac{4}{3} \times 3.14 \times (1.4 \times 10^{-15} \text{ m})^3 \times 4 = 4.6 \times 10^{-44} \text{ m}^3.$$

This volume is so small that the *density* ρ of the ^{4}He nucleus is enormous. Using the mass m_α given in Table 1 for this nucleus, we have

$$\rho = \frac{m_\alpha}{V_\alpha} = \frac{6.6 \times 10^{-27} \text{ Kg}}{4.6 \times 10^{-44} \text{ m}^3} = 1.4 \times 10^{17} \text{ kg/m}^3;$$

and, since 1 ton $= 10^3$ kg and 1 ton/m$^3 = 1$ g/cm^3, we have

$$\rho = 1.4 \times 10^{14} \text{ ton/m}^3 = 1.4 \times 10^{14} \text{ g/cm}^3.$$

Thus the density of a ^{4}He nucleus, and in fact that of all nuclear matter, is larger than one hundred million million times that of water.

1.2. RADIOACTIVE DECAY

Henri Becquerel (1896) observed that uranium salts emitted radiation, and 2 years later Pierre and Marie Curie noted that this *natural radioactivity* was characteristic of the uranium element and independent of its chemical or physical state. In fact, it was soon established that radioactivity was a nuclear phenomenon. We have mentioned the existence of stable and unstable nuclei; the unstable or radioactive nuclei tend to transform themselves into stable ones by spontaneous release of energy in the form of radiation, i.e. by *radioactive decay*. For example, radioactive tritium, $^3_1$H, decays *spontaneously* to stable $^3_2$He by emission of one electron:

$$^3_1\text{H} \rightarrow {}_{-1}^{\ 0}\text{e} + {}^3_2\text{He} + {}^0_0\nu + Q. \tag{2}$$

All radioactive decay processes are spontaneous *nuclear reactions*. We see that Eq. (2) is similar to that used for chemical reactions; here ${}_{-1}^{\ 0}$e represents an electron ($A \cong 0$, negligible; $Z = -1$, negative charge) and ${}^0_0\nu$ a neutrino (see below). Q is the energy released during the process; it is shared between the decay products in the form of kinetic energy. Clearly, the algebraic sum of the atomic numbers in the right-hand member is equal to 1, the Z of tritium in the left-hand member; the same balance is true for the mass numbers. We shall soon see (Section 1.3) that the actual weights of the nuclei and the energies are also balanced in both members.

Modes of decay. Radionuclides may decay by emission of alpha particles, beta particles (electrons), or gamma rays.

(a) *Alpha decay.* This results in a nuclide whose A and Z are respectively 4 and 2 units smaller than those of the parent nuclide:

$$^A_Z\text{E} \rightarrow {}^4_2\text{He} + {}^{A-4}_{Z-2}\text{E} + Q;$$

e.g.
$$^{226}_{88}\text{Ra} \rightarrow {}^4_2\text{He} + {}^{222}_{86}\text{Rn} + Q.$$

The energy released, Q, is shared between the alpha particle ($^4_2$He) and the daughter nucleus in the form of kinetic energy. All individual alpha disintegrations involve only two products, and the emitted alpha particles are thus monoenergetic in each particular case. Alpha particles emitted by different nuclides may have different kinetic energies, but, in general, they can be stopped by a thin cardboard sheet.

(b) *Beta decay.* This occurs when electrons are involved in the disintegration process. Besides negative electrons, or *negatrons*, there are also positive electrons, called *positrons*, whose properties are the same as those of negatrons except that they carry a positive elementary charge. Beta particles (negatrons or positrons) are more penetrating than alpha particles. They can be stopped by 1–3 mm of aluminum. There are three types of beta-decay.

Negatron emission. The Z of the product nuclide increases by 1 while A remains unchanged.

$$^A_Z E \rightarrow {}_{-1}^{\;0}e + {}_{z+1}^{\;\;A}E + {}_0^0\nu + Q;$$

e.g.
$$^{131}_{53}I \rightarrow {}_{-1}^{\;0}e + {}^{131}_{54}Xe + {}_0^0\nu + Q.$$

Equation (2) is also an example of negatron emission. We see that a third particle, $^0_0\nu$, is emitted in beta decay; it is called *neutrino*, and it has no charge and negligible mass. It carries momentum, however, and the beta particles emitted are not monoenergetic because the kinetic energy Q must now be shared among three different particles. Therefore there is a *spectrum* of emitted electron energies; the maximum beta particle energy is attained when the neutrino has zero kinetic energy. Only these maximum beta particle energies are normally listed in tables (Goldman, 1965; Strominger *et al.*, 1958).

Positron emission. The Z of the daughter nuclide decreases by 1 and A remains constant:

$$^A_Z E \rightarrow {}_{+1}^{\;0}e + {}_{z-1}^{\;\;A}E + {}_0^0\nu + Q;$$

e.g.
$$^{18}_{9}F \rightarrow {}_{+1}^{\;0}e + {}^{18}_{8}O + {}_0^0\nu + Q.$$

Like the negatrons, the positrons are not monoenergetic, and only their maximum energy is listed in tables.

Electron capture. If a nucleus $^A_Z E$ does not have enough excess energy to emit a positron, it may still decay to $_{z-1}^{\;\;A}E$ by reacting with the closest of the atomic (negative) electrons:

$$^A_Z E + {}_{-1}^{\;0}e \rightarrow {}_{z-1}^{\;\;A}E + {}_0^0\nu + Q;$$

e.g.
$$^{51}_{24}Cr + {}_{-1}^{\;0}e \rightarrow {}^{51}_{23}V + {}_0^0\nu + Q.$$

Obviously there is no particle emitted here except the almost undetectable neutrino.

(c) *Gamma-decay.* We have seen in Section 1.1 an example of isomeric transition:

$$^{60m}_{27}\text{Co} \rightarrow {}^{60}_{27}\text{Co} + {}^{0}_{0}\gamma + Q.$$

Gamma decay can also occur after alpha or beta decay (see Section 1.5) when the daughter nucleus is left in an excited state, i.e. it is left with an excess of internal energy. Though gamma rays are monoenergetic, often two or more are emitted simultaneously, and a discrete gamma-ray spectrum is obtained. During gamma decay there is no change of A or Z; only the internal energy of the nucleus decreases. The general equation then is

$$^{A}_{Z}\text{E} \rightarrow {}^{A}_{Z}\text{E} + {}^{0}_{0}\gamma + Q.$$

Gamma rays are high-energy *photons* (quanta of electromagnetic radiation), i.e. energetic X-rays; a beam of them *cannot* be completely stopped by a screen or shield as was the case with alpha and beta particles. In fact a particular gamma-ray shielding material can be described in terms of the thickness of it, $d_{\frac{1}{2}}$, needed to halve the intensity of a monoenergetic gamma-ray beam; $d_{\frac{1}{2}}$ is called the *half-thickness* of the material. Clearly, a thickness $2d_{\frac{1}{2}}$ will reduce the intensity by a factor of 4; $3d_{\frac{1}{2}}$ by a factor of 8, and so on; an infinite thickness would be necessary to reduce the gamma intensity to zero.

1.3. NUCLEAR REACTIONS

Artificial radioactivity. Rutherford (1919) had observed nuclear transmutations caused by bombardment of nitrogen with alpha particles of polonium, ^{214}Po; however, it was not until 1934 that artificially made radioisotopes began to be produced. In that year Joliot and Curie irradiated boron and aluminum with polonium alpha particles and obtained radioactive ^{13}N and ^{30}P; some particle accelerators were built as well, and they began to be applied to nuclear research. The nuclear reactions associated with the above discoveries can be expressed in the following manner (Section 1.2):

(a) $\quad ^{14}_{7}\text{N} + {}^{4}_{2}\text{He} \rightarrow {}^{17}_{8}\text{O} + {}^{1}_{1}\text{H} + Q_1;$

(b) $\quad ^{10}_{5}\text{B} + {}^{4}_{2}\text{He} \rightarrow {}^{13}_{7}\text{N} + {}^{1}_{0}\text{n} + Q_2;$ $\qquad$ (3)

(c) $\quad ^{27}_{13}\text{Al} + {}^{4}_{2}\text{He} \rightarrow {}^{30}_{15}\text{P} + {}^{1}_{0}\text{n} + Q_3;$

where $_0^1n$ represents a neutron, $_1^1H$ a proton, and $_2^4He$ an alpha particle. The latter two particles are often represented also by the symbols p and α, respectively (see Table 2); Eq. (3a) would then become

$$^{14}_7N + ^4_2\alpha \rightarrow ^1_1p + ^{17}_8O + Q_1.$$

Furthermore, nuclear reactions are frequently expressed in shorthand notation; the bombarding and the ejected particles, in that order, are written in parentheses and between the target and product nuclei. For Eqs. (3) we have : (a): $^{14}_7N(\alpha,p)^{17}_8O$; (b): $^{10}_5B(\alpha,n)^{13}_7N$; and (c): $^{27}_{13}Al(\alpha,n)^{30}_{15}P$. In general, a nuclear reaction takes place when a nucleus interacts with a neutron, a charged particle (see Table 2), or a gamma photon, yielding one or more other particles, or nuclei, or both.

Energetics. As in radioactive decay (see Section 1.2) the nuclear reaction Eqs. (3) show that the sum of the mass numbers A of the reactants is equal to the corresponding sum for the products; the same is true for the sums of atomic numbers Z. Furthermore, these equations are also balanced energetically. To understand this we must use Einstein's famous equation:

$$\Delta E = \Delta mc^2, \tag{4}$$

which gives the energy change ΔE suffered by a system when its total mass changes by an amount Δm; c is the speed of light. Let us take a simple reaction as an example:

$$^2_1H + ^3_1H \rightarrow ^4_2He + ^1_0n + Q. \tag{5}$$

Clearly, for Q to be positive (energy *release*) the sum of the exact masses* of the deuteron m_d and the triton m_t (Table 2) must be *larger* than the sum of the exact masses of the alpha particle m_α and the neutron m_n. In fact, $Q = \Delta E$ is the energy into which this mass excess, Δm, of the left-hand member of Eq. (5) is converted according to Eq. (4). We may write:

$$\Delta m = (m_d + m_t) - (m_\alpha + m_n), \tag{6}$$

$$Q = \Delta E = \Delta mc^2. \tag{7}$$

Many Q values, calculated by the above equations, may be found in tables (Everling *et al.*, 1960).

Energies of nuclear processes are usually measured in *electron-volts* (eV). One electron-volt is the kinetic energy which a free electron acquires in an

* The exact mass of a nucleus is its *actual* mass as given in Table 1. It should not be confused with the mass number A equal to the number of nucleons which form the nucleus.

electric field caused by a potential difference of 1 V. Multiples of 1 eV are 1 keV (1 kilo electron-volt) ($= 10^3$ eV), and 1 MeV (1 mega electron-volt) ($= 10^6$ eV). Although masses are measured in kilograms in the MKS system, a useful alternative unit, at the atomic and nuclear levels, is the *atomic mass unit* (amu) (See Table 1); in the literature atomic masses can be found tabulated in amu for all radioactive and stable isotopes (Sullivan, 1958; Mattauch *et al.*, 1965). The equivalence established by Eqs. (4) and (7), expressed in terms of MeV and amu is:

$$Q \text{ (in MeV)} = 931.478 \times \Delta m \text{ (in amu)}. \tag{8}$$

We can now calculate the value of Q for the reaction $^2_1\text{H}(t,n)\,^4_2\text{He}$ of Eq. (5). We first obtain m_d, m_t, m_α, and m_n:

Deuterium atom mass ($^2_1$H)	2.014740 amu (Sullivan, 1958)
electron mass, m_e (Table 1)	0.000549 amu
	————
deuteron mass, m_d	2.014191 amu
Tritium atom mass ($^3_1$H)	3.017005 amu
m_e	0.000549 amu
	————
triton mass, m_t	3.016456 amu
Helium atom mass ($^4_2$He)	4.003874 amu
$2 \times m_e$	0.001097 amu
	————
mass of nucleus m_α	4.002777 amu
Neutron mass, m_n	1.008986 amu

Thus by Eqs. (6) and (8):

$\Delta m = (2.014191 + 3.016456) - (4.002777 + 1.008986)$ amu,
$\Delta m = 0.018884$ amu,
Q (in MeV) $= 931.478$ MeV/amu $\times 0.018884$ amu,
$Q = 17.59$ MeV.

Since Q is positive, an energy of 17.59 MeV is *released* in each interaction. As with chemical reactions a nuclear reaction with positive Q (such as Eq. (5)) is called *exoergic*, while the term *endoergic* is reserved for reactions of negative Q. An example of the latter is Eq. (3a), for which $Q_1 = -1.19$ MeV; energy must be *added* to the system for this reaction to take place. The usual way to supply this energy is to accelerate particles at high kinetic energies and make them collide with nuclei contained in a target. We will describe a few particle accelerators in Section 2.3.

To be precise, a fraction of the energy of the bombarding particle must be used to impart momentum to the whole system during the collision (conservation of momentum); thus the minimum particle energy required, called the *threshold energy* E_T, should be greater than Q. Kinematic calculations show that (Weidner and Sells, 1960):

$$E_T = - Q \left(\frac{A_1 + A_2}{A_1} \right), \tag{9}$$

where A_1 and A_2 are the mass numbers of the target nucleus and the bombarding particle respectively. For Eq. (3a) the threshold energy is:

$$E_T = - (- 1.19 \text{ MeV}) \frac{14 + 4}{14} = 1.53 \text{ MeV}.$$

Nuclear Energy. It is interesting to calculate how much heat would be liberated if the small amount of deuterium contained in 1 g of the element hydrogen (a natural mixture of isotopes) underwent the reaction of Eq. (5). The number of atoms N of an isotope in **X** grams of the natural mixture that constitutes an element is

$$N = \omega \, N_0 f / M, \tag{10}$$

where N_0 is Avogadro's number (see Table 1), f is the fractional natural abundance of the isotope (Goldman, 1965; Strominger *et al.*, 1958; Sullivan, 1958), and M is the atomic weight of the element. In our example, $\omega = 1$ g, $M = 1.008$, and, since the percent natural abundance of deuterium in hydrogen is 0.015%, $f = 0.00015$. Thus $N = 1 \times 6.023 \times 10^{23} \times 0.00015 / 1.008 = 8.96 \times 10^{19}$ deuterium atoms. The heat released when one deuteron interacts is 17.6 MeV $\times$ 3.83 $\times$ 10^{-14} cal/MeV $= 6.74 \times 10^{-13}$ cal (see Table 1). The total heat released will be 6.74 $\times$ 10^{-13} cal/deuteron $\times$ 8.96 $\times$ 10^{19} deuterons $= 6.04 \times 10^7$ cal. This is about 1000 times the energy released by the most powerful chemical reaction. In fact, the reaction ^2_1H (t,n) ^4_2He is one of the processes used in the so-called "hydrogen (fusion) bomb". Of course, pure deuterium is used there, and f (Eq. (10)) becomes unity, i.e. 6667 times larger than before; the energy release in the bomb is 4.03 $\times$ 10^{11} cal.

Coulomb barrier. One might expect that this strongly exoergic nuclear reaction would proceed spontaneously by simply mixing tritium and deuterium ions (nuclei). This is not true, however, since for a nuclear reaction to take place the two reacting positive nuclei must be brought in contact despite the electrostatic (or Coulomb) force causing repulsion between them. From elementary physics we know that the energy V necessary to cause two charges of equal sign to approach from infinity to a given distance is proportional to the product of the charges divided by the distance. If we let subindex 1 correspond to the target nucleus and subindex 2 to the bombarding particle, their charges will be Z_1e and Z_2e, respectively

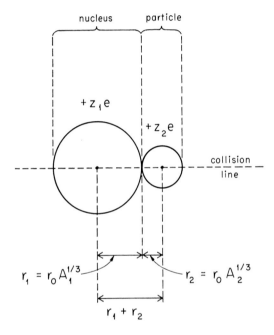

FIG. 2. Coulomb interaction in a nuclear reaction.

(Section 1.1 and Table 1). From Fig. 2 and Eq. (1) we find that the distance at contact is $r_1 + r_2 = r_0 (A_1^{1/3} + A_2^{1/3})$. Thus the energy V, called the *Coulomb barrier*, is:

$$V = K \frac{Z_1e\, Z_2e}{r_0(A_1^{1/3} + A_2^{1/3})} = K' \frac{Z_1 Z_2}{A_1^{1/3} + A_2^{1/3}}, \qquad (11)$$

where $K' = K(e^2/r_0) = 1.03$ MeV $=$ const. Thus, for example, in Eq. (5), for the deuteron (target) $Z_1 = 1$, $A_1 = 2$; and for the triton (particle) $Z_2 = 1$, and $A_2 = 3$. Using Eq. (11),

$$V = 1.03 \times \frac{1 \times 1}{\sqrt[3]{2} + \sqrt[3]{3}} \text{ MeV} = 0.38 \text{ MeV.}^*$$

Therefore, to make the reaction $_1^2\text{H(t,n)}_2^4\text{He}$ possible, energy must be supplied to the system even when this reaction is strongly exoergic. In fact, it is known that the hydrogen bomb must be triggered by a fission bomb; the latter provides the millions of degrees of temperature necessary to raise the kinetic energy of the deuterons and tritons to a value higher than V.

Nuclear fission. Hahn and Strassmann (1939) discovered that the bombardment of uranium with *thermal neutrons*† causes the uranium nucleus to split or undergo *fission* into two lighter nuclei. In the case of ^{235}U these nuclei, generally called *fission products* or *fission fragments*, may have Z numbers ranging from 30(zinc) to 65(terbium), and A numbers from 72 to 161. For example, the well-known radioisotopes $_{38}^{90}\text{Sr}$, $_{39}^{90}\text{Y}$, $_{53}^{131}\text{I}$, $_{55}^{137}\text{Cs}$, $_{56}^{140}\text{Ba}$, and $_{57}^{140}\text{La}$, are frequently obtained as fission products of ^{235}U. The fission of this nucleus may be represented as a nuclear reaction as follows:

$$^{235}_{92}\text{U} + {}_0^1\text{n} \rightarrow {}_Z^A\text{E} + {}_{Z'}^{A'}\text{E} + 2{}_0^1\text{n} + Q, \tag{12}$$

where $_Z^A\text{E}$ and $_{Z'}^{A'}\text{E}$ are the fission fragments, and $A' + A + 2 = 236$, $Z + Z' = 92$. Another expression used, though not very explicit, is ^{235}U (n,f) F.P. The fission process produces more neutrons than it absorbs; in fact, an average of 2.3–2.5 neutrons are produced by each fission. It is thus possible to establish a self-sustaining or *chain reaction* once fission is started. The Q value (Eq. (8)) for fission is about 200 MeV (strongly exoergic); the sum of the exact masses on the right-hand member is always much smaller than the sum on the left-hand member regardless of the identities of $_Z^A\text{E}$ and $_{Z'}^{A'}\text{E}$. Furthermore, these two fission fragments generally release even more energy in the form of a series of successive beta or neutron decays. All the above properties are very useful in the design of nuclear reactors (see Section 2.2) and of atomic (fission) bombs.

Besides ^{235}U, a number of heavy nuclei undergo fission when bombarded with slow neutrons; for example ^{232}U, ^{233}U, ^{239}Pu, and ^{242}Am. Fission has also been induced in nuclei, like ^{235}U, ^{238}U, and ^{232}Th, by accelerated protons, deuterons, and alpha particles, and by gamma rays. Finally, a number of the newly discovered heavy isotopes decay by *spontaneous fission*; examples are $_{95}^{241}\text{Am}$, $_{96}^{248}\text{Cm}$, $_{97}^{249}\text{Bk}$, and $_{98}^{252}\text{Cf}$. Many of the charac-

---

* This value is in fact too high for this reaction. In calculating rigorously, V should be obtained from quantum mechanics. Equation (11) is only an approximation whose error is relatively small when applied to reactions of heavier nuclei.

† Thermal neutrons are neutrons having the same kinetic energy as gas molecules at room temperature, i.e., 0.025 eV (see Section 2.2).

teristics described for the fission of ^{235}U are present in all these other examples.

1.4. LAWS OF RADIOACTIVE DECAY AND GROWTH

Units. The decay rate of a radionuclide, i.e. the number of its atoms (nuclei) which undergo radioactive decay in a unit of time, is also called its *activity or radioactivity A*; it is usually expressed in disintegrations per second (dps) or per minute (dpm).* Radioactivity is measured with special instruments called *radiation counters* or *detectors*. In general, their *detection efficiency* ϵ is less than unity; they thus count a number of events per unit time, $a = \epsilon A$, which is smaller than A but proportional to it. The *count-rate a* is measured in counts per unit time (cps or cpm). The unit of radio-activity is *the Curie* (Ci): $1c = 3.7 \times 10^{10}$ dps $= 2.22 \times 10^{12}$ dpm. Often multiples and submultiples are used, e.g.: 1 kilo-curie (kCi) $= 10^3$ Ci; 1 millicurie (mCi) $= 10^{-3}$ Ci; 1 microcurie (mcCi) $= 10^{-6}$ Ci; and so on.

Decay law. Two important facts have been observed experimentally. Firstly, the activity A of a radionuclide is directly proportional to the number N^* of radioactive atoms present at a given time:

$$A = \lambda N^*, \lambda = \text{decay constant.} \tag{13}$$

Secondly, the time required for the activity of a radionuclide to decrease to half its original value is a constant for that radionuclide; in other words, if the time $T_{\frac{1}{2}}$ is required for an initial activity A to decrease to a value $A/2$, an equal time $T_{\frac{1}{2}}$ will have to elapse before this latter activity, $A/2$, decreases to $A/4$. In fact, this time, $T_{\frac{1}{2}}$, called the *half-life* of the radionuclide, remains constant even if the radionuclide is subjected to extreme physical and chemical conditions. The property of half-life is due to the random mechanism of radioactivity (Friedlander *et al.*, 1964) and leads to a very useful expression that gives N^* at a given time t in terms of λ (Eq. (13)) and of N_0^*, the number of atoms present at time $t = 0$:

$$N^* = N_0^* \, e^{-\lambda t}.$$

If we multiply both members of this equation by λ, by Eq. (13) we have

$$A = A_0 \, e^{-\lambda t}. \tag{14}$$

---

* It should be noted that the expressions dps (or d/s) and dpm (or d/m) are equivalent to $\sec^{-1}$ and 1 $\min^{-1}$, respectively, since "disintegrations" or "atoms" are not strictly physical units.

This is the most important equation of radioactive decay; A_0 is the activity of the radionuclide at the initial time $t = 0$. Values for the exponential functions, e^x (in our case $x = -\lambda t$), can be found in a number of tables, some of them particularly devoted to radioactive decay (Harvey, 1962; U.S. Dept. of Health, Education and Welfare, 1960; National Bureau of Standards, 1961). Many slide rules are designed to compute exponentials. In fact the number

$$e = 1 + \frac{1}{1} + \frac{1}{1 \times 2} + \frac{1}{1 \times 2 \times 3} + \cdots \cong 2.71828,$$

is the well-known base for natural logarithms (Hodgman, 1962); if we apply natural logarithms to Eq. (14) we obtain the equation of a *straight line*:

$$\ln A = \ln A_0 - \lambda t. \tag{15}$$

It is interesting to find the value of the half-life $T_{\frac{1}{2}}$; by its definition, if $t = T_{\frac{1}{2}}$ in Eq. (15), A must be equal to $A_0/2$. Substituting,

$$\ln (A_0/2) = \ln A_0 - \lambda T_{\frac{1}{2}} = \ln A_0 - \ln 2;$$

then
$$- \ln 2 = - \lambda T_{\frac{1}{2}}$$

and
$$T_{\frac{1}{2}} = \frac{\ln 2}{\lambda} = \frac{0.693}{\lambda}. \tag{16}$$

Half-lives for all known radionuclides are given in tables (Friedlander *et al.*, 1964; Goldman, 1965; Strominger *et al.*, 1958; Sullivan, 1958; Way *et al.*, 1961). Substituting $\lambda = 0.693/T_{\frac{1}{2}}$ in Eqs. (14) and (15) we have

$$A = A_0 \, e^{-0.693 \, (t/T_{\frac{1}{2}})}, \tag{17}$$

$$\ln A = \ln A_0 - 0.693 \, (t/T_{\frac{1}{2}}). \tag{18}$$

The straight line A of Fig. 3 is a plot of Eq. (18) in semi-logarithmic scale.*

Radioactive daughters. We have observed (Section 1.3) that the fission process is always followed by chains of successive decays. Most natural radionuclides also give rise to radioactive series of this kind. The mathematical expression that gives the activity of a daughter radionuclide increases in complexity with the length of the chain involved (Friedlander *et al.*, 1964; Harvey, 1962). As an illustration, we will discuss only the case

---

* In this scale, although the numbers written at the left of the ordinate are the activities A, the actual *lengths* measured on this axis are the corresponding values of log A, i.e. decimal logarithms proportional to ln A.

of a very long-lived radioactive parent, which decays to a radioactive daughter of much shorter half-life; e.g.,

$$^{137}\text{Cs}(T_{\frac{1}{2}} = 30 \text{ years}) \xrightarrow{\beta^-} {}^{137}\text{Ba}(T_{\frac{1}{2}} = 2.6 \text{ min}).$$

Firstly, we see that the term $0.693 \, (t/T_{\frac{1}{2}})$ in Eq. (18) for ^{137}Cs is very small if t is of the order of days:

$$t/T_{\frac{1}{2}} = t(\text{days})/(30 \times 365 \text{ days}) = t/10{,}950.$$

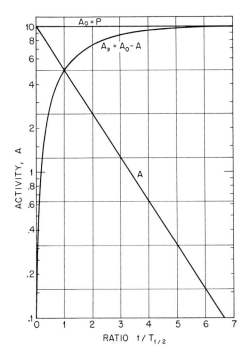

FIG. 3. Radioactive decay and growth: A = decay of daughter separated from parent of constant activity, A_o; A_p = growth of daughter in pure parent fraction.

During a great number of half-lives of ^{137}Ba (several days) the term 0.693 $(t/T_{\frac{1}{2}})$ can be neglected in Eq. (18). Thus $A = A_0 = \text{const.}$ Secondly, each disintegration of the parent produces one daughter atom; an equilibrium will therefore be reached when the numbers of daughter atoms formed and disintegrated per unit time are the same, i.e. when the radioactivity of the parent is *equal* to that of the daughter. This state is called *secular equilibrium*. In our example $A_{\text{Cs}} = A_{\text{Ba}}$, or (from Eq. (13)) $\lambda_{\text{Cs}} N_{\text{Cs}} = \lambda_{\text{Ba}} N_{\text{Ba}}$. Note that owing to the great difference between λ_{Cs} and λ_{Ba}, the numbers of atoms N_{Cs} and N_{Ba} differ by several orders of magnitude. In general, it is true that if a very long-lived parent (subindex 1) generates a chain of radioactive daughters (subindexes 2, 3, ..., n) of shorter half-life, a state of secular equilibrium will be reached where

$$A_1 = A_2 = A_3 = \cdots = A_n; \text{ or } \lambda_1 N_1 = \lambda_2 N_2 = \lambda_3 N_3 = \cdots \lambda_n N_n.$$

This phenomenon is very frequent in natural radioactivity.

Radioactive growth. Suppose that we have a radionuclide (activity $A_0 =$ const.), in secular equilibrium with a daughter (activity, also A_0), and that we *separate* chemically or physically the daughter at time $t = 0$. Let A be the activity of the separated daughter fraction at time t; this fraction will decay normally, according to Eqs. (17) or (18), and to curve A in Fig. 3. At the same time, new daughter material will begin to *grow* in the pure parent fraction; let A_p be the activity of this growing daughter material. Since the decay laws are independent of physico-chemical manipulations it must be at all times:

$$A_0 = A + A_p = \text{const.}$$

Thus, by Eq. (17),

$$A_p = A_0 - A = A_0 - A_0\, e^{-0.693\,(t/T_{\frac{1}{2}})},$$

$$A_p = A_0\, [1 - e^{-0.693\,(t/T_{\frac{1}{2}})}], \tag{19}$$

where $T_{\frac{1}{2}}$ corresponds to the daughter radionuclide. Curve A_p in Fig. 3 graphically represents Eq. (19).

1.5. DECAY SCHEMES

Since radionuclides may decay by several modes simultaneously, it is very helpful to have their decay parameters abstracted in graphical form. Diagrams of this kind are called decay schemes (Dzelepov and Peker, 1957; Strominger and Hollander, 1958; Way *et al.*, 1961), and are employed extensively by nuclear physicists and chemists. As an example, Fig. 4 shows the decay scheme of ^{64}Cu ($T_{\frac{1}{2}} = 12.8$ hr). It exhibits four different modes of decay: (a) 38% by negatron emission with a maximum β^- energy of 0.573 MeV; (b) 0.6% by electron capture followed by emission of a 1.34 MeV gamma photon (total energy jump = 0.34 MeV + 1.34 MeV = 1.68 MeV); (c) 42.4% by electron capture involving a full 1.68 MeV jump; and (d) 19% by positron emission with a maximum β^+ energy of 0.656

MeV. Negatron emission leads to stable ^{64}Zn, while electron capture and positron emission produce ^{64}Ni, also stable. The symbols $(2+)$, $0+$, etc., are related to *nuclear spin* and *parity* (Friedlander *et al.*, 1964; Harvey, 1962; Wiedner and Sells, 1960), and their explanation is beyond the scope of this chapter.

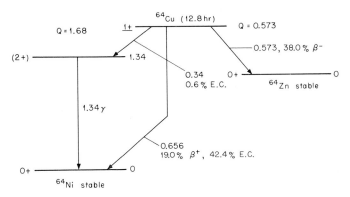

Fig. 4. Decay scheme of ^{64}Cu.

2. PRODUCTION OF RADIOACTIVITY

2.1. ACTIVATION

Equation (19) gives the growth in radioactivity A_p of a daughter related to the decay of a parent whose activity $A_0 = $ const. In fact, A_0 may be regarded in Eq. (19) as a *constant rate of production P* of the daughter radionuclide; thus $A_0 = P = $ const., and Eq. (19) becomes

$$A_p = P(1 - e^{-0.693\, t/T_{\frac{1}{2}}}). \qquad (20)$$

This equation continues to be valid if we generalize the rate P to *any* means of radioactivity production; for example, to nuclear reactions caused by particle bombardment (irradiation). As in Eq. (19) A_p will now be the activity of the product nuclide. Figure 3 shows that the radioactivity production process reaches *saturation*; i.e. 50% of the maximum activity obtainable is generated after bombardment during one half-life $T_{\frac{1}{2}}$ of the product, and 75% of the maximum after 2 $T_{\frac{1}{2}}$; but then the growth becomes very slow and finally practically stops when $A_p \cong P$. At this point ($\sim 7T_{\frac{1}{2}}$) further bombardment does not result in any significant increase of the activity A_p. The factor in parentheses in Eq. (20) is called the *saturation factor*. In practice, since irradiation time at nuclear reactors (neutron bombardment) and charged-particle accelerators is expensive, a sample is seldom irradiated during a time longer than one half-life.

Neutron activation. The *neutron flux* ϕ (inside a nuclear reactor, for example) is defined as the number of neutrons that cross an area of 1 cm² during 1 sec. In general, it is understood that the neutrons may be traveling in *any* direction in space; they do not necessarily form a beam.

The probability of occurrence of a nuclear reaction, usually called *cross-section* σ, is the number of individual reactions which take place in 1 sec (reaction rate) per unit of flux per target atom:

$$\sigma = \frac{P}{\phi N}, \tag{21}$$

where P is equal to the rate of production of Eq. (20) and N is the total number of target atoms, i.e. atoms that may undergo the nuclear reaction; N may be calculated by Eq. (10). The cross-section is measured in cm², or in *barns* (b) ($1b = 10^{-24}$ cm²); it is a constant which only depends on the nature of the nuclear reaction and on the kinetic energy of the bombarding particle.

Substituting the value of P given by Eq. (21) in Eq. (20), we obtain the very useful neutron-activation equation

$$A_p = N\phi\sigma\,(1 - e^{-0.693\,t/T_{\frac{1}{2}}}). \tag{22}$$

Nuclear reactions induced by photon (gamma-ray) irradiation are also ruled by Eq. (22).

Charged-particle activation. Accelerated protons, deuterons, α particles, ³He particles, and tritons are frequently used to produce radioactivity. During charged-particle bombardments the particle is gradually slowed down and finally stopped as it penetrates the target. The distance traveled by the charged particle in the target is called the *range*, and it depends on the nature of target and particle, and on the kinetic energy of the latter. Therefore, as the nuclear-reaction cross section depends on the kinetic energy of the bombarding particle, the cross-section of a charged-particle reaction may be considered a constant only if the target is a *thin foil* (negligible energy degradation). The activation equation for this case is similar to Eq. (22) but slightly modified to account for the small thickness τ (in cm), of the foil, and for the geometrical fact that the flux of charged particles is, in fact, a *beam* which carries I particles/sec:

$$A_p = nI\sigma\tau(1 - e^{-0.693\,t/T_{\frac{1}{2}}}); \tag{23}$$

the same symbols of Eq. (22) are used otherwise, except that n is the number of target atoms per cm^3:

$$n = cf N_0/M. \tag{24}$$

This equation is analogous to Eq. (10), but here c is the *concentration*, in g/cm^3, of the target element in the irradiated sample.

Many important applications of charged-particle activation involve bombardment of *thick targets*. Equation (23) can be integrated to account for the variation of σ with τ; though such a derivation is beyond our scope (Ricci and Hahn, 1964) the final thick-target equation is simple:

$$A_p = nI\bar{\sigma}R(1 - e^{-0.693\,t/T_{\frac{1}{2}}}), \tag{25}$$

where R is the range of the charged particle in the target and $\bar{\sigma}$ is the average cross-section, a complicated function of the particle kinetic energy.

2.2. NUCLEAR REACTORS

Nuclear reactors, or piles, are by far the most important generators of radioactivity. They are widely used to produce radioisotopes and to carry out activation analyses and other nuclear analytical techniques based on neutron reactions. Nuclear reactors use the principle of fission chain reaction (Section 1.3). Figure 5 shows schematically the main characteristics of a nuclear reactor. Thermal neutrons (see below) induce fission of ^{235}U in the graphite–uranium lattice, also called the reactor core; fission products and fast neutrons (0.1–15 MeV) are produced, and energy (heat) is released. The ^{235}U fission cross-section is relatively small for fast neutrons; thus they are slowed down by scattering collisions with the carbon nuclei of the graphite in the core. Graphite is a neutron *moderator*, i.e. a substance capable of slowing down neutrons without substantially absorbing them. Other good moderators are beryllium metal and heavy water (^2H_2O). The slowing-down process, called neutron *thermalization*, continues until most of the neutrons become *thermal*, i.e. until they reach the kinetic energy of the molecules of a gas at 20° (0.025 eV). Since at this energy the ^{235}U fission cross-section is maximum (580 b), the neutrons induce fission on new ^{235}U nuclei and the chain reaction proceeds.

The chain reaction would stop if the rate of neutron disappearance (by absorption or escape) were larger than the rate of neutron production. To maintain the neutron balance, the graphite reflector (Fig. 5) sends a substantial fraction of the escaping neutrons back to the core. On the other hand, the chain reaction would go out of control in a few milliseconds and the reactor would explode if the rate of neutron production were larger than that of neutron loss; the automatically operated control and safety rods guarantee that this does not happen. These rods are made of elements whose cross-section for thermal neutron absorption is very high, e.g. cadmium (20,000 b). The chain reaction diminishes and eventually stops as the control rods are driven gradually into the core.

The figure shows a sample irradiation hole which allows the simultaneous bombardment of a number of samples of relatively large size during extended periods of time; these holes are mainly used for radioisotope

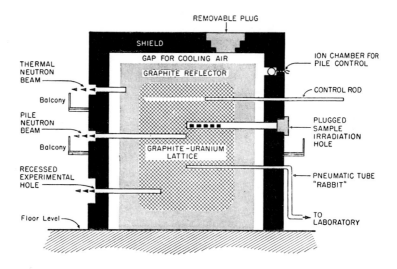

FIG. 5. Sketch of the Brookhaven National Laboratory nuclear reactor (from Hughes, D. J. (1953), *Pile Neutron Research*, Addison-Wesley, Cambridge, Mass.).

production. Short irradiations of individual small samples can be made at the pneumatic "rabbit" facility, also shown, which can transfer specimens from the core to the laboratory (and vice versa) in a few seconds; this facility is particularly appropriate for activation analysis. The neutron-beam holes are useful for physics experiments, and the external shielding is to provide radiological protection around the reactor.

Reactors may vary widely in technology, shape, and dimensions. Figure 5 shows a *heterogenous* reactor; the moderator and the fuel (uranium) are in a solid lattice. The core of a *homogenous* reactor consists, for example, of a solution of fuel (uranium salt) in a moderator (heavy or natural water).

Activation in nuclear reactors. Owing to the characteristics of their operation, nuclear reactors provide copious fluxes of neutrons of a wide range of energies. Figure 6 shows the neutron energy spectrum for a hypothetical reactor with typical flux values for energetically different neutron groups. Thermal neutrons are the most widely used for radio-isotope production and activation analysis, since the cross-sections for (n,γ) reactions and fission are highest for these energies; the thermal flux is

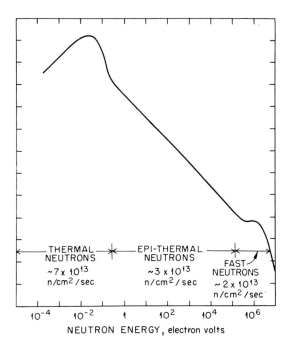

FIG. 6. General features of a reactor neutron spectrum (from Lyon, 1964). Ordinate (logarithmic) represents relative flux in units of $n/(cm^2 \, sec \, eV)$.

also the largest in most reactors. Most of the radionuclides employed today are produced by (n,γ) reactions or fission. Examples of the former are: $^{50}Cr(n,\gamma)^{51}Cr$, $^{23}Na(n,\gamma)^{24}Na$, $^{81}Br(n,\gamma)^{82}Br$, $^{58}Fe(n,\gamma)^{59}Fe$, ^{59}Co-$(n,\gamma)^{60}Co$, $^{84}Kr(n,\gamma)^{85}Kr$, $^{196}Hg(n,\gamma)^{197}Hg$, and $^{202}Hg(n,\gamma)^{203}Hg$. Examples of fission-produced radioisotopes were given in Section 1.3 (Nuclear fission).

Let us calculate the activity A_{th} of ^{51}Cr that may be produced by irradiating 1 g of chromium metal for 1 day with thermal neutrons in the reactor represented by Fig. 6. We should use Eq. (22), modified with the parameters of thermal activation,

$$A_{th} = N\phi_{th}\sigma_0 \, (1 - e^{-0.693 \, t/T_{\frac{1}{2}}}).\tag{26}$$

The *thermal flux* is $\phi_{th} = 7 \times 10^{13}$ n/(cm^2 sec) $= 7 \times 10^{13}$cm^{-2}sec^{-1}. The *thermal cross-section*, $\sigma_0 = 17.0$ b. Also, $t = 1$ day and $T_{\frac{1}{2}} = 27.8$ days (Goldman, 1965; Strominger *et al.*, 1958).

The number N may be evaluated by Eq. (10) by using the values: $\omega = 1$ g, $N_0 = 6.023 \times 10^{23}$, $f = 0.0431$, and $M = 51.996$ from the same references; thus the *yield* of ^{51}Cr for thermal neutrons is

$$A_{th} = \frac{1\text{g} \times 6.023 \times 10^{23} \times 0.0431}{51.996 \text{ g}} \times 7 \times 10^{13} \text{ cm}^{-1} \text{ sec}^{-2} \times 17.0$$

$$\times 10^{-24} \text{ cm}^2 \times (1 - e^{-0.693 \times 1d/27.8d}),$$

$$A_{th} = 1.46 \times 10^{10} \text{ sec}^{-1} = 1.46 \times 10^{10} \text{ dps},$$

which, according to Section 1.4, is equivalent to

$$A_{th} = \frac{1.46 \times 10^{10} \text{ dps}}{3.7 \times 10^{10} \text{ dps/Ci}} = 0.395 \text{ Ci} = 395 \text{ mCi}$$

in curie units. These calculations, which may be facilitated by the use of nomographs (Benson and Gleit, 1963; Ricci, 1964; Stehn and Clancy, 1955), are quite similar to those used to calculate sensitivities in activation analysis (Section 2.4).

It should be pointed out that epi-thermal or resonance neutrons do induce (n,γ) reactions also, and therefore their contribution should be added to the above calculated thermal activation. Resonance activation may be computed by the equation

$$A_r = N\phi_r I_0 (1 - e^{-0.693t/T_{\frac{1}{2}}}),\tag{27}$$

which is similar to Eq. (22) except for the parameters ϕ_r, the *resonance flux*, and I_0 the *resonance integral* (Drake, 1966; Lyon, 1964); the latter is an expression of the overall (n,γ) cross-section for resonance neutrons of a given element. The total (n,γ) activation is, then, by Eqs. (26) and (27):*

$$A = A_{th} + A_r = N(\phi_{th}\sigma_0 + \phi_r I_0) \, (1 - e^{-0.693 \, t/T_{\frac{1}{2}}}).\tag{28}$$

---

* The rigorous treatment of resonance activation is considerably more complex than it is given here, and lies beyond our scope. In consequence, Eq. (28) only represents a good approximation.

The fast or direct-fission neutrons of a reactor can also induce nuclear reactions. These are mainly (n,p), (n,α), and (n,2n) processes; a few typical examples are: ^{32}S (n,p)^{32}P, ^{56}Fe (n,p)^{56}Mn, ^{27}Al(n,α)^{24}Na, ^{35}Cl (n,α)^{32}P, ^{23}Na (n,2n)^{22}Na. Again, in this case, activation calculations can be made by using Eq. (22), properly modified:

$$A_f = N\phi_f \bar{\sigma}_f \left(1 - e^{-0.693\, t/T_{\frac{1}{2}}}\right). \tag{29}$$

Here, ϕ_f represents the *integrated fast neutron flux*, and $\bar{\sigma}_f$ the reaction cross-section averaged over the energy range of the reactor fast neutrons (see Fig. 6); values for $\bar{\sigma}_f$, also called fission-neutron *average cross section*, can be found in the literature (Hogg and Weber, 1963; Rochlin, 1959); generally, these values are orders of magnitude smaller than those for σ_0 or I_0. Because of this fact and because the fast neutron flux in a reactor is generally smaller than the thermal flux, fast neutron reactions are not as important in nuclear piles as (n,γ) reactions. However, the former have one advantage over the latter; most fast neutron reactions yield radioisotopes whose Z's are *different* from that of the irradiated target (different chemical elements), while (n,γ) reactions leave the Z of the target nuclide unchanged. This leads to the important consequence that radioisotopes produced by fast neutron reactions can be easily separated by chemical methods from the bulk of the irradiated target, whereas (n,γ) products cannot.

2.3. CHARGED-PARTICLE ACCELERATORS

A number of ingenious devices have been invented, which can raise the kinetic energy of ions and, thus, can provide beams of accelerated charged particles capable of inducing nuclear reactions by collision with adequate targets. Among these machines, the most useful in radioisotope production and activation analysis are the cyclotron and the Van de Graaff accelerator, both capable of producing energetic beams of protons, deuterons, ^{3}He particles, and alpha-particles.

Cyclotron. It was invented by Lawrence (1929); the first cyclotron produced 13 keV protons. Since then, important developments have taken place which led to the construction of a variety of models; they range from giant machines, capable of delivering, for example, 700 MeV protons for nuclear physics research, to relatively small, inexpensive, high beam-intensity cyclotrons, ideally suited for radioisotope production and activation analysis.

A cyclotron accelerates charged particles in a vacuum box by a combination of electrostatic and magnetic fields. A schematic view of a cyclotron is shown in Fig. 7. It consists of two hollow metal boxes, called "dees" because of their shape, located between the poles of an electromagnet. In the center of the gap, between the dees, positive (or at times negative) ions are formed by the ion source *S*. A large potential difference is established between the dees, whose polarities may be alternated by radio frequency. Suppose that a positive ion is formed at *S*; suppose also that the right dee happens to be negative at this instant. The dee will attract (and accelerate) the ion into it. When the ion is inside the dee it sees no electric field, but it

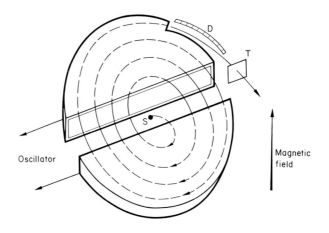

FIG. 7. The cyclotron principle (from Harvey, 1962).

will be acted upon by the magnetic field. Therefore, the velocity of the ion inside the dee is constant (no electric force) but its trajectory draws a half circle (magnetic force) which takes the ion back to the gap. The radio frequency is synchronized so as to cause the left dee to become negatively charged at this very moment, and the particle is then reaccelerated into the left dee. This process is repeated many times, and in general the ion describes a spiral because it is accelerated each time it crosses the gap. The particle kinetic energy is quite high by the time it reaches *D*, the electrostatic deflector that forces it out of the cyclotron, onto the target *T*. Rather high dee voltages (20,000 to 200,000 V) are generally used. Radio frequencies of about 11 or 12 Mc/s and magnetic fields of 15,000–17,000 G are typical for many cyclotrons.

Van de Graaff accelerator. It bears the name of the man who invented it in 1929. Its principle is simpler than that of the cyclotron because it is a purely electrostatic generator. Its operation is schematically shown in Fig. 8. A high potential is transferred to the upper sphere by an insulating belt made of silk or rubber. The belt passes through the gap *AB* where it receives a continuous discharge from the point *B* connected to a high-voltage d.c. source (10,000–30,000 V). Charges deposit and spread over the

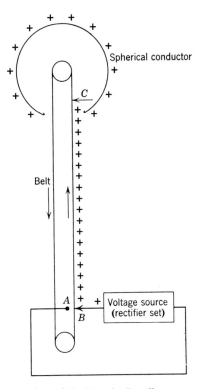

FIG. 8. Charging mechanism of the Van de Graaff generator (from Friedlander *et al.*, 1964).

belt; they are later picked up by a sharp-toothed comb *C* and finally spread over the upper sphere. This sphere will continue to charge up until an equilibrium is reached between its rate of charge and its rate of leakage by corona discharge and other effects. A vacuum tube, called the accelerating tube, runs from the upper sphere to ground (zero potential). Ions are produced in the sphere, by an ion source, and allowed to drift into the accelerating tube towards ground potential. These particles gain great amounts of kinetic energy in the process, and finally hit the target located at the zero-potential end of the drifting tube.

As in the case of cyclotrons, the sophistication and power of Van de Graaff accelerators have increased since 1929. The so-called Tandem Van de Graaff accelerators, for example, consist of two or even three Van de Graaff generators on line, capable of delivering 20 MeV and 30 MeV charged particles respectively.

Charged-particle reactions. Examples of reactions induced by charged particles, particularly useful in radioisotope production are:

$^7\text{Li}(p,n)^7\text{Be}$ $^{24}\text{Mg}(d,\alpha)^{22}\text{Na}$ $^{16}\text{O}(\alpha,pn)^{18}\text{F}$

$^{52}\text{Cr}(p,n)^{52}\text{Mn}$ $^{47}\text{Ti}(d,n)^{48}\text{V}$ $^{50}\text{Cr}(\alpha,2n)^{52}\text{Fe}$

$^{53}\text{Cr}(p,2n)^{52}\text{Mn}$ $^{56}\text{Fe}(d,\alpha)^{54}\text{Mn}$ $^{121}\text{Sb}(\alpha,n)^{124}\text{I}$

$^{65}\text{Cu}(p,n)^{65}\text{Zn}$ $^{58}\text{Fe}(d,2n)^{58}\text{Co}$ $^{123}\text{Sb}(\alpha,n)^{126}\text{I}$

$^{109}\text{Ag}(p,n)^{109}\text{Cd}$ $^{111}\text{Cd}(d,2n)^{111}\text{In}$

A number of the above reactions have also been used in charged-particle activation analysis. However, ^{3}He-activation has proven to be probably the most interesting technique for analysis of light elements. Useful reactions are:

$^9\text{Be}(^3\text{He},n)^{11}\text{C}$ $^{16}\text{O}(^3\text{He},\alpha)^{15}\text{O}$

$^{12}\text{C}(^3\text{He},\alpha)^{11}\text{C}$ $^{16}\text{O}(^3\text{He},p)^{18}\text{F}$

$^{14}\text{N}(^3\text{He},\alpha)^{13}\text{N}$ $^{16}\text{O}(^3\text{He},n)^{18}\text{Ne} \xrightarrow{\beta^+} {}^{18}\text{F}$

Although irradiations at charged-particle accelerators cannot be as lengthy as those performed in reactors, the radioactive yields and activation-analysis sensitivities (Section 2.4) normally obtained with the former are quite good. The main reason for this is that beam intensities of 10^{14} particles per second (I in Eqns. (23) and (25)) are common for charged-particle accelerators, while typical reactor fluxes are smaller (see Fig. 6). Equations (23) and (25) can be directly used to compute charged-particle reaction yields.

Finally, an interesting feature of these reactions is that most radioactive products correspond to elements different from the one bombarded. Thus the product can be easily separated from the bulk of the target by chemistry (see fast neutron reactions, Section 2.2). In fact, this characteristic of charged-particle bombardments is widely used to produce *carrier free* radioisotopes, i.e. radionuclides which contain no significant amounts of the corresponding stable elements of the same Z.

2.4. FAST-NEUTRON PRODUCTION

Among the examples of charged-particle reactions we saw a good number of processes where neutrons were emitted. Some reactions can, in fact, produce copious amounts of neutrons and are currently used for neutron generation.

The most important ones are listed below, followed by their corresponding energy-release value Q (Section 1.3):

$^7Li(p,n)^7Be$	-1.65	$^7Li(^3He,n)^9B$	$+9.35$
$^2H(d,n)^3He$	$+3.27$	$^9Be(^3He,n)^{11}C$	$+7.6$
$^3H(d,n)^4He$	$+17.6$	$^{11}B(^3He,n)^{13}N$	$+10.2$
$^7Li(d,n2\alpha)$	$+15.0$	$^9Be(\alpha,n)^{12}C$	$+5.71$
$^9Be(d,n)^{10}B$	$+3.79$		

Each of these reactions produces neutrons of various energies, depending on the Q-value and on the angle of the neutron trajectory with the direction of the bombarding particle beam. The neutrons emitted in the forward direction, i.e. in the same direction of the beam, are the most energetic.

Fast neutrons from accelerators induce reactions (n,p), (n,α), (n,2n), etc., as do reactor fast neutrons (Section 2.2). In fact, Eq. (29) can be directly used to calculate activation by accelerator fast neutrons, as long as $\bar{\sigma}_f$ is now defined as the average cross-section for the neutron-energy spectrum (different for each accelerator) seen by the irradiated sample; ϕ_f is again the neutron flux integrated over that spectrum. A good compilation of *excitation functions*, i.e. curves of reaction cross section vs. particle energy, for neutron-induced reactions may be found in the article of Jessen *et al.* (1966).

Among our examples, a particularly interesting reaction is ^3H (d, n)^4He, which we studied in detail in Section 1.3. The Coulomb barrier which the deuteron has to overcome is so small and this reaction is so exoergic ($Q = +17.6$ MeV) that it provides the working basis for the widely used 14 MeV *neutron generator*. This device consists of a small electrostatic (Cockroft–Walton) accelerator which produces a highly intense beam of 100–150 KeV deuterons; these particles produce neutrons by bombarding a titanium target saturated with tritium (^3H) by adsorption. In general these generators can produce about 10^{10} to 10^{11} neutrons/sec, within a narrow energy range (14–15 MeV). These accelerators are relatively inexpensive and are very common in activation-analysis laboratories. Their neutron energy is so well defined that tables of cross-sections for 14 MeV neutrons (Chatterjee, 1964 and 1965; Nuert and Pollehn, 1963) make yield calculations very simple in this case. Equation (29) can be quickly used in the form:

$$A_f = N\phi_{14}\sigma_{14}\,(1 - e^{-0.693\,t/T_{\frac{1}{2}}}), \tag{30}$$

where σ_{14} is the 14 MeV neutron cross-section (tables), and ϕ_{14} the 14 MeV neutron flux.

2.5. ACTIVATION ANALYSIS

Elemental chemical analysis by radioactivation, more commonly known as activation analysis, is one of the most sensitive analytical techniques presently available. It is based on the fact, clearly stated by the general Eqns. (22), (23), (25) (and their consequences, Eqns. (26)-(30)) that the radioactivity produced by bombardment of a given mass of element is directly proportional to that mass. The high sensitivity of activation analysis stems from the usually high yield of nuclear reactions and from the great efficiency for radiation detection displayed by present, and even old, instruments.

Procedure. The most common technique in activation analysis is the *comparator method* (Bowen and Gibbons, 1963; Lyon, 1964). It has the advantage that most parameters of Eqns. (22), (23), and (25) (and, there-fore, of Eqns. (26–30)) may be eliminated from the calculations. In neutron activation, for example, this prodcedure requires the simultaneous ir-radiation of the sample (or unknown) with a standard (or comparator) which contains a *known* amount of the element sought in the sample. Let us assume that a sample is being analyzed for chromium against a chro-mium metal standard, by using the reaction ^{50}Cr (n,γ) ^{51}Cr in a nuclear reactor. Chromium-51 ($T_{\frac{1}{2}} = 27.8$ days) is formed both in the sample and in the standard, reaching the absolute activities A_x and A_s, respectively, after an irradiation time t. But the irradiations are simul-taneous and the nuclear reaction is the same in both sample and standard; thus, when we take the ratio A_x/A_s of their activities according to Eqn. (26), the parameters ϕ_{th} and σ_0, and the saturation factor cancel, and we obtain*

$$\frac{A_x}{A_s} = \frac{N_x}{N_s}. \tag{31}$$

Furthermore, the counting efficiency, $\epsilon = a/A$ (Section 1.4), is the same in sample and standard; thus, $A_x/A_s = a_x/a_s$, where the a's are cpm directly

---

* In the general case of neutron activation analysis, Eq. (22) would be used and the reasoning would be analogous.

read on the radiation counter. Also, because in Eqn. (10) N_0, f, and M are the same for both sample and standard (they are just parameters of the natural element Cr) (Goldman, 1965; Strominger *et al.*, 1958), we have that $N_x/N_s = \omega_x/\omega_s$; as in Eq. (10), ω_x and ω_s are masses of Cr element in the unknown and the standard, respectively. Finally, then, Eq. (31) becomes

$$\frac{a_x}{a_s} = \frac{\omega_x}{\omega_s}, \tag{32}$$

where the only unknown is ω_x, the number of grams of chromium in the sample; the other three parameters can be easily obtained from the experiment. Equation (32) clearly shows the attractive simplicity of activation analysis. It should be stressed that this discussion is valid in general for neutron and photon activation analysis; the same reasoning applies, after choosing the proper expression among Eqns. (22), (26)–(30).

Sensitivity. Substituting Eq. (10) in the general equation (22) for neutron and photon activation,

$$A_p = \frac{\omega N_0 f}{M} \phi\sigma(1 - e^{-0.693\, t/T_{\frac{1}{2}}}).$$

The activation-analysis sensitivity may now be immediately defined as $S = A_p/\omega$. Thus,

$$S = (N_0 f/M)\, \phi\sigma(1 - e^{-0.693\, t/T_{\frac{1}{2}}}). \tag{33}$$

For example, let us determine the sensitivity for thermal neutron activation analysis of chromium, in the irradiation conditions of the yield calculation of Section 2.2. We will have $S = A_{th}/\omega$, or, using results of that calculation,

$$S = \frac{1.46 \times 10^{10} \text{ dps}}{1 \text{ g Cr}} = \frac{1.46 \times 10^{10} \text{ dps}}{10^6 \text{ mcg Cr}} = 14,600 \text{ dps/mcg}.$$

Clearly, the sensitivity may also be defined in terms of cpm; the value S' so obtained is proportional to S (Section 1.4):

$$S' = a/\omega = \epsilon A/\omega = \epsilon S.$$

As is shown by Eq. (33), S (or S') depends not only on the nature of the nuclear reaction but also on the flux ϕ and the irradiation time t.

Charged-particle activation analysis. The principles and the procedures are the same as for neutron or photon activation analysis. However, a practical difference is that charged particles have a limited range R in a target (Section 2.1) and, therefore Eq. (23) and particularly Eq. (25), should be used to calculate radioactivation. The expression corresponding to Eq. (31) (comparator method), obtained now from Eq. (25), includes also the ranges R_x and R_s of the charged particle in the sample and the standard, respectively (Ricci and Hahn, 1964).

$$\frac{A_x}{A_s} = \frac{n_x}{n_s}\frac{R_x}{R_s}. \tag{34}$$

Clearly, I, $\bar{\sigma}$, t and $T_{\frac{1}{2}}$ (Eq. (25)) are the same for sample and standard and cancel. Proceeding in the same manner used to obtain Eq. (32), by Eq. (24) we first have $n_x/n_s = c_x/c_s$, where c_x and c_s are the concentrations of the sought element in the unknown and the standard, respectively. Changing now to cpm, Eq. (34) becomes

$$\frac{a_x}{a_s} = \frac{c_x}{c_s}\frac{R_x}{R_s}. \tag{35}$$

The sensitivity in charged-particle activation analysis may simply be defined as $S = A_p/c$; combining Eqns. (24) and (25) we obtain

$$S = (N_0 f/M) I \bar{\sigma} R (1 - e^{-0.693\,t/T_{\frac{1}{2}}}).$$

In terms of cpm we now have $S' = a/c = \epsilon A/c = \epsilon S$. Besides depending on the irradiation conditions (I and t) and on the nature of the nuclear reaction, as in neutron activation, the sensitivity here also varies with the range R.

Bio-pharmacological applications. Activation analysis has been and is being applied widely in numerous fields, including biology and pharmacology. For example, oxygen-18 has been followed in bio-pharmacological studies by charged-particle activation (Roth, 1965) while neutron activation of 43 other stable tracers has been suggested with the same purpose. The use of this method in bio-pharmaceutical research is, in fact, so wide and diversified (I.A.E.A., 1967) that even *in vivo* activation analysis of humans has been recently reported.

2.6. PRODUCTION OF RADIOISOTOPES

Irradiation. Radioactive tracers are produced by irradiation of stable elements, isotopes, or compounds in reactors or accelerators, using techniques very similar to those used in activation analysis. In fact, the procedure is generally simpler in radioisotope production because irradiation conditions are not so critical. In general, the irradiated sample is chemically stable under bombardment, and it contains a large percentage of the stable element or isotope capable of yielding the sought radioisotope. Calculations of radioisotope yields are made by using Eq. (22) (or the corresponding Eqs. (26)–(30)) if neutron or photon irradiations are used, or Eqs. (23) and (25) if the bombardment is with charged particles.

Chemical separations. Frequently the radioisotope must be isolated chemically from other radioactivities, also produced during the irradiation, to achieve *radiochemical purity*. Very often radiochemical separation is necessary also in activation analysis to avoid radioactive *interferences* which preclude a good counting procedure. Naturally, when radiochemical separation is applied, both radioisotope yield and activation analysis calculations should be corrected for chemical separation yields.

REFERENCES

(A) BOOKS, REVIEWS AND MONOGRAPHS

BOWEN, H. J. M. and GIBBONS, D. (1963) *Radioactivation Analysis*, Oxford University Press, London, England.

CHATTERJEE, A. (1964) Alpha reaction cross sections for 14-MeV neutrons. *Neucleonics* **22**: No. 8, 108–9.

CHATTERJEE, A. (1965) Proton, deuteron and triton reaction cross sections for 14-MeV neutrons. *Nucleonics*, **23**: No. 8, 112–18.

CHOPPIN, G. R. (1964) *Nuclei and Radioactivity*. W. A. Benjamin, New York, U.S.A.

DRAKE, M. K. (1966) A compilation of resonance integrals. *Nucleonics*, **24**:No. 8, 108–11.

DZELEPOV, V. S. and PEKER, L. K. (1957) *Decay Schemes of Radioactive Isotopes*. Rpt. AECL-457, Atomic Energy of Canada.

EVERLING, F., KOENIG, L. A., MATTAUCH, J. H. E., and WAPSTRA, A. H. (1960) *Nuclear Data Tables—Consistent Set of Q-Values*: I. $A \leqslant 66$; II. $67 \leqslant A \leqslant 199$. U.S.A.E.C. Rpts., National Academy of Sciences—National Research Council.

FRIEDLANDER, G., KENNEDY, J. W. and MILLER, J. M. (1964) *Nuclear and Radiochemistry*, 2nd ed. John Wiley, New York, U.S.A.

GOLDMAN, D. T. (1965) *Chart of the Nuclides*. 8th ed., Knolls Atomic Power Laboratory, General Electric Company, Schenectady, N.Y., U.S.A.

HARVEY, B. G. (1962) *Introduction to Nuclear Physics and Chemistry*. Prentice-Hall, Englewood Cliffs, N.J., U.S.A.

HARVEY, B. G. (1965) *Nuclear Chemistry*. Prentice-Hall, Englewood Cliffs, N.J., U.S.A.

HODGMAN, C. D. (ed.), (1962) *Handbook of Mathematical Tables*. Chemical Rubber Publishing Co., Cleveland, Ohio, U.S.A.

HOGG, C. H. and WEBER, L. D. (1963) Fast-neutron dosimetry at the MTR-ETR site. *Symposium on Radiation Effects on Metals and Neutron Dosimetry*. Los Angeles 1962, ASTM Special Technical Publication No. 341, 133–40, ASTM Philadelphia, Penn., U.S.A.

INTERNATIONAL ATOMIC ENERGY AGENCY (1967) *Proceedings Symposium on Nuclear Activation Techniques in the Life Sciences*. Amsterdam, 8–12 May.

JESSEN, P., BORMANN, M., DREYER, F. and NEUERT, H. (1966) Experimental excitation functions for (n,p), (n,t), (n,α), (n,2n), (n,np), and (n,nα) reactions. *Nuclear Data*, **1**:Sec. A, 103–202.

LYON, JR., W. S. (ed.), (1964) *Guide to Activation Analysis*. D. Van Nostrand, Princeton, N.J., U.S.A.

MATTAUCH, J. H. E., THIELE, W. and WAPSTRA, A. H. (1965) 1964 atomic mass table, *Nuclear Phys.*, **67**:1–31.

NATIONAL BUREAU OF STANDARDS (1961) *Tables of the Exponential Function e^x*, 4th edn. Applied Mathematics Series 14, U.S. Government Printing Office, Washington, D.C., U.S.A.

NEUERT, H. and POLLEHN, H. (1963) *Tables of Cross Sections of Nuclear Reactions with Neutrons in the 14–15 MeV Energy Range*. Rpt. EUR 122.e, Euratom.

ROCHLIN, R. S. (1959) Fission-neutron cross sections for threshold reactions. *Nucleonics*, **17**: No. 1, 54–5.

ROTH, L. J. (ed.), (1965) *Isotopes in Experimental Pharmacology*, The University of Chicago Press, Chicago, Ill., U.S.A.

STROMINGER, D. and HOLLANDER, J. M. (1958) *Decay Schemes*. Rpt. UCRL-8289, University of California, Radiation Laboratory.

STROMINGER, D., HOLLANDER, J. M. and SEABO G, G. T. (1958) Table of isotopes. *Rev. Modern Phys.*, **30**:585–904.

SULLIVAN, W. H. (1958) *Trilinear Chart of the Nuclides*. Oak Ridge National Laboratory.

U.S. DEPARTMENT OF HEALTH, EDUCATION AND WELFARE (1960), *Radiological Health Handbook*. U.S. Government Printing Office, Washington, D.C., U.S.A.

WAY, K. *et al.* (1961 to date) *Nuclear Data Sheets*. Nuclear Data Group, National Academy of Science, National Research Council.

WEIDNER, R. T. and SELLS, R. L. (1960) *Elementary Modern Physics*, Allyn & Bacon, Boston, Mass., U.S.A.

(B) ORIGINAL PAPERS

BENSON, P. A. and GLEIT, C. E. (1963) Nomograph for determination of neutron-induced activities, *Nucleonics*, **21**: No. 8, 148–50.

RICCI, E. (1964) Nomographs for calculating induced radioactivity and decay. *Nucleonics*, **22**: No. 8, 105–7.

RICCI, E. and HAHN, R. L. (1964) Theory and experiment in rapid, sensitive ^{3}He activation analysis, *Anal. Chem.*, **37**:742–8.

STEHN, J. R. and CLANCY, E. F. (1955) Nomogram for radioisotope buildup and decay, *Nucleonics*, **13**: No. 4, 27.

CHAPTER 3

PREPARATION OF
INORGANIC TRACERS

Howard J. Glenn*

Abbott Laboratories, North Chicago, Illinois, U.S.A.

1. INTRODUCTION

FOR approximately 40 years after the Curies' first isolation of radium the principal radiation resources of the world consisted of a few kilograms of radium and members of its series that had been isolated by laborious extraction from pitchblend and other minerals. There were also small amounts of radioactive thorium and members of its series obtainable from minerals such as monazite. Artificial radioactivity had been known since 1934, and in the late 1930's it was possible to make limited but useful quantities of radioactive isotopes with the then existing cyclotrons. The use of isotopes was limited essentially to physicists at those very few institutions wealthy and fortunate enough to possess a cyclotron. The first reactor-produced isotopes were prepared in 1946 in the United States and announced in the journal *Science*.† Radioisotopes were available shortly thereafter in 1948 from Harwell, England. Major producing reactors are now also in operation in France (Fisher, 1966–7), Belgium, Holland, Norway, Japan, Canada, Egypt, the Soviet Union, and several other countries throughout the world. There are almost 200 species of radioactive isotopes available today from primary or secondary suppliers. The number seems small since over 1000 radioactive isotopes have been isolated and over 1500 have been identified. However, there are now accessible tracer isotopes with usable half-lives for most of the stable elements. The two most important isotopes not having suitable radioactive counterparts are those which would undoubtedly be most important in pharmacological work—oxygen and nitrogen. Generally speaking, though, there are ample

*Present address: The University of Texas, M. D. Anderson Hospital and Tumor Institute at Houston, Houston, Texas, 77025.
† *Science*, **103**:697–705 (1946).

radioisotopes available for most aspects of biological, pharmacological, and medical work.

It is difficult, if not impossible, to limit the scope of this chapter to the preparation of inorganic tracer isotopes for use in pharmacology only. The various disciplines are so interrelated. For example, all pharmaceutical manufacturers now producing radiopharmaceuticals for medical use (Silver, 1965; Wagner, 1966; Fowler, 1965) do extensive radiation and standard pharmacology in new product development. Some of the most exciting work in recent veterinary science is pharmacological in nature (Kallfelz and Wasserman, 1966; Leng and West, 1966–7). Some of the reported pharmacological work using isotopes is essentially biochemical in nature (Chain, 1965). The aim of this chapter is, therefore, to cover the preparation of the most common and available inorganic tracers used in the life-sciences that have a definite relationship to pharmacology. In isotopes, the pharmacologist has a tool that is constantly opening new areas of endeavor, experimentation, and understanding.

There are three stages in the process of making a radioactive chemical (Grove, 1965). The first is the making of the required radioisotope by means of a nuclear transformation in a reactor or cyclotron. The second is the separation in purification of the isotope from the irradiated target material. The third is the use of the raw isotope in the synthesis of a definite chemical product by chemical or biological means. This chapter will deal largely with the first two aspects, but a limited number of inorganic chemical transformations will be given whereby the isotope appears in the final product in a different form than the raw isotope.

2. THE MANUFACTURE OF INORGANIC ISOTOPES

For all practical purposes, the naturally occurring radioisotopes are present in such small quantities or have such unsatisfactory half-lives or radiation characteristics that they are little used as tracers in the life-sciences. There are two general sources (Baker, 1966) for the manufacturing of radioisotopes. These are: (1) the reactor, and (2) the cyclotron. The reactor furnishes a source of neutrons which either can irradiate stable elements bringing about nuclear transformations or can bring about fission of the fuel elements to isotopes of smaller atomic weight. The cyclotron furnishes a source of accelerated charged particles such as the proton (p), the deuteron (d), or the alpha particle (α) which can be beamed

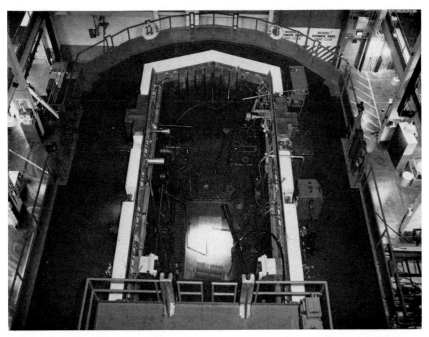

FIG. 1. Oak Ridge research reactor for isotope production, Oak Ridge National Laboratories, Oak Ridge, Tennessee.

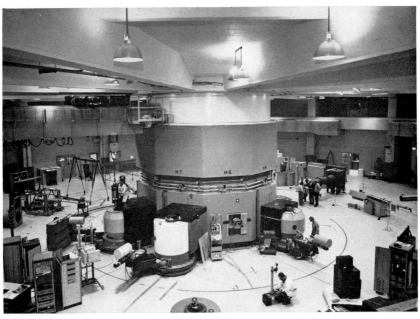

FIG. 2. High flux beam research reactor, Brookhaven National Laboratories, Upton, Long Island, New York.

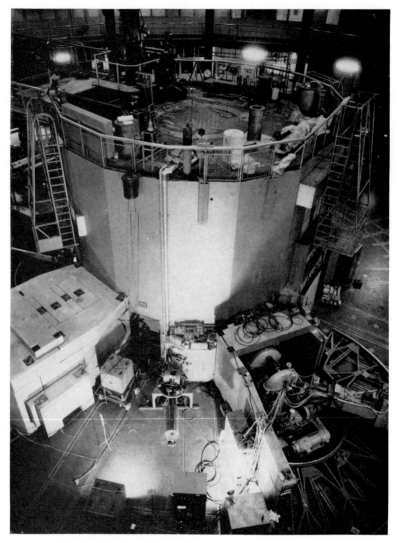

FIG. 3. EL3 reactor for isotope production, Saclay, France.

at the nucleus of a stable element bringing about a nuclear transformation. There are approximately 175 radionuclides in common use today of which about 120–5 are derived from neutron irradiated targets, about 15–20 from fission products, about 30–35 from cyclotrons, and a few from naturally occurring minerals. These figures are only approximate since there are several nuclides that can be obtained from more than one source or by more than one means.

2.2. REACTOR–PRODUCED ISOTOPES

Reactors account for the bulk (in numbers and in quantities) of isotopes produced in the world. Early reactors were powered by natural uranium and were graphite-moderated. They had neutron fluxes ranging from approximately 10^{10} to 10^{13} n/cm² sec. Newer reactors are powered by enriched ^{235}U and may have fluxes in excess of 10^{15} n/cm² sec. Pictures of some of the isotope production reactors are shown in Figs. 1–3. Figure 1 is the Oak Ridge Research Reactor located at the Oak Ridge National Laboratories, Oak Ridge, Tennessee. Figure 2 is the High Flux Beam Research Reactor, Brookhaven National Laboratory, Upton, Long Island, New York. Figure 3 is the EL3 reactor, Saclay, France. The production reactor furnishes as high a neutron flux as possible for neutron activation. Neither the theory nor the energetics of neutron activation, however, will be discussed here because they are covered in the preceding chapter. Neutron bombardment usually gives rise to the "neutron rich" isotopes in which the nucleus of the newly formed isotope has a greater number of neutrons than the stable isotopes of the same element. These unstable isotopes usually decay, often with the emission of a charged beta particle, and often accompanied also by gamma radiation (Leddicott and Reynolds, 1951).

2.2.1. *Nuclear reactions*

When neutrons react with target nuclei, several different nuclear processes can produce radionuclides. There are five common nuclear reactions:

(1) *The* (n,γ) *reaction.* In this nuclear reaction, the target nucleus captures a neutron and gamma radiation is given off. This is the most common type of neutron-induced reaction, and more than half the isotopes in general use are produced by this reaction. Since the isotope produced is of the same chemical nature, a chemical separation cannot be carried out;

thus the specific activity of the resulting radioisotope is limited. Examples
of this nuclear process are:

$$^{197}Au\ (n,\gamma)^{198}Au;$$
$$^{23}Na\ (n,\gamma)^{24}Na;$$
$$^{202}Hg\ (n,\gamma)^{203}Hg.$$

Occasionally a Szilard–Chalmers (1934) reaction takes place during this
nuclear process whereby the recoil of a nucleus after capturing a neutron
results in the product radioisotope being in a different chemical state from
that of the target element. This permits chemical separation with ultimate
improvement in specific activity. For example,

$$^{37}Cl \quad (n,\gamma) \quad ^{38}Cl.$$
Chlorate   Chloride

(2) *The* (n, p) *reaction.* In this nuclear reaction, the target nucleus captures a neutron and gives off a proton. In general, fast neutrons are
required for this reaction, and the cross-section for such a reaction is very
small. Since the nuclide produced by the reaction is of a different chemical
nature from the target element, high specific activity material can be
obtained by chemical separations. Examples of this nuclear process are:

$$^{32}S\ (n,p)^{32}P;$$
$$^{35}Cl\ (n,p)^{35}S;$$
$$^{14}N\ (n,p)^{14}C.$$

(3) *The* (n,α) *reaction.* In this nuclear reaction, the target nucleus
captures a neutron and gives off an alpha particle. Again, the product
nuclide differs chemically from the target nuclide and high specific activity
material results from a chemical separation of the nuclide from the target
material. Examples of this nuclear process are:

$$^{6}Li\ (n,\alpha)^{3}H;$$
$$^{27}Al\ (n,\alpha)^{24}Na;$$
$$^{40}Ca\ (n,\alpha)^{37}Ar.$$

(4) *The* (n, γ)-*decay reaction.* In this nuclear reaction, the target nucleus
captures a neutron and gamma radiation is given off. The new radioactive
nuclide then undergoes radioactive decay and a daughter nuclide is
formed. Since the daughter is usually of a different chemical nature, this is
a useful method of producing a carrier-free isotope. This principle will be
discussed in greater detail in Section 2.4. Examples of this type of nuclear
process are:

$$^{130}\text{Te (n,}\gamma\text{)}\ ^{131}\text{Te} \xrightarrow[\text{decay}]{\beta}\ ^{131}\text{I};$$

$$^{124}\text{Xe (n,}\gamma\text{)}\ ^{125}\text{Xe} \xrightarrow[\text{decay}]{\text{E.C.}}\ ^{125}\text{I};$$

$$^{198}\text{Pt (n,}\gamma\text{)}\ ^{199}\text{Pt} \xrightarrow[\text{decay}]{\beta}\ ^{199}\text{Au}.$$

(5) *The neutron-fission* (n,f) *reaction.* When the reactor fuel nuclei (^{235}U or ^{239}Pu) capture a neutron, fission may take place leading to a wide variety of radioactive fission products. These radioisotopes may accumulate in the reactor fuel and later be processed to give curies of isotopes; or small amounts of the nuclide may be irradiated for certain short-lived isotopes. High specific activity material results on chemical separation. Examples of the neutron-fission process are:

$$^{235}\text{U (n,f)}^{131}\text{I};$$
$$^{235}\text{U (n,f)}^{90}\text{Sr};$$
$$^{235}\text{U (n,f)}^{137}\text{Cs};$$
$$^{235}\text{U (n,f)}^{133}\text{Xe}.$$

The availability of the newer reactors with their resulting high flux has introduced a complicating factor in the production of radioactive inorganic isotopes in the reactor. This complication is known as secondary neutron capture or secondary burnup. The newly formed radioisotope in the reactor itself becomes a target for subsequent neutron capture, and a new radioactive isotopic impurity is produced. The higher the flux, the greater the statistical probability of the secondary neutron capture, and thus the more serious the effect. This factor must now be evaluated carefully for the production of each isotope. For example, 60-day ^{125}I can be produced in a reactor by an (n,γ-decay reaction on ^{124}Xe (cross-section about 200 b). A secondary (n,γ) reaction on the ^{125}I (cross-section about 1200 b) formed leads to 14-day ^{126}I. This unwanted ^{126}I has undesirable radiation characteristics, and the impurity—since it is of identical chemical nature—can only be removed by its more rapid decay. This results in great loss of ^{125}I since it is decaying at the same time. The amount of ^{126}I can be kept below 1% by using short batch irradiations, by the use of a circulating loop process whereby the ^{125}Xe intermediate can be removed from the irradiation zone, or by the use of enriched ^{124}Xe. The products of these manufacturing techniques are then permitted to decay for a short time until the desired low quantity of ^{126}I impurity is reached. Baker *et al.* (1963–4a) discuss this problem of secondary burnup in the production of ^{125}I.

Secondary neutron capture also limits the production of many radio-isotopes in the rare earth series since the cross-sections of the desired radioisotopes are high.

The advantage of using a high neutron flux in the manufacture of ^{131}I has been pointed out by Grove (1965). When a reactor with a flux of 10^{12} n/cm^2 sec was used at the Radiochemical Centre, Amersham, England, it was necessary to irradiate 6 kg of tellurium dioxide each week to produce 40 Ci of ^{131}I. When production was shifted to a reactor with 10^{14} n/cm^2 sec, it was only necessary to irradiate 200 g of tellurium dioxide for one month to obtain 200 c.

2.2.2. *Target considerations*

In this general discussion of the production of inorganic radioisotopic tracers by reactors, a few words must be said about the use of proper target material for the irradiation. The choice of a target material must be made with several considerations in mind. The target must be safe to use in the reactor; it must be of unusual purity; it must be in a form suitable for subsequent processing; and the stable isotope irradiated may be enriched for better yields. Target preparation has become a highly specialized procedure (Baker *et al.*, 1964a).

High flux reactors generate a considerable amount of heat. Thus the target must be cooled, and this usually necessitates complex and expensive means of cooling, and means of inserting and withdrawing sample targets into and from the reactor. No target can be used that could contaminate or harm the reactor or the accessory attachments. For example, there is some reluctance to use ortho or meta telluric acid as a target material for the preparation of ^{131}I (Gleason, 1962). The heat generated in a high flux reactor without adequate cooling means is sufficient to break down the telluric acids to oxides and water, and the resulting steam could burst the capsule containing the newly formed radioactive material. Target materials which undergo heat and radiation decomposition to give gases are usually avoided. In general, the best forms of the target material usually acceptable for radiation in reactors are the metals, their oxides or their anhydrous inorganic salts. It should also be noted that many substances normally considered inert become more reactive under conditions of neutron flux and heat. For example, nitrogen and moisture interreact to form nitric acid which can be highly corrosive.

The ideal target is one that is completely chemically inert under reactor conditions. A target such as this would undoubtedly be so resistant to chemical reaction that the additional chemical processing necessary to convert the target into a usable isotopic form would be very difficult. A few targets can be used directly. Examples of this class are cobalt, gold, and iridium. Most targets for the preparation of inorganic isotopes require chemical solution and purification, and the isotopes are furnished in solution.

A second aspect of target consideration is the importance of target purity. It is probably more important to have absolutely pure target material in this field than in any other field of chemistry. Grove (1965) gives an example of spectroscopically pure rubidium used in the preparation of ^{86}Rb which gave rise to 0.5% ^{134}Cs in the final product due to a trace impurity of cesium present in the starting rubidium. Spectroscopically pure nickel may contain traces of natural cobalt, and this natural cobalt may give unacceptable amounts of ^{60}Co as a contaminant in the ^{58}Co formed by ^{58}Ni (n,p)^{58}Co reaction. The best way of determining the purity of a sample prior to irradiation is to submit a small portion of the target material to irradiation and determine the impurities by activation analysis. The target material should also be checked for impurities of the same chemical material as the isotope sought. For example, if natural iodine is an impurity in the starting material, or is formed in a fission reaction, the specific activity of the radioactive iodine formed will be greatly decreased.

Radiation yield of the desired radioisotope is greatly increased by the use of an enriched stable isotope starting material. This should be taken into consideration in the choice and preparation of target material for the production of inorganic isotopes. This aspect is discussed by Baker (1966) for the production of ^{55}Fe and ^{59}Fe. In general, as one nuclide is enriched, others are depleted. If normal iron is irradiated, a product containing about 10% ^{59}Fe and 90% ^{55}Fe will result. If iron with the stable isotope ^{54}Fe enriched to 98% is irradiated, the radioactive product will be almost pure ^{55}Fe. Conversely, if the target consists of iron enriched to 85% with ^{58}Fe, the ^{55}Fe formed on irradiation is less than 5% of the ^{59}Fe formed.

Baker *et al.* (1963–4b) emphasize the importance of using enriched target material in the preparation of ^{47}Ca. Natural calcium contains about 600 times as much ^{44}Ca as ^{46}Ca and thus largely ^{45}Ca results from neutron irradiation of natural calcium due to the ^{44}Ca (n,γ)^{45}Ca reaction. The calutron enrichment process developed at Oak Ridge National Laboratories makes possible a 10,000-fold enrichment factor of ^{46}Ca. The irradiation of an enriched target containing ^{46}Ca/^{44}Ca in a ratio of 6:1 gives mainly ^{47}Ca by the ^{46}Ca (n,γ)^{47}Ca reaction. The ^{47}Ca/^{45}Ca ratio is greater than 20:1. If target material enriched to 40 % ^{46}Ca is used, the ^{45}Ca impurity content of the final product is less than 1 % at time out of pile.

2.2.3. *Short-lived isotopes*

The increasing demand for the medium short-lived isotope (half-life equals 1–75 hr) has generated much reactor research aimed at their production. The production of short-lived radionuclides is rather difficult in a

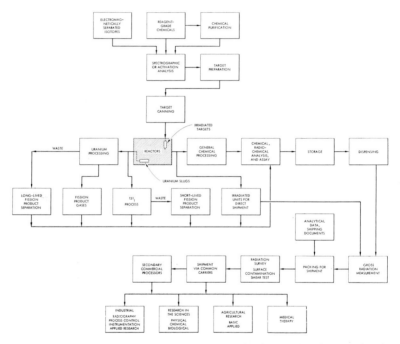

Fig. 4. Flow diagram, inorganic isotope production, Oak Ridge National Laboratories, Oak Ridge, Tennessee.

reactor since the rate of nuclide decay soon equals the rate of nuclide production. However, the use of high flux reactors and enriched targets has made available many short-lived isotopes for common use. The greater number of reactors located in various geographic locations has simplified to some extent the logistics of supply. The techniques of reactor preparation, purification, and uses of these short-lived isotopes are discussed by Baker *et al.* (1964b). These authors list 24 short-lived isotopes available from the neutron-fission reaction in a reactor and 43 short-lived

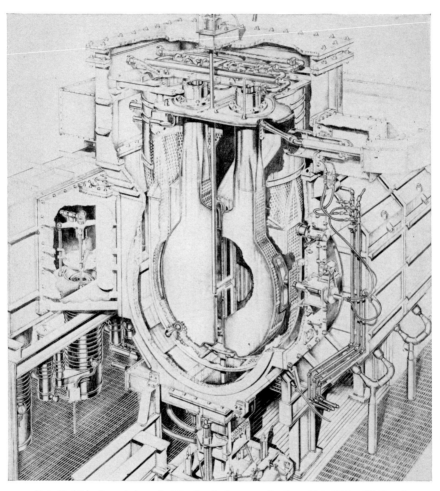

FIG. 5. 86-inch cyclotron facility for isotope production, Oak Ridge National
Laboratories, Oak Ridge, Tennessee.

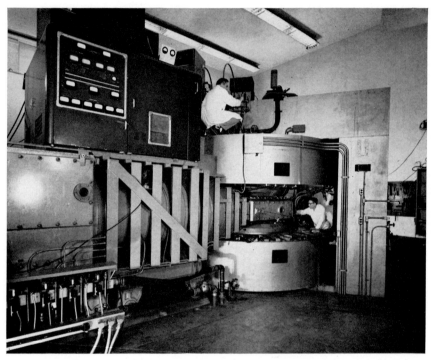

FIG. 6. Sector focusing, variable-energy accelerator, Brookhaven National Laboratories, Upton, Long Island, New York.

isotopes available from neutron activation in the reactor. Nelson and Krause (1963) have described the preparation of such short-lived isotopes as ^{24}Na, ^{31}Si, ^{42}K, ^{64}Cu, ^{65}Ni, ^{82}Br, and ^{109}Pd from neutron-irradiated targets, and ^{99}Mo, ^{132}Te, and ^{140}La from fission products.

Figure 4 is a flow diagram relating to the reactor production of inorganic isotopes as done at Oak Ridge National Laboratories, Oak Ridge, Tennessee.

2.3. CYCLOTRON–PRODUCED ISOTOPES

In many branches of physics, chemistry, engineering, biology, pharmacology, and medicine, isotopes not available from reactors are constantly needed. The other common means of producing inorganic radioisotopes is by means of the particle accelerator. There are various kinds of particle accelerators. Among these should be listed the cyclotron, the synchrocyclotron, the betatron, the synchrotron, the Cockcroft–Walton and Van de Graaf electrostatic generators, and the linear accelerator. There is neither time nor space to describe the physical principles or components of the accelerators. These are amply described by Glasstone (1958), Lanzl (1964), Pinajian (1966a), Pinajian and Butler (1963–4), and others. The instrument usually used in the production of isotopic tracers is the cyclotron.

The science of producing radio elements by charged particles began in 1934 with the discovery of artificial radioactivity when Joliot and Curie used 100 mCi of polonium as a source of α-particles. Accelerators are now available with energies in the billions of electron volts and with beam currents in the milliampere range. Figure 5 is a picture of the 86-inch cyclotron facility at Oak Ridge National Laboratories, Oak Ridge, Tennessee. Figure 6 is a picture of the sector-focusing, variable-energy accelerator at Brookhaven National Laboratories, Upton, Long Island, New York. These accelerators are used to produce neutron-deficient nuclides which cannot, in general, be produced in reactors. These neutron-deficient nuclides are produced by bombarding suitable target materials with accelerated protons, deuterons, tritons, or α-particles. The charged particles add to the nucleus of the target material, and the nucleus then usually decays through proton transformation into a neutron by the emission of a positron or by electron capture.

The use of the cyclotron in isotope production is also discussed by Conzett and Harvey (1966). Often the only isotope of an element available is the one that can be made in the cyclotron. As stated previously, there are no good isotopes of nitrogen and oxygen for pharmacological work. The longest-lived isotopes available from reactor production are ^{16}N with a half-life of 7.4 sec and ^{19}O with a half-life of 29 sec. The pharmacological work that has been done has been with the cyclotron produced isotopes of ^{12}N with a half-life of 10 min and of ^{15}O with a half-life of 2 min. In a similar manner, although long-lived ^{14}C (half-life 5.730 years) is available from a reactor, it is often advantageous to use in biological systems large amounts of cyclotron-produced ^{11}C (half-life 20.5 min). This isotope can be produced by several cyclotron-induced reactions including the ^{11}B (p,n)^{11}C reaction. Sometimes the desired isotopes can be made practically, only in a cyclotron. Important examples of these useful isotopes are ^{22}Na made by the ^{24}Mg (d,α)^{22}Na reaction, ^{57}Co made by the ^{58}Ni (p,pn)^{57}Ni → ^{57}Co reaction, ^{7}Be made by the ^{12}C (p,3p,3n)^{7}Be reaction, and ^{52}Fe made by the ^{52}Cr (α,4n)^{52}Fe reaction or by the ^{50}Cr (α,2n) ^{52}Fe reaction. Considerable information on the use of accelerated deuterons in the production of inorganic isotopes is given by Allen and Cohen (1965–6). Other general papers relating to cyclotron production of inorganic radioisotopic tracers are by Gruverman and Kruger (1959), Martin *et al.* (1955), and Gleason *et al.* (1962).

2.3.1. *Positron emitters*

One of the most fascinating aspects of cyclotron-produced isotopes is the fact that many of the neutron-deficient nuclides decay with positron ($\beta+$) emission. This has given rise to the development of the "positron camera" (Anger, 1963). Use of scintillation counters in coincidence makes possible the detection of the coincident 0.51 MeV photons arising from the positron annihilation. This leads to accurate spacial location of the nucleus at the moment of decay. By the use of ^{18}F (made by the ^{16}O (α,pn)^{18}F reaction) the uptake of fluorine into bones and teeth has been studied. Brain tumors have been localized using ^{74}As made by the ^{74}Ge (d,2n)^{74}As reaction. Also used in brain tumor localizations is ^{68}Ga made by the ^{69}Ga (p,2n) ^{68}Ge → ^{68}Ga (Pinajian, 1964). Coronary flow has been studied in animals and humans by Bing *et al.* (1965a, b) and McHenry and Knoebel (1967) using ^{84}Rb made by the ^{84}Kr(d,2n)^{84}Rb reaction. The nuclide ^{52}Fe (made by the ^{50}Cr(α, 2n)^{52}Fe reaction has been used to study the uptake and location of iron in bone marrow.

2.3.2. *Carrier-free isotopes*

One of the most important aspects of cyclotron-produced nuclides is the fact that the desired isotope is usually produced in a carrier-free state. This is usually not possible in a reactor-produced isotope. In certain trace-element studies it is necessary to use the carrier-free material. For example, ^{65}Zn may be produced in a reactor by a $^{64}Zn (n,\gamma)^{65}Zn$ reaction to a specific activity of about 500 mCi per gram of zinc. Carrier-free material may be produced in a cyclotron by a $^{65}Cu (d,2n)^{65}Zn$ reaction or a $^{65}Cu (p,n)^{65}Zn$ reaction. Also, ^{51}Cr may be produced in a reactor by a $^{50}Cr (n,\gamma)^{51}Cr$ reaction to a specific activity of about 100 Ci per gram of Cr. High as this specific activity is, it may be produced essentially carrier-free in a cyclotron by a $^{51}V (d,2n)^{51}Cr$ reaction.

2.3.3. Target considerations

Target preparation for cyclotron bombardment is a highly developed science unto itself. No effort will be made to discuss the subject in detail in this chapter. All the comments made under targets for reactor irradiation are pertinent with emphasis on target stability to heat and on the extreme importance of target purity. In addition, there are more complex engineering and fabrication problems necessary to adapt the target to the particular cyclotron used. There are many published references to target preparation for cyclotron use. Among these are Martin and Green (1956), Baker *et al.* (1960), and Kobisk (1966).

2.3.4. Short-lived isotopes

The cyclotron is unsurpassed in the preparation of short-lived isotopes. Pinajian (1966b) shows that the 1207 radionuclides of elements with atomic numbers 1 through 83 (hydrogen through bismuth) are mostly of the short-lived variety. The most common half-life is about 1 hr. About 49% of the nuclides have half-lives less than 1 hr; about 24% have half-lives from 1 hr to 1 day; about 20% have half-lives of from 1 day to 1 year; and about 7% have half lives longer than 1 year. Approximately one-half of each group is on the neutron-excess side (reactor produced) of the stability line, and about one-half on the neutron deficient side (cyclotron produced). Thus as many cyclotron-produced isotopes should be usable as reactor-produced, and the number of short-lived isotopes theoretically available should be far greater than the number of longer lived ones. However, Silver (1965) in a recent survey showed that only 34 nuclides of 26 elements have been used to study over 70 body functions. Of these, over 70% of the types of study were carried out with only 9 nuclides of 6 elements: ^{131}I, ^{51}Cr, ^{125}I, ^{99m}Tc, ^{132}I, ^{22}Na, ^{85}Kr, ^{197}Hg, and ^{203}Hg. Thus, considering the special characteristics of the short-lived isotopes along with the greatly reduced radiation to the living organism, it is apparent that the short-lived radio-nuclides offer great promise as tracers in pharmacology, biology, and medicine. The best source of supply seems to be the cyclotron. This possibility is thoroughly discussed by Ter-Pogossian and Wagner (1966).

2.4. NUCLIDE GENERATORS (RADIOACTIVE COWS)

Much has been said of the growing importance of the short-lived iso-topes in biology, pharmacology, and nuclear medicine. The problems of routine production purification and transportation of the very short-lived isotopes are easily understandable when one considers that the half-lives of the desired isotopes are usually measured in hours. These problems relating to time were considered insurmountable until the advent of the nuclide generator or "radioactive cow". The nuclide generator is a con-venient way of making short-lived isotopes available at long distances from the source of production. It is essentially, in its most practical form, a column-milking system for separating two genetically related radionuclides from each other. The idea is usually applied to systems in which a longer-lived parent radionuclide continually decays to a shorter-lived daughter nuclide although other systems have been described. The parent radio-nuclide is usually absorbed in an ion exchange material within a column and permitted to decay. The daughter is separated by fluid elution (milked) and the parent left to generate a new supply of daughter element. This principle of inorganic tracer preparation has been discussed in several articles by Richards (1966), Brucer (1965, 1966), and Greene *et al.* (1963–4) and Stang and Richards (1964).

The most comprehensive discussions on nuclide generators have been by Brucer (1965, 1966). In these references he described 118 possible nuclide generators. Although there are many ways of classifying generators, the most convenient manner divides the nuclide generators into three classifi-cations.

(1) *Converse generators.* In this type of generator, a longer-lived isotope gives rise to a shorter-lived daughter. Most of the practical generators are of this type since it is the shorter-lived isotope generally desired. The im-portant examples of this type will be discussed in greater detail later.

(2) *Reverse generators.* In this generator a shorter-lived isotope decays to generate a longer-lived isotope. Examples of this type of generator are the 6.4-day parent ^{56}Ni, which decays to the 77-day daughter ^{56}Co, and the 85-day parent ^{88}Zr, which produces the 105-day daughter ^{88}Y.

(3) *Isomer generators.* In this system the parent and the daughter are

of the same chemical element. Frequently the radiation of this decay is useful, as in ^{197m}Hg decaying to ^{197}Hg. However, if this type of generator is to be used as a source of specific nuclide, a further decay must take place to produce a different element to make separation possible. For example, ^{129m}Te generates ^{129}Te as a daughter which, in turn decays to generate the granddaughter ^{129}I, which can be separated.

The radiation and physical relationships of parent–daughter radioisotope systems are well known. These have been discussed in detail by Lapp and

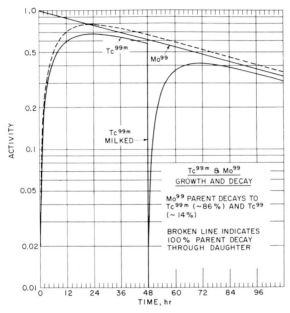

FIG. 7. Growth and decay curves of ^{99}Mo and ^{99m}Tc illustrating parent–daughter relationship made use of in the converse nuclide generator (cow).

Andrews (1954) and Friedlander *et al.* (1964), and others. These relationships are based on the rates of decay of the two isotopes involved. This may be better understood by reference to Fig. 7. This figure shows a growth–decay system for a typical and much-used system—the ^{99}Mo–^{99m}Tc generator. The daughter ^{99m}Tc activity grows in from the decay of the parent ^{99}Mo until the two activities are equal. The maximum growth of the daughter activity is always at this point. From this point on, the daughter activity usually exceeds the parent activity until they reach a state of "equilibrium" where the ratio of the two activities remains constant and both isotopes appear to decay with the half-life of the parent. When the daughter is milked from the parent, the process is repeated. The separated daughter, of course, decays with its own half-life. Once a growth–decay curve of a nuclide generator system is known, it is easy to estimate the period of time required for daughter regeneration for maximum yield. In Fig. 7 it can be seen that the optimum time between milking for the ^{99}Mo–^{99m}Tc cow is about four daughter half-lives or 24 hr.

Radioisotope users are accustomed to receiving isotopes in a ready-to-use precalibrated form. If a nuclide generator is to be used, additional effort must be extended to confirm the purity and to establish the radio assay of the product. Therefore, to be of value as a research tool, a generator must be simple, convenient, dependable, and rapid to operate. The product separated must be of a high degree of purity both as to the radioactive component and the stable nonradioactive components. It is the non-radioactive components of a generator that are frequently overlooked. A frequent contaminant, for example, from nuclide generators based on alumina packing is aluminum ion. Thus purity checks must be made for all possible contaminants.

The eluted or separated product should also be in a form convenient for use or for further processing. Frequently the short half-life of the eluted daughter isotope does not permit extensive purification procedures or considerable additional chemical manipulation. Various separation procedures such as distillation, solvent extraction, precipitation, and ion exchange techniques have been used to separate daughter nuclide from parent nuclide. Of these, the ion exchange procedure, because of its inherent ease and simplicity, has proved to be the method of choice and is used wherever possible. Usually, other methods are used only when ion exchange techniques cannot be used. However, one must be aware of the problems always associated with ion-exchange columns. Precautions must be taken to prevent the introduction into the separated product of foreign material arising from the organic ion exchange material either from the natural or radiation-induced decomposition of the organic material. Organic ion-exchange materials have also been known to support bacterial growth and contain highly pyrogenic materials. Therefore, as a basic principle, the use of inorganic exchange materials such as Al_2O_3 (alumina) or ZrO_2 are preferred where feasible because of their resistance to radiation damage, their greater stability to sterilizing procedures, and their less likelihood of contamination with pyrogenic materials.

Finally, the device (generator or cow) should be of simple and rugged construction which permits easy shielding for use and packaging for transportation. Figure 8 shows a simple generator developed at Brookhaven National Laboratories which has been successfully used for the preparation and separation of short-lived ^{132}I, ^{99m}Tc, and ^{68}Ga from their respective parents. A modified version has been used for the separation of ^{87m}Sr from ^{87}Y. This generator meets all basic requirements for the production of a radiochemical, but not necessarily a radiopharmaceutical. Additional steps leading to a sterile, pyrogen-free product are necessary before a product suitable for parenteral use in humans is obtained. Several commercial modifications of this generator which give a sterile product are now available.

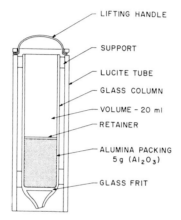

FIG. 8. Suitable radionuclide generator (cow) as developed by Brookhaven National Laboratories, Upton, Long Island, New York.

From a historical standpoint, the first commercially available nuclide generator in a convenient package was the $^{132}Te-^{132}I$ system described by Winsche *et al.* (1951) and modified by Stang *et al.* (1958) and Tucker *et al.* (1958). Various other methods of daughter separation and purification have been reported by Cook *et al.* (1956) and Arnott and Peruma (1957). In the best system, 3.2-day ^{132}Te is suspended on an alumina column and the 2.3-hr ^{132}I is eluted usually with 0.01 M ammonium hydroxide solution in the form of iodide. Unfortunately the radiation characteristics of ^{132}I are not the best since it decays with numerous hard beta and gamma rays. This short-lived isotope has been more widely used in Europe than in North America.

To date the most important nuclide generator is the $^{99}Mo-^{99m}Tc$ system which is widely used in the nuclear medicine field. The short half-life and the clean 140 keV gamma ray of the ^{99m}Tc make this a particularly good scanning isotope in humans (Harper *et al.*, 1964a, b; Harper *et al.*, 1965; Stern *et al.*, 1965). The generator has been described in numerous articles by Richards (1965a, b), Tucker *et al.* (1958), Allen (1965), Pinajian (1966b), and others. The parent 2.8-day ^{99}Mo is deposited on an alumina column. The ^{99}Mo is prepared either by the neutron-fission process or by a neutron-gamma reaction on ^{98}Mo. The 6-hr daughter ^{99m}Tc is milked from the column using 0.1 M nitric acid, 0.1 M hydrochloric acid, or an isotonic solution of sodium chloride. For parenteral use, the latter solution is preferable. Usually, 70–80% of the expected activity is separated. If the parent ^{99}Mo is of fission origin, it may be necessary to remove other radiation contaminants such as ^{103}Ru and ^{106}Ru by an extraction process with methyl ethyl ketone as described by Harper (1964b). The chemical form of the ^{99m}Tc as milked from the column is the pertechnetate, and in this form it has some of the same biological distribution and activities as I^-, ReO_4^-, and ClO_4^-. It is usually used directly in this form, but other inorganic preparations and uses in the thiocyanate (Harper *et al.*, 1964b) and in the sulfide–sulfur colloid (Tc_2S_7–S) (Larson and Nelp, 1966) (Patton *et al.*, 1966) forms have been described.

Another nuclide generator coming into more common use is the ^{113}Sn–^{113m}In cow (Subramanian and McAfee, 1967). The 118-day ^{113}Sn is suspended on a hydrogen-reduced zirconium oxide column. The daughter, 1.7-hr ^{113m}In is eluted with very dilute hydrochloric acid solution, pH 1.1–1.5, as ^{113m}In Cl in 84–86% yield. The nuclide has been used largely as a gelatin stabilized colloid of ^{113m}In OH or gelatin stabilized iron-^{113m}In hydroxide suspension. The column and the preparation and use of the ^{113m}In components have been described by Stern *et al.* (1966, 1967) Goodwin *et al.* (1966), and Castronovo and Stern (1967). The nuclide has been used thus far for lung, liver, brain, and blood pool scanning. Its short 1.7-hr half-life and its clean 390 keV gamma ray make the isotope an excellent nuclide for *in vivo* biomedical and pharmacological studies.

It has long been recognized that in biological systems a nuclide tracer suitable for bone studies would be highly desirable. The readily available ^{45}Ca is only a weak beta emitter and not suitable for studies requiring gamma radiation. The more recent availability of ^{47}Ca has aided the situation somewhat in certain studies, but the hard gamma energy of ^{47}Ca does not adapt itself to radioisotopic scanning. It has long been realized that there are definite differences, but also certain similarities in the metabolism of calcium and strontium. However, the radiation characteristics of the available strontium isotopes (^{90}Sr and ^{85}Sr) were not considered ideal for the intended uses either. Recently, a nuclide generator system has been developed which makes available the short-lived ^{87m}Sr with a half-life of 2.8 hr and a 388 keV gamma ray. In the method of Allen and Pinajian (1965) the parent nuclide, 80-hr ^{87}Y, is prepared by bombarding ^{87}Sr in a cyclotron with protons using a 95.4% enriched ^{87}Sr target in the form of strontium carbonate. A $^{87}Sr (pn)^{87}Y$ reaction ensues. The ^{87}Y parent is absorbed on a Bio-Rad AGl, X-10 resin in the carbonate form and the daughter ^{87m}Sr eluted with 0.1 M ammonium carbonate solution. The milked solution is then evaporated to dryness to remove the volatile ammonium carbonate and the residue dissolved in isotonic saline for use.

The nuclide generator system developed by Hillman *et al.* (1966) prepares the parent ^{87}Y by bombarding natural rubidium chloride with α-particles in a Rb (α,xn)Y reaction. The parent nuclide is absorbed on a Dowex-1 column in the carbonate form and the daughter separated by milking the column with a 0.005% citric acid solution, pH 5.0.

The value of ^{87m}Sr in human clinical studies has been explored by Charkes *et al.* (1964) and Mecklenburg (1964).

The nuclide generator system $^{68}Ge–^{68}Ga$ has been used for the preparation of ^{68}Ga, half-life 68 min, for pharmacological and medical studies. A solvent extraction system was first described by Gleason (1960). The long-lived ^{68}Ge was prepared by the $^{69}Ga (p,2n)^{68}Ge$ reaction and separated from the gallium by a distillation and precipitation technique. After returning to solution, the short-lived daughter ^{68}Ga was separated from the parent by solvent extraction at a pH of 4.5 with 25% acetylacetone in cyclohexane. By re-extracting the organic phase with 0.1 N hydrochloric acid, 96% of the ^{68}Ga could be returned to the aqueous phase.

An improved ^{68}Ga cow was described by Greene and Tucker (1961) whereby the parent ^{68}Ge is suspended on a column made of chromatographic alumina and the daughter ^{68}Ga is separated by eluting (milking) with 0.005 M EDTA (ethylenediamine tetra-acetic acid) solution, pH 7. A similar cow has been described by Yano and Anger (1964) for medical use, and the use of ^{68}Ga in the form of gallium citrate has been described as a bone-scanning agent in animals by Hayes *et al.* (1965).

The use of a nuclide generator to separate 2.6-min ^{137m}Ba from the 30-year half-life parent ^{137}Cs has been described by Blau *et al.* (1966). The parent ^{137}Cs is adsorbed on ammonium molybdophosphate ion exchange crystals and the daughter ^{137m}Ba is separated by eluting with a 0.1 N hydrochloric acid–0.1 N ammonium chloride solution. After several milkings, the ^{137}Cs content is less than one part per billion. The extremely short half-life of the ^{137}Ba makes possible the giving of multimillicurie doses, and the repetition of the study every few minutes. This short-lived isotope has been used successfully in studies of vascular dynamics and renal and portal blood flow.

A ^{188}W–^{188}Re cow has been described by Lewis and Eldridge (1966). The parent tungsten isotope, ^{188}W, is prepared by double neutron capture in ^{186}W targets. The nuclide generator was prepared by absorbing the ^{188}W as tungstate on the chloride form of Bio-Rad HZO-1, a hydrous zirconium oxide ion exchanger. The ^{188}Re elution and separation is best achieved for pharmacological purposes by the use of isotonic saline solution. The principle advantage of this generator is the 70-day half-life of the parent ^{188}W. The radiation properties of the 17-hr daughter ^{188}Re are not the best, but are acceptable. Hayes and Rafter (1966) have reported on the pharmacological properties of this isotope in animals. Perrhenate in animals behaves similarly to pertechnetate and iodide.

Many other nuclide generator possibilities have been envisioned. Among these, as suggested by Stang and Richard (1964), are the following:

Parent (half life)	Daughter (half life)
^{28}Mg (21.3 hr)	^{28}Al (2.3 min)
^{42}Ar (3.5 year)	^{42}K (12.4 hr)
^{140}Ba (2.8 days)	^{140}La (40.2 hr)
^{144}Ce (285 days)	^{144}Pr (17.3 min)
^{103}Pd (17 days)	^{103m}Rh (57 min)
^{44}Ti (10 years)	^{44}Sc (3.9 hr)

3. THE SEPARATION AND PURIFICATION OF INORGANIC ISOTOPES

The second stage in the process of making a radioactive chemical for tracer purposes, whether it is made in a reactor, in a cyclotron, or by a nuclide generator, is the separation, purification, or refinement of the desired radioisotope from the target material or from other generated radiation impurities. There are two broad classifications of purification problems according to whether or not the product is of the same atomic number as the target and thus chemically indistinguishable from it, or of a differing atomic number and thus able to be separated chemically.

It was pointed out earlier that the neutron–gamma (n–γ) reaction yields products of the same atomic number. Thus the specific activity of products produced from this reaction is always of a lower order of magnitude because of the impossibility of chemically separating the radioactive nuclide from the nonradioactive target material of the same element. Simply bringing target into solution is usually not sufficient purification because of the necessity of separating the other radiation impurities. For example, in the preparation of ^{55}Fe from the reaction ^{54}Fe(n,γ)^{55}Fe, a small amount of ^{54}Mn may be formed from the reaction ^{54}Fe(n,p)^{54}Mn. Thus the ^{54}Mn must be separated from the ^{55}Fe by chemical means.

Or, radio-impurities may arise from the irradiation of trace impurities in the target material. Unless purification steps are taken, ^{51}Cr prepared by the reaction ^{50}Cr(n,γ)^{51}Cr may be contaminated by trace amounts of ^{60}Co arising from the reaction ^{59}Co(n,γ)^{60}Co on almost immeasurable amounts of cobalt impurity in the chromium. Thus a chemical separation of cobalt from chromium brings about a radionuclide purification also.

If the radiation impurities are of the same atomic number (same chemical element the impurities cannot be separated. It is therefore necessary, if possible, to rely on a difference between the decay rates of the isotopes to bring about a radiation purification. For example, several arsenic isotopes are frequently formed together, and the radio purity of ^{74}As is increased on standing in comparison with ^{72}As because the ^{72}As with a half-life of 26 hr decays away at a faster rate than ^{74}As with a half life of 18 days. Conversely, the radio purity of ^{74}As decreases on standing in comparison with ^{73}As due to the longer half-life of 76 days for ^{73}As.

Frequently, the presence of radiation impurities of the same atomic number are best "removed" by minimizing their formation in the first place. Wilson (1966a) gives what is probably a classical example of this when he discusses the presence of ^{203}Hg contamination in ^{197}Hg. If natural mercury is irradiated for about 1 week at optimum flux, ^{197}Hg (half-life of 65 hr) is produced which contains about 2% ^{203}Hg (half-life of 47 days) at time out of pile. If a target enriched in ^{196}Hg to an isotopic abundance of 25% (instead of the normal 0.146%) is used, ^{197}Hg essentially free of ^{203}Hg can be produced. The competing reactions are ^{196}Hg(n,γ)^{197}Hg and ^{202}Hg(n,γ)-^{203}Hg.

If the desired radioisotope is produced by any one of a number of nuclear reactions in which there is a change in atomic number, then the radioisotope is in a different chemical form than is the target, and a chemical separation may be effected as a means of purification. Chemical separation of any two or more species is based on differences in their physical and chemical properties, and takes advantage of preferential distribution between two easily separated phases. The phases may be solid–liquid, liquid–liquid, solid–gas, or liquid–gas. The ratio of distribution in the phases between the radioisotope desired and the impurity is called the "separation factor" and is a measure of the separation efficiency. Obviously, high separation factors are desirable, and, if the separation factor is high enough, purification may be effected in one stage. If not, several stages may be necessary to effect adequate purification.

The methods for separating and purifying radioisotopic tracers include such techniques as ion exchange (Orr, 1964), solvent extraction, precipitation, and distillation. The preparative process for each isotope must be studied in order to determine the best purification scheme. The principal difference between isolating radionuclides and ordinary compounds lies in the exceedingly small quantities involved in radiochemistry. One is dealing with only trace amounts of chemical even though relatively large amounts of radiation may be present; thus procedures must be adapted to trace quantity recovery, and phenomena like surface absorption, physical hold-up, mechanical loss, etc., become of paramount importance. Originally, the term "carrier-free" was applied to a radioisotope if no additional non-radioactive carrier element of the same chemical composition was added during the processing. Now this term is being reevaluated in a more realistic manner and a specific activity approaching that of the theoretical is now being recommended before the term "carrier-free" is used (Grove, 1965).

The theoretical weight of one curie of carrier-free radioisotope may be closely approximated by the formula:

$$\frac{\text{grams}}{\text{curie}} = \frac{M \times T_{\frac{1}{2}} \text{ (days)}}{1.3 \times 10^8},$$

where M is the mass number (atomic weight) of the radioisotope and $T_{\frac{1}{2}}$ is the half-life of the radioisotope in days. For ^{131}I, for example, one can calculate the approximate grams per curie of carrier-free material to be:

$$\frac{131 \times 8.05}{1.3 \times 10^8} = 8.1 \times 10^{-6} \text{ g/ci.}$$

In a like manner, it can be shown that 1 Ci of ^{32}P weighs only 3.5×10^{-6} g; 1 Ci of ^{60}Co weighs only 8.8×10^{-4} g; and 1 Ci of ^{14}C weighs only 0.22 g. The theoretical weights of 1 Ci of other radioactive isotopes are correspondingly small. Therefore, any procedure used, chemical or otherwise, must be effective in the handling of microgram or sub-microgram amounts of material, and all the skills of a microanalytical chemist must be employed if "carrier-free" quantities are to be isolated.

It is also necessary that a radionuclide tracer, after preparation and purification, be quantified as to the amount of radioactivity present. Radioactive tracers are always prepared, specified, and distributed on the basis of activity. The special unit of activity is defined as the curie, which is 3.7×10^{10} nuclear disintegrations or transformations per second, or subunits such as the millicurie (10^{-3} Ci) or the microcurie (10^{-6} Ci). It is not the purpose of this chapter to discuss the measurement and quantification of radioactivity other than to affirm that this is a necessary step in the preparation of an inorganic radioactive tracer and that its preparation is not complete until the activity has been quantitated in terms of specific activity (mCi/mg or mCi/milliatom) and/or assay (mCi/ml) if a solution is involved. This aspect has been covered by Wilson (1966b), Mann and Garfinkel (1966), Lyon *et al.* (1966), Parr (1965), and others.

For excellent directions for the complete preparation and purification of many of the commercially available inorganic tracers, one should refer to Stang (1964) and Case (1964). Excellent information on product specifications, testing, and chemical and radiation quantification is available in the Oak Ridge National Laboratory (Tennessee) Master Analytical Manual, TID-7015, Sections 1, 2, 3, 5, and 9, Supplements 1–8.

4. THE SYNTHESES OF COMPLEX INORGANIC ISOTOPES

The third area to be covered briefly in this chapter is the use of the commercially available simple inorganic radiochemicals in the syntheses of more complex inorganic tracer substances. Admittedly much of the tracer work in pharmacology, biochemistry, and medicine has been done with labeled organic molecules, the syntheses of which will be covered in the following chapter. However, certain more complex labeled inorganic compounds have been important in pharmacology and medicine. As the use of labeled compounds increases, so will the use of the more complex inorganic tracers.

4.1. EXCHANGE REACTIONS

Although exchange reactions are common ways of preparing tritium, iodine, and some carbon labeled organic compounds, it is not common to prepare inorganic compounds in this manner. A covalent or coordinate–covalent type of bonding within the molecule is usually considered a prerequisite for this manner of synthesis. The ionic or polar bonding present in most of the simpler inorganic molecules is too labile a bond for molecular labeling. The high degree of ionization resulting from the ionic bonding brings about separation between the radioactive ion and the rest of the molecule. There is immediate and complete exchange between $^{23}Na^+$ and $^{22}Na^+$ in sodium chloride; but because of the high degree of ionization, it is more of an isotope dilution effect whereby the $^{22}Na^+$ is diluted by and distributed with the nonradioactive $^{23}Na^+$. In any physiological system, an ionic-labeled ion should not be used to trace a more complex molecule because of ionic separation. For example, $^{22}Na^+$ cannot be used to trace sodium chromate because ionization will separate the sodium ions from the chromate ion.

In certain cases of inorganic molecules with largely covalent or coordinate–covalent bonding, the exchange technique can be used to prepare the labeled compound. An example is the preparation of ^{125}I or ^{131}I labeled iodine monochloride. It is not necessary to prepare by rigorous synthetic means labeled iodine monochloride. There is immediate exchange between free iodine labeled with ^{125}I or ^{131}I and the ^{127}I in iodine monochloride in an organic solvent such as carbon tetrachloride, or there is immediate exchange between labeled iodide ion and the ^{127}I in iodine monochloride in acetic acid or dilute (3 N) hydrochloric acid.

There is usually very little or very limited exchange between a simple ion and the same species within a radical. There is, to illustrate, essentially no exchange between arsenic ion and the arsenic in the arsenate radical or between the chromium ion and the chromium in the chromate radical. Exchange rates studies such as this may be of theoretical interest, but have little practical synthetic value.

4.2. CHELATED OR COMPLEXED INORGANIC ISOTOPES

A second means of labeling compounds with inorganic ions should be mentioned briefly even though it brings us to the fringes of labeled organic compounds. This involves the chelation reaction. In this process, the inorganic ion is bound tightly to or complexed with, usually, an organic molecule through a combination of polar and nonpolar bonds in such a manner that, within certain ranges of hydrogen ion concentration, the ionic properties of the inorganic ion are lost or changed. The primary purpose is not to label the organic chelating agent but to modify the properties of the inorganic ion.

One of the outstanding examples of a change in pharmacological properties of an inorganic ion brought about by the use of this technique is illustrated with ^{51}Cr. Chromic chloride Cr-51 ($^{51}CrCl_3$) binds tightly to serum proteins and has been used to measure gastric enteropathies (Walker-

Smith *et al.*, 1967). Sodium chromate Cr-51 ($Na_2{}^{51}CrO_4$) labels red blood cells and has been widely used to measure red blood cell mass and erythrocite survival time (Albert, 1963). However, if ^{51}Cr is chelated with ethylene-diamine tetra-acetate (EDTA), its physiological properties are completely changed (Winter and Meyers, 1962). Stacy and Thorburn (1966) also synthesized ^{51}Cr-EDTA and showed that in sheep, only 1.5–2% of the material was bound to plasma and that the substance could be used to estimate the kidney glomerular filtration rate.

^{68}Ga chelated with EDTA (Yano and Anger, 1964) and ^{113m}In chelated with EDTA (Stern *et al.*, 1967) behave pharmacologically quite different from their ionic counterparts.

Most cations can be chelated with EDTA or other common chelating agents. Citric acid, an organic acid, is often used as a complexing agent. The inorganic cation is bound in a different manner than what one would expect from a simple carboxylic acid. Since ferrous citrate is often used in hematological studies in pharmacology, and since the material is not available from commercial suppliers, its preparation is described by Glenn (1966). Ferrous sulfate is made alkaline with sodium hydroxide to precipitate the ferrous hydroxide. The precipitate is washed well and dissolved in a stoichiometric amount of citric acid and kept in a reduced state by a small amount of ascorbic acid. The radioactive ferrous citrate ^{59}Fe or ^{55}Fe may be made by adding the radioactive iron to any desired assay at the beginning of the preparation. Tauxe (1961) describes a method of preparing ferric ammonium citrate labeled with ^{59}Fe. This product is suitable for the determination of serum iron binding capacity.

The use of ^{68}Ga complexed with citrate is described by Hayes *et al.* (1965).

4.3. INORGANIC CHEMICAL REACTIONS

Essentially any standard inorganic reaction can be duplicated in the radioisotope laboratory in the preparation of inorganic tracer compounds for use in pharmacology. It must always be borne in mind, however, that the use of very small quantities may bring about handling problems not usually encountered in the laboratory. For example, the volatility of iodine or hydrogen iodide is a real hazard in an isotope laboratory unless elaborate precautions are taken to trap the minute amount of evolved gases. Large amounts of ^{131}I radiation may be released in a very small volume of gas. All isotope reactions must, therefore, be run in an adequate fume hood and special precautions used to trap volatile components. Trouble may also be encountered if one is attempting to purify a carrier-free material by precipitation. The solubility product of the substance may not be exceeded and no precipitation may result. It is possible, however, that the material in the resulting clear solution may not act ionic; it may act colloidal in nature. The pharmacology and chemistry of [113m]In as reported by Stern *et al.* (1967) is an excellent example of this phenomenon. It is shown that the distribution of carrier-free [113m]In in organs varies greatly with the chemical form of the [113m]In as determined by pH.

Surface absorption of the active material is also usually a problem. One must take precautions against losing much of the activity on the surface of the glassware or other substances used in purification such as ion exchange resin, filter papers, etc. It is customary to soak glassware in hot phosphoric acid before working with ^{32}P, or hot sulfuric acid before working with ^{35}S, or with sodium iodide before working with ^{131}I or [125]I. The resulting products cannot be considered carrier-free, but reaction yields are improved. The addition of a few milligrams of the proper carrier ion will also prevent surface absorption. Frequently the surface of all glassware can be siliconized to prevent surface absorption of the isotope (Petroff *et al.*, 1964).

One should carefully read the articles of Bonner and Kahn (1951) in which some aspects and the behavior of carrier-free radioisotopic tracers are discussed.

Following are selected examples of inorganic syntheses on simpler starting materials yielding products of value to the pharmacologist in tracer studies.

Sodium chromate Cr-51 (Abbott, 1966a). The chemical form in which ^{51}Cr is available from direct reactor processing is usually chromic chloride Cr-51. It is often contaminated with ^{60}Co due to trace impurities of cobalt present in the irradiated chromium. In processing, then, the chromic chloride Cr-51 is usually made alkaline in the presence of an added small quantity of ferric iron salt. The cobalt impurity co-precipitates with the ferric hydroxide and the amphoteric chromium remains in alkaline solution. The chromium is then oxidized to chromate by hydrogen peroxide or sodium peroxide and the solution neutralized to a pH of 7–8. The sodium chromate Cr-51 is usually used to label red blood cells to do red blood cell mass studies or red blood cell survival studies.

Colloidal gold Au-198. The chemical form in which [198]Au is available from direct reactor processing is usually in the form of metallic gold foil or auric chloride Au-198. Colloidal gold Au-198 is available from commercial radiopharmaceutical suppliers, but only in limited colloidal sizes. It thus may become necessary to prepare a stable colloidal solution for pharmacological work. A good preparation has been described by Henry *et al.* (1957) and modified by Douis (1963). The gold foil is dissolved in aqua regia and evaporated to dryness in the presence of excess hydrochloric acid. The chlorauric acid Au-198 is reduced to colloidal gold in the presence of gelatin at 70° by ascorbic acid in the presence of a small amount of "seed" inactive gold colloid. The colloidal size of the "seed" colloid determines the size of the product colloid. Colloidal gold Au-198 has been used in cancer studies, RES studies, liver studies, bone marrow studies, and flow studies in pharmacology and medicine.

A further chemical reaction has been performed on radioactive colloidal gold by Hahn (1967). He treats the ^{198}Au colloid with aqueous silver nitrate solution to prepare silver-coated radioactive gold colloid.

Chromic phosphate P-32. The chemical form in which ^{32}P is usually available from the reactor is labeled orthophosphate. This is suitable for many tracer studies involving phosphate, but occasionally an insoluble form is wanted. To satisfy this need, two chromic phosphates P-32 have been developed. The first is a true colloidal dispersion of chromic phosphate P-32 as recently described by Anghileri and Marquis (1967).

The second is a particulate suspension (Abbott, 1966b) which is made in a very insoluble form in order to resist enzymatic and microbial attack in biological systems. In this preparation, the ^{32}P in the form of phosphate is precipitated and heated at an elevated temperature for several hours to convert to an "ignited" and more insoluble form. The residue is then ground to a fine powder and suspended in 25% glucose for administration.

The preparation of both a true colloid and a suspension of chromic phosphate P-32 has also been described by Burg and Chevallier (1958).

The preparation of condensed phosphate (polymetaphosphate) labeled with ^{32}P and used in therapy of carcinoma of the prostate has been described by Kaplan *et al.* (1960). Its preparation is based on the careful and controlled heating of sodium dihydrogen phosphate as described by Jones (1942).

Sulfur-35 and phosphorus-32 inorganic compounds. A large amount of pharmacological and biochemical work has been done with labeled ^{32}P and ^{35}S compounds, most of them organic compounds. However, certain basic inorganic ^{32}P and ^{35}S compounds are required in the syntheses of the compounds, and these inorganic starting materials must be synthesized. Some of these syntheses are very difficult and require a high degree of laboratory skill. Among the more common inorganic compounds are labeled $^{32}PCl_3$, $^{32}POCl_3$, $^{32}PSCL_3$, $^{32}PCl_5$, $^{32}P_2S_5$, ^{35}S, $^{35}SO_2$, $H_2{}^{35}S$, and $K^{35}SH$.

^{35}S is now usually available commercially in three forms as sulfuric acid, as barium sulfide, and as elemental sulfur in a solvent such as benzene. However, sometimes circumstances demand other forms or special states of purity. Thus much simple inorganic chemistry has been done with ^{35}S. Tarver and Schmidt (1939) wanted labeled hydrogen sulfide and potassium hydrogen sulfide as starting materials for a series of organic syntheses. They fused elemental ^{35}S with iron to form pure ferrous sulfide ^{35}S. When this was treated with dilute acid, hydrogen sulfide-^{35}S was generated for use. When the hydrogen sulfide-^{35}S was trapped in dilute potassium hydroxide solution, potassium hydrogen sulfide,^{35}S resulted. These products were then used in the syntheses of ^{35}S-labeled organic compounds.

A new direct laboratory method of preparing carrier-free $H_2{}^{35}SO_4$ from reactor irradiated potassium chloride has been reported by Suarez (1966). The radioactive sulfur constituents are reduced to $^{35}SO_2$ by a hot mercury–phosphoric acid combination. The distilled $^{35}SO_2$ is oxidized to $H_2{}^{35}SO_4$ by hydrogen peroxide. Hard beta radiation impurities are reported to be less than 0.01 %.

Seligman *et al.* (1943) have also prepared purified simple ^{35}S compounds. Starting with sulfuric acid-^{35}S, they precipitated barium sulfate-^{35}S. This was reduced in 98 % yield to barium sulfide-^{35}S by heating at 750° in a stream of hydrogen. Hydrogen sulfide-^{35}S was freed by treating the sulfide with phosphoric acid. The hydrogen sulfide-^{35}S was then either converted to elemental sulfur-^{35}S by oxidation with iodine or was changed to potassium hydrogen sulfide-^{35}S by dilute potassium hydroxide solution. These inorganic products were then used in the more complex organic syntheses of methionine-^{35}S, cystine-^{35}S, and homocystine-^{35}S.

Koski (1950) wanted very high specific activity hydrogen sulfide-^{35}S and prepared it in 95 % yield in a rather unusual way. The ^{35}S was prepared by the $^{35}Cl(n,p)^{35}S$ reaction on potassium chloride. The potassium chloride containing the ^{35}S was then heated in an atmosphere of hydrogen in a quartz container at 1100°C for 3 hr and then at 550° overnight.

The preparation of sulfur dioxide-^{35}S has been reported by Johnson and Huston (1950). A mixture of barium sulfate-^{35}S and red phosphorus was ignited electrically in a stream of oxygen. A pure sulfur dioxide-^{35}S was secured in good yield.

Considerable synthetic work has also been done with ^{32}P; since phosphoric acid-^{32}P is usually the only labeled form commercially available, other inorganic forms must be synthesized. Once again, the inorganic compounds prepared are usually only the starting material for more complex labeled organic compounds. Therefore the degree of purity must be high.

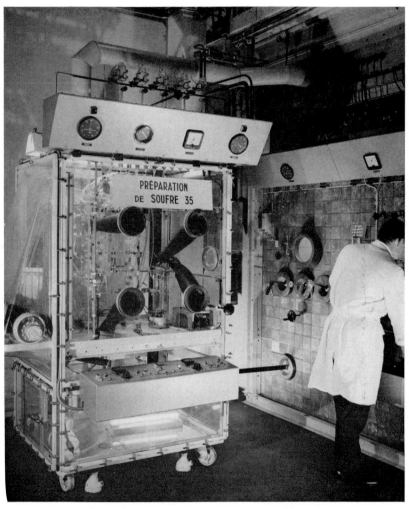

FIG. 9. Enclosure unit for the preparation of ^{35}S, Saclay, France.

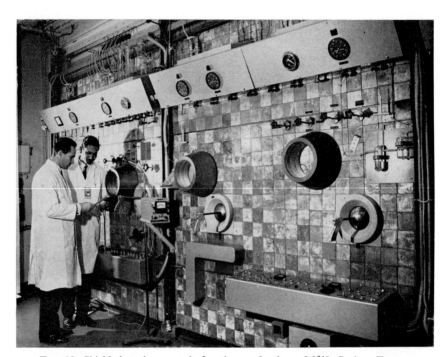

FIG. 10. Shielded enclosure unit for the production of ^{131}I, Saclay, France.

Axelrod (1948) and Kalinsky and Weinstein (1954) have prepared phosphorus oxychloride by heating phosphoric acid-^{32}P with nonradioactive phosphorus pentachloride according to the following equation:

$$H_3PO_4 + 3PCl_5 \rightarrow 4POCl_3 + 3HCl.$$

A purified product resulted in about 95% yield by the improved method of Kalinsky and Weinstein.

Fukuto and Metcalf (1954) have prepared thiophosphoryl-^{32}P chloride by reacting phosphoryl-^{32}P chloride with sulfur in the presence of aluminum chloride as follows:

$$2^{32}POCl_3 + 3S \rightarrow 2^{32}PSCl_3 + SO_2.$$

Their yield was about 62%.

Probably the most complete study on the preparation of high specific activity inorganic labeled ^{32}P compounds has been made by Bebesel and Turcanu (1966). They found that compounds labeled with ^{32}P such as P_2S_5, PCl_3, $PSCl_3$, $POCl_3$, and H_3PO_4 could be obtained by simple methods with good yields and high specific activities. Carrier-free ^{32}P from the ^{32}S(n,p)^{32}P reaction on elemental sulfur was concentrated on red phosphorus or activated carbon. Then simple inorganic chemical reactions led to the desired labeled product. Their work can be summarized by the flow diagram of Fig. 8a. Figure yields are given in parentheses.

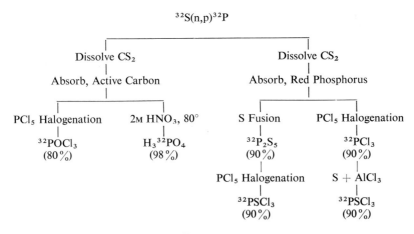

Fig. 8a.

5. RADIATION SAFETY AND HEALTH PHYSICS

A brief word should be said about the safe handling of radioisotopes during synthetic procedures. All isotopes should be handled under the rules and regulations of the governmental atomic energy regulating authority and with the cooperation of a person trained in radiation health physics. No work should be done with radioisotopes unless the individual has had proper training in the safe handling of radioactive materials and is fully informed as to the potential dangers associated with radiation. On the low level scale of operation, all reactions should be run within a good fume hood behind shielding, and all volatile radioactive components collected in a trapping system designed for that particular isotopic synthesis. All high level syntheses should be run in enclosed systems with adequate shielding and air flow. All exit gases from the fume hood or closed system should be passed through particulate and absolute filters to prevent the release of radioactive materials to the atmosphere. Figure 9 shows an enclosed plastic unit used in the synthesis of ^{35}S compounds, and Fig. 10 shows an enclosed heavily shielded unit used in the production of ^{131}I, at Saclay, France.

The hands should be protected by suitable gloves at all times, and the eyes by safety glasses. No radioactive material should be ingested; this means there should be no eating or smoking in a radioisotope laboratory. Laboratory workers should wear individual radiation badges and dosimeters at all times within the laboratory, and these should be read at routine intervals by the health physicist to assure that permissible radiation doses are not exceeded. Sufficient clothing should be on hand so that immediate changes can be made in case of contamination. Decontamination showers and areas should be available to personnel. Continuous care must be taken at all steps of the synthetic process to avoid the spillage or scattering of radioactive material, and all dry and liquid radioactive waste should be disposed of in the proper manner as prescribed by local law. All procedures should be monitored by the radiation health physicist.

REFERENCES

(A) BOOKS, REVIEWS AND MONOGRAPHS

BEHRENS, C. F. and KING, E. R. (1964) *Atomic Medicine*, 4th edn. Williams & Wilkins, Baltimore, Maryland.

BLAHD, W. H. (1965) *Nuclear Medicine*. McGraw-Hill, New York, U.S.A.

CASE, F. N. (coordinator), (1964) *ORNL Radioisotopes Procedures Manual*. ORNL-3633, June, Oak Ridge National Laboratories, Oak Ridge, Tenn., U.S.A.

GRAUL, E. H. (ed.), (1957) *Fortschritte der angewandten Radioisotopie und Grenzgebiete*. Dr. Alfred Hutig, Verlag, Heidelberg, Germany.

STANG, L. G. (coordinator), (1964) *Manual of Isotope Production Processes in use at Brookhaven National Laboratory*, BNL 864(T-347), August. Brookhaven National Laboratory, Upton, New York, U.S.A.
WAY, K. *et al.* (1966) *Nuclear Data Sheets.* Academic Press, New York, U.S.A.
WILSON, B. J. (ed.), (1966) *The Radiochemical Manual*, 2nd edn. Radiochemical Centre, Amersham, England.
WILSON, D. W., NIER, A. O. C., and REIMANN, S. P. (1946) *Preparation and Measurement of Isotopic Tracers.* J. W. Edwards, Ann Arbor, Michigan, U.S.A.

Bulletin d'Informations Scientifique et Techniques, No. 51 (1961). Published by Commissariat à l'Energie Atomique, Centre d'Études Nucléaires de Saclay, France.
Processed Isotopes. Catalog for Brookhaven National Laboratory, Upton, Long Island, New York, U.S.A.
Radio and Stable Isotopes. Catalog for Isotopes Development Center, Oak Ridge National Laboratory, Oak Ridge, Tenn., U.S.A.
Radioactive Products. Catalog for the Radiochemical Centre, Amersham, England.
Radioactive Materials. Catalog for Nuclear Science and Engineering Corporation, Pittsburg, Penn., U.S.A.
Radio-Isotopes and Labelled Compounds. Catalog for Le Commissariat à l'Energie Atomique, France; Le Centre d'Étude de l'Energie Nucléaire, Belgium; and La Societa Ricerche Impianti Nucleari, Italy.
Radio-Isotopes. Catalog for Institutt for Atomenergi, Kjeller, Norway.
Radioisotope and Nuclear Services Technical Data Sheets. Union Carbide Corporation Research Center, Tuxedo, New York, U.S.A.
Radioisotope Sample Measurement Techniques in Medicine and Biology, Proceedings of a Symposium held by the International Atomic Energy Commission in Vienna, May 24–28, 1965. IAEA, Vienna, 1965.

(B) ORIGINAL PAPERS

ABBOTT (1966a) Rachromate-51, sodium chromate Cr-51 injection. *Radiopharmaceutical Product Literature*, 01-3024/R5-12 Rev. June 1966. Abbott Laboratories, North Chicago, Ill., U.S.A., 1–24.
ABBOTT (1966b) Chromic phosphate P-32. *Radiopharmaceutical Product Literature*, 01-3623/R5-12 Rev. April 1966, Abbott Laboratories, North Chicago, Ill., U.S.A., 1–11.
ALBERT, S. N. (1963) *Blood Volume.* Thomas, Springfield, Ill., U.S.A.
ALLEN, A. J. and COHEN, B. L. (1965–6) Production of carrier-free radioisotopes with the University of Pittsburg cyclotron. *Isotopes Radiat. Technol.* 3:85–87.
ALLEN, J. F. (1965) An improved technetium-99m generator for medical applications. *Int. J. Appl. Radiat. Isotopes*, 16:332–4.
ALLEN, J. F. and PINAJIAN, J. J. (1965) A Sr[87m] generator for medical applications. *Int. J. Appl. Radiat. Isotopes*, 16:319–25.
ANGER, H. O. (1963) Gamma-ray and positron scintillation camera. *Nucleonics*, 21 (10): 56–9.
ANGHILERI, L. J. and MARQUIS, R. (1967) New colloidal chromic phosphate (P32) for local irradiation of the central nervous system. *Int. J. Appl. Radiat. Isotopes*, 18:97–100.
ARNOTT, D. G. and PERUMA, C. P. (1957) An emanating source for I[132]. *Int. J. Appl. Radiat. Isotopes*, 2:85–86.
AXELROD, B. (1948) A study of the mechanism of "phosphotransferase" activity by the use of radioactive phosphorus. *J. Biol. Chem.*, 176:295–8.

BAKER, P. S. (1966) Reactor-produced radionuclides, in *Radioactive Pharmaceuticals*, Proc. Symposium held in Oak Ridge, Tenn., November, 1965, CONF-651111, U.S. AEC Division of Technical Information Extension, Oak Ridge, Tenn., U.S.A. pp. 129–39.

BAKER, P. S., DUNCAN, F. R. and LOVE, L. O. (1960) Cyclotron targets using enriched stable isotopes. *Nucl. Sci. Eng.*, 7:325–32.

BAKER, P. S., RUPP, A. F., and ASSOCIATES (1963–4a) Iodine-125 production. *Isotopes Radiat. Technol.* 1:143–6, 155–7.

BAKER, P. S., RUPP, A. F., and ASSOCIATES (1963–1964b). Calcium-47 production at ORNL. *Isotopes Radiat. Technol.*, 1:146–9, 157–8.

BAKER, P. S., RUPP, A. F., and ASSOCIATES (1964a) ORNL Target Fabrication Center. *Isotopes Radiat. Technol.*, 2:5–8, 16–17.

BAKER, P. S., RUPP, A. F. and ASSOCIATES (1964b) Production and application of short-lived radioisotopes. *Isotopes Radiat. Technol.*, 1:207–24.

BEBESEL, P. I. and TURCANU, C. N. (1966). New possibilities to obtain ^{32}P-labeled inorganic compounds of high specific activity. *J. Labeled Comp.*, 2:314–16.

BING, R. J., COHEN, A., GALLAGHER, J. P., LUEBS, E. D., VARGA, Z., YAMANAKA, J. and ZALESKI, E. J. (1965a) The quantitative determination of coronary flow with a positron emitter (rubidium 84). *Circulation*, 32:636.

BING, R. J., COHEN, A., ZALESKI, E. J., and LUEBS, E. D. (1965b) The use of a positron emitter in the determination of coronary blood flow in man. *J. Nucl. Med.* 6:651.

BLAU, M., ZIELINSKI, R. R., and BENDER, M. A. (1966) Ba^{137m} cow—a new short-lived isotope generator. *Nucleonics*, 24(10):60–2.

BONNER, N. A. and KAHN, M. (1951) Some aspects and behavior of carrier-free tracers, I. *Nucleonics*, 8(2):46–59; II, *Nucleonics*, 8(3):40–61.

BRUCER, M. (1965) 118 medical radioisotope cows. *Isotopes Radiat. Technol.* 3:1–12.

BRUCER, M. (1966) A herd of radioisotope cows. *Vignettes in Nuclear Medicine*, No. 3. Published by Nuclear Consultants Division of Mallinckrodt Chemical Works, St. Louis, Miss., U.S.A.

BURG, C. and CHEVALLIER, A. (1958) New method for the preparation of very active chromium radiophosphate for therapeutic use. Proceedings of the Second United Nations International Conference on the Peaceful Uses of Atomic Energy, Geneva, Switzerland, September 1–13, 26:424–6.

CASE, F. N. (coordinator). (1964) *ORNL Radioisotopes Procedure Manual*. ORNL-3633, June.

CASTRONOVO, F. P. and STERN, H. S. (1967) Experiences with the Sn^{113}–In^{113m} generator. *Nucleonics*, 25(2):64–5.

CHAIN, E. B. (1965) Use of radioisotopes in general biochemistry. *Chem. Ind.* 1352–3.

CHARKES, N. D., SKLAROFF, D. M. and BIERLY, J. (1964) Detection of metastasis to bone by strontium 87m. *Amer. J. Roentg. Rad. Ther. Nucl. Med.*, 91:1121–7.

CONZETT, H. E. and HARVEY, B. G. (1966) Role of the modern cyclotron in nuclear research. *Nucleonics*, 24(2):48–57.

COOK, G. B., EAKINS, J., and VEALL, N. (1956) The production and clinical applications of iodine-132. *Int. J. Appl. Radiat. Isotopes*, 1:85–93.

DOUIS, M. (1963) Préparation de l'or colloidal 198. *Minerva Nucleare*, 7:448–50.

FISHER, C. (1966–7) Production and use of radioisotopes in France. *Isotopes Radiat. Technol.*, 4:189–94.

FOWLER, J. F. (1965) Radioisotopes in medical diagnosis. *Chem. Ind.*, 1353–5.

FRIEDLANDER, G., KENNEDY, J. W. and MILLER, J. M. (1964) *Nuclear and Radiochemistry*, 2nd edn. John Wiley, New York, U.S.A., pp. 69–77.

FUKUTO, T. R. and METCALF, R. L. (1954) Isomerization of β-ethylmercaptoethyl diethyl thionophosphate (Saptox). *J. Amer. Chem. Soc.*, 76:5103–6.

GLASSTONE, S. (1958) *Sourcebook on Atomic Energy*, 2nd edn. D. Van Nostrand, New York, U.S.A. pp. 252–72.

GLEASON, G. I. (1960) A positron cow. *Int. J. Appl. Radiat. Isotopes*, 8:90–4.

GLEASON, G. I. (1962) U.S. Patent 3,033,652, May 8, 1962.

GLEASON, G. I., GRUVERMAN, I. J. and NEED, J. L. (1962) Practical production yields of radionuclides with 17- and 21-MeV protons. *Int. J. Appl. Radiat. Isotopes*, 13:223–8.

GLENN, H. J. (1966) *Iron-59 Preparations*. Abbott Laboratories Radiopharmaceutical Product Literature, 97-0259/R4-13, North Chicago, Illinois, U.S.A.

GOODWIN, D. A., STERN, H. S., WAGNER, JR., H. N., and KRAMER, H. H. (1966) A new radio-pharmaceutical for liver scanning. *Nucleonics*, 24(11):65–8.

GREENE, M. W., DOERING, R. F., and HILLMAN, M. (1963–4) Milking systems: status of the art. *Isotopes Radiat. Technol.* 1:152–9.

GREENE, M. W. and TUCKER, W. D. (1961) An improved gallium-68 cow. *Int. J. Appl. Radiat. Isotopes*, 12:62–3.

GROVE, W. P. (1965) Recent progress in radioactive chemical manufacture. *Chem. Ind.*, 128–34.

GRUVERMAN, I. J. and KRUGER, P. (1959) Cyclotron-produced carrier-free radioisotopes. *Int. J. Appl. Radiat. Isotopes*, 5:21–31.

HAHN, P. F. (1967) Production and use of silver-coated radioactive gold colloids. *Int. J. Appl. Radiat. Isotopes*, 18:177–81.

HARPER, P. V., BECK, R., CHARLESTON, D., and LATHROP, K. A. (1964a) Optimization of a scanning method using ^{99m}Tc. *Nucleonics*, 22(1):50–4.

HARPER, P. V., LATHROP, K. A., McCARDLE, R. J. and ANDROS, G. (1964b) The use of ^{99m}Tc as a clinical scanning agent for thyroid, liver, and brain. Second International Atomic Energy Agency Symposium on Medical Radioisotope Scanning, Athens, Greece, April 20–24, 2:33–45.

HARPER, P. V., LATHROP, K. A., ANDROS, G., McCARDLE, R., GOODMAN, A. and COVELL, J. (1965) Technetium-99m as a clinical tracer material. Sixth International Symposium on Radioactive Isotopes in Clinical Medicine and Research, Badgastein, Austria. In: 9–11, 1964, *Radioaktive Isotope Klinik Forschung*, 6:136–45.

HAYES, R. L., CARLTON, J. E. and BYRD, B. L. (1965) Bone scanning with gallium-68: A carrier effect. *J. Nucl. Med.*, 6:605–10.

HAYES, R. L. and RAFTER, J. J. (1966) Renium-188 as a possible diagnostic agent. *J. Nucl. Med.*, 7:797.

HENRY, R., HERCZEG, C. and FISHER, C. (1957) Une nouvelle méthode de préparation d'or colloidal radioactif. *Int. J. Appl. Radiat. Isotopes*, 2:136–9.

HILLMAN, M., GREENE, M. W., BISHOP, W. N. and RICHARDS, P. (1966) Production of Y^{87} and a Sr^{87m} generator. *Int. J. Appl. Radiat. Isotopes*, 17:9–12.

JOHNSON, R. E. and HUSTON, J. L. (1950) Preparation of radioactive sulfur dioxide from barium sulfate, *J. Amer. Chem. Soc.* 72:1841–2.

JOLIOT, F. and CURIE, I. (1934) Artificial production of a new kind of radio-element. *Nature, Lond.*, 133:201–2.

JONES, L. T. (1942) Estimation of ortho-, pyro, meta-, and polyphosphates in the presence of one another. *Ind. Eng. Chem. Analyt. Ed.*, 14:536–42.

KALINSKY, J. L. and WEINSTEIN, A. (1954) Improved procedure for synthesis of P-32 phosphorus oxytrichloride. *J. Amer. Chem. Soc.*, 76:5882.

KALLFELZ, F. A. and WASSERMAN, R. H. (1966) Radioisotopes in Veterinary Medicine. *Isotopes Radiat. Technol.*, 3:382–3.

KAPLAN, E., FELS, G., KOTLOWSKI, B. R., GRECO, J. and WALSH, W. S. (1960) Therapy of carcinoma of the prostate metastatic to bone with P^{32} labeled condensed phosphate. *J. Nucl. Med.*, 1:1–13.

KOBISK, E. H. (1966) Isotope targets for nuclear research. *Nucleonics*, 24(8):122–4.

KOSKI, W. S. (1950) Preparation of high specific activity hydrogen sulfide (H_2S^{35}) from neutron-irradiated potassium chloride. *Nature, Lond.*, 165:565–6.

LANZL, L. H. (1964) Particle accelerators, in Behrens, C. F. and KING, E. R., *Atomic Medicine*, 4th ed., Williams & Wilkins, pp. 615–50.

LAPP, R. E. and ANDREWS, H. L. (1954) *Nuclear radiation physics*, 2nd ed. Prentice-Hall, New York, pp. 92–96.

LARSON, S. M. and NELP, W. B. (1966) Radiopharmacology of a simplified technetium-99m—colloid preparation for photoscanning. *J. Nucl. Med.*, 7:817–26.

LEDDICOTT, G. W. and REYNOLDS, S. A. (1951) Activation analysis with the Oak Ridge reactor. *Nucleonics*, 8(3):62–5.

LENG, R. A. and WEST, C. E. (1966–67) Investigation of metabolic processes with radioisotopes. *Isotopes Radiat. Technol.*, 4:186–8.

LEWIS, R. E. and ELDRIDGE, J. S. (1966) Production of 70-day tungsten-188 and development of a 17-hour rhenium-188 radioisotope generator. *J. Nucl. Med.*, 7:804–5.

LYON, W. S., REYNOLDS, S. A. and WYATT, E. I. (1966) Methods for assay of radioisotopes. *Nucleonics*, 24:(8), 116–17.

MANN, W. B. and GARFINKEL, S. B. (1966) *Radioactivity and its Measurement*. D. Van Nostrand, Princeton, N.J., U.S.A.

MARTIN, J. A. and GREEN, F. L. (1956) Cyclotron target for the irradiation of chemical compounds. *Nucl. Sci. Eng.*, 1:185–90.

MARTIN, J. A., LIVINGSTON, R. S., MURRAY, R. L. and RANKIN, M. (1955) Radioisotope production rates in a 22-Mev cyclotron. *Nucleonics*, 13(3):28–32.

McHENRY, P. L. and KNOEBEL, S. B. (1967) Measurement of coronary blood flow by coincidence counting and a bolus of ^{84}Rb Cl. *J. Appl. Physiol.*, 22:495–500.

MECKLENBURG, R. L. (1964) Clinical value of generator produced 87m strontium. *J. Nucl. Med.*, 5:929–35.

NELSON, F. and KRAUS, K. A. (1963) Some techniques for isolating and using short-lived radioisotopes, in *Production and Use of Short-lived Radioisotopes from Reactors*, Report STI/PUB/64, 1:pp. 191–213. Proceedings of a Seminar held in Vienna, November 5–9, 1962. International Atomic Energy Agency, Vienna, March 1963.

ORR, P. B. (1964) Ion-exchange purification of radioisotopes at the ORNL Isotopes Development Center. *Isotopes Radiat. Technol.*, 2:1–5, 16.

PARR, R. M. (1965) Measuring radioisotopes in biomedical samples. *Nucleonics*, 23(9):56–62.

PATTON, D. D., GARCIA, E. N. and WEBBER, M. M. (1966) Simplified preparation of technetium-99m sulfide colloid for liver scanning. *Amer. J. Roentg. Rad. Ther. Nucl. Med.*, 97:880–5.

PETROFF, C. P., NAIR, P. P. and TURNER, D. A. (1964) The use of siliconized glass vials in preventing wall adsorption of some inorganic radioactive compounds in liquid scintillation counting. *Int. J. Appl. Radiat. Isotopes*, 15:491–4.

PINAJIAN, J. J. (1964) Production and medical uses of ^{67}Ga, ^{68}Ga and ^{72}Ga. *Isotopes Radiat. Technol.*, 1:34–343, 345.

PINAJIAN, J. J. (1966a) ORNL 86-in cyclotron, in *Radioactive Pharmaceuticals*, Proceedings Symposium held in Oak Ridge, Tennessee, November 1965, CONF-651111, U.S.A.E.C. Division of Technical Information Extension, Oak Ridge, Tenn., U.S.A., pp. 143–54.

PINAJIAN, J. J. (1966b) A technetium-99m generator using hydrous zirconium oxide. *Int. J. Appl. Radiat. Isotopes*, 17:664–6.

PINAJIAN, J. J. and BUTLER, T. A. (1963–4) ORNL 86-in cyclotron facility for isotope production. *Isotopes Radiat. Technol.*, 1:136–43, 155.

Production and Use of Short-Lived Radioisotopes from Reactor, Report STI/PUB/64. Proceedings of a Seminar held in Vienna, November 5–9, 1962. International Atomic Energy Agency, Vienna, March 1963, 2:3–146.

RICHARDS, P. (1965a) Nuclide generators, in *Radioactive Pharmaceuticals*, Proceedings Symposium held in Oak Ridge, Tennessee, November 1965, CONF-651111. U.S.A.E.C. Division of Technical Information Extension, Oak Ridge, Tenn, U.S.A., pp. 155–63.
RICHARDS, P. (1965b) *The Technetium-99m Generator*. Brookhaven National Laboratory Report No. 9601 (1965).
SELIGMAN, A. M., RUTENBERG, A. M. and BANKS, H. (1943) Preparation of amino acids containing radioactive sulfur. *J. Clin. Invest.*, 22:275–9.
SILVER, S. (1965) Use of radioisotopes in medicine. *Nucleonics*, 23(8):106–11.
STACY, B. D. and THORNBURN, G. D. (1966) Chromium-51 ethylenediamine-tetracetate for estimation of glomerular filtration rate. *Science*, 152:1076–7.
STANG, JR., L. G. (coordinator), (1964) *Manual of Isotope Production Processes in Use at Brookhaven National Laboratory*, BNL 864(T-347), August.
STANG, JR., L. G. and RICHARDS, P. (1964) Tailoring the isotope to the need. *Nucleonics*, 22(1):46–49.
STANG, JR., L. G., TUCKER, W. D., DOERING, R. F., WEISS, A. J., GREENE, M. W., and BANKS, H. O. (1958) Development of methods for the production of certain short-lived radioisotopes in *Radioisotopes in Scientific Research*, Proceedings of the First UNESCO International Conference, Paris, 1957. Pergamon Press, 1:50–70.
STERN, H. S., ZOLLE, I. and McAFEE, J. G. (1965) Preparation of technetium (^{99m}Tc)–labeled serum albumin (human). *Int. J. Appl. Radiat. Isotopes*, 16:283–8.
STERN, H. S., GOODWIN, D. A., WAGNER, JR., H. N. and KRAMER, H. H. (1966) In^{113m}—A short-lived isotope for lung scanning. *Nucleonics*, 24(10):57–9.
STERN, H. S., GOODWIN, D. A., SCHEFFEE, U., WAGNER, JR., H. N. and KRAMER, H. H. (1967) In^{113m} for blood-pool and brain scanning. *Nucleonics*, 25(2):62–5, 68.
SUAREZ, C. (1966) A new direct method for preparing carrier-free $H_2S^{34}O_4$ from reactor irradiated potassium chloride. *Int. J. Appl. Radiat. Isotopes*, 15:491–3.
SUBRAMANIAN, G. and McAFEE, J. G. (1967) A radioisotope generator of indium-113m. *Int. J. Appl. Radiat. Isotopes*, 18:215–21.
SZILARD, L. and CHALMERS, T. A. (1934) Chemical separation of the radioactive element from its bombarded isotope in the Fermi effect. *Nature, Lond.*, 134:462, 494–5.
TARVER, H. and SCHMIDT, C. L. A. (1939) Radioactive sulfur. *J. Biol. Chem.*, 130:67–80.
TAUXE, W. N. (1961) A rapid radioactive method for the determination of the serum iron-binding capacity. *Amer. J. Clin. Path.*, 35:403–6.
TER-POGOSSIAN, M. M. and WAGNER, JR., H. N. (1966) A new look at the cyclotron for making short-lived isotopes. *Nucleonics*, 24 (10): 50–6, 62.
TUCKER, W. D., GREENE, M. W., WEISS, A. J. and MURRENHOFF, A. (1958) *Methods of Preparation of Some Carrier-free Radioisotopes Involving Sorption on Alumina*, U.S.A.E.C. Report BNL-3746, Brookhaven National Laboratory, May 29.
WAGNER, H. (1966) Nuclear medicine: Present and future. *Radiology*, 86:601–14.
WALKER-SMITH, J. A., SKYRING, A. P. and MISTILIS, S. P. (1967) Use of $^{51}CrCl_3$ in the diagnosis of protein-losing enteropathy, *Gut*, 8:166–8.
WILSON, B. J. (ed.), (1966a) *The Radiochemical Manual*, 2nd ed. Radiochemical Centre, Amersham, England, pp. 26, (1966b) pp. 109–20.
WINSCHE, W. E., STANG, JR., L. G. and TUCKER, W. D. (1951) Production of iodine-132. *Nucleonics*, 8(3):14–18, 94.
WINTER, C. C. and MYERS, W. G. (1962) Three new test agents for the radioisotope renogram: DISA-I^{131}; EDTA-Cr^{51}; and Hippuran-I^{125}. *J. Nucl. Med.*, 3:273–81.
YANO, Y. and ANGER, H. O. (1964) A gallium positron cow for medical use. *J. Nucl. Med.*, 5:484–7.

CHAPTER 4

PREPARATION OF RADIOACTIVE TRACERS: SYNTHETIC ORGANIC TRACERS

J. R. Catch

The Radiochemical Centre, Amersham, Buckinghamshire, England

1. DEFINITIONS

THE reader may find it useful to have the following definitions of terms used in this section.

Carrier-free. A preparation of a radioisotope to which no carrier has been added and for which precautions have been taken to minimize contamination with other isotopes. Material of high specific activity is often loosely referred to as "carrier-free", but more correctly this should be termed material of high isotopic abundance.

Isotopes. Nuclides having the same atomic number but different mass numbers.

Labeled compound. Usually a compound in which one or more of the atoms of a proportion of the molecules is replaced by a radioactive isotope.

Milliatom. One-thousandth part of the atomic weight of the element in grams.

Millimole (mM). One-thousandth part of a mole, which is the molecular weight of a compound in grams.

Nuclide. A species of atom characterized by its mass number, atomic number, and nuclear energy state, provided that the mean life in that state is long enough to be observable.

Radiochemical purity. Of a radioactive material, the proportion of the total activity that is present in the stated chemical form.

Radioisotope. An isotope which is radioactive.

Specific activity. The activity per unit mass of an element or compound containing a radioactive nuclide.

Uniform labeling. Labeling (usually with carbon-14) distributed with statistical uniformity throughout all the atoms of the element concerned, without further definition of the molecular species present.

General labeling. Labeling probably on all the atoms concerned, known or suspected to be nonuniform.

2. INTRODUCTION

When tracer isotopes were novel, research workers in the biological sciences who wished to use them had of necessity to prepare their own labeled compounds.

The remarkable development of tracer methods in the last two decades has stimulated the production of isotopic chemicals by commercial and national laboratories, and a very wide range is now available. This, inevitably, concentrates on tracer compounds of general biochemical interest, and on those of established value in diagnostic medicine.

The pharmacologist using labeled substrates (such as intermediary metabolites) to study the effects of unlabeled drugs (see, for example, Skosey, 1966) has therefore an extensive range of useful tracer compounds at his disposal. But many pharmacologists require tracers primarily for studying the metabolism of drugs, partly for attempts to explain modes of action in terms of localization, biochemistry, and kinetics, partly to help assess the safety of new drugs before their release for general use. No organized supply (commercial or otherwise) has gone far to produce such labeled drugs, and the individual research worker must often still do so for himself.

There are, of course, reasons for this. If the drug is new and promising, only the manufacturer is interested in it, and he may be unwilling to give away information to others. Although radioisotope manufacturers sometimes prepare compounds to order, the demand is much greater (and, in particular, more varied) than they can economically meet. After the initial investigation there will probably be little further interest in any one labeled drug, and the costs for such special preparations are inevitably higher than for tracer compounds in wide and regular demand. Many pharmaceutical manufacturers therefore operate their own preparative laboratories for labeled compounds, with staff specializing in the work, purchasing suitable labeled intermediates when appropriate; and this appears to be sensible practice. This solution is not so easily adopted by academic research workers.

For drugs already in use there are different problems, notably diversity and cost. Study of a single drug (whether of its pharmacology or metabolism) is of much less use than comparative study of a number of related drugs (including many which are not clinically acceptable) and analogous chemical compounds. But the enterprise of chemists during nearly a century has provided an embarrassingly large range of drugs to be studied. Research workers therefore ask for a very wide range of labeled drugs; but each is needed only in small quantity and perhaps for one investigation. Here then is the problem; as with other highly specialized chemical reagents, it seems to be uneconomic to prepare these compounds commercially. In any attempt to produce them noncommercially (e.g. by a co-operative scheme, as has been proposed from time to time) there will always be great difficulty in selection of topics from the almost infinite number available.

The problem may be put in another way. The effort required to prepare labeled compounds for a research project is by no means negligible. It may be a substantial part of the whole work. The total demand for labeled drugs represents a significant fractional addition to the world's effort in pharmacological research. It is not surprising that this is not quickly and easily found.

Many research workers will therefore need to prepare their own labeled drugs. The present review is intended to give them some guidance on general principles. A comprehensive, detailed treatment cannot be given in the space available.

Clinical isotope users are rather better served. The supply industry has grown up with the speciality, and has not (as with synthetic drugs) a huge backlog of work needing to be reevaluated. The area of development has, so far, proved to be limited, by comparison with synthetic drugs. But it is still important for the clinician developing the use of these materials to have some knowledge of how they are produced. Without such knowledge, developments may get out of touch with practical realities.

3. GENERAL PRINCIPLES

The preparation of labeled compounds is subject to certain general conditions, whatever the use to be made of the compounds. The nuclide (or isotope, as it is more commonly if less correctly termed) is first prepared in a simple chemical form, which is then incorporated into the required compound by chemical, biochemical, or radiation-catalyzed synthesis. More direct labeling by simple irradiation procedures is useful only in most exceptional cases. Readers needing a fairly full discussion in general terms may be referred to the *Radiochemical Manual* of the Radiochemical Centre, 1966.

Radionuclides in Pharmacology

TABLE 1. IMPORTANT NUCLIDES

Isotope	Half-life	Type of decay and particle energies (MeV)		Gamma energies (MeV)	Toxicity
Carbon-14	5730 y	β^-	0.159–100%		Medium Lower B
Hydrogen-3 (Tritium)	12.26 y	β^-	0.018–100%		Low
Sulphur-35	87.2 d	β^-	0.167–100%		Medium Lower B
Iodine-131	8.04 d	β^-	0.25–2.8%	0.08–2.2%	Medium Upper A
			0.33–9.3%	0.28–6.3%	
			0.61–87.2%	0.36–79%	
			0.81–0.7%	0.64–9.3%	
				0.72–2.8%	
0.7% of ^{131}I decays to 12 d ^{131m}Xe					
Iodine-132	2.3 h	β^-	0.80–21%	0.38–4.8%	Medium Lower B
			1.04–15%	0.52–21.5%	
			1.22–12%	0.62–5.2%	
			1.49–12%	0.65–26.0%	
			1.61–21%	0.67–100%	
			2.14–18%	0.72–6.5%	
				0.78–84.0%	
				0.95–21.0%	
				1.14–5%	
				1.30–4%	
				1.39–8.5%	
				Many others of <2% intensity	
Iodine-125	60 d	EC	100%	0.035–7%	—
				0.027–	
				Te X-rays (138%)	
Phosphorus-32	14.3 d	β^-	1.71–100%		Medium Lower B
Bromine-82	35.4 h	β^-	0.44–100%	0.55–65%	Medium Lower B
				0.62–42%	
				0.70–28%	
				0.78–83%	
				0.83–23%	
				1.04–29%	
				1.32–28%	
				1.48–17%	
Cobalt-57	270 d	EC	100%	0.014–8.2%	Medium Lower B
				0.122–88.8%	
				0.136–8.8%	
				0.7–0.2%	

Toxicity classification from the International Atomic Energy Agency, Vienna, 1963. Technical Reports Series No. 15.

TABLE 1—*cont.*

Isotope	Half-life	Type of decay and particle energies (MeV)		Gamma energies (MeV)	Toxicity
Mercury-197	65 h	EC	100%	0.077–19.3% 0.19–0.5% 0.069–Au X-rays (74.5%)	Medium Lower B
Mercury-203	47 d	β⁻	0.21–100%	0.279–81.5%	Medium Lower B
Selenium-75	121 d	EC	100%	0.024–0% 0.066–1% 0.096–3% 0.12–15% 0.14–54% 0.20–1.5% 0.27–56% 0.28–23% 0.31–1.4% 0.40–12.5%	Medium Lower B
Technetium-99 m	6 h	IT	100%	0.002–0% 0.140–90.1% 0.142–0.04%	Low

The way in which a problem is approached does, however, vary according to the prospective use. In academic biochemistry the chemical or biochemical requirements come first, and the radiation characteristics and half-life are secondary. For diagnostic and therapeutic chemicals the reverse has generally been true. The nuclide is first selected and a suitable chemical or physical form then sought (Bayly, 1966) (Table 1).

Preparative methods are most usefully classified according to the nuclide used, but some general features of the three classes of use may first be discussed.

3.1. LABELED DRUGS

Carbon-14, tritium, and sulphur-35 are the most important tracers for these; others are used much more rarely. Carbon-14 gives unambiguous evidence on metabolism of carbon atoms. The β-energy is low enough to give good resolution in autoradiography, and the specific activities attainable (now up to 55–60 mc/mAtom carbon) are amply high enough for most work in this group. Higher levels are needed for only a small proportion of drugs having very high pharmacological activity; some elegant and sensitive work has been done even with curare alkaloids using carbon-14 (Waser and Lüthi, 1956).

With increasing production, the prime cost of carbon-14 has fallen during the last 10 years, but it is still an expensive nuclide. This becomes particularly important if the overall yield in a synthesis is poor. Recovery of carbon-14 from residues, even when nominally possible, is often un-rewarding in practice. Experiments in large animals may therefore be expensive with carbon-14. This handicaps the academic worker rather than the pharmaceutical manufacturer, for whom carbon-14 labeling is likely to be a small part of the cost of developing a new drug.

Tritium labeling can provide specific activities 500 times greater than for carbon-14, the low β-energy is excellent for autoradiography, and the primary isotope is cheap. But tritium is used almost invariably as a tracer for a carbon atom or a molecular fragment, so that the interpretation of the results depend fundamentally on knowledge of the integrity of the car-bon–hydrogen bond. Such knowledge is often lacking, and special care is therefore needed in using tritium as a metabolic tracer.

Both carbon-14 and tritium are versatile tracers, applicable to almost all organic compounds, and providing a variety of possibilities for position labeling. Sulfur-35 can be used only for sulfur-containing drugs and will trace only sulfur-containing metabolites. The half-life is convenient in some respects, as activities will decay reasonably quickly, but for extended experimental programmes it is troublesome, as preparations may have to be repeated.

Rather few drugs are iodine compounds, so that iodine isotopes are little used as strictly isotopic tracers. Because of the choice available, simple labeling procedures, useful characteristics and low cost, they have in the past been widely used for non-isotopic labeling. With the special exception of proteins and polypeptides, this use is now declining. In small molecules, substitution with iodine (or even a smaller atom) produces virtually a different compound which is likely to be metabolized differently. This appears to be so even for triglycerides and fatty acids (Weiss *et al.*, 1963). Non-isotopic labeling in general (including non-isotopic labeling with inorganic ions (chromium-51) or organic radicals (acetyl), which is used rather rarely) can often be used for physical parameters (volume, flow rate, or turnover rates), but is rarely if ever used in studies of intermediary metabolism.

For proteins and large polypeptides, and for macromolecules generally, iodine-labeling is very useful in this limited sense, but needs to be used carefully and critically. The chemical and biochemical behavior of the iodine-labeled compound may depend critically on the exact method of iodination as well as the level and uniformity of substitution (see, for example, European Atomic Energy Agency, 1966). Moreover, it appears unsafe to generalize too readily. For example, it is generally assumed for plasma proteins that, the longer the half-life, the more nearly it will approximate to the true value for unsubstituted native protein. Although this may be true for plasma proteins it is not true for peptide hormones. Iodine-131 labeled parathyroid hormone is metabolically degraded *in vivo* at a slower rate than the unlabeled hormone (Yalow and Berson, 1966), and successive iodinations of insulin lengthens its biological half-life (private communication between Professor U. Rosa of Sorin, Saluggia, and Dr. J. S. Glover of the Radiochemical Centre, 1967).

Isotopes other than carbon-14, tritium, sulfur, and iodine are little used except as specialized diagnostic tracers.

3.2. INTERMEDIARY METABOLITES

Carbon-14 is inevitably the most important isotope. Tritium, used with care, is valuable. Other isotopes find only limited, special uses.

3.3. DIAGNOSTIC AND THERAPEUTIC COMPOUNDS

These are used either as *in vitro* biochemical reagents, or *in vivo*. Examples of reagents used *in vitro* are acetic anhydride (carbon-14 or tritium), glucose-^{14}C, L-histidine-^{14}C, insulin-^{125}I and pipsyl chloride (^{125}I or ^{35}S). Labeling for such reagents is chosen on the basis of convenience (including reasonably long half-life), sensitivity, and cost.

For *in vivo* use, the choice tends to be determined by the radiological dose to the patient and the radiation characteristics of the nuclide (for example, for scanning). There is a strong preference for short-lived tracers, and these in turn are, for convenience, sought as "daughter" elements in decay chains, which may be obtained from "cow" systems. These conditions restrict the choice of available isotopes. Even when a convenient "cow" system provides a valuable nuclide (for example, technetium-99m) the preparation and testing of labeled compounds presents difficult problems because of the short half-life. Reagents of this kind must, however, also satisfy certain physiological or biochemical criteria. It is difficult to reconcile all these requirements. Carbon-14 (for example) is an extremely versatile tracer, but it has a very long half-life and no gamma-radiation to make external scanning possible. Carbon-11 emits a useful gamma-ray (0.51 MeV, from positron emission), but the half-life of 20 min makes it impossible to synthesize any but the simplest compounds of carbon-11.

In these circumstances it is inevitable that attention should be concentrated on compounds of iodine isotopes. There is a wide choice of these, and they may be incorporated quickly into many compounds. One may, however, regret that the concentration of interest on scanning procedures may be leading to comparative neglect of diagnostic tests on a rational biochemical basis, for which tracer isotopes (and especially carbon-14 and tritium) seem admirably suited.

4. LABELING WITH CARBON-14

4.1. SYNTHESIS

Carbon-14 is extracted from irradiated targets of aluminum or beryllium nitride. The yield is only 2.5 mCi per annum per gram nitrogen at a flux of 10^{13} n/cm² sec. Annual world requirements are now measured in hundreds of curies, so that long irradiations of large quantities of target are necessary. The isotopic abundance of the carbon-14 is dependent mainly on the carbon-12 content of the target. By keeping this to a low value, and by long irradiations, abundances of 90–95% are now attainable. At 100% abundance 14 mg of elementary carbon-14 is equivalent to 62 mCi.

The most convenient form for primary extraction is carbon dioxide and this is the starting point for all syntheses. Attempts to use direct syntheses from "hot atom" reactions such as

have proved of very limited use because only low specific activities and small quantities can be produced in this way. Synthesis with carbon-14 is systematic; there are twelve possible primary stages:

(1) Carboxylation of an organo-metallic compound to give a carboxyl-labeled acid.
(2) Reduction to methanol.

(3) Reduction to cyanide.
(4) Reduction to carbide, for acetylene preparation.
(5) Reduction to formate.
(6) Reduction to cyanamide.
(7) Reduction to carbon monoxide.
(8) Conversion to urea via ammonium carbonate.
(9) Reduction to methane.
(10) Reduction to formaldehyde.
(11) Reduction to elementary carbon.
(12) Conversion to an alkyl carbonate via silver carbonate.

Of these only the first six are of much importance. The manner in which these are exploited is best shown by Tables 2–8 (reproduced by permission from the *Radiochemical Manual*, Radiochemical Centre, 1966).

The need to start from carbon dioxide is the most fundamental controlling factor in carbon-14 labeling, but a wide range of carbon-14 labeled synthetic intermediates may now be purchased commercially, and there is an extensive and useful literature of carbon-14 preparations (Calvin *et al.*, 1949; Catch, 1961; Ronzio, 1954; Murray and Williams, 1958; Nevenzel *et al.*, 1954, 1957; Bubner and Schmidt, 1966; Weygand and Simon, 1955). The research worker preparing a special compound for his own use should nevertheless be aware of the various approaches, even if he only completes a synthesis from a purchased intermediate. It will help to choose the best route, it will show the possibilities for alternative labeling, and may give information on likely trace impurities.

The two most important factors in practice are the small scale of working and the rather high cost of the isotope. Synthetic drugs are not commonly of very high potency, so that extremely high specific activities are (speaking generally) less important than in some other biochemical applications of tracers. It follows that syntheses need not be on a mass scale very different from that of experimental unlabeled syntheses in a pharmaceutical research laboratory.

Yields are most important. Unlabeled synthetic reagents are cheap, and time spent on the synthesis is expensive. It is often best to accept a very poor yield, at the experimental stage, for the sake of speed. In some measure this may be true even for carbon-14 syntheses, but beyond a certain point poor yields become intolerably expensive in isotope. Unreliable yields are in some respects even more troublesome than poor yields.

The position of labeling by chemical synthesis is highly specific. The activity will normally be confined to one position in the molecule unless

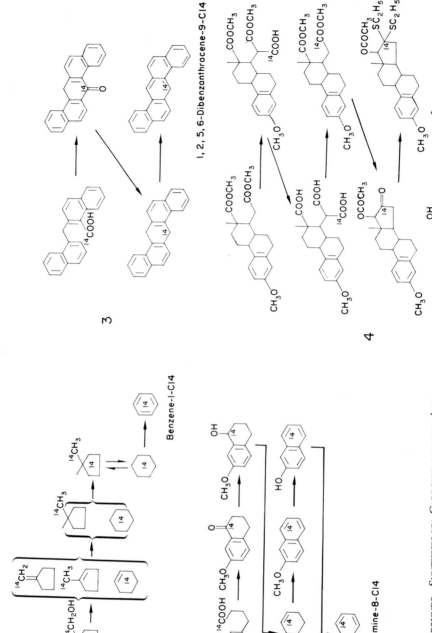

TABLE 2. CARBON-14 COMPOUNDS—SYNTHESES VIA CARBOXYL-LABELED ACIDS

Reproduced by permission from the *Radiochemical Manual* (Radiochemical Centre, 1966).

TABLE 2. *(continued)*

5

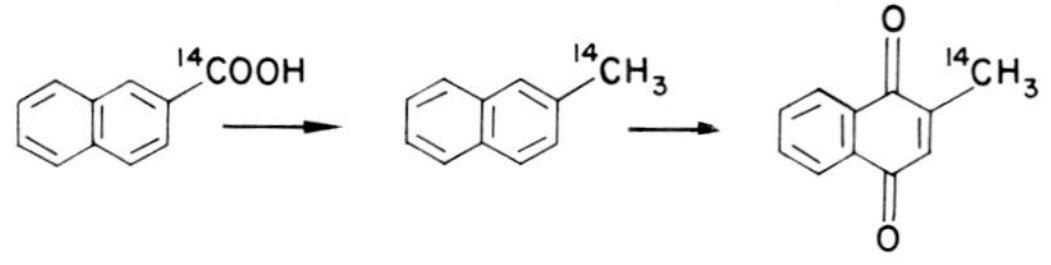

8   2(Methyl[C14])-1,4-naphthoquinone

3-Phenyl (alanine-3-Cl4)

Styrene-β-Cl4

9

6

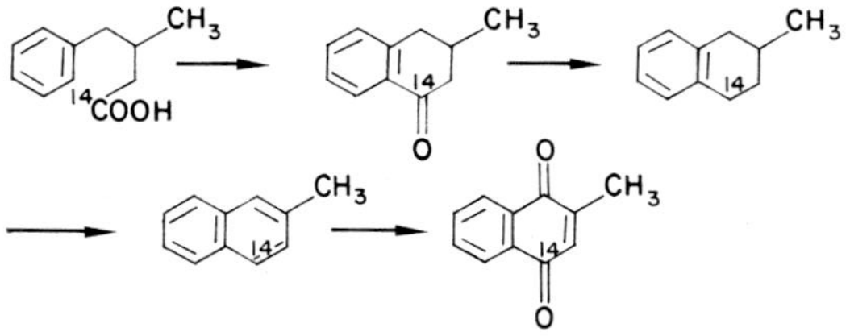

2-Methyl-1,4(naphthoquinone-4-Cl4)

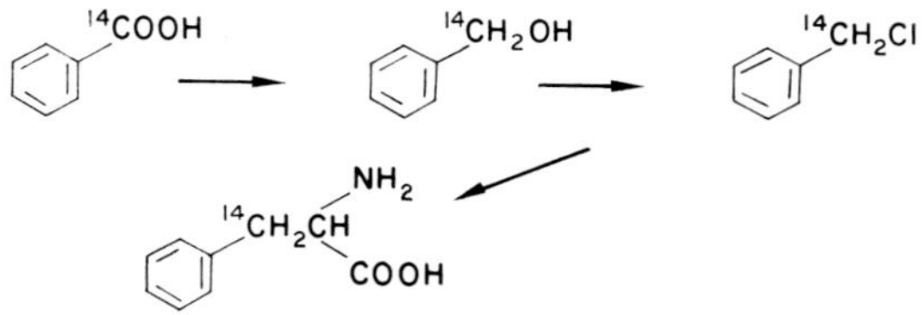

10

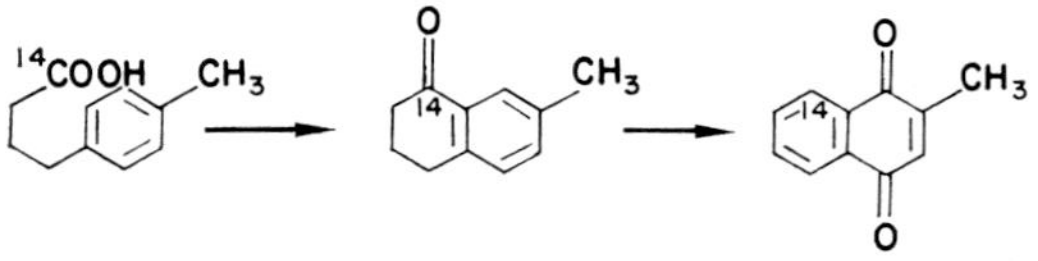

2-Methyl-1,4-(naphthoquinone-8-C14)

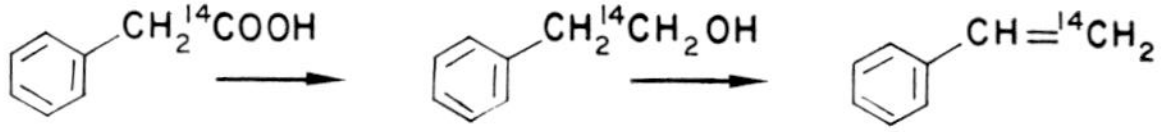

7

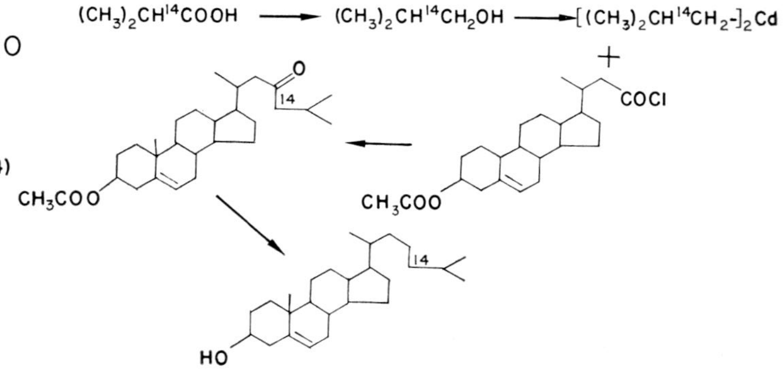

Cholesterol-24-Cl4

Reproduced by permission from the *Radiochemical Manual* (Radiochemical Centre, 1966).

Radionuclides in Pharmacology

symmetry at some stage (such as labeled ethylene or benzene) produces (effectively) multiple labeling. Some positions in the molecule may be relatively easy to label, others extremely difficult. The importance of labeling any particular position depends on the information needed, and this may depend on some knowledge of labeling to ensure a significant result. But in fact the extreme difficulty (or inefficiency) of labeling in many positions in complex molecules is often prohibitive.

Penicillins have, for example, been labeled only in the side-chain

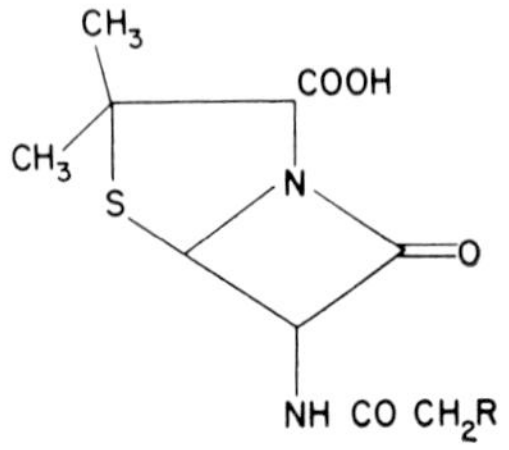

CH_3

CH_3

COOH

S

N

O

NH CO CH$_2$R

derived from phenylacetic acid, or in the S atom; steroids are commonly labeled, by partial synthesis, in carbon 4 of ring A, other positions in the ring system being much more difficult. Imipramine ("Tofranil") has been labeled in the side-chain and in the methylene bridge carbons;

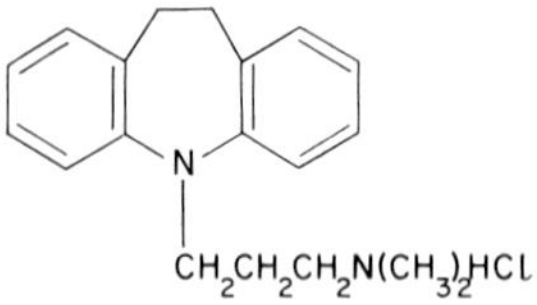

N

$CH_2CH_2CH_2N(CH_3)_2HCl$

labeling in the aromatic rings would require preparation of ring-labeled *o*-nitrotoluene-C14, and has not yet been done.

It is not easy to produce uniform labeling by synthesis, because all the carbon units would need to be uniformly labeled at the same specific activity and this increases greatly the amount of synthetic work. This is unfortunate, since uniform labeling gives a valuable overall picture of the metabolism of a drug. Imipramine may again serve as an example; uniform labeling would require the following basic components, both uniformly labeled:

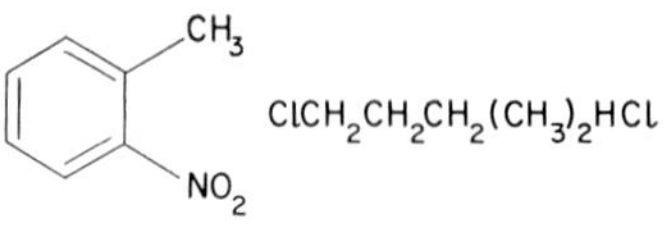

CH_3

$ClCH_2CH_2CH_2(CH_3)_2HCl$

NO_2

Although formally possible, it would be extremely tedious to prepare these, and the risk of failure in a single synthetic stage would be discouraging. It would be quicker, more efficient, and safer to synthesize all the separately labeled forms (or as many as are thought necessary) and mix them if desired. This has the advantage that the individual labelings may be studied separately.

It may be noted that to prepare all the forms labelled in *specific* carbon atoms would be especially difficult. The *N*-methyl and methylene carbons of the side chain, and the methyl carbon of *o*-nitrotoluene, are reasonably accessible. Uniform labeling in the benzene rings, or in *o*-nitrotoluene, will be more troublesome and inefficient, but not wholly impracticable. But specific position labeling of aromatic compounds is discouragingly difficult. The work of Swan and Wright (1956) illustrates this point. 3,4-Dihydroxyphenylethylamine was successfully labeled in carbon atoms 3, 4 and 5 of the ring (separately), but specific activities were low and yields were from 0.4 to 1.3%.

Space does not permit a discussion of the techniques peculiar to carbon-14 synthesis. They are well documented (Calvin *et al.*, 1949; Catch, 1961; Ronzio, 1954; Murray and Williams, 1958; Bubner and Schmidt, 1966; Weygand and Simon, 1955). One practical point may be noted; the need to check a synthesis throughout with *representative materials*. Yields at successive stages may be checked with pure reagents, but when the whole synthesis is carried through from carbon dioxide the overall yield is likely to be lower, sometimes much lower, since yields at some stages may be greatly affected by small amounts of impurity. In small-scale total synthesis it is not always possible to purify thoroughly at intermediate stages.

4.2. BIOSYNTHESIS

Biosynthetic methods are important for labeling common intermediary metabolites. They are less important for labeling drugs because most drugs are synthetic.

It is difficult to discuss biosynthesis systematically. The use of more or less purified enzymes to perform specific reactions is really a valuable accessory to chemical synthesis. Approaches to biosynthesis may be classified according to their use of an *inorganic* (carbonate) substrate or an *organic* substrate, which itself may be synthetic or biosynthetic in origin.

4.2.1. *Inorganic Substrate*

Although important for producing carbon-14 labeled carbohydrates, amino acids, nucleosides, and nucleotides, this approach offers little or nothing to drug labeling. It has been tried for penicillin (Martin *et al.*, 1953) and streptomycin (Hunter *et al.*, 1954) but predictably the yields are very poor.

Certain plant products, such as alkaloids and cardiac glycosides, have been labeled in small quantities and at rather low specific activities by growing the plants in carbon-14 dioxide. This aspect of "isotope farming" has been disappointing, the most serious problem being the sensitivity of plants to radiation; pronounced abnormalities appear at a level of 1 mCi/g carbon (12 mCi/mAtom). If it were not for this, the second major difficulty, which is the very small conversion of carbon dioxide into the desired product, might possibly have been overcome by using and recycling large amounts of carbon-14. The yield of digitoxin, for example, appears to have been about 0.02 % of the carbon-14 dioxide used (Okita *et al.*, 1954). For accounts of the pioneering work at the Argonne National Laboratory, and subsequent publications on plant growth chambers for carbon-14 labeling, the reader may be referred to the original publications (Okita *et al.*, 1954; Scully *et al.*, 1955; Kuzin and Tokarskaya, 1959; Grossbard and Barton, 1963; Smith *et al.*, 1963; Sauerbeck, 1960; Merenova, 1954; Alworth *et al.*, 1964).

4.2.2. *Organic substrate*

This approach is more favorable, and a few examples are summarized in Table 9.

A more detailed knowledge of biogenetic pathways would no doubt provide much more efficient biosyntheses from highly specific (probably synthetic) organic substrates. At the present time, little has been achieved in this way in practice.

5. LABELING WITH TRITIUM

As already observed, the user must never forget that tritium is a tracer for hydrogen; to trace a carbon atom one must have knowledge of the stability of the carbon-tritium bond. It is usually much easier to introduce tritium into an organic molecule than to introduce a carbon isotope. Unfortunately, the tritium often comes out again relatively easily.

The question of the stability of a tritium atom is sometimes over-simplified. In hydroxyl, carboxyl, amino, and imino groups there will obviously be rapid exchange with hydrogen ions, and therefore in water. The hydrogen atoms in benzene, by contrast, are very stable in neutral conditions. Between these extremes there is a great diversity of behavior

TABLE 9. LABELING WITH CARBON-14: BIOSYNTHESIS: ORGANIC SUBSTRATE

Product	Substrate	Yield (%)	Organism	Reference
Chlorotetracycline	Glycine-2-^{14}C	52	*Streptomyces aureofaciens*	Miller *et al.*, 1965
Dextran	Sucrose	8–12	*Leuconostoc mesenteroides*	Scully *et al.*, 1952
Neomycin	D-Glucose (U)	19.5	*Streptomyces fradiae*	Sebek, 1955
Penicillin	Various	Up to 1–2	*Penicillium notatum*	Martin *et al.*, 1953 Arnstein and Clubb, 1957
Penicillin	Phenyl (acetic acid-1-^{14}C)	(?)	*Penicillium notatum*	Gordon *et al.*, 1953
Streptomycin	D-Glucose (U)	1	*Streptomyces griseus*	Karow *et al.*, 1952 Hunter and Hockenhull, 1955
Streptomycin	Acetates, glycines	0.2–1	*Streptomyces griseus*	Numerof, *et al.*, 1953
Terramycin (oxytetracycline)	Acetate-2-^{14}C	Up to 6	*Streptomyces rimosus*	Snell *et al.*, 1956

which may be dependent on detailed conditions (pH, temperature, catalyst) which may affect equilibrium of tautomeric forms. Careful thought must always be given to the use of tritium in any particular tracer experiment. For a more thorough discussion, including methods of verifying stabilities experimentally, Evans's book (Evans, 1966) may be consulted.

Biosynthetic labeling with tritium, except by efficient specific enzyme syntheses, has proved of little use. Problems of radiation dose limit the specific activity which can be used (Porter and Watson, 1954) with tritiated water as a substrate. Biosynthesis from specific precursors should be more promising. Examples are aldosterone-16-T and other steroids (Ayres *et al.*, 1958) and actinomycin (Ciferri *et al.*, 1964).

The primary labeling processes with tritium are:

(1) Exchange with heterogeneous catalysis.
(2) Exchange with homogeneous catalysis.
(3) Exchange catalyzed by radiation.
(4) Substitution by chemical reduction.
(5) Addition (hydrogenation).

5.1. EXCHANGE WITH HETEROGENEOUS CATALYSIS

This is generally the easiest and quickest method of tritium labeling. The unlabeled organic substance is heated, with, for example, tritium labeled water or acetic acid and a catalyst such as palladium or platinum. After disposal of the excess solvent, labile tritium is removed by repeated equilibration with water or other appropriate solvents and the product purified by suitable methods. Chemically catalyzed exchange can give quite high specific activities (1–20 c/mM). It results in labeling which is general but rarely uniform, and the precise determination of labeling is usually so laborious that it is not often attempted. The method is not, of course, applicable to compounds which are unstable under the conditions used, and it is not often possible to obtain a theoretical equilibrium concentration without excessive breakdown of the starting material. Purification of the products is not usually too difficult, and the method, although rather unpredictable, is generally useful. The erratic results of these exchange reactions are suspected to be due to variation in the activity of the catalyst used, and greater reliability could no doubt be attained by more thorough investigation.

5.2. EXCHANGE WITH HOMOGENEOUS CATALYSIS

Hydrogen atoms in "labile" positions undergo rapid exchange and equilibration with tritium oxide. Examples are 2-naphthoic acid and malonic acid.

$$CH_2(COOH)_2 + 3T_2O \rightleftharpoons CHT(COOT)_2 + 3THO$$

The products are not of much interest in themselves, because the label will exchange off again equally readily in aqueous solution; but by reaction of the substituted naphthoic acid with diazomethane, followed by hydrolysis tritium labeled methanol is readily obtained.

Similarly, by decarboxylation of the labeled malonic acid

$$CHT(COOT)_2 \xrightarrow{\text{heat}} CHT_2COOT + CO_2$$

$$\downarrow NaOH$$

$$CHT_2COOH \longleftarrow CHT_2COONa + THO$$

followed by removal of the labile tritium, one obtains acetic acid labeled with tritium in the methyl group. Exchanges of this kind are necessarily possible only in particular cases, but, as in the examples quoted, can be useful practical methods.

Hydrogen exchanges catalysed by acid reagents, although extensively studied for their theoretical interest, are not much used in practical tritium labeling. This no doubt is because the conditions required for a high degree of substitution are rather drastic, so that relatively few compounds will survive them; and for those which will, for example the simpler aromatic compounds, more efficient alternative methods of labeling are already available.

5.3. EXCHANGE CATALYZED BY RADIATION

Radiation-induced labeling as described by Wilzbach and others (Dorfman and Wilzbach, 1959; Wilzbach, 1962, 1957; Wenzel and Schulze, 1962) often appeals to the beginner in tracer work because of its superficial simplicity. In its simplest form—there are elaborations of the method—the finely divided organic compound is exposed to elementary tritium. Hydrogen exchange occurs in some measure with most compounds, but is complicated by side reactions such as additions to unsaturated centres (Dutton *et al.*, 1958; Bradlow *et al.*, 1959; Evans, 1961) and, above all, by extensive radiation decomposition. This decomposition seriously limits the specific activities attainable, and unfortunately is most marked with large and sensitive molecules for which the method would otherwise be particularly valuable. As a consequence a very complex mixture of labeled compounds results, and special care is necessary in purification (Jellinck and Smyth, 1958; Chadha *et al.*, 1962). On really rigorous purification and analysis, it will often be found that the desired product is present only in very small concentration compared with labeled impurities. Observations published at the Brussels Conference in 1963 (European Atomic Energy Community, 1964), two of them dealing with lysozyme, show interesting differences of opinion on the success of the Wilzbach labeling of protein materials, and suggest that much care is necessary in using it. The success of labeling by the Wilzbach method or its variants is very unpredictable, although it can occasionally score a pronounced success as in the example of atropine (Evans, 1961). The method is, however, at least relatively simple to try, although it is not often that of choice.

Labeling by recoil tritons, e.g. by neutron irradiation of a mixture of an organic substance with a lithium salt, may also be mentioned under this heading. As a means of preparing labeled compounds it is less useful than the Wilzbach method, and is at present of academic interest only. This academic interest is considerable, but it should not mislead the reader into overestimating the value of this approach to tritium labeling for practical tracer uses.

5.4. SUBSTITUTION BY CHEMICAL REDUCTION

Reduction of a halogen compound by a metal, such as zinc, in the presence of tritium oxide or tritium labeled acetic acid, of the general type

$$RX + M^{++} + T_2O \rightarrow RT + MOTX$$

will produce a compound with a tritium atom in place of the original halogen.

Reductions of this kind, although sometimes used for labeling, require a large excess of tritium in the water, acetic acid, or other comparable solvent used. This large excess is avoided by converting the halide RX into an organo-metallic compound such as a Grignard reagent, and reacting this with an equivalent quantity of tritium oxide,

$$RMgX + T_2O \rightarrow RT + MgOTX.$$

The method obviously lends itself to high specific activities and work on a small scale. A comparable method of chemical reduction uses sodium borotritide for reduction of carbonyl compounds

$$4R_2CO + NaBT_4 + 2H_2O \rightarrow 4R_2CTOH + NaBO_2.$$

while reductions with tritiated lithium borohydride are often used for labeling carbohydrates (Isbell *et al.*, 1960). These chemical reductions can usually be relied upon to give completely specific labeling, although isotope effects and exchange reactions often reduce the specific activity of the product as it would be predicted from the simple equation.

Another variant is reduction using elementary tritium and a catalyst such as platinum or palladium:

$$RX + T_2 \xrightarrow{\text{Pd or Pt}} RT + TX.$$

This is often a very efficient method, but it should not be assumed that the labeling by this means is completely specific, since hydrogen migration can occur in the presence of catalysts. As in labeling by addition of tritium, care is needed in the selection of solvents and other conditions such as pH (Nystrom, 1962). Elementary tritium in the presence of platinum or palladium exchanges rapidly with water, ethanol, acetic acid, and many other solvents that are used for catalytic hydrogenations or reductions. Ethers (particularly dioxan), and esters have proved particularly useful as solvents, since they exchange less readily.

5.5. ADDITION (HYDROGENATION)

Addition to unsaturated centers (particularly carbon–carbon double and triple bonds) catalyzed by platinum or palladium is a generally useful and efficient method of tritium labeling. There is always some risk that exchange or hydrogen migration will occur at the same time, and it cannot be assumed that tritium will be located only at places indicated by simple addition to the double or triple bond. Another source of trouble is tritium exchange with solvent, which has been referred to in the preceding paragraph.

Uniform labeling with tritium is hardly ever possible because hydrogen atoms vary so much in stability; conversely, completely specific labeling is not always easy. Only purely chemical (not catalytic) methods may be relied upon with confidence.

The value of the various methods may be summarized briefly; for more complete discussion see *Tritium and its Compounds* (Evans, 1966).

1. Although easy, the method is not always reliable or reproducible and may not give very high specific activities. Its use is probably declining.
2. This method is only of limited use.
3. Radiation-induced labeling is very widely practised, but difficulties of purification and low specific activities are serious handicaps.
4. These methods, especially halogen–tritium exchange, are increasingly important. They are clean, give very high specific activities and more or less specific labeling.
5. Hydrogen addition is also very valuable for the high specific activities it can give.

Formerly most tritium-labeling was carried out directly on the product to be labeled, but chemical or biochemical synthetic steps are becoming more common. These trends arise from greater demands for high specific activities, specific position labeling, and more exact information on stability of the tracer atom.

5.6. LABELING WITH SULFUR-35

Sulfur-35 is usually extracted at high specific activity from neutron-irradiated potassium chloride. Very high specific activities are possible (up to 1 Ci/mM), but in practice the limit may be set by the chemical scale of the preparation. In its primary form of sulfate the isotope is cheap, but the half-life of 87 days may be inconvenient for extended experiments.

As with carbon-14, the approaches to ^{35}S labeling are systematic.

Table 10 shows the primary stages. Table 11 provides examples of further syntheses based on sulfur dioxide.

5.7. LABELING WITH IODINE ISOTOPES

For ^{131}I, and even more for ^{132}I, methods must be rapid and simple. The basic reactions used are exchange ($^{127}I \rightleftharpoons {}^{131}I$) oxidative iodination ($H \rightleftharpoons {}^{131}I$) or addition

$$(H \; \underline{\quad\quad} \; {}^{131}I) \; \text{or addition} \; (\overset{\diagdown}{\diagup} \rightleftharpoons \; \longrightarrow \; \overset{I}{\underset{I}{\diagup\diagdown}} \;)$$

Most iodine labeling is "non-isotopic"; that is to say, the tracer compound is an iodine-substituted analog of the compound to be studied. Iodinated tyrosines and thyroxine derivatives provide one of the few exceptions. "Non-isotopic" labeling is best used only when true isotopic labeling is, for one reason or another, impracticable. Labeling of fats for clinical study of fat absorption is an example. Although carbon-14 or even tritium would be a more valid tracer (Weiss *et al.*, 1963) the short half-life and easy measurement of ^{131}I, and the apparent ease of labeling, are attractive. In fact, the labeling of unsaturated fats is not quite simple. The fat itself is likely to be a complex mixture of mixed glycerides, of variously unsaturated fatty acids, and may well contain also quite unrelated unsaturated impurities. When reacted with a limited amount of iodine or iodine monochloride, a complex mixture of labeled products is likely to be produced. If the quantity of iodinating agent is very small, it may be taken up entirely by irrelevant impurities. Even if a pure fat (such as pure monolein) is iodinated carefully to produce only one labeled molecular species, it remains open to question how closely this will parallel the behavior of the fat for which it is used as a tracer.

Problems of this kind need to be considered in all "non-isotopic" labeling with iodine or other "foreign" labels. They have been studied most extensively for proteins (see, for example, European Atomic Energy Agency, 1966), and include denaturation of the protein by excessive substitution with iodine, denaturation by the chemical conditions of iodination, and loss of labeling from iodination in an unstable position of the molecule, or from decomposition on storage (the greater stability of ^{125}I labeled compounds, compared with ^{131}I compounds, should be remembered in this connection). How important these are depends very much on the use of the product. Labeling of albumin for determination of blood or plasma volume is not very critical. Labeling for metabolic study is extremely critical. Immunological reactions appear to have requirements somewhere between these extremes. It has been shown that the properties of an iodinated protein may depend not only on the degree of substitution (Campbell *et al.*, 1956; Cohen *et al.*, 1956; McFarlane, 1958), but the exact method of producing it (Rosa *et al.*, 1966) and the specific positions in the molecule. It is important for the research user to be aware of the problems in iodine-labeling of proteins.

An irritating practical difficulty is the occasional failure of iodination reactions. "Carrier-free" iodine, without an added reducing agent, is needed for many iodinations. At the low concentrations sometimes used (mCi quantities) traces of impurity (which have not yet been identified, and remain entirely unknown) may interfere. The problem seems to arise with all iodine isotopes extracted and processed in various ways. The chloramine oxidation method (Greenwood *et al.*, 1962) is one of the least erratic of those generally used, but is not always acceptable on other grounds.

Of the iodine isotopes available, ^{131}I is cheap, easy to measure, and has a convenient half-life; ^{125}I is more costly, but the longer half-life is a great advantage, and the radiological and scanning characteristics are sometimes favorable; ^{125}I compounds are more stable than those of ^{131}I, since there is no β-radiation. ^{132}I has so short a half-life that preparation (and testing) of labeled compounds is troublesome, although some laboratories use it.

Problems of radiological protection can easily arise in preparing iodine compounds, particularly with ^{131}I. Quite large quantities may be used because of the short half-life, there are energetic β- and γ-rays, volatile chemical forms are employed, and the "maximum permissible total body burden" is low (0.7 μc, thyroid). Special precautions become increasingly necessary in the range 1–10 mCi, and complex syntheses with larger quantities require much care and special equipment.

5.8. SPECIAL COMPOUNDS

As already observed, a number of compounds are used clinically to study either function or local uptake of various organs. They are extremely varied in character, for example:

Cyanocobalamin	(^{57}Co, ^{58}Co)

Chlormerodrin
Bromomercurihydroxypropane } (^{197}Hg, ^{203}Hg)
Mersalyl

Diisopropyl phosphofluoridate	(^{32}P)
Selenomethionine	(^{75}Se)
Human serum albumin	(^{131}I, ^{125}I, ^{99m}Tc)
Insulin, human growth hormone, etc.	(^{125}I)

Triopac
Iodipamide
Sodium diatrizoate
Diodone
Oleic acid
"Fats"   } (^{131}I, ^{125}I)
Hippuran
Thyroxine, iodo-tyrosines and iodo-thyronines
"Rose Bengal"
Polyvinylpyrrolidone

Some of these have been discussed briefly above. Others will be treated in more detail elsewhere in this *Encyclopedia*.

Brief notes are given on the methods of preparation of others in the list. Detailed methods are not always to be found in the published literature, no doubt because they have commercial value to isotope producers.

Cyanocobalamin. Fermentation of a *Streptomyces* on a medium containing ^{58}Co^{++} or ^{57}Co^{++}, but low in cobalt (Rosenblum and Woodbury, 1951; Smith, 1952; Bradley *et al.*, 1954).

The stability of solutions of radioactive cyanocobalamins is greatly improved by a low concentration of benzyl alcohol (0.9% is used at the Radiochemical Centre).

Chlormerodrin. 3-chloromercuri-2-methoxypropylurea

$$NH_2CONHCH_2CHCH_2HgCl$$
$$|$$
$$OCH_3$$

Prepared by reaction between allylurea and mercuric chloride in methanol solution (Rowland *et al.*, 1950).

Bromomercuri-2-hydroxypropane (BMHP)

$$CH_3CHCH_2HgBr$$
$$|$$
$$OH$$

Prepared by reaction between propylene and mercuric bromide in aqueous solution (Sand and Hofmann, 1900).

Mersalyl. O-l[3-hydroxymercuri-2-methoxypropyl)-carbamyl]phenoxy-acetic acid, sodium salt.

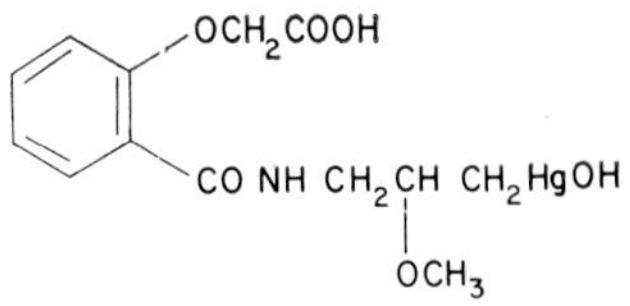

Prepared by reaction between *n*-allyl-*o*-carboxymethyl-salicylamide and mercuric acetate

Diisopropylphosphofluoridate (DFP)

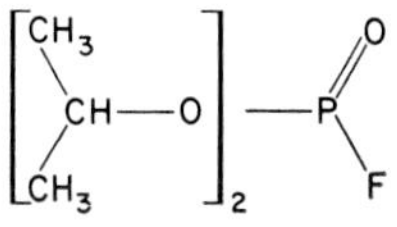

Prepared from PCl_3 via the route

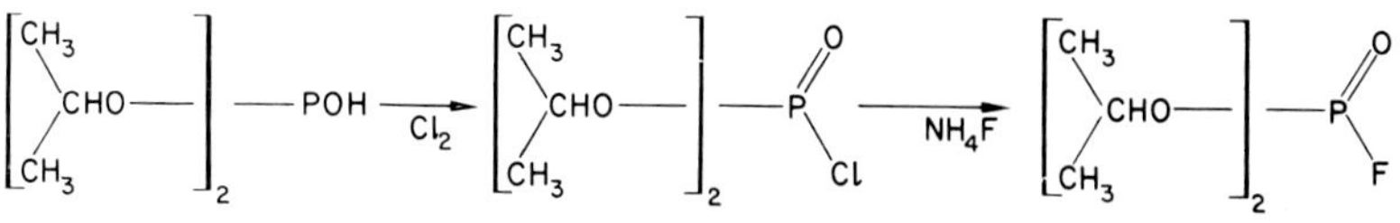

L-*Selenomethionine*

$$CH_3SeCH_2CH_2CHCOOH$$
$$|$$
$$NH_2$$

This compound is prepared biosynthetically (Blau, 1961).

Human serum albumin, insulin, human growth hormone, etc. It would be misleading to give references to methods of iodinating proteins without reference also to the prospective use and criteria of quality (European Atomic Energy Agency, 1966).

A special problem of proteins labeled by iodination is that the properties will depend on the history of the protein before iodination. Human proteins, for example, may be heat-treated to destroy the virus of homologous serum jaundice, and are sometimes processed by solvent precipitation. Such treatment may affect the metabolic properties of the protein. The purity of proteins is also often uncertain.

Sodium acetriozate ("Triopac"). 2,4,6-Triiodo-3-acetaminobenzoic acid, sodium salt.

Prepared by iodination of *m*-aminobenzoic acid and acetylation; or by exchange (Liebster *et al.*, 1959).

Iodipamide ("Biligrafin"). Adipoyl *bis*(*N*-3-amino-2,4,6-triiodobenzoic acid)

This compound is labeled by exchange.

Sodium diatrizoate ("Hypaque"). 2,4,6-Triiodo-3,5-diacetaminobenzoic acid

Labeled by exchange (Liebster *et al.*, 1959).

Diodone ("Diodrast"). 3,5-Diiodo-4-pyridone-*N*-acetic acid

Prepared by the route

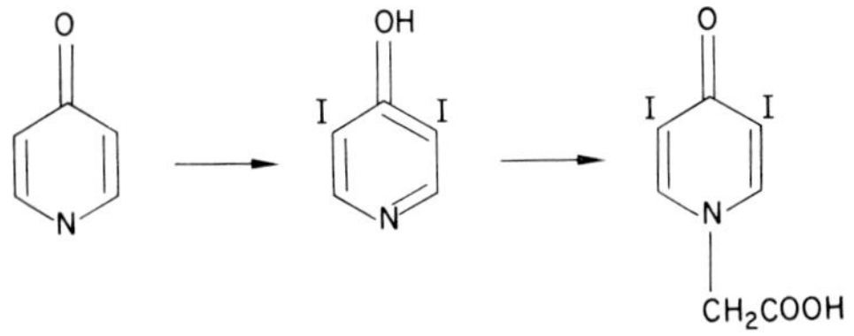

and may be labeled by exchange (Liebster *et al.*, 1959).

Hippuran. *o*-Iodohippuric acid

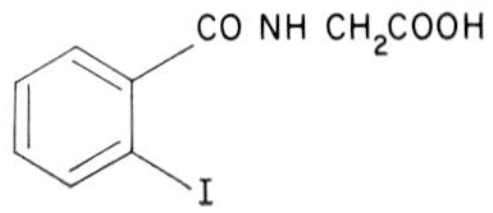

Labeled by exchange (see, for example, Mitta *et al.*, 1961).
"*Rose Bengal*". Tetrachlorotetraiodofluorescein

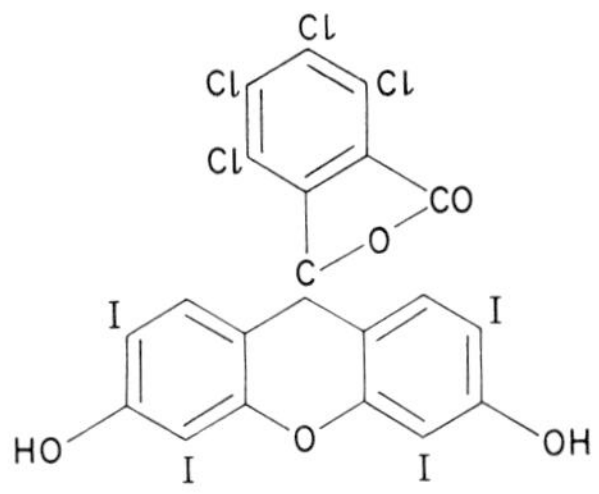

Prepared by iodination of tetrachlorofluorescein, although methods of labeling by exchange have been described.

Polyvinylpyrrolidone (PVP)

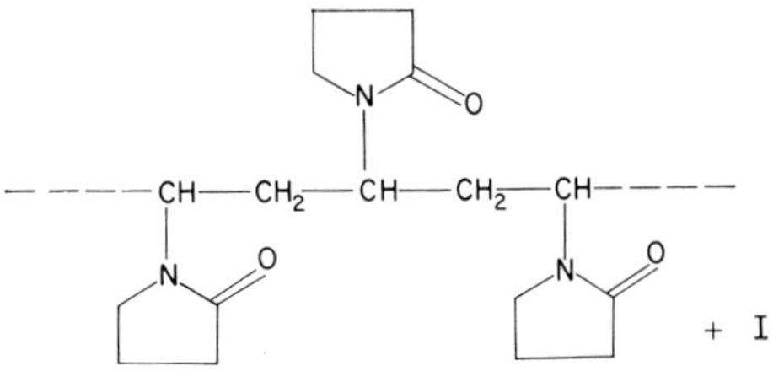

Prepared by the iodination of polyvinyl pyrrolidone. The position of labeling is uncertain, but is believed to be in the pyrrolidone ring (Briner, 1961).

L-3-*Iodotyrosine* (MIT). L-3,5-*Diiodotyrosine* (DIT)

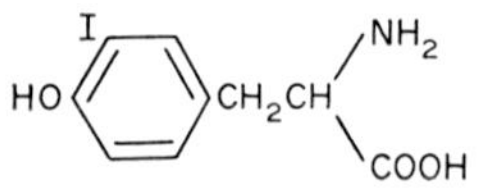

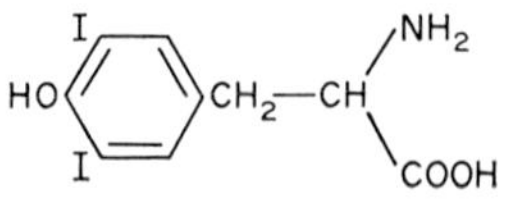

These are prepared by iodination of L-tyrosine and separation of the two above products by paper chromatography (Lemmon *et al.*, 1950: see also Murray and Williams, 1958, p. 1205). Exchange reactions have also been described (Miller *et al.*, 1944).

Thyroxine (T4)

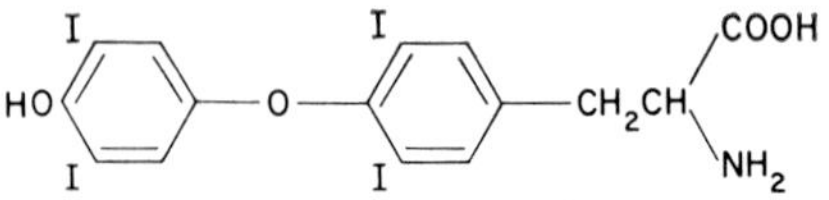

Thyroxine exists in D- and L-forms and various isomers may be prepared by iodination of mono- and diiodothyronines, of ethyl *N*-acetyl-3-(3,5-diamino-4-(4-methoxyphenoxy)phenyl)alanine, or triiodothyronine (see, for example, Murray and Williams, 1958, Vol. II, pp. 1212 ff; Roche and Michel, 1961).

Labeling is commonly, however, in the 3′,5′ positions, which is readily achieved by exchange (Gleason, 1955).

Triiodothyronine (T3)

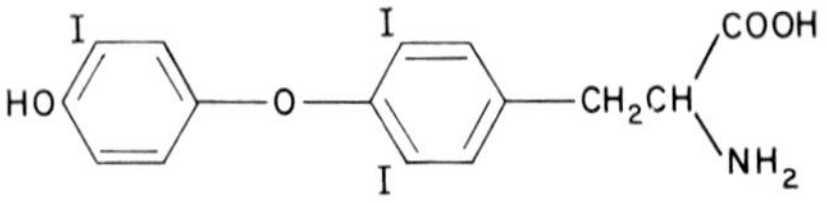

Of the various isomers possible, that shown, with labelling in position 3′, is the usual one. It is prepared by controlled iodination of 3,5-diiodo-thyronine and chromatographic separation from the thyroxine which is also formed, or by exchange (Gleason, 1955).

5.9. ANALYSIS OF RADIOACTIVE COMPOUNDS

The following definitions are used:

Radionuclidic purity. The proportion of the total radioactivity which is in the form of the stated radionuclide.

Radiochemical purity. The proportion of the total activity which is present in the specified chemical form (this term cannot be applied precisely to non-isotopic labeling: see below).

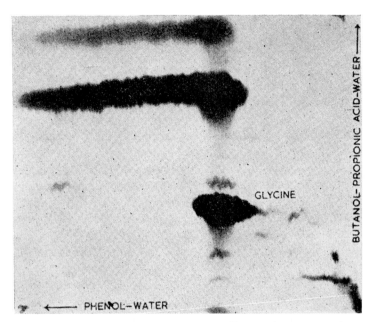

FIG. 1. Radioautogram of chromatogram of (2-^{14}C) glycine. Paper: Whatman No. 4 pretreated with oxalic acid. Solvents: Phenol/water (first dimension): n-butanol/propionic acid/water (second dimension).

Chemical purity. The proportion of the material in the specified chemical form regardless of any isotopic substitution.

Present standards of isotope production are such that radionuclidic purity is rarely in question unless short-lived isotopes are allowed to decay for long periods so that minute amounts of long-lived impurities are detectable.

It is most important to distinguish between chemical and radiochemical purity, which may not in fact be related to each other.

For most users, radiochemical purity is most important. It is best determined directly; usually by chromatographic and/or reverse isotope dilution analysis. Indirect evidence (from chemical purity, or behavior in an experiment) is often valuable but can be misleading. This is because dilution with carrier can raise the chemical purity without altering the radiochemical purity, so that it is important to know the whole history of the compound if chemical purity is used to estimate radiochemical purity. In Wilzbach and other radiation-induced labeling there is usually a large excess of carrier and radiochemical impurities may be "carrier-free". Evidence on chemical purity, biological potency, etc., has therefore very limited significance for such products. Indirect evidence may also be misleading in other ways. Infrared spectra for carboxylic acids are an example; at high isotopic abundances carbon-14 can differ considerably from carbon-12 (Baxter and Horsler, 1964).

Very small quantities (mass) of labeled compounds are sometimes analyzed, and misleading results (artefacts) in chromatography are not uncommon. Examples are oxidation, hydrolysis, adsorption, and ester exchange with eluting solvents. A simple but striking case has been reported by Huggins and Moses (1961).

Figure 1 shows what appears to be gross impurity in a sample of labeled glycine which was, in fact, quite pure.

An example recently observed at the Radiochemical Centre and still not fully explained may be given. Diethylstilboestrol, on thin layer chromatography on silica gel G and in the solvent system chloroform:acetone 4:1 separated into a major and a minor spot. The major spot, on being again chromatographed in the same system, separated again in the same way; while the minor spot appeared to revert in some degree to diethylstilboestrol. In other chromatographic systems which were tried these phenomena did not occur with diethylstilboestrol (unpublished observation by Dr. D. J. Thomas of the Radiochemical Centre, 1967). Such phenomena are by no means uncommon.

Subject to this warning, paper and thin-layer chromatography are most valuable methods in conjunction with scanning, autoradiography, or dissection and sample counting. The sensitivity of detection is very high (1 ppm is quite common) and often extends to all the decomposition products, unlike chemical methods of detection which are often specific. Dissection and sample counting is the most sensitive when low levels of impurities are being studied, but scanning is quicker and easier, and often sufficiently informative. Paper electrophoresis is also valuable and convenient. Gas–liquid chromatography, with radioactive scanning, is invaluable for compounds which are sufficiently volatile.

Reverse isotope dilution analysis is specific for the carrier used and not therefore sensitive to small amounts of impurity, found by difference. It is very sensitive for small impurities determined directly. In examining histidine-^{14}C, for example, for traces of histamine-^{14}C, unlabeled histidine as a carrier will detect histamine-^{14}C only by a difference of specific activities; but if histamine is used as a carrier, histamine-^{14}C may be determined with great sensitivity and good accuracy.

Experience at the Radiochemical Centre has revealed a number of examples in which dilution analysis for the major component has shown a substantial impurity which had escaped detection in several chromatographic systems.

Purity, and analytical results, should be expressed quantitatively. The impurity found should be related to the quantity of sample examined, and this in turn to the acceptable limits. It is easy to find 1 ppm impurity, but difficult to purify and keep organic compounds better than 99–99.9 % pure.

Higher standards of purity are required for labeled compounds than for ordinary reagents and drugs. The efficacy and safety of an unlabeled drug in clinical use is not usually affected by a few percent of impurity. Metabolic studies by older, chemical methods rarely accounted for the whole of a given dose, and for these also some degree of impurity may not always have been very important. The same will often be true of pharmacological and physiological experiments; small amounts of impurity will often not affect the results (unless the impurity itself is biologically active) and may not be suspected or observed. But in metabolic experiments with tracers it is possible to account for all the administered tracer and quite small amounts of labeled impurity may invalidate the experiment completely. This should be remembered, for example, when sterilizing labeled drugs by autoclaving. A small degree of decomposition, which would be negligible on pharmacological grounds, may be unacceptable for a tracer compound.

When non-isotopic labeling is used the ordinary definitions of purity lose their precise meaning; iodinated oleic acid, for example, is not oleic acid, and iodinated insulin is not insulin. It is often not possible at present to define exactly what a material such as an iodinated protein should be in precise chemical terms. The quality can therefore be defined only in terms of a specific property or use of such a material. Iodinated insulin, for example, may be specified for immuno-assay or for metabolic study, and a product suitable for one use may not be satisfactory for the other.

Readers for whom the analysis of labeled compounds is novel may find the booklets *Radioactive Tracers in Chemical Analysis* (Gorsuch, 1966a) and *Radioactive Isotope Dilution Analysis* (Gorsuch, 1966b) useful.

Sterility and freedom from pyrogens are required for compounds used in medicine or administered experimentally to humans. For the limited number of compounds in routine clinical use the commercial supplier will be responsible in the first place, although users must also exercise care. Experience has shown that local "re-dispensing" of isotope preparations may concentrate on radiological safety to the extent that aseptic precautions are insufficiently observed.

For compounds (such as labeled drugs) in occasional experimental use, responsibility must remain with the user. Pyrogens, generally speaking, are not a high risk with synthetic drugs unless solutions are stored.

The presence of potential substrate materials (carbohydrates, amino acids, etc.) increases the risk of microbiological growth. Storage at $0°$ is not a complete safeguard.

To ensure sterility, autoclaving is to be preferred if possible. It is always wise to check the purity of the compound after autoclaving, for the reasons given above.

5.10. INSTABILITY OF RADIOACTIVE ORGANIC CHEMICALS

Because of the small quantities used, purely chemical decomposition of tracer compounds probably occurs more often than is suspected; but the problem is aggravated by self-irradiation.

Knowledge of this decomposition is still very empirical, although much information has been published (Catch, 1966; Bayly and Evans, 1966). For labeled drugs, in general, there is little information.

The diversity and complexity of labeled compounds is so great that one cannot expect detailed investigation of their radiation chemistry. Some advice may be given in general terms, but with the warning that many exceptions may be found for recommendations 6–9.

(1) Review the origin, preparation, age, and history of the compound, its specific activity and its chemical character.

(2) If in doubt, re-analyze it for radiochemical purity, paying special attention to impurities which will interfere in the experimental use.

(3) Remember the possibility of unexpected behavior at low concentrations or in small quantities, which may also obscure analytical results.

(4) Be alert to the risks of chemical decomposition, e.g. by heat, light, or microbiological infection, independently of radiation.

(5) Ensure that storage vessels or ampoules are perfectly clean, neutral, and chemically inert.

(6) Dissolve the compound in benzene or in a solvent consisting largely of benzene if that is possible. The radioactive concentration should be low, and it is probably wise to free it from oxygen.

(7) If benzene is unsuitable, consider the use of alcohol, water, or other such solvents, or filter paper (which should then be dehydrated as thoroughly as possible). Again, freedom from oxygen is advisable.

(8) If the sample is stored in a dry solid state (and this is often the best form, especially at moderate specific activities) the quantities should be as small as convenient to reduce self-absorption. For carbon-14 compounds, quantities of a few milligrams or less are suggested; the expedient is of course valueless for tritium compounds. The material should be dehydrated and freed from oxygen as completely as possible.

(9) Store samples at the lowest convenient temperature unless there are known reasons to the contrary.

It is sometimes possible to choose between two isotopic labels, one of which may give a more stable product because there is less self-absorption of energy. Examples are insulin-^{125}I or albumin-^{125}I (more stable than ^{131}I) and cyanocobalamins-^{57}Co (more stable than ^{58}Co).

For a more detailed discussion of radiation decomposition the reader may be referred to monographs and publications on the subject (Catch, 1966; Bayly and Evans, 1966) which provide a more extensive bibliography.

REFERENCES

(A) BOOKS, REVIEWS AND MONOGRAPHS

BUBNER, M. and SCHMIDT, L. (1966) *Die Syntheses Kohlenstoff-14-markierter organischer Verbindungen*, 1st ed. Georg Thieme, Leipzig.

CALVIN, M., HEIDELBERGER, C., REID, J. C., TOLBERT, B. M. and YANKWICH, P. F. (1949) *Isotopic Carbon. Techniques in its Measurement and Chemical Manipulation.* 1st ed. John Wiley, New York, U.S.A.

CATCH, J. R. (1961) *Carbon-14 Compounds*, 1st ed., Butterworths, London.

CATCH, J. R. (1966) *The Stability of Labelled Organic Compounds*, rev. ed. Radiochemical Centre, Amersham (RCC Review 3).

EUROPEAN ATOMIC ENERGY AGENCY (1966) *Labelled Proteins in Tracer Studies*, 1st ed. Proceedings of the Conference, Pisa, January 17–19, 1966. Donato, L., Milhaud, G. and Sirchis, J. (eds.). Euratom, Brussels (EUR 2950 d, f, e).

EUROPEAN ATOMIC ENERGY COMMUNITY (1964) *Proceedings Conference on Methods of Preparing and Storing Marked Molecules, Brussels*, 1963. 1st ed. European Atomic Energy Community, Brussels.

EVANS, E. A. (1966) *Tritium and its Compounds*, 1st ed., Butterworths, London.

GORSUCH, T. T. (1966a) *Radioactive Tracers in Chemical Analysis*, 1st ed. Radiochemical Centre, Amersham (RCC Review 5).

GORSUCH, T. T. (1966b) *Radioactive Isotope Dilution Analysis*, rev. ed. Radiochemical Centre, Amersham, England (RCC Review 2).

MURRAY, A. and WILLIAMS, D. L. (1958) *Organic Synthesis with Isotopes*, Parts 1 and 2, 1st ed. Interscience Publishers, New York.

NEVENZEL, J. C., RILEY, R. F., HOWTON, D. R. and STEINBERG, G. (1954) *Bibliography of Syntheses with Carbon Isotopes*, 1st ed. University of California, School of Medicine, Los Angeles, U.S.A. (Report No. UCLA 316).

NEVENZEL, J. C., HOWTON, D. R., RILEY, R. F. and STEINBERG, G. (1957) *A Bibliography of Syntheses with Carbon Isotopes*, 1953–54, 1st ed. University of California, School of Medicine, Los Angeles, U.S.A. (Report No. UCLA 395).

RADIOCHEMICAL CENTRE (1966) *The Radiochemical Manual*, 2nd ed. Wilson, B. J. (ed.). Radiochemical Centre, Amersham, England.

ROCHE, J. and MICHEL, R. (1961) Biochimie des hormones thyroidiennes, in *Künstliche radioaktive Isotope in Physiologie, Diagnostik und Therapie*, Vol. 1 Schweigk, H. and Turba, F. (eds.). Springer-Verlag, Berlin, pp. 1197–1222.

RONZIO, A. R. (1954) Microsyntheses with tracer elements, in *Technique of Organic Chemistry*, Vol. 6. Weissberger, A. (ed.). pp. 367–409 *Micro and Semimicro Methods*, (1st ed.) by Cheronis, N. D., Ronzio, A. R. and Ma, T. S. Interscience Publishers, New York, U.S.A.

WEISS, A. G., GRENIER, J. F., and HATANO, M. (1963) Les tests de l'absorption intestinale par les graisses marquées aux halogènes, leurs incertitudes, in *Radioaktive Isotope in Klinik und Forschung*, Band, V., Fellinger, K. and Höfer, R. (eds.). Urban und Schwarzenberg, Munich–Berlin, pp. 443–53.

WENZEL, M. and SCHULZE, P. E. (1962) *Tritium-markierung. Darstellung, Messung und Anwendung nach Wilzbach ³H-markierter Verbindungen*, 1st ed. Walter de Gruyter, Berlin.

WEYGAND, F. and SIMON, H. (1955) Herstellung isotopenhaltiger organisher Verbindungen, in *Methoden der organischen Chemie*, 1st ed. Weyl, Th. and Houben, J. George Thieme, Stuttgart, vol. 4, part 2.

(B) ORIGINAL PAPERS

ALWORTH, W. L., DE SELMS, R. C. and RAPOPORT, H. (1964) The biosynthesis of nicotine in *Nicotiana glutinosa* from carbon-14 dioxide. *J. Amer. Chem. Soc.*, **86**:1608–16.

ARNSTEIN, H. R. V. and CLUBB, M. E. (1957) The biosynthesis of penicillin. 5: Comparison of valine and hydroxyvaline as penicillin precursors. *Biochem. J.*, **65**:618–27.

AYRES, P. J., PEARLMAN, W. H., TAIT, J. F. and TAIT, S. A. S. (1958) The biosynthetic preparation of (16-^{3}H) aldosterone and (16-^{3}H) corticosterone. *Biochem. J.*, **70**:230–6.

BAXTER, B. H. and HORSLER, A. F. C. (1964) Isotope effects in the infra-red spectra of some carbon-14 labelled acids, an ester and sodium salt. *Nature, Lond.*, **204**:675–6.

BAYLY, R. J. (1966) Labeled compounds in medical diagnosis. *Nucleonics*, **24**(6):46–53.

BAYLY, R. J. and EVANS, E. A. (1966) Stability and storage of compounds labelled with radioisotopes. *J. Labelled Comp.*, **2**:1–34.

BLAU, M. (1961) Biosynthesis of (^{75}Se)selenomethionine and (^{75}Se)selenocystine. *Biochim. Biophys. Acta*, **49**:389–90.

BRADLEY, J. E., SMITH, E. L., BAKER, S. J. and MOLLIN, D. L. (1954) The use of radioactive isotope of cobalt Co^{58} for the preparation of labelled vitamin B12. *Lancet*, **267**:476–7.

BRADLOW, H. L., FUKUSHIMA, D. K. and GALLAGHER, T. F. (1959) Stereospecific incorporation of tritium by unsaturated steroids. *Atomlight*, **9**:2–3.

BRINER, W. H. (1961) A note of the formulation of iodine-131 labelled polyvinyl-pyrrolidone for intravenous administration. *J. Nucl. Med.*, **2**:94–8.

CAMPBELL, R. M., CUTHBERTSON, D. P., MATTHEWS, C. M. and McFARLANE, A. S. (1956) Behaviour of ^{14}C and ^{131}I-labelled plasma proteins in the rat. *Int. J. Appl. Radiat. Isotopes*, **1**:66–84.

CHADHA, M. S., WOELLER, F. H. and LEMMON, R. M. (1962) Experiments on Wilzbach tritium labeling accompanied by charcoal absorption and electric discharge, in *Bio-organic Chemistry Quarterly Report, September through November 1961*. University of California, Ernest O. Lawrence Radiation Laboratory, Berkeley, California (Report No. UCRL 10032), pp. 94–101.

CIFERRI, O., FRACCARO, M., ALBERTINI, A., CASSANI, G., MANNINI, A., and TIEPOLO, L. (1964) Tritium-labeled actinomycin. Preparation and cytological distribution in human cells cultured *in vitro*, in *Proceedings Symposium on Preparation and Biochemical Application of Labeled Molecules*, Venice, 1964, Sirchis, J. (ed.). European Atomic Energy Community, Brussels, pp. 147–63.

COHEN, S., HOLLOWAY, R. C., MATHEWS, C. and McFARLANE, A. S. (1956) Distribution and elimination of ^{131}I and ^{14}C-labelled plasma proteins in the rabbit. *Biochem. J.*, **62**:143–54.

DORFMAN, L. M. and WILZBACH, K. E. (1959) Tritium labeling of organic compounds by means of electric discharge. *J. Phys. Chem. Ithaca*, **63**:799–801.

DUTTON, H. J., JONES, E. P., MASON, L. H. and NYSTROM, R. F. (1958) The labelling of fatty acids by exposure to tritium gas. *Chem. Ind.*, **36**:1176–7.

EVANS, E. A. (1961) Preparation of tritium-labelled atropine at high specific activity. *Chem. Ind.*, **51**:2097.

GLEASON, G. I. (1955) Some notes on the exchange of iodine with thyroxine homologues. *J. Biol. Chem.*, **213**:837–41.

GORDON, M., PAN, S. C., VIRGONA, A. and NUMEROF, P. (1953) Biosynthesis of penicillin. I: Role of phenylacetic acid. *Science, N.Y.*, **118**:43.

GREENWOOD, F. C., HUNTER, W. M. and GLOVER, J. S. (1962) The preparation of ^{131}I-labelled human growth hormone of high specific radioactivity. *Biochem. J.*, **89**:114–23.

GROSSBARD, E. and BARTON, G. E. (1963) A low-cost growth chamber for the cultivation from seeds of grasses labelled with carbon-14. *Int. J. Appl. Radiat. Isotopes*, **14**:517–25.

HUGGINS, A. K. and MOSES, V. (1961) Breakdown of (2-^{14}C)-glycine during paper chromatography. *Nature, Lond.*, **191**:668–70.

HUNTER, G. D., HERBERT, M. and HOCKENHULL, D. J. D. (1954) Actimomycete meta bolism: Origin of the guanidine groups in streptomycin. *Biochem. J.*, **58**:249–54.

HUNTER, G. D. and HOCKENHULL, D. J. D. (1955) Actimomycete metabolism. Incorporation of ^{14}C-labelled compounds into streptomycin. *Biochem. J.*, **59**:268–72.

ISBELL, H. S., FRUSH, H. L. and MOYER, J. D. (1960) Tritium-labeled compounds. IV: D-Glucose-6-*t*, D-xylose-5-*t* and D-mannitol-1-*t*. *J. Res. Natn. Bur. Stand.*, **64A**: 359–62.

JELLINCK, P. H. and SMYTH, D. G. (1958) Molecular changes in exchange labelling with tritium. *Nature, Lond.*, **182**:46.

KAROW, E. O., PECK, R. L., ROSENBLUM, C. and WOODBURY, D. T. (1952) Microbiological synthesis of C^{14}-labeled streptomycin. *J. Amer. Chem. Soc.*, **74**:3056–9.

KUZIN, A. M. and TOKARSKAYA, V. I. (1959) Complete labeling of the organic substances of plants by radioactive carbon as a method for studying metabolic disturbances. *Biochemistry (USSR)*, **24**:71–7.

LEMMON, R. M., TARPEY, W. and SCOTT, K. G. (1950) Paper chromatography in synthetic organic chemistry. Microgram scale syntheses of labeled monoiodotyrosine, diiodotyrosine and thyroxine. *J. Amer. Chem. Soc.*, **72**:758–61.

LIEBSTER, J., KACL, J., and BABICKY, A. (1959) Labelling of radiographic contrast media with iodine-131. *Nature, Lond.*, **182**:1474–5.

MCFARLANE, A. S. (1958) Efficient trace-labelling of proteins with iodine. *Nature, Lond.*, **182**:53.

MARTIN, E., BERKY, J., GODZESKY, C., MILLER, P., TOME, J. and STONE, R. W. (1953) Biosynthesis of penicillin in the presence of C^{14}. *J. Biol. Chem.*, **203**:239–50.

MERENOVA, V. I. (1954) Biosynthesis of chlorophyll, atropine, glucose and proteins having labelled carbon (in Russian). *Biokhimiya*, **19**:698–701.

MILLER, W. H., ANDERSON, G. W., MADISON, R. K. and SALLEY, D. J. (1944) Exchange reactions of diiodotyrosine. *Science, N.Y.*, **100**:340–1.

MILLER, P. A., MCCORMICK, J. R. D. and DOERSCHUK, A. P. (1956) Studies of chlorotetracycline biosynthesis and the preparation of chlorotetracycline-C^{14}. *Science, N.Y.*, **123**:1030–1.

MITTA, A. E. A., FRAGA, A. and VEALL, N. (1961) A simplified method for preparing I^{131} labelled Hippuran. *Int. J. Appl. Radiat. Isotopes*, **12**:146–7.

NUMEROF, P., GORDON, M., VIRGONA, A. and O'BRIEN, E. (1953) Biosynthesis of streptomycin. I: Studies with C-14-labeled glycine and acetate. *J. Amer. Chem. Soc.*, **76**:1341–4.

NYSTROM, R. F. (1962) The radiation induced addition of tritium to unsaturated systems. *Atomlight*, **23**:508.

OKITA, G. T., KELSEY, F. E., WALASZEK, E. J. and GEILING, E. M. K. (1954) Biosynthesis and isolation of carbon-14 labeled digitoxin. *J. Pharmacol. Exp. Ther.*, **110**:244–50.

PORTER, J. W. and WATSON, M. S. (1954) Gross effects of growth-inhibiting levels of tritium oxide on *Chlorella pyrenoidosa*. *Amer. J. Bot.*, **41**:550–5.

ROSA, U., PENNISI, G. F., SCASSELLATI, G. A., BIANCHI, R., FEDERIGHI, G., DONATO, L., ROSSI, C. A. and AMBROSINO, C. (1966) Factors affecting proteins iodination, in *Labelled Proteins in Tracer Studies*, 1st ed. Proceedings of the Conference, Pisa, January 17–19, 1966. Donato, L., Milhaud, G. and Sirchis, J. (eds.). Euratom, Brussels (EUR 2950, d, f, e), pp. 17–30.

ROSENBLUM, C. and WOODBURY, D. T. (1951) Cobalt 60 labeled vitamin B12 of high specific activity. *Science, N.Y.*, **113**:215.

ROWLAND, R. L., PERRY, W. L., FOREMAN, E. L., and FRIEDMAN, H. L. (1950) Mercurial diuretics. I: Addition of mercuric acetate to allyl urea. *J. Amer. Chem. Soc.*, **72**: 3595–8.

SAND, J. and HOFMANN, K. A. (1900) Einwirkung von Propylen und Butylene auf Mercurisalze. *Ber. dt. chem. Ges.*, **33**:1353–8.

SAUERBECK, D. (1960) Zur Markierung von Pflanzen mit ^{14}C. *Atompraxis*, 6:221–5.

SCULLY, N. J., STAVELY, H. E., SKOK, J., STANLEY, A. R., DALE, J. K., CRAIG, J. T., HODGE, E. B., CHORNEY, W., WATANABE, R. and BALDWIN, R. (1952) Biosynthesis of the C^{14}-labeled form of dextran. *Science, N.Y.*, 116:87–9.

SCULLY, N. J., CHORNEY, W., KOSTAL, G., WATANABE, R., SKOK, J. and GLATTFELD, J. W. (1955) Biosynthesis in C^{14}-labeled plants; their use in agricultural and biological research, in Proceedings of the First International Conference on the Peaceful Uses of Atomic Energy, Geneva, 1955, vol. 12. United Nations, New York, U.S.A., pp. 377–85.

SEBEK, O. K. (1955) The synthesis of neomycin-C^{14} by *Steptomyces fradiae*. *Archs. Biochem. Biophys.* 57:71–9.

SKOSEY, J. L. (1966) Effect of adrenocorticotropin and other hormone preparations upon the metabolism of acetate-1-^{14}C and other ^{14}C-labeled substrates by adipose tissue *in vitro. J. Biol. Chem.*, 241:5108–13.

SMITH, J. H., ALLISON, F. E. and MULLINS, J. F. (1963) A biosynthesis chamber for producing plants labeled with carbon-14. *Atompraxis*, 9:73–5.

SMITH, E. L. (1952) Radioactive penicillin and vitamin B12. *Brit. Med. Bull.*, 8:203–5.

SNELL, J. F., WAGNER, R. L. and HOCHSTEIN, F. A. (1956) Radioactive oxytetracycline (Terramycin). I: Mode of synthesis and properties of the radioactive compound, in Proceedings of the First International Conference on the Peaceful Uses of Atomic Energy, Geneva, 1955, vol. 12. United Nations, New York, U.S.A., pp. 431–4.

SWAN, G. A. and WRIGHT, D. (1956) A study of melanin formation by use of 2-(3:4-dihydroxy(3-^{14}C)phenyl)-, 2-(3:4-dihydroxy(4-^{14}C)phenyl)-, and 2-(3:4,dihydroxy-(5-^{14}C)phenyl)-ethylamine. *J. Chem. Soc.*, 1549–57.

WASER, P. G. and LÜTHI, U. (1956) Autoradiography of end-plates with carbon-14-calabash-curarine 1 and carbon-14-decamethonium. *Nature, Lond.*, 178:981.

WILZBACH, K. E. (1957) Tritium-labeling by exposure of organic compounds to tritium gas. *J. Amer. Chem. Soc.*, 79:1013.

WILZBACH, K. E. (1962) Gas exposure method for tritium labelling, in Proceedings. Symposium on the Detection and Use of Tritium in the Physical and Biological Sciences, Vienna, 1961, vol. 2. International Atomic Energy Agency, Vienna, pp. 3–10.

WOLF, A. P. (1964) Recoil labeling of organic molecules with special reference to compounds of biological and biochemical significance, in Proceedings Symposium on Preparation and Bio-medical Application of Labeled Molecules, Venice, 1964, Sirchis, J. (ed.). European Atomic Energy Community, Brussels, pp. 423–5.

YALOW, R. S. and BERSON, S. A. (1966) Labelling of proteins–problems and practices, *Trans. N.Y. Acad. Sci.*, Series II, 29:1033–44.

CHAPTER 5

ORGANIC TRACERS OF BIOLOGICAL ORIGIN

J. Ingrand and U. Rosa

Laboratoire de Physique Medicale, Faculté de Medicine,
Cochin–Port Royal, Paris, France, and SORIN, Saluggia, Italy

INTRODUCTION

THE extreme sensitivity of techniques based on the detection of radio-activity has made the use of tracers a current practice in pharmacology.

The special field of organic tracers of biological origin (animal or vegetal) is an immense one, covering chemical compounds of simple structure such as amino acids, aliphatic acids, and monosaccharides, as well as more complex molecules such as the nucleic acids, proteins, vitamins, alkaloids, antibiotics, secretion products such as snake venom and toxins, and even cells and microorganisms.

Faced with so many tracers and their heterogeneous nature, the present study is largely confined to interesting compounds in biochemical pharmacology without considering derivatives of bacterial origin (microorganisms, toxins, and vaccines), and cells and multicellular organisms (blood cells, cancerous cells, parasites, and so on).

Typical examples will be taken from the chemical class of proteins that have been the subject of very many papers.

The first section deals with the radioisotopes used for labeling, since their radioactive characteristics must be considered in planning experiments. Section 2 successively considers three methods of preparation of organic tracers: the introduction of radioisotopes into molecules by biosynthesis, by exchange, and by addition of foreign atoms. In the final section the emphasis is on the precautions to be taken by the experimenter in selecting the mode of labeling, and in performing the control tests to justify the use of the tracer for the experiment in hand.

1. ISOTOPES USED FOR LABELING

Advances in nuclear technology have made it possible to produce most of the isotopes which are constituents of the living organism. However, a

131

radioisotope is used in pharmacology only if it has characteristics that suit the experiment being planned. It is very rare for an isotope to have no disadvantages, and generally the inconveniences inherent in radioactivity have to be anticipated.

It is basic to the use of labeled compounds that the stable isotope of an element naturally present in a molecule may be replaced by a radioactive isotope of the same element. Thus, in particular, $^{12}_{6}C$ is replaced by $^{14}_{6}C$, $^{1}_{1}H$ is replaced by $^{3}_{1}H$, $^{32}_{16}S$ by $^{35}_{16}S$, and $^{127}_{53}I$ by $^{125}_{53}I$ or by $^{131}_{53}I$. This principle fully applies to the methods of labeling by synthesis, biosynthesis, and exchange; but the method in which a radioactive isotope of an element not naturally occurring in the molecule is added to this molecule has many advantages, and, assuming that the necessary precautions are taken, this technique can produce excellent results too.

But whatever method is used, the choice of isotope depends on its particular characteristics, namely the half-life, mode of disintegration, radiation energy, availability, and production cost.

1.1. HALF-LIFE

The isotope should have a long enough life for experiments to be performed without haste, and the labeled product should keep well in storage. In particular circumstances short-lived isotopes are used: e.g. iodine-132, (2 hr), technetium-99m (6 hr), and copper-64 (12 hr) (the figures in brackets denoting half-lives).

1.2. MODE OF DECAY AND RADIATION ENERGY

The low-energy pure beta emitters long posed practical problems of detection, while sample preparation for final counting was a tiresome task. Since 1958, however, a satisfactory solution has been obtainable by liquid scintillation techniques combined with improved methods of mineralization.

In autoradiography, on the other hand, the reduced mean range of the low-energy beta emitters (^{14}C, ^{35}S, ^{3}H) has always been an advantage. In particular, the weak energy of tritium enables the tritiated products to be localized with very great precision; in fact, in a medium of unit density, the high-energy electrons (18 keV) travel 8 mcm and the medium-energy electrons (5.69 keV) 1.3 mcm (Verly, 1960).

The electromagnetic ray emitters (X-ray and gamma-ray) have the advantage of easy detection, even externally, and this permits certain studies on the living animal, but it does not enable autohistoradiograms of high resolution to be obtained.

1.3. SPECIFIC ACTIVITY

A high specific activity (activity per unit of mass) is very often essential for biological research with radioactive tracers, since the introduction of an excessive amount of the labeled compound can affect the natural metabolism. The specific activity of a labeled product depends in the first place on the nature of the radioactive element used for the labeling. As a first approximation, the specific activity of the labeled product is higher the higher the specific activity of original radioactive element. In general, the radioactive isotopes that can be prepared by neutron bombardment and nuclear reactions other than (n,γ) are exceptions. Among these, we find radiocarbon ^{14}C, radiosulfur ^{35}S, radiohydrogen ^{3}H, and radiophosphorus ^{32}P, the stable isotopes of which are the most important components of natural substances. Since these radioisotopes are all prepared by nuclear reactions using chemically different targets, they can be produced at a very high specific activity (carrier-free). A special case is radioiodine ^{131}I, which is formed by decay of the radioactive parent ^{131}Te, which in its turn is obtained from $^{130}Te\ (n,\gamma)^{131}Te$ reaction.

Radioisotopes of high specific activity are prepared in accelerators using nuclear reactions other than (n,γ). However, it should be stressed that labeled compounds are subject to an autoirradiation effect, and the damage which results depends, *inter alia*, on the specific activity. The specific activity of a labeled product is therefore a reasonable compromise between the need to use a small quantity of tracer, on the one hand, and the need to limit the destructive effect of the radiations on the product itself (see *Effects of Autoradiolysis*), Section 3.1.2.

1.4. AVAILABILITY

There are also practical considerations which should never be overlooked, i.e. the cost of the isotope and the proximity to a nuclear reactor. One may mention, for instance, the relatively low cost of tritiated molecules. A nearby nuclear power station is a particularly important factor in the case of short-lived isotopes of infrequent usage, such as the reactor-produced ^{64}Cu.

The main characteristics of the radioisotopes most currently used in pharmacology for labeling biological compounds are shown in Table 1.

TABLE 1. CHARACTERISTICS OF RADIOISOTOPES USED IN PHARMACOLOGY

Atomic number	Symbol	Mass number	Mode of decay	Particle energy (MeV)	Photon energy (MeV)	Half-life
1	H	3	β^-	0.018	—	12.3 yr
6	C	14	β^-	0.155	—	5.760 yr
15	P	32	β^-	1.71	—	14.3 days
16	S	35	β^-	0.167	—	87.2 days
24	Cr	51	K, γ		0.32	27.8 days
26	Fe	55	K		0.006	2.9 yr
26	Fe	59	β^-, γ	0.46	1.3	45 days
27	Co	57	K, γ		0.12	270 days
27	Co	58	K, γ, β^+		0.81	71 days
27	Co	60	β^-, γ	0.31	1.17–1.3	5.2 yr
29	Cu	64	β^-, β^+, γ	0.66	0.51	12.9 hr
29	Cu	67	β^-, γ	0.40	0.18	61.0 hr
34	Se	75	K, γ		0.4	120 days
35	Br	82	β^-, γ	0.46	0.55–0.78	35.5 hr
43	Tc	99m	I.T., γ		0.14	6 hr
53	I	125	K, γ		0.035	60 days
53	I	131	β^-, γ	0.61	0.36	8 days

1.5. GENERAL CONSIDERATIONS

In the following pages we shall see that the choice of radioisotope is influenced by the technique adopted for labeling. The procedure in turn depends on the properties of the substance to be labeled, and especially on its chemical stability and structural complexity. With substances of biological origin, the range of choice is rather limited to the substances formed, particularly from hydrogen, carbon, sulfur, nitrogen, and oxygen, of which only the first three elements have radioactive isotopes that can be used in practice.

Later it will also be seen that the number of usable radioisotopes can be increased by the attachment of foreign atoms (labeling by addition). Even in this case the number of radioisotopes used in practice is relatively small.

After considering problems in isotope selection, we pass on to the different methods of production of organic tracers of biological origin.

2. METHODS OF LABELING

For producing tracers the pharmacologist has a variety of methods at his disposal. In many respects the most satisfactory method is chemical synthesis, but this can only be employed if the compounds structure is known and if the efficiency of synthesis is satisfactory. On the other hand, the relatively high production cost and the relatively low specific activity are at times a very serious drawback. In all such unfavorable cases it is necessary to call upon other methods of labeling—biosynthesis, isotopic exchange, and the addition of foreign atoms—which are the subject of the present section.

2.1. BIOSYNTHESIS

The methods of organic synthesis can be used to produce a very large number of labeled molecules in which the position of the isotope is determined with precision. However, there are other compounds such as proteins, polysaccharides, and most of the antibiotics and alkaloids, which still cannot be synthesized by the methods of organic chemistry. In these cases, radioisotopes can be introduced into the test molecules by the use of living organisms (Woodruff and Fowler, 1950; Catch, 1964; Laufer *et al.*, 1964). Biosynthesis is simple in principle and wide in scope, making it possible to obtain not only simple chemical compounds (glucides, amino acids, alcohol acids, and polyols), but also more complex molecules (lipoïds, thioglucosides, vitamins, antibiotics, enzymes, and alkaloids).

Among the isotopes most used at the present time, one finds carbon-14, tritium, and sulfur-35, but certain isotopes of selenium (^{75}Se), cobalt (^{57}Co), iodine (^{131}I), phosphorus (^{32}P), iron (^{55}Fe), and even short-lived isotopes like copper (^{67}Cu) (Sternlieb *et al.*, 1961; Waldmann and Wochner, 1965b) may also be used.

After we have considered the advantages and disadvantages of bio-synthesis, we shall illustrate by some examples the choice of biosynthetic methods at the disposal of the research worker.

2.1.1. *Characteristics of biosynthetic methods*

Biosynthesis, by definition, is the formation of molecules following an *in vivo* or *in vitro* reaction of a substrate (precursor) with all or part of a living organism.

The use of biological material immediately implies perfect knowledge of the biochemical processes of metabolism of the particular material concerned. Since it is very difficult to realise the induction of a living cell in the sense of a modification of the chemical composition of the metabolites, the researcher is only left with the choice of substrate most appropriate to preparing the known compound for concentrating in the biological element.

From this statement, it will be clear that biosynthetic techniques have certain advantages but equally serious limitations.

(*a*) *Advantages.* Biosynthesis enables very important biological compounds to be obtained which would not be forthcoming by chemical synthesis. It should immediately be said that the compounds so obtained, unlike those produced by isotopic exchange or addition of foreign atoms, behave exactly the same as the "original" compounds in physico-chemical and biological respects. The plasma proteins labeled with ^{14}C are the best example, since they serve as a reference in metabolic studies (Campbell *et al.*, 1956; Cohen *et al.*, 1956; Masouredis and Beeckmans, 1955).

With the amino acids, biosynthesis makes it possible to isolate not only the racemic compounds but also the *l* form, which is generally the biologically most active form.

In other respects it is possible in certain cases to adopt simple, and therefore cheap, chemical precursors at the start of biosynthesis.

The efficiency of the preparation, often expressed as the percentage of radioisotope incorporated into the labeled molecule, is very variable. It ranges from 1% for gibberelline (Parisi *et al.*, 1964) to 40% for seleno-methionine (Blau, 1961), and for the proteins (Erb and Maurer, 1960).

(*b*) *Disadvantages.* For several reasons, the specific activity of the compounds obtained is with few exceptions weak or medium. In the first place, the radiosensitivity of the biological substrate restricts the amount of radioactivity to a maximum limit. The radiosensitivity of the substrate varies with the isotope, the living cell, and the medium (Table 2). Secondly, the substrate is generally not entirely used up in forming the molecule at which the researcher is aiming, and numerous other products are obtained at the same time. For example, less than 2 % of the radioactivity of the precursor amino acid is found in the protein extracted at the end.

TABLE 2. COMPARATIVE RADIOSENSITIVITY AS A FUNCTION OF BIOLOGICAL SUBSTRATE, ISOTOPE AND THE MEDIUM

Biological substrate	Isotope	Medium	Maximum tolerated radioactivity	Reference
Higher vegetables	^{14}C	Air	1 mCi/g of carbon	Catch, 1964
Malt yeast	^{14}C	Solution	5 mCi/mg of yeast	Laufer *et al.*, 1964
Chlorella	^{3}H	Solution	20 mCi/ml	Catch, 1964
Malt yeast	^{75}Se	Solution	10 mCi/l	Blau, 1961
Brassica	^{35}S	Air	1.7 mCi/l	Kutacek *et al.*, 1966

Table 3 shows the specific activity obtained by biosynthesis considered as an end in itself (commercial production), and as an intermediary stage (pure or applied research). The presence of impurities, other than the required compound, makes it necessary to undertake often increasingly delicate extractions and purifications which add to the cost of the preparation.

After biosynthesis, the position of the radioisotope within the molecule is generally not determined with certainty (Table 4). However, an induction can be considered, as shown by Cifferi *et al.* (1965).

As the final disadvantage, it should not be overlooked that medical ethics prohibit the use of biosynthesis in man.

2.1.2. *Biosynthetic methods*

If the chemistry of the compound being prepared conditions the choice of precursor, the metabolic characteristics of the biological substrate are finally decisive. For the sake of convenience we have arbitrarily classed the methods of biosynthesis according to the substrate used: entire animals,

TABLE 3. SOME SPECIFIC ACTIVITIES OBTAINED BY BIOSYNTHESIS

Compound	Isotope	Specific activity	Reference
Vitamin B[12]	[57]Co	50–200 mCi/mg	Catch, 1964
ATP[a]	[32]P	2 mCi/m$_M$	Vanderheiden and Boszormenyi-Nagy, 1965
γ-globulins	[3]H	5 mCi/g	Crawhall *et al.*, 1958
Glucose-fructose	[3]H	500 mCi/g	Hasan, 1962
Glucose-mannose	[14]C	40 mCi/g	Laufer *et al.*, 1964
Proteins	[14]C	0.4 mCi/mg	Erb and Maurer, 1960
Gibberelline	[14]C	1 mCi/m$_M$	Parisi *et al.*, 1964
Lysozyme	[3]H	23 mCi/m$_M$	Schnek *et al.*, 1964
Ovomucoid	[3]H	15.7 mCi/m$_M$	Schnek *et al.*, 1964
Ovalbumin	[3]H	42.3 mCi/m$_M$	Schnek *et al.*, 1964
Conalbumin	[3]H	86 mCi/m$_M$	Schnek *et al.*, 1964
Lactic acid	[3]H	0.64 mCi/m$_M$	Wenzel and Günther, 1964
DNA[b]	[3]H	1.5 mCi/g	Paoletti and Lamonthezie, 1964
Galactose	[14]C	8 mCi/m$_M$	Aubert and Milhaud, 1964
Glycerol	[14]C	4 mCi/m$_M$	Aubert and Milhaud 1964

[a] Adenosine triphosphosphoric acid.
[b] Deoxyribonucleic acid.

TABLE 4. LOCALIZATION OF RADIOACTIVITY IN ACTINOMYCIN BY PRECURSORS
(CIFFERI *et al.*, 1965)

Precursor	Radioactivity refound on
Tryptophan-(benzene-^{14}C)	Chromophoric group
Protein hydrolysate	Whole of the molecule
Valine-proline-[14]C	Polypeptide chain
Methionine-(methyl-^{14}C)	Methyl group of chromophore

organs or organites separated from animals, plants, algae, microorganisms, yeasts, fungi, and enzymatic systems.

(*a*) *Entire animals.* In spite of the low efficiency, particular labeled molecules have been prepared by the administration of a precursor to entire animals followed by extraction of the blood or an organ. Labeled plasma proteins are obtained in this way from animals fed with yeast containing sulfur amino acids [35]S (Waldschandt, 1958).

Table 5 shows some examples of tracers produced on the same principle.

TABLE 5. EXAMPLES OF TRACERS EXTRACTED FROM THE BLOOD OR ORGANS OF AN ANIMAL AFTER A RADIOACTIVE PRECURSOR IS INTRODUCED

Labeled molecule	Precursor	Animal	Organ	Reference
Antibody γ-globulins	Valine-^{3}H	Rabbit	Plasma	Crawhall *et al.*, 1958
Thyroglobulin	Na ^{131}I	Rat	Thyroid	Brown and Jackson, 1956
Vasopressine	Cystine-^{35}S	Dog	Hypophysis	Sachs, 1959
Heparin	Na$_2$^{35}SO$_4$	Dog	Liver	Eiber and Danishefsky, 1957, 1959
Cytochrome c	^{55}Fe Cl$_2$	Rat	Muscle	Beinert, 1948, 1950
Heparin	Glucose-^{14}C	Dog	Liver	Danishefsky and Eiber, 1957
Serumalbumin	Leucine-^{3}H	Rat	Plasma	Done and Payne, 1956
Plasma proteins	Lysine ^{14}C Cystine ^{35}S	Dog	Plasma	Goldsworthy and Vol-wiler, 1958

(*b*) *Animal organs or organelles.* Instead of the entire animal it is preferable, whenever possible, to leave the precursor in incubation with sections or homogenates of organs conserved in a correctly selected medium (Table 6). Thus, for instance, for the biological preparation of steroids (Ayres, 1962) 200 mg progesterone (16-^{3}H) with 8.5 Ci of tritium, were set to incubate with 4 kg of bovine suprarenal cortex with the fascicular layer as far as possible removed. Incubation was in a bicarbonated Krebs–Ringer solution equilibrated with oxygen 95% and carbon dioxide 5%. The tissue was agitated for 30 min in this solution, which was then replaced by a fresh saline solution containing progesterone. After contact for a 2 hr period, and purification 3.9 mg of hydrocortisone (cortisol), 14.3 mg of corticosterone, and 2.7 mg of aldosterone were obtained with specific activities 5.2, 10.9, and 5.8 mCi/mg respectively.

(*c*) *Enzymes.* After whole animals, isolated organs, and intracellular organelles, it was to be foreseen that research would turn to purified enzymatic systems in order to prepare particular labeled molecules. The high specificity of these techniques holds such interest that their complexity may be unrealized. For example, it should be mentioned that l-amino acids

TABLE 6. MOLECULES LABELED BY BIOSYNTHESIS *in vitro* USING ISOLATED ORGANS

Labeled molecule	Precursor	Organ	Reference
Lipoids and sterols	Acetate and mevalonate-^{14}C	Liver	Fumagalli and Paoletti, 1964
Insulin	Leucine-^{14}C	Pancreas	Light and Simpson 1956
	Valine-^{14}C	Pancreas	Bauer, 1964
	Leucine-^{3}H	Pancreas	
17-β-ostradiol	Aminoacids^{14}-C	Testicle	Rabinowitz, 1959
Insulin	Glycine-^{14}C	Pancreas	Vaughan and Anfinsen, 1954
Ribonuclease	Phenyl alanine -^{14}C	Pancreas	Vaughan and Anfinsen, 1954
ACTH	Phenyl alanine -^{14}C	Antehypophysis	Wool *et al.*, 1961
Cytochrome C	Valine-^{14}C	Cardiac mitochondria	Bates and Simpson 1959
Insulin	Methionine-^{35}S	Pancreas	Petting and Rice 1952

are prepared from racemics using d-aminoxydase; thymidine (Sekiguchi and Yoshikawa, 1959), is produced by a hepatic enzyme, and triphosphate ribonucleosides are obtained from phosphate and nucleosides present in the hemolysates of human erythrocytes (Vanderheiden and Boszormenyi-Nagy, 1965).

We will consider in more detail the preparation of l-lactic acid by enzymatic conversion in the presence of tritiated water (Wenzel and Günther, 1964). The principle consists in reducing the pyruvate by an appropriate tritiated co-enzyme—NADT (nicotinamide–adenine–dinucleotide), itself formed after incubation in water of fumarate, of fumarate hydratase, of NAD^+ (oxidized) and of malate dehydrogenase. At the end of the reaction, fumaric, malic, and lactic acids are isolated with specific activities of 0.37, 0.93, and 0.64 mCi/mM respectively.

(*d*) *Entire plants and isolated leaves.* Not only animals but also plants are supplying substrates for biosynthesis. Interest in the alkaloids and other vegetal compounds, and the difficulty, if not the impossibility, of synthesizing them, has led botanists and pharmacologists to cultivate particular plants in liquid or gaseous media containing radioactive precursors (Ilyin, 1958; Scully *et al.*, 1956; Lette, 1959).

Although the idea is attractive in principle, biosynthesis by "isotope farming" (Catch, 1964) is not still practiced on a large scale owing to the high cost of the installations. However, many semiquantitative tests have been performed by individual research workers (Table 7).

(*e*) *Microorganisms, algae, and fungi.* The low cost of the culture of microorganisms, algae and fungi accounts for the many publications concerning biosynthesis by means of such substrates. In a review published in 1950, Woodruff and Fowler already referred to the use of *Pseudomonas saccharophila, Aerobacter aerogenes, Clostridium lactoacetophilum, C. acidi urici, Lactobacillus arabinosus, Escherichia coli, Rhizopus nigricans,* and *Torula utilis.*

TABLE 7. MOLECULES LABELED BY BIOSYNTHESIS USING PLANTS (EXAMPLES)

Labeled molecule	Species	Precursor	Reference
Nicotine	*Nicotiana rustica*	$^{14}CO_2$	Tso, 1965
Holaphyllin	*Holarrhena floribunda*	Cholesterol-^{14}C	Bennett and Heftmann, 1965
Glucobrassicin	*Brassica oleracea*	$^{35}SO_2$	Kutacek, 1966
Alkaloids	Ergot of rye	$^{14}CO_2$	Weygand *et al.*, 1964
Thebain, codeine and morphine	*Papaveraceae*	$^{14}CO_2$	Battersby *et al.*, 1964
Lecithin, cephalin	Soya	^{32}P-phosphate	Hölzl *et al.*, 1964
Atropine	*Solanaceae*	$^{14}CO_2$	Evertsbuch and Geiling, 1953
Digitoxin	*Scrofulariaceae*	$^{14}CO_2$	Geiling *et al.*, 1948
Morphine	*Papaveraceae*	$^{14}CO_2$	Achor and Geiling, 1954

Malt yeast (*Saccharomyces cerevisiae* and *T. utilis*) is used very frequently for the preparation of labeled molecules (Table 8).

Several marine algae are also of interest in biosynthesis, e.g. *Chlorella pyrenoidosa* (Erb, 1959; Liebster *et al.*, 1961), and *Rhodimenia palmata* (Aubert and Milhaud, 1964). In this latter case, photosynthesis in the presence of $^{14}CO_2$ terminates in an α-glycerol galactoside which, subjected to enzymatic hydrolysis, yields galactose and glycerol of suitable specific activity. The efficiency of the operation is satisfactory, since about 9 mCi of galactose and 4.5 mCi of glycerol are obtained from 10 g of algae and 28 mCi of $Ba^{14}CO_3$.

It has been possible to prepare sulfolipids by using *Euglena gracilis* (Davies *et al.*, 1966).

Fungi also rank highly in the context of biosynthesis for the production of antibiotics (Cooper and Rowley, 1959), vitamines, and various other products (Table 9).

In concluding this quick survey of the scope for biosynthetic methods, it should be mentioned that, in the general case, biosynthesis by labeled precursors is very often considered, not as an end in itself, but for elucidat-

TABLE 8. SOME LABELED COMPOUNDS PREPARED WITH MALT YEAST

Labeled compound	Precursor	Reference
Selenomethionine and selenocystine	Selenite-^{75}Se	Blau, 1961
RNA[a]	$^{14}CO_2$ and $^{32}PO_4H_3$	Ebel, 1964
Methionine, taurine	$^{35}SO_3H^-$	Schram *et al.*, 1964
Ribonucleotides	$^{14}CO_2$	Laufer *et al.*, 1964
Amino acids	$^{14}CO_2$	Laufer *et al.*, 1964 Strassman, 1960
Glucose, mannose	$^{14}CO_2$	Laufer *et al.*, 1964
Thiamine	$^{14}CO_2$	Johnson *et al.*, 1966

[a] Ribonucleic acid.

TABLE 9. BIOSYNTHESIS FROM FUNGI

Labeled molecule	Species	Precursor	Reference
Vitamin B12	*Streptomyces* sp.	^{60}Co	Chaiet *et al.*, 1950
β-carotene	*Phycomyces, Blakesleeanus*	^{14}C-acetate	Huang and De Witt 1965; Lilly *et al.*, 1958
Gibberelline	*Fusarium moniliforme*	^{14}C-glucose	Parisi *et al.*, 1964; Zeig *et al.*, 1958, McComb, 1964
Terramycin	*Streptomyces rimosus*	^{14}C-acetate	Snell *et al.*, 1956
Penicillin	*Penicillium* sp.	$^{35}SO_4^{2-}$	Howell and Thayer, 1948
Actinomycin	*Streptomyces antibioticus*	$^{14}CO_3^{2-}$	Cifferi *et al.*, 1964
Penicillin	*Penicillium chrysogenum*	$^{35}SO_4^{2-}$	Ullberg, 1954
Penicillin	*Penicillium* sp.	$^{14}CO_3^{2-}$	Martin *et al.*, 1953
Streptomycin	*Streptomyces* sp.	$^{14}CO_3^{2-}$	Numerof *et al.*, 1954
Chlortetracycline	*Streptomyces* sp.	$^{14}CO_3^{2-}$	Mendenwald, and Haberland 1957
Paromomycine	*Streptomyces* sp.	^3H (water)	Ober, 1962

ing particular metabolic pathways. But biological tracer production is a valid technique whenever an efficacious precursor is available. The use of entire animals and plants will long remain uneconomic, in contrast to the controlled use of organs, enzymes, and isolated microorganisms.

2.2. ISOTOPIC EXCHANGE

In suitable experimental conditions an appropriate radioactive isotope can be exchanged for one or several atoms of an organic molecule; less frequently the exchange is made between groups of atoms.

In the theoretical study of exchange reactions, it is assumed that the isotopes are chemically identical. One may therefore wonder about the thermodynamic justification of exchange reactions, considering that the enthalpy of the process is zero. However, it should be borne in mind that the entropy of the system of exchange at equilibrium, when the radioactive isotope is uniformly distributed between the reagents, is greater than at the beginning when the isotope is distributed in a nonuniform manner. Hence, as soon as the exchange starts, the entropy S of the system increases and the free energy F decreases according to the relation

$$F = - T \Delta S.$$

From the kinetic standpoint, exchange reactions are a very special case since the concentrations of the various reagents remain constant. The rate of the reaction, as measured using the variation of the specific radioactivity of one of the chemical species which are reacting, is governed by a first-order law, independently of the molecularity of the reaction. Thus for an exchange-reaction schematically represented as follows,

$$A X + B X° \underset{k_2}{\overset{k_1}{\rightleftarrows}} A X° + B X,$$

where X° is the radioactive isotope, at equilibrium the radioactive isotope will be statistically distributed between AX and BX ($k_1 = k_2$).

The foregoing considerations apply only if one neglects the isotopic effect (see Section 3 below), which is a very important factor whenever the exchange is made between isotopes of the light elements (e.g. hydrogen exchange with deuterium or tritium). Thus, for instance, the following exchange reaction (Myers and Prestwood, 1951),

$$HT + H_2O \underset{k_2}{\overset{k_1}{\rightleftarrows}} H_2 + HTO$$

has an actual equilibrium constant k_1 which is very different to its equilibrium constant k_2 when the isotopic effect is neglected ($k_1/k_2 = 6.194$). On the other hand, the isotopic effect is negligible for the exchange reaction

$$^{127}I + {}^{129}I + {}^{127}IO_3^{\ominus} \overset{k_1}{\underset{k_2}{\rightleftharpoons}} {}^{127}I_2 + {}^{129}IO_3^{\ominus},$$

for which the ratio k_1/k_2 is 1.002.

The exchange reactions can be regulated by several mechanisms. Often the rate-determining step is the reversible dissociation of the molecule subjected to the exchange

$$AX \rightleftharpoons A^{\oplus} + X^{\ominus}; A^{\oplus} + {}^{\circ}X^{\ominus} \rightleftharpoons A^{\circ}X$$

where $^{\circ}X$ is the radioactive isotope of X. The rate of the exchange reaction is correspondingly greater for a lower A–X binding energy. For example, the exchange between the aromatic halides and radioactive halogen in ionic form is favored if a group —NO_2 is bound to the aromatic nucleus in an ortho or para position in relation to the halogen atom. Clearly, any factor capable of favoring dissociation, for example a polar solvent, increases the rate of exchange.

Several exchange reactions are processes of homolytic substitution of the following type:

$$AX \rightleftharpoons A^{\circ} + X^{\circ}; A^{\circ} + {}^{\circ}X_2 \rightarrow A^{\circ}X + {}^{\circ}X; \ldots,$$

e.g. for several exchange reactions with tritium, deuterium, and iodine in its molecular state. Homolytic breaking of the A–X bond can be favored by an external source of energy (e.g. ultraviolet radiations).

In practice it is rare to meet with a simple exchange reaction, the mechanism of which is known. It has to be emphasized that the exchange is often verified on several sites in the same molecule. If the sites are not equivalent, the labeling proceeds by parallel exchange reactions, the rates of which are different; and in certain cases the mechanisms are different too.

The exchange labeling of a given molecular species cannot be envisaged unless the introduced radioactive atom is not susceptible to further change in the course of later experiences. For instance, it would be pointless to label the hydrogen of alcohol hydroxyl or of the amino group by exchange, for the ^3H hydrogen atoms are unstable in an aqueous solution in most test conditions.

In general, the atoms which form heteropolar (ion) bonds can be displaced without difficulty by exchange, while the atoms bound by stable homopolar (covalent) bonds only with difficulty present sufficient reactivity for the exchange. For instance, organic thio compounds exchange their sulfur atoms with very great difficulty; the same applies to the phosphoric esters as far as the phosphorus atom is concerned.

Also in practice the exchange reaction occurs in conditions different to those under which the labeled product is used. Thus, for instance, the purine ring will exchange its hydrogens with tritium only if a platinum catalyst is present; otherwise the exchange is irreversible, which enables the labeled product to be used with success as a tracer in pharmacology.

Under certain test conditions the errors due to exchange may be neglected. However, the need to effectuate exchange reactions in conditions different to those of utilization undoubtedly limits the use of this method of labeling as far as the preparation of tracers of biological origin is concerned.

We will now consider the main applications of the exchange method of labeling, the principles of which have been described in the papers by Myers and Prestwood (1951) and Murray and Williams (1958).

The two isotopes which have particularly held the attention of research workers are tritium and radioiodine. Sulfur exchange is only noted in passing (Moravek and Nejedly, 1960).

2.2.1. *Introduction of tritium*

Labeling by exchange of the hydrogen present in the molecule to be labeled with tritium has given rise to very many papers and reviews, among which reference should be made to Wilzbach (1957, 1962), Verly (1960), and Wenzel and Schultze (1962).

Several hundred thermolabile and nonsynthetizable products have been prepared in this way; particularly favorable results have been obtained with the steroids and other aromatic derivatives. The specific activity can be very high, even permitting the study of the hexestrol distribution after administration of oestrogen in physiological doses; hitherto this has not been practicable with carbon-14 (Glascock, 1962).

The main inconvenience of the tritium exchange technique is the need for a high degree of purification of the product of the exchange reaction. Numerous side reactions can occur, e.g. fragmentation, addition of fragments, polymerization, addition of tritium on nonsaturated bonds, isomerization, and racemization. The tritiated impurities thus produced can on occasion have a very high specific activity, and they can be eliminated only after lengthy operations.

Unlike chemical synthesis, the exchange method does not place the tritium in a single and predictable position. But preferential labeling of the aromatic compounds has often been reported (Ache *et al.*, 1962).

The exchange of hydrogen $_1^1H$ by tritium $_1^3H$ can be accomplished with or without a catalyst and in the absence or presence of an external source of energy.

(*a*) *Catalysis.* The compound to be labeled is dissolved in tritiated water or tritiated acetic acid, in the presence of platinum or palladium as catalyst. This method, which is very much akin to classical organic synthesis, has enabled steroids, purines, pyrimidines, and hydrocarbons to be labeled (Garnett *et al.*, 1962).

As an example of catalytic exchange, we will describe the preparation of tritiated thymidine (Verly, 1960). The thymidine is dissolved in tritiated water to which freshly reduced Adams' catalyzer is added; after heating in sealed tube, the water and catalyzer are removed. To remove labile atoms of tritium from the thymidine, the residue is heated in soda; after neutralization with sulfuric acid, the solution is evaporated to dryness. The residue is then extracted with boiling butanol (in which sodium sulfate is insoluble), and treated with charcoal. The labeled thymidine, which is partially hydrolyzed during the exchange, is purified by chromatography and crystallization.

(*b*) *Tritiated hydrogen.* The method of exchange with tritiated hydrogen (Wilzbach, 1957) permits labeling of many hydrogenated substances which cannot be prepared by chemical synthesis.

The exchange of a C–H bond for a C–T bond takes place by absorption of the energy of disintegration of the tritium nucleus, the tritium here occupying a site which has become vacant after the break of the bond between the hydrogen atom and the rest of the molecule.

Tritium is generally used directly in the gaseous form (Table 10), but it can also be generated from uranium tritide (Felter and Currie, 1962; Wenzel and Schultze, 1962).

Since the mean range of the β^- particle of the tritium is on average about 0.7 mg/cm², the complete absorption of the energy is within a layer of 7 μ in a medium of unit density. Under these conditions labeling by exchange is confined to the surface of the organic compound. This fundamental observation has led some authors to carry out the exchange on organic substrates absorbed on a thin layer of charcoal (Wenzel *et al.*, 1962b; Karlson *et al.*, 1963; Maurer *et al.*, 1964).

Many efforts have been made to improve the labeling yield, in particular by the use of an external source of energy (Lemmon *et al.*, 1959; Ghanem and Westermark, 1960; Cacace *et al.*, 1961), such as ionizing radiations

TABLE 10. SOME EXPERIMENTAL CONDITIONS IN EXCHANGE BY TRITIUM GAS

Compound	Weight (mg)	Quantity of tritium (curies)	Pressure (atm)	Duration of contact	Specific activity	Reference
Digitoxigenin	25	2	0.2	$7\frac{1}{2}$ hr	0.07 mCi/g	Maurer et al., 1964
Tetanic toxin	—	5	0.38	$2\frac{1}{2}$ days	—	Speirs, 1962
Norcocaine	100	2	—	15 days	2.5 mCi/mM	Schmidt and Werner, 1962
Atropin	100	2	—	15 days	16.5 mCi/mM	Schmidt and Werner, 1962
Lysozyme	110	2.5	0.17–0.29	92 hr	27–60 mCi/mM	Leonis, 1964
Ribonuclease	180	6	0.37	92 hr	110–190 mCi/mM	Leonis, 1964

(^{60}Co), ultraviolet radiations, high-frequency microwaves, electric discharge, and photosensitization by mercury.

In certain cases these techniques succeed in considerably increasing the incorporation of tritium, but often the destruction of the hydrogenated compound progresses more rapidly than the gain in exchange yield. The lower consumption of tritium and the time gained for incubation do not constitute a sufficient advantage compared with the complications in purification.

Nevertheless, the list of molecules tritiated by exchange is continually growing, and we cannot consider compiling a complete list here. We shall confine ourselves to mentioning some examples: sugars (Simon *et al.*, 1964); proteins (Vaughan *et al.*, 1957); antibodies (Cardinaud *et al.*, 1964; Jeejeeboy *et al.*, 1964); alkaloids—morphine (Misra and Woods, 1960), atropin and norcocaine (Schmidt and Werner, 1962), and digitoxigenin (Maurer *et al.*, 1964, Malamos, 1965); hormones—vasopressin (Fong *et al.*, 1960), growth hormone (Collipp *et al.*, 1966), insulin (von Holt *et al.*, 1960); enzymes—ribonuclease (Steinberg *et al.*, 1957); steroids (Wilzbach, 1957; Karlson *et al.*, 1963); and antibiotics—penicillins G and V, tetracyclins, streptomycin, chloramphenicol (Giovannozzi-Sermanni and Possagno, 1960), and pristinamycin (Benazet and Bourat, 1965).

(*c*) *Irradiation with recoil tritons.* This method has found few pharmacological applications, and it will only be described for its theoretical value (Rowland and Wolfgang, 1956; Rowland and Numerof, 1957). It consists in irradiating with slow neutrons a target containing a mixture of lithium salt and of the hydrogenated compound which is to be labeled. The tritons that are formed in the reaction

$$^6_3\text{Li} + {}^1_0\text{n} \rightarrow {}^3_1\text{H} + {}^4_2\text{He}$$

bombard the substance where they can replace the protons.

The purification problems are of the same order as those arising when gaseous tritium is used.

(*d*) *Other forms of exchange.* The C–H bond is not the only one affected by the absorption of the disintegration energy of tritium. In particular, the C–I bonds are very sensitive to radiation. This has enabled various organic derivatives to be prepared (Fong and Greenlee, 1962; Roche *et al.*, 1964b), e.g. thyronines.

2.2.2. *Introduction of radioactive iodine* (^{131}I)

This method has especially been used for labeling the iodine derivatives of thyronine (thyroxine and tri-iodothyronine) and of tyrosine (mono- and di-iodotyrosine).

Radioactive iodine can be used in the iodide state, but in most cases the active agent of the exchange is elementary iodine. In the case of di-iodo-tyrosine, for instance, it has been found that the exchange is blocked in the presence of substances capable of reducing the elementary iodine (Miller *et al.*, 1944); the same observation was made by Gleason (1955) for thyroxine.

As an example we will describe the labeling of tri-iodo-thyronine with radioiodine (Gleason, 1955). The tri-iodo-thyronine is dissolved in tertiary butyl alcohol. A solution of labeled elementary iodine is prepared separately in the same solvent. The two solutions are then quickly mixed, and the pH is brought to 7–8 with a phosphate buffer. After approximately 10 sec the exchange is rapidly blocked with sulfite.

In these conditions the exchange yield is of about 35–40 %; the tri-iodo-thyronine is always accompanied with a small quantity of thyroxine formed by addition of the iodine to the tri-iodo-thyronine. The duration of the reaction is about 10 sec in order to minimize the importance of this side effect.

If the molecule undergoing the exchange contains several iodine atoms, the rate of the exchange reaction can be different according to the position of the iodine atom in the molecular structure. This leads to heterogeneous labeling which in turn may cause a false interpretation of the results when the labeled product is used as tracer. This seems to be the case for tri-iodo-thyronine and thyroxine labeled by exchange.

Gleason (1955) observed that in the conditions described above, the (3,5)-di-iodo-thyronine does not exchange its iodine atoms; since, however, the thyroxine and the tri-iodo-thyronine undergo the exchange, it is inferred that only the iodine atoms in the ortho position relative to the hydroxyl group of the thyronine are capable of reacting.

2.3. ADDITION OF FOREIGN ATOMS

For products of complex structure, a widely used method of labeling is to add to the original product one or several radioactive atoms, or a radical containing a radioactive atom.

Labeling by addition of foreign atoms has the serious disadvantage that the chemical composition of the original product is modified by the method. The general consequence is that this method of labeling is used only for substances of very high molecular weight where the addition of foreign atoms may cause no modification in the biological behavior.

Proteins, plasma proteins, antibodies, protein hormones, enzymes, gluco-proteins, etc., are among the substances of biological origin that are most often subjected to labeling by addition. Only very rarely has labeling by addition been used to produce nonprotein biological tracers (Tubis, 1965).

The chemical reaction most often adopted is iodination. Iodine shows considerable reactivity in regard to the tyrosine residues contained in the proteins. Furthermore, the two radioactive isotopes currently being used (^{125}I and ^{131}I; see Table 1) have very favorable nuclear characteristics.

Radioactive chromium (^{51}Cr) has also been used for labeling proteins.

As we have already pointed out, the use of this method of labeling is based on the hypothesis that a protein will not be substantially modified if a small number of iodine or chromium atoms is bound to the molecule in question. This hypothesis has therefore to be carefully verified in every case.

In spite of these limitations, labeling by addition is widely used. The reason is that the chemical procedures are quite simple compared, for instance, with biosynthesis, and the efficiency of the method is quite high.

It should also be stressed that products labeled by addition simplify the study of metabolism, the radioactive atom not being recycled once it leaves the labeled molecule after metabolic degradation.

2.3.1. *Labeling protein substances with radioiodine*

The labeling of protein substances with radioiodine is based on the high reactivity of the tyrosine residues toward the elementary iodine. According to the iodine concentration and the number of tyrosine residues reacting in the protein, the end product will contain variable amounts of mono-iodinated and di-iodinated tyrosyl groups.

The kinetics of the reaction have been studied by Mayberry *et al.* (1965) on acetyl-tyrosine and mono-iodo-acetyl-tyrosine:

$$\text{(1)}$$

$$\text{(2)}$$

According to these authors, reaction (2) is the one which controls the process. This mechanism is in very good agreement with the experimental results and explains why the reaction rate depends on the concentration of the $OH^{\ominus}$ and of the $I^{\ominus}$. Mayberry and his co-workers also measured the rate constant for the iodination of the mono-iodo-acetyl-tyrosine; this reaction is 30 times slower than for acetyl-tyrosine when the measurement of the rate is based on the respective concentrations of the phenolate ions. It should be noted, however, that with neutral pH the tyrosine and mono-iodo-tyrosine appear in an undissociated form; under these conditions, the rates of iodination should be approximately the same, the values of pK here being 10.2 and 8.8 respectively (Hughes, 1966). So one should expect the partial iodination of the proteins to give rise to the formation of radicals either of mono-iodo-tyrosine or of di-iodo-tyrosine.

The iodination reaction of tyrosine is often accompanied by other reactions. Among these, the iodination of histidine and the oxidation of the cysteine residues should be mentioned (Hughes and Straessle, 1950; Rosa *et al.*, 1967,a). The oxidation of the —SH groups must be regarded as an inevitable effect of iodination, and this implies that whenever the intactness of the —SH play an essential role in the biological function of the protein, the labeling leads to inactivation.

In the case of albumin the iodine-induced oxidation of the —SH groups does not, however, seem to lead to any modification in metabolic behavior (Freeman, 1957; Rosa *et al.*, 1967a).

In general, the reaction of the iodine with the —SH groups produces different results according to the type of protein. For albumin (Hughes and Straessle, 1950), the —SH are probably oxidized to the highest valence states. In the case of the tobacco mosaic virus (TMV), the formation of the iodo-sulfenyl group has been demonstrated.

The side reactions can generally be limited (excepting, of course, the oxidation of —SH) by reducing to a very low level the concentration of the iodine which reacts with the protein. For example, the iodination of histidyl residues is normally avoided in the labeling of albumin, but it becomes appreciable if the degree of substitution reaches 8–10 atoms of iodine per molecule of protein. With insulin the iodination is selective on the tyrosyl residues up to a degree of substitution of the order 4–5 iodine atoms per molecule of hormone (MW 6000); further iodination also affects the histidyl residues (Wolff and Covelli, 1967).

The reactivity toward iodine of the various residues depends on their intramolecular localization; it may happen that tyrosyl groups which are "buried" in the molecular structure will react only with difficulty, thereby allowing parallel reactions to compete with the principal one.

TABLE 11. REACTIONS OF IODINE WITH THE PROTEINS (AFTER HUGHES, 1966)

(1) $HOI + RSH \longrightarrow RSI + H_2O$

(2) $RSH + RSI \longrightarrow RSSR + H^{\oplus} + I^{\ominus}$

(3)

(4)

(5)

The reactions observed in labeling proteins are given in Table 11, namely oxidation of —SH groups (1, 2), iodination of histidine (3), and iodination of tyrosine (4, 5). In particular cases, oxidation of the tryptophan residues can also take place.

Techniques of labeling. Radioiodine is supplied in the form of sodium or potassium iodide in aqueous solution.

Iodination is generally carried out at slightly alkaline pH so as to increase the rate of the reaction (see Section 2.3.1). A common method of labeling proteins is to add the radioiodine in iodide form to an aqueous solution of elementary iodine and potassium iodide. The exchange reactions convert the radioactive iodide into elementary iodine. The solution is then placed in contact with the protein dissolved in a borate buffer at pH 8–8.5. The use of this technique is limited owing to the fact that any reducing agent present in the radioactive iodine solution is capable of reducing a non-negligible quantity of elementary iodine, of which only a part can still be used for labeling. To neutralize this effect, the amount of carrier iodine must be quite large. We shall see that this addition is not always practicable. Special procedures have to be used in every case where the quantity of carrier must remain slight.

The most used method of labeling (McFarlane, 1956, 1958) consists in using as iodinating agent the iodine monochloride instead of the elementary iodine. ICl is labeled with the radioiodine by direct exchange. If the radio-iodine is in fact carrier-free, the exchange manifests itself by a rapid quantitative conversion of the radioactive iodine into labeled ICl, which in turn reacts with the protein. It should be noted that for the labeling reaction by elementary iodine the theoretical yield is only 50 % whereas for ICl the theoretical yield is 100 %. The efficiency of the elementary iodine is low since two iodine atoms must react to enable one iodine atom to be incorporated in the tyrosine (see Table 11); when using ICl, the reaction is as follows:

$$\text{ICl} + \text{R} - \langle \varphi \rangle \overset{\text{H}}{-} \text{OH} \rightarrow \text{R} - \langle \varphi \rangle \overset{\text{I}}{-} \text{OH} + \text{H}^{\oplus} + \text{Cl}^{\ominus}$$

By way of illustration we describe the labeling of albumin by the method of iodine monochloride.

Preparation of the labeled ICl. The standard solution of ICl (0.02 M in ICl, 2.0 M in NaCl, 0.02 M in KCl, and 0.1 M in HCl) is purified of traces of elementary iodine by extraction with carbon tetrachloride (1 ml of this solution corresponds to 2.55 mg of iodine). Then 0.015 ml of the standard ICl solution is added to 3 mCi of iodine ^{131}I contained in 2 ml of neutral solution.

Labeling of the albumin. 100 mg of human albumin is dissolved in 4 ml of glycine buffer (2 M, pH 9). The labeled ICl solution is then added quickly and without agitation to the albumin solution. Iodine in inorganic form is separated by elution on a column of Sephadex G-25 with a 0.1 M glycine buffer, pH 9. Some methods are based on the use of a large quantity of oxidizing agent with the aim of ensuring quantitative conversion of the radioactive iodine into elementary iodine. According to Pressman *et al.*

(1950), oxidation can take place with sodium nitrite in an acid medium. The iodine solution, brought to pH 8, is then mixed with the protein dissolved in a borate buffer. Providing a suitable quantity of sodium nitrite is used, the oxidation of the radioiodine into elementary iodine is practically quantitative even if a relatively large quantity of reducing agent is present originally.

In other methods the radioactive iodine is directly oxidized into elementary iodine in the presence of the protein to be labeled; in this way Gilmore *et al.* (1954) have labeled antibodies using an excess of ammonium persulfate as an oxidizing agent. This method gives a labeling yield close to 100%, the I^- ions which form from the iodination reaction of the tyrosine being re-oxidized into iodine by the excess of persulfate. The same principle has been applied in using chloramine-T as the oxidant according to a method developed by Greenwood and Glover (1963) for the preparation of labeled hormones with very high specific activity (0.5–0.8 Ci/mg).

Hypochlorous acid has also been used as the oxidizing agent for labeling albumin (Steinfeld *et al.*, 1958). In general, however, the use of an excess of the oxidizing agents in the presence of the protein must be avoided. The occurrence of damages to the protein is demonstrated for albumin when the labeling is carried out with chloramine-T (McFarlane, 1965).

In order to minimize damage to the protein, special methods of labeling have been proposed. In one instance, use is made of anodic oxidation of the iodide into elementary iodine in an electrolytic cell (Rosa *et al.*, 1964, 1965, 1967a). The elementary iodine is liberated at the anode and reacts with the protein which is present in aqueous solution at pH 7. The advantage of this method is that the rate at which the elementary iodine is formed can be controlled by the current of electrolysis (constant-current electrolysis). The efficiency of labeling is very high since the iodide ions formed in the tyrosine iodination reaction are recycled at the anode. For albumin, fibrinogen, and insulin (Rosa *et al.*, 1967b), it has been demonstrated that electrolysis introduces no further damage to the protein.

Nunez and Pommier (1965) have proposed an enzymatic method which has been applied to albumin (Protein + peroxydase + glucose-oxidase system + KI). Banerjee *et al.* (1963) have used a Conway diffusion unit for labeling insulin. The protein is introduced into the central part of the diffusion unit. The iodine forms in the external part of the unit and passes into the protein solution by diffusion.

Many products of biological origin, mostly proteins, have been labeled with radioiodine. Some of them are listed in Table 12.

Table 12. Some Products of Biological Origin Labeled with Iodine by Addition[a]

Nucleic acids	Ascoli and Kahan, 1966
Growth hormone	Sonenberg *et al.*, 1954; Hunter and Greenwood, 1962
Prolactin	Sonenberg, 1951b
Corticostimuline	Sonenberg *et al.*, 1951a; Galskov, 1966; Felber, 1965
Insulin	Pearson, 1959; Izzo *et al.*, 1964; d'Addabo *et al.*, 1960; Berson *et al.*, 1956
Glucagon	McCall *et al.*, 1962; Berson *et al.*, 1957b; 1958; Cox *et al.*, 1957
Trypsin	Bogner *et al.*, 1959; Miller, 1960
Cytochrome-*c*	Reichlin, 1966
Parathormone	Melick *et al.*, 1965
Casein	Lavik *et al.*, 1952; Afifi *et al.*, 1963
Vasopressin	Permutt *et al.*, 1966
Histones	Hupka *et al.*, 1958
Transferrin	Gitlin, 1965
Coeruloplasmin	Kekki *et al.*, 1966
Coccidioidine	Sawaki *et al.*, 1966
Snake venom	Gennaro and Ramsey, 1959
Antibodies	Pressman and Eisen, 1950
Chylomicrons	Hoffman, 1960
Ribonuclease	Inman and Nisonoff, 1966
Diphteric toxin	Masouredis, 1959
Tetracyclin	Dunn *et al.*, 1960

[a] The plasma proteins are omitted owing to the large number of publications dealing with them.

2.3.2. *Addition of chromium-51*

Chromium-51 can be used for the labeling of proteins. All proteins are capable of binding metal ions, but the strength and stability of the bond vary greatly with the type of ion and protein, and also with the charge of the protein. The transition elements generally have a very great affinity for the proteins and form the most stable combinations.

The theoretical study of chromation is much more intricate than is that of iodination. The experience gained with tanning, where cutaneous collagen is treated by chromium salts at nonphysiological pH and concentrations, cannot be extended without safeguards to the study of the chromium–protein bonds formed in less severe conditions.

The formation of coordination complexes is accepted by many authors (Gray and Sterling, 1950; Gustavson, 1958; Naismith, 1958; Rollinson, 1966). According to Gray, in particular, the linkage would imply polar attraction of the metal by the protein carboxyles, followed by the formation of bonds of the "chromihexamine" type with the basic residues: lysine, histidine, or arginine.

Besides the conceptions of tanning theory (McLaughlin and Theis, 1945; O'Flaherty, 1958), numerous useful indications for the use of chromium-51 have been obtained with the aid of nonradioactive chromium. Ways of avoiding the denaturation of the protein have been particularly studied.

Michael (1939) has shown that the anion complexes of chromium precipitate the proteins on the acidic side of the isoelectric point, and the cation complexes on the alkaline side. The precipitate is a salt formed between the complex ion and the protein of opposite charge. This author suggests that the reaction is not accompanied by denaturation since the precipitates re-dissolve when the pH is modified.

On the other hand, Thomas and Norris (1925) have drawn attention to the fact that even if the metals at low concentration do not induce protein denaturation, this has been observed to occur at higher concentration; in this case, the rate of the process depends on the concentration of metal, pH, and temperature.

More recently, studies *in vitro* have been made on bovine serum albumin (Baetjer *et al.*, 1955; Grogan and Oppenheimer, 1955; Clark, 1959) in contact with sodium chromate or chromium chloride at different pH. The results obtained by these authors all agree perfectly and revealed that:

(1) for sodium chromate at pH greater than 5.4, no precipitation or denaturation associated with partial reduction of chromium VI take place;

(2) for sodium chromate at pH less than 5.4, a white precipitate appears, containing one chromium molecule for every protein molecule; the protein molecule undergoes denaturation to an extent dependent upon temperature and duration of the reaction;

(3) for chromium chloride at pH greater than 5.4, a white precipitate is formed—a complex mixture of protein and chromium hydroxide; as a result of this co-precipitation, it is difficult to regard protein denaturation as conclusive, but the formation of chromium III–protein complexes is effective at the pH studied (Grogan and Oppenheimer, 1955);

(4) for chromium chloride at pH less than 5.4, no precipitate appears, but by other means denaturation of the protein molecule occurs which can include up to 18 chromium molecules.

In a practical sense these results are a guide to the choice of pH for the *in vitro* labeling of proteins; pH values below the isoelectric point should be avoided owing to the risk of altering the protein.

Since 1950, the year in which Gray and Sterling recommended the use of chromium-51 for labeling red corpuscles, this isotope has been increasingly used. Yet, as pointed out by Frank and Gray (1953), it is well to bear in mind that the capacity of the chromium to bind to the proteins depends on the chemical form of the tracer.

In its hexavalent form, as in sodium chromate, chromium-51 is used especially for labeling blood cells (red cells, leucocytes, and platelets). It can, however, be used for labeling molecules in solution such as hemoglobin (Gray and Sterling, 1950), dextran (Kubat, 1963), pepsin (Cohen *et al.*, 1966), casein (Ritz and Rubin, 1964), and endotoxin of *Escherichia coli* (Braude *et al.*, 1955a, b). It seems that the reducing power of the substrate in relation to chromium VI may be a determining cause of labeling (Ingrand, 1964).

Very often the molecules in solution are labeled by trivalent chromium, generally in the form of chromium chloride, and sometimes as chromium perchlorate (Schultze and Hughes, 1965).

Labeling with chromium-51 has the advantage of extreme simplicity; a good example is the preparation of serum albumin-^{51}Cr (Waldmann, 1961, 1965a). Radiochromium chloride of high specific activity is set to incubate at pH 4, in the presence of glucose, with an aqueous solution of 25 % serum albumin. After a period of 30 min the protein is purified by dialysis and passage over ion-exchange resin.

The disadvantages of this technique are of a theoretical and practical nature. In the first place, the position of the chromium in the labeled molecule is not known with certainty; moreover, the degree of substitution very quickly varies with the relative concentration of chromium, which implies that different sites are liable to fix the chromium. Thus, in blood serum, for a small amount of chromium (1–2 mcg per gram of protein) the β-globulins retain the major part of the element, but with 10–75 mcg of chromium per gram of protein the proportion of chromium fixed on the α-globulins increases notably (Cohen *et al.*, 1965). In addition, the aging of $CrCl_3$ solutions affects the labeling yield (Frank and Gray, 1953); Naismith, 1958).

Except in special cases (Waldmann, 1961; Mabry *et al.*, 1965), a plasma protein-^{131}I is to be preferred to a protein-^{51}Cr which has a significantly lower plasmatic half-life (Sterling, 1951; Waldmann, 1965a). However, several products of pharmacological interest have been labeled with trivalent ^{51}Cr: ribonuclease (Schultze and Hughes, 1965), siderophilin (Hopkins and Schnurz, 1964), endotoxin of *Escherichia coli* (Braude *et al.*, 1955a; Noyes *et al.*, 1959), and cytochrome-*c* (Ingrand, 1966).

2.3.3. *Addition of other isotopes*

Besides the addition of iodine-131 and chromium-51, reference should also be made to the addition of sulfur-35, tritium, carbon-14, technetium-99m, and bromine-82.

(*a*) *Sulfur*-35. Sulfur-35 can be bound to the protein by reaction with yperite molecules, sulfate molecules, or molecules of diazotized arylsulfonic acid.

The first type of reaction involves the amino groups, and it has seldom been employed (Boursnell *et al.*, 1946; Francis *et al.*, 1951, 1955).

The second type of reaction consists in the reaction between the ^{35}S-labeled sulfuric acid and the aliphatic hydroxyl groups of serine and threonine (Glendening *et al.*, 1947); it has served to label thyreostimulin (Sonenberg and Money, 1955) and insulin (Stadie, 1952).

The third type of reaction leads to an azo-protein by coupling of the diazonium sulfanilate with the nucleus of tyrosine or histidine (Garvey and Campbell 1954; Garvey *et al.*, 1960; Ingraham, 1951); it has been used with advantage in producing a radioactive thyreostimulin (Sonenberg *et al.*, 1952; Wegelius, 1960).

Reaction with sulfite has been also used to label deshydrogenases (Mohring *et al.*, 1960).

(*b*) *Tritium.* The addition of tritium occurs on double bonds with the advantage that the radioisotope is placed in a known position. It has been used for the preparation of steroids (Osinski, 1962), antibodies (Rosen *et al.*, 1964), tyrosine (Roche *et al.*, 1964a), fatty acids (Dutton *et al.*, 1958), and prostaglandins (Hansson and Samuelsson, 1965).

(*c*) *Others.* Carbon 14 has been bound to albumin by labeled tosyl-amino acids or oxalyl-amino acids (Margen and Tarver, 1963).

Technetium-99m, despite its short life, has been recommended for labeling serum albumin (McAfee *et al.*, 1964; Stern *et al.*, 1965).

2.3.4. *Problems in labeling by addition*

When working with tracers it is often essential for the labeled product to behave exactly like the original product. The most common causes of discrepancies are briefly discussed in Section 3 below, but labeling by addition introduces a special factor of its own, in that the labeled product is not chemically identical to the original product. In practice, each time a product labeled by addition is used it is necessary to check that the implanting of foreign atoms in the molecule of the original product has not at all altered the biological and chemical properties that will be involved in the experiment in hand (see, for instance, Johnson *et al.*, 1960; Freeman, 1959;

Izzo *et al.*, 1964b; Margen and Tarver, 1963; Steinfeld *et al.*, 1958). Here we shall confine ourselves to the problems arising in metabolic studies in connection with the iodination of proteins.

One method of controlling whether iodination of the protein leads to important changes (Hughes, 1957, Lee *et al.*, 1959) is to study the modifications of the biological properties as a function of the degree of substitution (i.e. the number of iodine atoms bound to the protein molecule). An example of this method is illustrated in Fig. 1, which shows the variation of

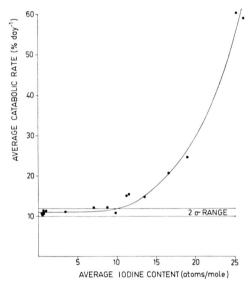

Fig. 1. Dependence of the fractional catabolic rate (average on 7 days' experiments) of human albumin on the extent of the iodination (from Cohen *et al.*, 1956).

the fractional catabolic rate (cf. subsection 3.2.2(b)) of human albumin as a function of the quantity of iodine bound to the protein. The rate remains approximately constant up to iodination of about 10 bound iodine atoms per albumin molecule. This result leads to the conclusion that iodination does not modify the amount of degradation of the albumin (except in the case of a massive substitution); hence iodinated albumin can be recommended as a correct tracer of endogenous albumin.

Another way of demonstrating that a protein labeled with radioiodine can validly be used as tracer is to compare the behavior of the protein *in vivo* with that of similar protein labeled by biosynthesis with ^{35}S or ^{14}C.

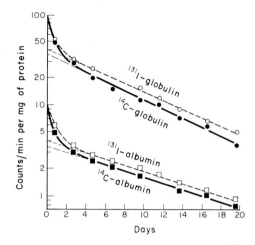

FIG. 2. Elimination of ^{131}I and ^{14}C labeled albumin and γ-globulin administered simultaneously by i.v. injection in the rabbit (from Cohen *et al.*, 1956).

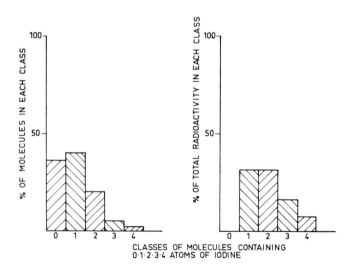

FIG. 3. Intramolecular distribution of iodine in human albumin containing on average 1 iodine atom per molecule, according to a binomial type distribution law (from Rosa *et al.*, 1966a).

Cohen *et al.* (1956) have thus proved that human albumin labeled with iodine is a good tracer of native albumin (Fig. 2).

When the inconveniences associated with labeling by addition are examined in detail, one must never neglect the possibility of a hetero-geneous distribution of the tracer among the molecules of the compound to be marked. The protein albumin, for instance, has 12 tyrosine radicals which are accessible to iodine; in all probability albumin labeled with iodine is composed of a population of molecules which contain different numbers of iodine atoms. According to the hypothesis that the distribution of the iodine among the tyrosine radicals is defined by a binomial type probability law (Oncley, 1957), an iodized albumin containing on average one iodine atom per molecule will have the composition represented schematically in Fig. 3.

Assuming, for instance, that all albumin molecules with two or more iodine atoms are altered biologically, 20–30% of the tracer molecules will behave differently from the original ones. If the distribution of the radio-activity is considered (Fig. 3), the situation is still more serious; since the heavily iodized molecules are the most radioactive, 50–60% of the total radioactivity is associated with the changed molecules. This example is not an actual case because albumin, as we have seen, can bear a high degree of substitution without its metabolic properties being altered; but the example does show that the heterogeneity of labeling could be an important source of error. In general, an attempt is made to minimize this heterogeneity by deliberately introducing the least possible iodine into the protein, which reduces to the minimum the probability of heavily iodized molecules being formed. All the same, this leads to certain practical difficulties in carrying out the labeling. Clearly the degree of iodination depends on the quantity of iodine used at the start. If this quantity is small, it will be the same for the degree of iodination of the protein, but the efficiency of labeling will be reduced (see the foregoing section). If methods of labeling which use an excess of oxidant are adopted, there is a risk of denaturation of the protein owing to the excessively destructive conditions of labeling. A reasonable compromise must always be found between the amount of iodination and the protection of the protein.

The fact of reduction of the amount of iodination can lead to mis-interpretation of the results of biological control tests. If, for instance, an iodized insulin preparation containing on average 0.1 iodine atom per molecule conserves all its biological activity (as measured by the isolated rat diaphragm method for example), this is by no means sufficient to prove that the iodination has not modified the hormone (Fig. 4). In fact, even if a homogeneous distribution of the iodine is assumed, no more than 10% of the insulin molecules will actually include an iodine atom. But since the accuracy of the biological test is less than 10%, all the iodized insulin molecules could be completely inactivated without this degradation being indicated by the test.

The example of insulin can further serve to show that the possibility of whether or not a particular product of biological origin labeled by addition can be used depends on the type of response desired. Thus Izzo *et al.*(1964b)

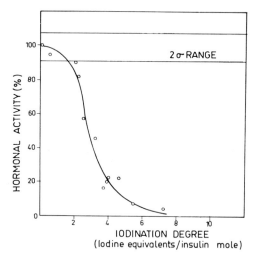

Fig. 4. Effect of incorporation of increasing number of iodine atoms into insulin on its biological activity, as measured by CO_2 production on rat epididymal fat pad. The $2 \times$ S.D. (standard deviation range) evaluated on 20 assays of native insulin is taken as the criterion to establish the significance of the biological activity decrease (from Rosa *et al.*, 1967b).

and Rosa *et al.* (1966b, 1967b) have demonstrated that the introduction of one extra iodine atom in the hormone molecule probably leads to a loss of biological activity (see Fig. 4). In these conditions, insulin iodized to an average degree of one iodine atom per molecule (MW 6000) is not a good tracer of endogenous insulin for studies on metabolism, since there are certainly iodized molecules with two or more iodine atoms. On the other hand, the immunological properties of the insulin are not modified even if larger quantities of iodine are introduced. Insulin iodized with an average substitution of one iodine atom per molecule is fully satisfactory for immunological dosages. This is a factor of considerable importance as regards the technique of labeling, since radioimmunological doses demand a very high specific activity of the labeled hormone (from 100 mCi/mg to 500 mCi/mg according to the method applied). Labeling is therefore accomplished with very small quantities of protein; if the degree of iodination had to be reduced still further the labeling would be almost impossible to carry out. The point is clearer if one considers that even in using carrier-free radioactive iodine for the iodination of growth hormone by the chloramine-T method (see previous section), the final degree of iodination is found to be 0.5–1 iodine atom per molecule of hormone.

These examples illustrate how a critical analysis of the experimental conditions will guide the research worker in the choice of the method of labeling. To conclude our commentary on the limits of labeling by addition, it is useful to recall that introducing of foreign atoms into a protein molecule will always lead to a modification of the biological properties. Iodine, for example, has approximately the same dimensions as the aromatic nucleus of tyrosine; it would be imprudent not to provide for certain "modifications of conformation" of the protein when several tyrosine radicals have been subjected to iodination. However, experience shows that in several cases there is a limiting degree of substitution where the alteration of the protein molecule can be considered negligible.

3. VALIDATION OF TRACERS AND PRECAUTIONS IN USE

The utilization of a labeled compound as a tracer is possible whenever it possesses the properties of the original unlabeled compound. As we have already seen, such a requirement is theoretically satisfied by all the methods of labeling, except in labeling by addition which by definition leads to a modification of the chemical composition of the original product. Some aspects of this problem have already been discussed.

In practice it can happen that the labeled product is a mixture of original (radioactive) product and of radioactive impurities. These impurities can be an important source of error.

The poor radiochemical purity of a labeled compound can have two principal causes: either the original product is not pure enough and labeled products different to the original product are formed from the impurities; or else labeled impurities are formed by the decomposition of the labeled product, even though this labeled product was pure originally. The decomposition can be verified during labeling by the effect of secondary chemical reactions or during storage by the autoirradiation of the labeled product (radiolysis). We will now briefly examine the different causes of alteration of the labeled product.

3.1. CAUSES OF ALTERATION

3.1.1. *Impurity of original compounds*

The presence of radioactive impurities in compounds of biological origin must very often be attributed to insufficient purity of the original compound. This is one of the greatest obstacles to the labeling of this class of products since in the majority of cases selective labeling of the principal compound is impossible. Furthermore, the impurities can often have a greater reactivity towards the radioactive isotope than that displayed by the original product. This has the effect of increasing the influence of the impurities on the results obtained with the tracer. The traces of globulins which very often accompany albumin are a typical example. When the albumin is iodized, the globulins react with the iodine more rapidly than does the albumin itself. This type of problem is common with protein substances. In certain cases the fact that the impurities are labeled facilitates the detection and extraction of these impurities. Thus traces of glucagon can be identified in insulin after labeling with radioiodine; the traces of globulins which often accompany albumin can be identified by radio-electrophoresis, even if the traces are insufficient in quantity to be detected by the normal methods of staining.

3.1.2. *Effect of autoradiolysis*

Labeled products are always subject to the destructive action of the radiations from the radioactive atoms that form part of the molecular structure of the products in question. The gamma-ray photons and beta particles lose a large part of their energy by interaction with the orbital electrons of the atoms of the matter which they traverse. This gives rise to the formation of secondary electrons with a broad energy spectrum which, in turn, react with other atoms. In radiation chemistry it is conventional to express the rate of decomposition by values of G which indicates the number of molecules (atoms or ions) destroyed for 100 eV (electron-volts) absorbed by the system.

The changes of a labeled product due to autoradiolysis arise either from a direct reaction with the radiation (primary effect) or from a reaction with the products that are formed from solvent molecules (secondary effect).

The secondary effect is due to the reaction of the molecules of the labeled substance with the reactive fragments formed as a result of the primary effect on the solvent molecules. The changes that are detected in a compound during storage are almost exclusively due to the secondary effect. In an aqueous solution, for instance, most of the dissipated energy is absorbed by the water molecules, giving rise to the formation of reactive radicals which react with the molecules of the labeled compound.

Several measures should be taken to reduce the damage caused by the secondary effect:

(a) Since the stability of a labeled product in solution is approximately proportional to the radioactive concentration (radioactivity per unit of volume)—at least in the case of low-energy beta emitters such as ^{35}S, ^{14}C, and ^{3}H—dilution of this solution is often the best way of protecting the labeled compound.

(b) The type of solvent plays an important part; some aromatic compounds such as benzene can dissipate the absorbed energy without reactive radicals being produced. Unfortunately, such compounds can rarely be used for products of biological origin which tolerate no other solvent than water.

(c) Since the secondary effects are purely chemical in nature, they depend on the temperature; conservation at a low temperature, if this is compatible with the nature of the labeled compound, has the effect of minimizing the variations caused by autoradiolysis.

(d) One very efficacious protective measure is to store the product in the solid state, preferably in thin-layer form (see Primary effect). In this case it is of the greatest importance that the sample is fully dehydrated because small pockets of solvent in the solid matter hasten the decomposition.

Decomposition and methods of protection have been the subject of many studies, among which reference should be made to the works of Tolbert *et al.* (1964), Evans and Stanford (1963), McCall and Camp (1961), Osinski and Deconinck (1964), Bayly and Evans (1966), and Bloom *et al.* (1958).

Proteins undergo appreciable degradation when the absorbed dose reaches 45,000 r (Berson and Yalow, 1957a; Steinfeld *et al.*, 1958; Cohen, 1959; Yalow and Berson, 1960). Some products are particularly sensitive to the effects of irradiation. For example, with a dose as low as 37 mrads, lysozyme loses about a third of its enzymatic activity (Tolbert *et al.*, 1964).

As pointed out above, the effect of autoradiolysis should be taken into account in selecting the radioisotope for labeling a given compound and in specifying the specific activity. In the case of labeling with iodine, for example, the choice of radioisotope (^{125}I or ^{131}I) conditions the stability of the labeled product. Iodine ^{125}I, a low-energy isotope, gives rise to minimal autoradiolysis compared with that of ^{131}I.

3.1.3. *Chemical effects of labeling operations*

One cause of variation may be the chemical treatment to which the compound is subjected during the processes of labeling and purification. For example, the structural modifications caused by oxidation and polymerization, and the denaturation owing to the effect of solvents, of heat (Merchant *et al.*, 1957) and of superficial phenomena, are to be feared; a special case is the deliberate implanting of foreign atoms in the molecule by the experimenter, but this can be the source of serious inconvenience (see Section 2).

It should not be overlooked that labeling may aggravate changes which existed in the original product. Different lots of human albumin, for example, even though nondifferentiated by analytical controls (ultracentrifugation, electrophoresis, etc.) can behave in a different way after labeling (Bianchi *et al.*, 1966).

3.1.4. *Isotopic effect*

Other factors may have consequences that modify the behavior of the labeled product in relation to the original product, e.g. the isotopic effect. The difference in chemical behavior in isotopes of high atomic mass can be neglected; but it is not the same for tritium, where the mass difference with the stable isotope is very important. The isotopic effect normally manifests itself by reaction rate differences (Jellinck and Smyth, 1958; Rachele *et al.*, 1959) between the C–T bond and the C–H bond. For instance, if a mixture of C–H and C–T (^{3}H) bonds is acted upon by an oxidative enzyme, the former will be broken statistically more frequently than the others; hence the specific activity of the substance set in action and of the product of the reaction will be modified before equilibrium is achieved. In this particular case, tritium could not serve to measure the rate of the reaction in which the unlabeled product is involved (Verly, 1960).

In the case of isotopes with carbons-12, -13, and -14, the corresponding isotopic effect is much less important, and is practically negligible.

3.2. METHODS OF CONTROL

It has already been mentioned that the methods of synthesis and biosynthesis generally enable structural similarity between the tracer and the original compound to be obtained. In this case the controls over the initial product are also valid for the labeled product; in practice, a physico-chemical analysis is generally made. But these synthetic methods have disadvantages in being limited to the preparation of compounds of relatively simple structure or in providing often a low specific activity, while the proceedings are very laborious.

In most cases, therefore, organic tracers of biological origin are molecules obtained by a reaction of exchange or addition. Here the risks of degradation and of metabolic modifications are more serious, and more specific biological tests are required in addition to the physico-chemical controls.

3.2.1. *Physico-chemical control tests*

Various analytical methods are readily available to test the chemical and radiochemical purity of the tracer solutions. Typical examples will be given for each method.

(*a*) *Chromatography and electrophoresis.* These two techniques are employed on a wide variety of substrates: paper, silica, diethylaminoethyl-cellulose (DEAE), sephadex, gelose, starch, cellulose acetate, and so on.

Cohen (1959) has analysed labeled serum albumin on a column of DEAE cellulose; Schultze and Hughes (1965) separated various polymers of albumin on a column of sephadex G-200; Hügli (1965) studied the purity of iodinated serum albumin by Whatman 1 paper chromatography; Scott *et al.* (1965) verified the composition of radioactive vitamin D_3 by chromatography on thin-layer silica gel; Glick *et al.* (1963) analyzed somathormone by starch gel electrophoresis.

(*b*) *Titration of functional groups.* The appearing or disappearing of functional groups can testify to a change taking place. The case of the sulfhydryl groups can be quoted as an example (Yalow and Berson, 1957).

(*c*) *Spectroscopy.* Amongst the nondestructive methods of analysis, spectroscopy takes first place. A reference should be made to the study of visible, ultraviolet, and infrared spectra (e.g. vitamin D_3: Scott *et al.*, 1965); and even of electron-spin resonance (Tolbert *et al.*, 1964), and nuclear magnetic resonance.

(*d*) *Ultracentrifugation.* The method of ultracentrifugation enabled Schultze and Hughes (1965) to observe the aggregation of serum albumin in the course of treatment by chromium-51, as previously indicated by Naismith (1958) using conarachin and stable chromium (Fig. 5). Similarly, Rajam and Jackson (1960) have analyzed antibodies labeled by exchange with tritium.

(*e*) *Other techniques.* The technique of isotopic dilution and the conventional methods of analysis currently in use should be mentioned, as well as the determination of physico-chemical constants such as the melting point.

The physico-chemical controls are indispensable. Generally they are sufficient to establish structural similarity between the original compound and its tracer whenever the tracer has been prepared by chemical synthesis or biosynthesis; but they are found to be lacking in the case of products labeled by exchange or addition. In these latter cases one must have resort to the techniques of biological tests, the results of which alone will warrant the use of the tracer in the proposed experiment.

It should also be mentioned that the results of physico-chemical analysis are not always in agreement with the biological test results. In the first

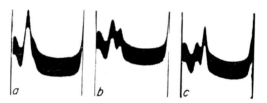

FIG. 5. Sedimentation diagrams of conarachin II after reaction with an anionic chromium complex at pH 5.3. The metal to protein molar ratio in the reaction mixture is 20.2. At different time intervals after the addition of chromium, samples were removed and submitted to ultracentrifugation: (a) after 1 hr; (b) after 5 hr; (c) after 20 hr (from Naismith, 1958).

place, the fact of observing a normal sedimentation diagram after ultracentrifugation gives no indication as to the presence of altered compounds which would be degraded excessively fast *in vivo* (Berson *et al.*, 1953). Conversely, a significant difference between the electrophoretic mobilities of the labeled and unlabeled albumin will not in every case prohibit the use of labeled albumin in systems where the electrophoretic mobility is not involved (Gabrieli *et al.*, 1954; Bennhold and Kallee, 1959).

Finally, artefacts due to the application of control tests should be borne in mind, such as the detection of quinones during chromatography of the thyronines, or the appearance of several spots when *pure* albumin is subjected to starch gel electrophoresis with an acetoborate buffer.

3.2.2. *Biological control tests*

Biological controls are needed for compounds labeled by addition since a foreign atom has been added to the molecule. However, it must immediately be said that in this case the requirements are necessarily less formal. For the proteins labeled by addition, it only matters that the tracer should be indistinguishable from the compound being studied *in a given system* (Berson and Yalow, 1965). Thus, for instance, in radioimmunology the behavior of the labeled hormone need not necessarily be identical to that of the unlabeled hormone when it is desired to use hormones labeled with iodine-131. In fact the radioimmunological test depends on the competitive inhibition of the hormone–antibody bond, in which a certain degree of alteration of the labeled hormone is without influence (Berson and Yalow, 1965).

Various biological tests in current usage will now be reviewed.

(*a*) *Comparison of behavior.* The behavior of compounds labeled by addition can be compared with the behavior of others labeled by chemical synthesis or biosynthesis. Many authors have measured the blood half-life of the plasma proteins (Cohen *et al.*, 1956; Campbell *et al.*, 1956; Schulze, 1957; Humphrey and McFarlane, 1954; Goldsworthy and Volwiler, 1957; Walter *et al.*, 1957; Haurowitz *et al.*, 1958, Armstrong *et al.*, 1955; Friedberg *et al.*, 1955; Masouredis and Beeckmans, 1955; Volwiller *et al.*, 1955) (see Fig. 2).

(*b*) *Determination of the catabolic rate.* The catabolic rate is defined as the quantity of radioactivity eliminated daily in the urines expressed as a fraction of the radioactivity remaining in the intravascular compartment.

It is useful to know this index is useful for plasma proteins with a sufficiently long biological half-life. A higher value on the first day than on the following days unquestionably indicates heterogeneity of the labeled preparation (McFarlane, 1965).

On the other hand, the catabolic rate cannot be measured as a biological test for hormones with too short a plasma half-life. In the case of iodized insulin, for example, where the plasma half-life is 20–50 min, the degradation of the hormone is complete after a few hours, and all the radioiodine is in the pool of iodides that then begin to appear in the urines.

(*c*) *Biological activity test.* Particular specific tests make it possible to verify that biological activity has been maintained in spite of the labeling: e.g. the isolated-rat diaphragm test on insulin-[131]I (Joiner, 1959; Izzo *et al.*, 1964b); the test of antibodies tritiated by a complement-fixation reaction (Rajam and Jackson, 1960); the study of endotoxin-^{51}Cr by the determination of its toxicity on the animal (Braude *et al.*, 1955b); and the test of cytochrome *c*-^{51}Cr by an enzymatic system (Ingrand, 1966). A reminder is given that the results of biological control tests can be falsified by heterogeneity of labeling.

(*d*) *Other tests*. Plasma protein denaturation can be assessed by an isolated liver preparation, which has the property that denatured proteins are preferentially captured (Gordon, 1957).

The test for human plasma proteins is a special problem. It can be resolved by the use of animals that have been maintained since birth in a state of tolerance with regard to human protein by frequently repeated injections (Freeman, 1959).

As we have seen, the labeled proteins form a homogeneous group of tracers obtained by the addition of foreign atoms. The various biological tests mentioned above will apply to them.

Other molecules besides proteins can be studied by *in vivo* methods.

For exogenous compounds that undergo no isotopic dilution by the endogenous compound, it is important to show that the specific activity does not decrease when the labeled compound is isolated from extracts of biological organs or fluids (Okita and Spratt, 1962). Thus morphine-^{3}H, purified until its specific activity was constant at 8.32 mcCi, has been administered to rats to be isolated later in the urines with exactly the same specific activity (Achor, 1958).

Once in possession of the results of the various physico-chemical and biological control tests, the pharmacologist is justified in using the labeled molecule, and taking advantage of the sensitivity of the techniques employing radioactivity.

CONCLUSION

In the light of the present study, it can be stated that techniques are now available for preparing any molecule that pharmacologists may wish to study.

When the chemical structure is known, a chemical synthesis can be considered; otherwise, if the compound can be suitably isolated, labeling by biosynthesis, exchange, or addition of foreign atoms, can be undertaken.

Secondly, it is clear that the mode of labeling must be carefully chosen. In effect, the resulting tracer must be indistinguishable from the non-radioactive compound in the experiment in hand, whether a complex biological system is concerned, or only a more simple *in vitro* reaction. In other respects, it is well to avoid a method of labeling that would produce insufficient specific activity, leading to the administration of toxic or non-physiological doses. Finally, we have drawn attention to the problems arising in the storage of labeled molecules and to the need for control tests before the experiment.

In any case, the results obtained up to the present concerning the metabolism and mechanism of action of biological tracers are on the whole very encouraging, and point to an increasingly frequent application of labeled molecules in the pharmacological field in future.

ACKNOWLEDGMENTS

The authors wish to thank Miss M. Hazouard for her assistance in the preparation of this manuscript.

REFERENCES

(A) BOOKS, REVIEWS AND MONOGRAPHS

ACHE, H. J., HERR, W., and THIEMANN, A. (1962) Study on the position of tritium in aromatic molecules labelled by different methods, in *Tritium in the Physical and Biological Sciences*. IAEA, Vienna, Vol. 2, pp. 21–36.

AUBERT, J. P. and MILHAUD, G. (1964) Préparation de galactose et de glycérol-^{14}C uniformement marquées. Proc. Conf. Methods Preparing and Storing Labeled Molecules. Bruxelles, Euratom, pp. 105–8.

AYRES, P. J. (1962) The biosynthesis of (16-H^3) steroid by isolated adrenal cortex tissue, in *Tritium in the Physical and Biological Sciences*. IAEA, Vienna, Vol. 2, pp. 131–7.

BERSON, S. A. and YALOW, R. S. (1965) *Considerations in the Preparation of I^{131} labelled Hormones. Radioisotopes Techniques in the Study of Proteins Metabolism*, IAEA, Vienna, pp. 29–33.

BIANCHI, R., ROSA, U., FEDERIGHI, G. and DONATO, L. (1966) Iodinated albumin as tracer, Proc. 1st Conf. Labelled Proteins in Tracer Studies, Euratom, Bruxelles, Eur 2950 d, f, e, pp. 61–9.

BANERJEE, R., EKINS, R. P., ELLIS, J., LOWY, C. and O'RIORDAN, J. (1963) Iodination of proteins to high specific activity, Proc. Conf. on Methods of Preparing and Storing Marked Molecules, Bruxelles, pp. 481–92.

CATCH, J. R. (1961) *Carbon 14 Compounds*. Butterworths, London.

CATCH, J. R. (1964) Biological preparation of labelled compounds, Proc. Conf. Methods Preparing and Storing Marked Molecules, Euratom, Bruxelles, pp. 293–300.

CIFERRI, O., ALBERTINI, A. and CASSANI, G. (1964) Produzione di attinomicine specificamente marcate, Proc. Conf. Methods Preparing and Storing Marked Molecules. Euratom, Bruxelles, pp. 243–50.

COMAR, C. L. (1955) *Radioisotopes in Biology and Agriculture*. Academic Press, New York, London.

DOVEY, A. (1954) Preparation and some uses of high specific activity plasma proteins, Proc. 2nd Radioisotope Conf. Oxford, Vol. I, p. 337, Butterworths, London, England.

EBEL, J. P. (1964) Sur la preparation et la purification des acides ribonucléiques de la levure marqués au ^{32}P et au ^{14}C, Proc. Conf. Methods Preparing and Storing Marked Molecules. Euratom, Bruxelles, pp. 133–49.

FELTER, R. E. and CURRIE, L. A. (1962) Tritium labelling by means of uranium hydride, in *Tritium in the Physical and Biological Sciences*, IAEA, Vienna, Vol. 2, pp. 61–7.

FENG, P. Y. and GREENLEE, T. W. (1962) Specific tritium labelling of organic compounds by the gas exposure method, in *Tritium in the Physical and Biological Sciences*, IAEA, Vienna, Vol. 2, pp. 11–17.

FUMAGALLI, R. and PAOLETTI, R. (1964) Preparazione di lipidi e steroli per biosintesi di precursori marcati, in Proc. Conf. Methods Preparing and Storing Marked Molecules. Euratom, Bruxelles, pp. 365–76.

GARNETT, J. L., HENDERSON, L. and SOLLICH, W. A. (1962) The synthesis of tritium-labelled aromatic compounds by platinum-catalyzed exchange with tritium oxide, in *Tritium in the Physical and Biological Sciences.* IAEA, Vienna, Vol. 2, pp. 47–57.

GITLIN, D. (1965) Observations on the selective permeability of the human placenta to plasma proteins and protein hormones, in *Radioisotope Techniques in the Study of Protein Metabolism.* IAEA, Vienna, pp. 197–204.

GLASCOCK, R. F. (1962) Some examples of the use of radioisotopes in biochemistry, in *Use of Radioisotopes in Animal Biology and the Medical Sciences,* Academic Press, London, England, Vol. 1, pp. 52–6.

HASAN, P. (1962) Discussion, in *Tritium in the Physical and Biological Sciences,* AIEA, Vienna, Vol. 2, p. 67.

HAUROWITZ, F., FLEISCHER, S., WALTER, H. and LEITZE, A. (1958) The metabolism of isotopically labeled plasma proteins, U.N. 2nd Conf. Genève, Vol. 25 (P–837), 111–14.

HUGHES, W. L. (1966) Chemical requirements of a satisfactory label, Proc. 1st Conf. Labelled Proteins in Tracer Studies. Euratom, Bruxelles. EUR 2950 d, f, e, pp. 3–14.

HUPKA, S., HNILICA, L. and GREGUSOVA, V. (1958) Labelling of calf thymus histone with radioiodine, U.N. 2nd Conf. Genève, Vol. 25 (P 2479), pp. 170–2.

INGRAND, J. (1964) Contribution à l'étude des propriétés biologiques des composés marqués au radiochrome ^{51}Cr. Thèse Doctorat Etat Pharmacie Paris, France. Rapport CEA No. R 2585 Centre d'Études Nucleaires de Saclay.

LEONIS, J. (1964) Tritiation de protéines et de peptides par échange, Proc. Conf. Methods Preparing and Storing Marked Molecules, Euratom, Bruxelles, pp. 269–81.

LETTE, E. (1959) *Biogenesis of Natural Substances,* M. Gates (ed.). Chap. 8. Univ. Minnesota, Minn., U.S.A.

MCCORMICK, J. A. (1959) *Utilization of Radioisotopes in Physical and Biological Sciences.* General topics TID 35/9, U.S.A.E.C. Technical Information Service.

MCFARLANE, A. S. (1963b) Metabolism of plasma proteins, in *Mammalian Protein Metabolism.* Academic Press, New York, U.S.A., Vol. 1, p. 297.

MCFARLANE, A. S. (1965) The preparation of I^{131} and I^{125} labelled plasma proteins, in *Radioisotope Techniques in the Study of Protein Metabolism.* IAEA, Vienna, pp. 3–6.

MCLAUGHLIN, G. D. and THEIS, E. R. (1945) Chemistry of chromium salts, chrome tanning, in *The Chemistry of Leather Manufacture.* Reinhold Publishing Co., New York, U.S.A., pp. 411–547.

MARGEN, S. and TARVER, H. (1963) The preparation of labelled albumin for turnover studies, 7th Symposium on Advances in Tracer Methodology, in *Advances in Tracer Methodology.* Plenum Press, New York (1965), Vol. 2, pp. 61–72.

MURRAY, A. and WILLIAMS, D. L. (1958) *Organic Synthesis with Isotopes,* Pt. 2. Interscience Publ., New York, U.S.A., pp. 1252–8.

MYERS, O. E. and PRESTWOOD, R. J. (1951) Isotopic exchange reactions-homogenous and heterogenous, in *Radioactivity Applied to Chemistry,* Wahl, A. S. and Bonner, N. A. (eds.). John Wiley, New York, U.S.A., pp. 323–64.

O'FLAHERTY, F. (1958) *Chemistry and Technology of Leather,* Vol. 2. Reinhold, New York, U.S.A.

OKITA, G. T. and SPRATT, J. L. (1962) Determination of radiotracer stability of tritium labeled compounds in biological studies, in *Tritium in the Physical and Biological Sciences.* IAEA, Vienna, Vol. 2, pp. 85–91.

OSINSKI, P. A. (1962) The synthesis of tritium labelled adrenal and gonadal hormones, in *Tritium in the Physical and Biological Sciences.* IAEA, Vienna, Vol. 2, pp. 113–18.

OSINSKI, P. A. and DECONINCK, J. M. (1964) Autoradiolyse des stéroides tritiés de haute activité spécifique, Proc. Conf. Methods Preparing and Storing Labeled Molecules. Euratom, Bruxelles, pp. 213–20.

NUNEZ, J. and POMMIER, J. (1965) New method of iodination and tritiation of proteins, in 10th Symposium on Advances in Tracer Methodology, Zürich, 1965.

PAOLETTI, C. and LAMONTHEZIE, N. (1964) Preparation biosynthetique de DNA tritié, Proc. Conf. Preparing and Storing Marked Molecules. Euratom, Bruxelles, pp. 121–31.

PARISI, B., LUCCHINI, G. and MARRE, E. (1964) Biosintesi di acido gibberellico marcato con ^{14}C, Proc. Conf. Methods Preparing and Storing Marked Molecules. Euratom, Bruxelles, pp. 389–98.

ROCHE, J., NUNEZ, J., JACQUEMIN, C., and POMMIER, J. (1964a) Saturation de doubles liaisons par l'acide iodhydrique tritié: préparation de thyroxine et de ses analogues tritiés, Proc. Conf. Methods Preparing and Storing Marked Molecules. Euratom Bruxelles, pp. 79–89.

ROCHE, J., NUNEZ, J., JACQUEMIN, C. and POMMIER, J. (1964b) Hydrogénolyse de phénols tritiés: préparation de thyronines tritiées, Proc. Conf. Methodes Preparing and Storing Marked Molecules. Euratom, Bruxelles, pp. 327–33.

ROLLINSON, C. L. (1966) Problems of chromium reactions, in Andrews, G. A., Kniseley, R. M. and Wagner, H. N. (eds.). *Radioactive Pharmaceuticals*. AEC Symposium Series, Oak Ridge Conference 651 111, National Bureau of Standards, Springfield, Virginia, U.S.A., pp. 429–46.

ROSA, U., PENNISI, G. F., SCASSELATI, G. A., BIANCHI, R., FEDERICHI, G., DONATO, L., ROSSI, C. A. and AMBROSINO, C. (1966a) Factors affecting protein iodination. *Proc. 1st Conf. Labelled Proteins in Tracer Studies*, Euratom, Bruxelles, EUR 2950 d, f, e, pp. 17–28.

ROSA, U., MASSAGLIA, A., PENNISI, F. and ROSSI, C. A. (1966b) Correlation of chemical changes with insulin biological activity. Proc. 1st Conf. Labelled Proteins in Tracer Studies. Euratom, Bruxelles, EUR 2950, d, f, e, pp. 225–34.

SCHNEK, A. G., LEONIS, J., LEDOUX, L., and RAPPAPORT, M. (1964) Marquage biosynthétique des protéines de l'oeuf de poule, Proc. Conf. Methods Preparing and Storing Marked Molecules. Euratom, Bruxelles, pp. 377–88.

SCHRAM, E., CAPE-GOLDFINGER, M. and MAYER, T. (1964) Préparation de dérivés biologiques marqués au soufre 35 de haute activité spécifique, in Proc. Conf. Methods Preparing and Storing Marked Molecules. Euratom, Bruxelles, pp. 399–407.

SCULLY, N. J. (1956) Biosynthesis in ^{14}C labeled plants, their use in agricultural and biological research, Proc. Int. Conf. Peaceful Uses of Atomic Energy. U.N. New York, U.S.A., Vol. 12, pp. 377–85.

SIMON, H., MÜLHOFER, G., and DORRER, H. D. (1964). Die Markierung von Zuckern und einigen Dicarbonsäuren mit Tritium durch Enzymreaktionen und/oder Wilzbachmarkierung. Proc. Conf. Methods Preparing and Storing Marked Molecules, Euratom, Bruxelles, pp. 283–92.

SNELL, J. F. (1956) Radioactive oxytetracycline (Terramycine). I: Mode of synthesis and properties of the radioactive compounds. Proc. Int. Conf. Peaceful Uses of Atomic Energy. U.N. New York, U.S.A., Vol. 12, pp. 431–4.

SPEIRS, R. S. (1962) Distribution of tritiated tetanus toxin following an intraperitoneal injection in immunized and non-immunized mice, in *Tritium in the Physical and Biological Sciences*, IAEA, Vienna, Vol. 2, pp. 419–28.

TARVER, H. (1957) *Methods in Enzymology*, Vol. 4. Academic Press, New York, U.S.A.

TOLBERT, B. M., KRINKS, M. H. and STEVENS, C. O. (1964) Radiation chemistry of aminoacides and proteins, *Proc. Conf. Methods Preparing and Storing Marked Molecules*. Euratom, Bruxelles, pp. 671–98.

TUBIS, M. (1966) Special iodinated compounds for biology and medicine, in *Radioactive Pharmaceuticals*, Andrews, G. A., Kiseley, R. M. and Wagner, H. N. (eds.). AEC Symposium series, Oak Ridge Conference 651 111, National Bureau of Standards, Springfield, Virginia, U.S.A., pp. 281–304.

VERLY, W. G. (1960) *Tritium: dosage, preparation de molécules marquées et applications biologiques.* IAEA Review Series No. 2, Vienna.

WALDMANN, T. A. (1965) The preparation of Cr^{51}-albumin, in *Radioisotopes Techniques in the Study of Proteins Metabolism.* IAEA, Vienna, pp. 35–40.

WALDMANN, T. A. and WOCHNER, R. D. (1965) The measurement of gastrointestinal protein loss by means of Cr^{51} albumin and Cu^{67} coeruloplasmin, in *Radioisotopes Techniques in the Study of Protein Metabolism.* IAEA, Vienna, pp. 171–81.

WENZEL, M. and GÜNTHER, TH. (1964) Enzymatic conversion in tritium water. I: Enzymatic synthesis of specifically tritiated *l*-lactic acid from HTO, *Proc. Conf. Methods Preparing and Storing Marked Molecules.* Euratom, Bruxelles, pp. 971–82.

WENZEL, M. and SCHULTZE, P. E. (1962) *Tritium Markierung.* Walter de Gruyter, Berlin.

WENZEL, M., WOLLENBERG, H. and SCHULZE, P. E. (1962) Specific activity of charcoal absorbed compounds after H^3 labeling by the Wilzbach procedure, in *Tritium in the Physical and Biological Sciences.* IAEA, Vienna, Vol. 2, pp. 37–45.

WILZBACH, K. E. (1962) Gas exposure method for tritium labelling, in *Tritium in the Physical and Biological Sciences.* IAEA, Vienna, Vol. 2, pp. 3–10.

(B) ORIGINAL WORKS

ACHOR, L. B. (1958) The preparation of biologically stable tritium labelled morphine. *J. Pharmacol. Exp. Therap.*, **122**:1A.

ACHOR, L. B. and GEILING, E. M. K. (1954) Isolation and purification of semimicroquantities of morphine. *Anal. Chem.*, **26**:1061–2.

D'ADDABBO, A., KALLEE, E. and LOHSS, F. (1960) Über I^{131} signiertes Insulin IV. immunologische Studien und Prednisolonwirkung. *Sonderband Strahlentherapie*, **45**:279–92.

AFIFI, F., HARTMANN, L., LOVERDO, A. and FAUVERT, R. (1963) Exploration des fonctions digestives au moyen de la caséïne marquée à l'iode radioactif ^{131}I. *Ann. Nutr., Fr.*, **17**:263–79.

ARMSTRONG, S. H., BRONSKY, D. and HERSHMAN, J. (1955) The persistance in the blood of the radioactive label of albumin, gamma globulin and globulins of intermediate mobility. *J. Lab. Clin. Med.*, **46**:857.

ASCOLI, F. and KAHAN, F. M. (1966) Iodination of nucleic acids in organic solvents with (I^{125} labelled) iodine monochloride. *J. Biol. Chem.*, **241**:428–31.

BAETJER, A. M., DAMRON, C. M., CLARK, J. H. and BUDACZ, W. (1955) Reaction of chromium compounds with body tissues and their constituents. *Arch. Ind. Health*, **12**:258–61.

BATES, H. M. and SIMPSON, M. V. (1959) The net synthesis of cytochrome *c* in calf heart mitochondria. *Biochim. Biophys. Acta*, **32**:597.

BATTERSBY, A. R., BINKS, R., FRANCIS, R. J., McCALDIN, D. J. and RAMUZ, H. (1964) Alkaloïd biosynthesis. IV: *l*-benzyliso-quinoleines as precursors of thebaine, codeine and morphine. *J. Chem. Soc.*, **4**:3600.

BAUER, G. E. (1964) The biosynthesis of ^{14}C and ^{3}H labeled insulin. *Atomlight*, **38**:1–7.

BAYLY, R. J. and EVANS, E. A. (1966) Stability and storage of compounds labelled with radioisotopes. *J. Labelled Compounds*, **2**:1–34.

BEINERT, H. (1948) Cytochrome *c* labelled with radioactive iron. *Science*, **108**:634.

BEINERT, H. (1950) Studies on the metabolism of administered cytochrome C. by the aid of iron labelled cytochrome, *Science*, **111**:469.

BENAZET, F. and BOURAT, G. (1965) Étude autoradiographique de la repartition du constituant I.A. de la pristinamycine chez la souris. *C. R. Acad. Sci.*, **260**:2622.

BENNETT, R. D. and HEFTMANN, E. (1965) Biosynthesis of holarrhena alkaloids from cholesterol. *Arch. Biochem. Biophys.*, **112**:616–20.

BERSON, S. A., YALOW, R. S., POST, J., LAWRENCE, H., NEWERLY, K. N., VILLAZON, M. J., and VAZQUEZ, O. N. (1953) Distribution and fate of intravenously administered modified human globin and its effect on blood volume. Studies utilizing I^{131} tagged globin. *J. Clin. Invest.*, **32**:22.

BERSON, S. A., YALOW, R. S., BAUMAN, A., ROTHSCHILD, M. A. and NEWERLY, K. (1956) Insulin I^{131} metabolism in human subjects; demonstration of insulin treated subjects. *J. Clin. Invest.*, **35**:170.

BERSON, S. A. and YALOW, R. S. (1957) Radiochemical and radiobiological alteration of I^{131} labeled proteins in solution. *Ann. N.Y. Acad. Sci.*, **70**:56.

BERSON, S. A., YALOW, R. S. and VOLK, B. W. (1957) *In vivo* and *in vitro* metabolism of insulin—I^{131} and glucagon. I^{131} in normal and cortisone treated rabbits. *J. Lab. Clin. Med.*, **49**:331.

BERSON, S. A. and YALOW, R. S. (1958) Isotopic tracers in the study of diabetes. *Adv. Biol. Med. Phys.*, **6**:349.

BENNHOLD, H. and KALLEE, E. (1959) Comparative studies on the half life of I^{131} labeled albumins and non radioactive human serum albumin in a case of analbuminemia. *J. Clin. Invest.*, **38**:863.

BLAU, M. (1961) Biosynthesis of ^{75}Se-selenomethionine and ^{75}Se-selenocystine. *Biochim. Biophys. Acta*, **49**:389–90.

BLOOM, H. J. G., CROCKETT, D. J. and STEWART, F. S. (1958) The effect of radiation on the stability of radiodinated human serum albumin. *Brit. J. Radiol.*, **31**:377.

BOCCI, V. (1964) Efficient labelling of serum protein with I^{131} using chloramine T. *Int. J. Appl. Rad. Isotopes*, **15**:449–56.

BOGNER, R. L., EDELMAN, A. and MARTIN, G. J. (1959) *In vivo* observations with radioactive trypsin. *Arch. Int. Pharmacodyn.*, **118**:122.

BOURSNELL, J. C., FRANCIS, C. E. and WORMALL, A. (1946) The immunological properties of proteins treated with muted gas and some related compounds. *Biochem. J.*, **40**:768.

BRAUDE, A. F., CAREY, F. J., SUTHERLAND, D. and ZALESKY, M. (1955a) Studies with radioactive endotoxin. I: The use of ^{51}Cr to label endotoxin of *Escherichia Coli*. *J. Clin. Invest.*, **34**:850–7.

BRAUDE, A. F., CAREY, F. J. and ZALESKY, M. (1955b) Studies with radioactive endotoxin. II: Correlation of physiologic effects with distribution of radioactivity in rabbits injected with lethal doses of *E. Coli* endotoxin labeled with radioactive sodium chromate. *J. Clin. Invest.*, **34**:858–66.

BROWN, F. and JACKSON, H. (1956) The fate of ^{131}I labeled homologous and heterologous thyroglobulins in the rat, dog, monkey and rabbit. *Biochem. J.*, **62**:295.

CACACE, F., GUARINO, A. and MONTEFINALE, G. (1961) Labelling of organic compounds by mercury photosensitized reaction with tritium gas. *Nature, Lond.*, **189**:54–5.

CAMPBELL, R. M., CUTHBERTSON, D. P., MATTHEWS, C. M. and McFARLANE, A. S. (1956) Behaviour of ^{14}C- and ^{131}I labelled plasma proteins in the rat. *Int. J. Appl. Rad. Isotopes*, **1**:66–84.

CARDINAUD, R., TAKASHIMA, K., DAUSSET, J. and FROMAGEOT, P. (1964) Tritiation d'une anti-γ-globuline et dosage radiochimique. *Int. J. Appl. Rad. Isotopes*, **15**:1.

CHAIET, L., ROSENBLUM, C. and WOODBURY, D. T. (1950) Biosynthesis of radioactive vitamin B_{12} containing ^{60}Co. *Science*, **111**:601.

CLARK, J. H. (1959) The denaturation of proteins by chromium salts. *Arch. Ind. Health*, **20**:117–23.

COLLIPP, P. J., PATRICK, J. R., GOODHEART, C. and KAPLAN, S. A. (1966) Distribution of tritium labelled human growth hormone in rats and guinea-pigs. *Proc. Soc. Exp. Biol. Med.*, **121**:173–7.

COHEN, S., HOLLOWAY, R. C., MATTHEWS, C. M. and McFARLANE, A. S. (1956) Distribution and elimination of ^{131}I and ^{14}C labeled plasma proteins in the rabbit. *Biochem. J.*, **62**:143.

COHEN, S. (1959) Chromatographic behaviour of human albumin labeled with iodine 131. *Nature*, **183**:393.

COHEN, Y., WEPIERRE, J. and PONTY, D. (1965) Fixation du chrome 51 sur les fractions protéiques du serum sanguin. *Sonderband Strahlentherapie*, **60**:273–86.

COHEN, Y., BLANCHARD-PELLETIER, D. and BONFILS, S. (1966) Le marquage de la pepsine par le chlorure du chrome ^{51}Cr. Choix des conditions techniques et des contrôles. *C. R. Soc. Biol.*, **160**:2272–6.

COOPER, P. D. and ROWLEY, D. (1949) Radioactive penicillin. *Nature, Lond.*, **163**:480.

COX, R. W., HENLEY, E. D., NARAHARA, H. T., VAN ARSDEL, P. and WILLIAMS, R. H. (1957) Studies on the metabolism of glucagon I^{131} in rats. *Endocrinology*, **60**:277.

CRAWHALL, J. C., HAWKINS, J. D. and SMYTH, D. G. (1958) The synthesis of tritiovaline and its incorporation into rat visceral proteins. Addendum, the biosynthesis of a tritium labeled antibody. *Biochem. J.*, **69**:286–7.

DANISHEFSKY, I. and EIBER, H. B. (1957) Utilization of glucose in the biosynthesis of heparin. *Amer. Chem. Soc. Abst.*, **131**:72C.

DAVIES, W. H., MERCER, E. I. and GOODWIN, T. W. (1966) Some observations on the biosynthesis of the plant sulpholipid by *Euglenia gracilis*. *Biochem. J.*, **98**:369–73.

DONE, J. and PAYNE, P. R. (1956) Investigations on rat serumalbumin marked with tritium labeled leucine. *Biochem. J.*, **64**:266.

DUNN, A. L., ESKELSON, C. D., McLEAY, J. F. and OGBORN, R. E. (1960) Preliminary study of radioactive product obtained from iodinating tetracycline. *Proc. Soc. Exp. Biol. Med.*, **104**:12–13.

DUTTON, H. J., JONES, E. P. and MASON, L. H. (1958) The labelling of fatty acids by exposure to tritium gas. *Chem. Ind., G.B.*, **36**:1176.

EIBER, H. B. and DANISHEFSKY, I. (1957) The incorporation of S^{35} sulfate into heparin. *J. Biol. Chem.*, **226**:721.

EIBER, H. B. and DANISHEFSKY, I. (1959) Distribution of injected heparin in different blood fractions. *Proc. Soc. Exp. Biol. Med.*, **102**:18.

ERB, W. and MAURER, W. (1960) Biosynthese von C^{14} markiertem Eiweiss mit *Chlorella pyrenoidosa*. *Biochem. Z.*, **332**:388–95.

EVANS, E. A. and STANFORD, F. G. (1963) Decomposition of tritium labeled organic compounds. *Nature, Lond.*, **197**:551–5.

EVERTSBUSCH, V. and GEILING, E. M. K. (1953) Distribution and excretion of radioactivity in mice following the administration of ^{14}C-labelled atropine. *Fed. Proc.*, **12**:319.

FELBER, J. P. (1965) Détermination de l'ACTH par une méthode radioimmunologique. *Sonderband Strahlentherapie*, **60**:368–77.

FONG, C. T. O., SILVER, L., CHRISTMAN, D. R. and SCHWARTZ, I. L. (1960) On the mechanism of action of the antidiuretic hormone (vasopressin). *Proc. Nat. Acad. Sci.*, **46**:1273.

FRANCIS, G. E., MULLIGAN, W. and WORMALL, A. (1951) Labelling of proteins with iodine 131, sulphur 35 and phosphorus 32. *Nature, Lond.*, **167**:148.

FRANCIS, G. E., MULLIGAN, W. and WORMALL, A. (1955) The use of radioactive isotopes in immunological investigations. 8. Labeling antibodies with ^{131}I and ^{35}S. *Biochem. J.*, **60**:363.

FRANK, H. and GRAY, S. J. (1953) The determination of plasma volume in man with radioactive chromic chloride. *J. Clin. Invest.*, **32**:991–9.

FREEMAN, T. (1959) The biological behaviour of normal and denaturated human plasma albumin. *Clin. Chim. Acta*, **4**:788.

FRIEDBERG, W., WALTER, H. and HAUROWITZ, F. (1955) The fate in rats of internally and externally labelled heterologous proteins. *J. Immunol.*, **75**:315.

GABRIELI, E. R., GOULIAN, D., KINERSLY, T. and COLLET, R. (1954) Zone paper electrophoresis studies on radioiodinated human serumalbumin. *J. Clin. Invest.*, **33**:136.

GALSKOV, A. (1966) Labelling of corticotropin with iodine 125. *Experientia*, **21**:1–4.

GARVEY, J. S. and CAMPBELL, D. H. (1954) The relation of circulating antibody concentration to localization of labeled (S^{35}) antigen. *J. Immunol.*, **72**:131.

GARVEY, J. S., EITZMAN, D. V. and SMITH, R. T. (1960) The distribution of S^{35} labeled bovine serumalbumin in newborn and immunologically tolerant adult rabbits. *J. Exp. Med.*, **112**:553–58.

GEILING, E. M. K., KELSEY, F. E., MCINTOSH, B. J. and GANZ, A. (1948) Biosynthesis of radioactive drugs using carbon 14. *Science*, **108**:558–9.

GENNARO, J. F. and RAMSEY, H. W. (1959) Distribution in the mouse of lethal and sublethal doses of cottonmouth moccasin venom labelled with iodine 131. *Nature, Lond.*, **184**:1244–5.

GHANEM, N. A. and WESTERMARK, T. (1960) Unspecific tritium labelling accelerated by microwave, alternating current and direct current electric discharge and by ultraviolet radiation. *J. Amer. Chem. Soc.*, **82**:4432–3.

GILLILAND, P. F. and PROUT, T. E. (1965) Radio-iodination of oxytocin. *Metabolism*, **14**:912–17.

GILMORE, R. C., ROBBINS, M. C. and REID, A. F. (1954) Labeling bovine and human albumin with iodine-131. *Nucleonics*, **12**(2):65.

GIOVANNOZZI-SERMANNI, G. and POSSAGNO, E. (1960) Preparation of tritium labelled antibiotics. *Energ. Nucl.*, **7**:797–800.

GLEASON, G. I. (1955) Some notes on the exchange of iodine with thyroxine homologues. *J. Biol. Chem.* **213**:837–41.

GLENDENING, M. D., GREENBERG, D. M. and FRAENKEL-CONRAT, H. (1947) Biologically active insulin sulfate. *J. Biol. Chem.*, **167**:125.

GLICK, S. M., ROTH, J., YALOW, R. S. and BERSON, S. A. (1963) Immuno assay of human growth hormone in plasma. *Nature, Lond.* **199**:784.

GOLDSWORTHY, P. D. and VOLWILER, W. (1957) Comparative metabolic fate of chemically (I^{131}) and biosynthetically (C^{14} or S^{35}) labeled proteins. *Ann. N.Y. Acad. Sci.*, **70**:26.

GOLDSWORTHY, P. D. and VOLWILER, W. (1958) Mechanism of protein turnover studies with cystine—S^{35} lysine C^{14} doubly labeled plasma proteins of the dog. *J. Biol. Chem.*, **230**:817–31.

GORDON, A. H. (1957) The use of the isolated perfused liver to detect alterations to plasma proteins. *Biochem. J.*, **66**:255.

GRAY, S. J. and STERLING, K. (1950) The tagging of red cells and plasma proteins with radioactive chromium. *J. Clin. Invest.*, **29**, 1604–13.

GREENWOOD, F. C., HUNTER, W. M. and GLOVER, C. (1963) The preparation of ^{131}I labelled human growth hormone of high specific activity. *Biochem. J.*, **89**:114.

GROGAN, C. H. and OPPENHEIMER, H. (1955) Experimental studies in metal cancerigenesis. V: Interaction of Cr III and Cr VI compounds with proteins. *Arch. Biochem. Biophys.*, **56**:204–21.

GUSTAVSON, K. H. (1958) A novel type of metal protein compounds. *Nature, Lond.*, **182**:1125–8.

HANSSON, E. and SAMUELSSON, B. (1965) Autoradiographic distribution studies of ^{3}H labeled prostaglandin El in mice. *Biochem. Biophys. Acta*, **106**:379–85.

HOFMANN, A. F. (1960) Exchange of iodine 131 labeled chylomicron protein *in vivo*. *Amer. J. Physiol.*, **199**:433–6.

HÖLZL, J., CHATTERJEE, M. and HORHAMMER, L. (1964) Über die Herstellung von ^{32}P-Lecithin und ^{32}P-Cephalin. *Biochem. Z.*, **340**:400–2.

HOPKINS, L. L. and SCHWARZ, K. (1964) Chromium III binding to serum proteins, specifically siderophilin. *Biochim. Biophys. Acta*, **90**:484.

HOWELL, S. F. and THAYER, J. D. (1948) Introduction of radioactive sulfur (S^{35}) into the penicillin molecule by biosynthesis, *Science*, **107**:299.

HUANG, H. S. and DE WITT, S. G. (1965) Vitamin A and carotenoids. I: Intestinal absorption and metabolism of ^{14}C labeled vitamin A alcohol and carotene in the rat. *J. Biol. Chem.*, **240**:2839–47.

HUGHES, W. L. (1957) The chemistry of iodination. *Ann. N.Y. Acad. Sci.*, **70**:3.

HUGHES, W. L. and STRAESSLE, R. (1950). Preparation and properties of serum and plasma proteins. *J. Amer. Chem. Soc.*, **72**:452.

HÜGLI, H. (1965) The labelling of proteins with I^{131}, in *Radioisotope Techniques in the Study of Protein Metabolism*. IAEA, Vienna, pp. 7–8.

HUMPHREY, J. H. and McFARLANE, A. S. (1954) Rate of elimination of homologous globulins from the circulation, *Biochem. J.*, **57**:186.

HUNTER, W. M. and GREENWOOD, F. C. (1962) Preparation of iodine-131 labeled human growth hormone of high specific activity. *Nature, Lond.*, **194**:495.

ILYIN, G. (1958) The biosynthesis of nicotine ^{14}C (in Russian). *Dokl. Akad. Nauk. SSSR*, **119**:540.

INGRAHAM, J. S. (1951) Artificial radioactive antigens. I: Preparation and evaluation and ^{35}S sulfanilic acid, azobovine-γ-globulin. *J. Infect. Dis.*, **89**:109.

INGRAND, J. (1966) Le cytochrome c marqué au chrome 51, I. et II. *Biochem. Pharmacol.*, **15**:1649–58.

INMAN, F. P. and NISONOFF, A. (1966) Reversible dissociation of fragment Fc of rabbit γG-immunoglobulin. *J. Biol. Chem.*, **241**:322–9.

IZZO, J. L., BALE, W. F., IZZO, M. J. and RONCONE, A. (1964a) High specific activity labeling of insulin with ^{131}I. *J. Biol. Chem.*, **239**:3743–8.

IZZO, J. L., RONCONE, A., IZZO, M. J. and BALE, W. F. (1964b) Relationship between degree of iodination of insulin and its biological, electrophoretic and immuno-chemical properties. *J. Biol. Chem.*, **239**:3749–54.

JEEJEEBHOY, K. N., STEWART, J. M., EVANS, E. A. and BOOTH, C. C. (1964) On the use of tritium labeled albumin for studies of intestinal absorption. *Gut*, **5**:346.

JELLINK, P. H. and SMYTH, D. G. (1958) Molecular changes in exchange labeling with tritium. *Nature, Lond.*, **182**,:46.

JOHNSON, A. (1960) The effect of iodination antibody activity. *J. Immunol.* **84**:213.

JOHNSON, D. B., HOWELLS, D. J. and GOODWIN, T. W. (1966) Observations on the biosynthesis of thiamine in yeast. *Biochem. J.*, **98**:30–37.

JOINER, C. L. (1959) Rate of clearance of insulin labeled with ^{131}I from the subcutaneous tissues in normal and diabetic subjects. *Lancet*, **1**:964.

KARLSON, P., MAURER, R. and WENZEL, M. (1963) A micromethod for the tritium labeling of steroids and ecdysone. *Z. Naturforsch.*, **18b**:219–24.

KEKKI, M., KOSKELO, P. and NIKKILA, E. A. (1966) Turnover of iodine 131-labeled coeruloplasmin in human beings. *Nature*, **209**:1252–3.

KUBAT, A. (1963) Eine Verbesserung der Etikettierung von Dextran mit ^{51}Cr durch Einwirkung von Askorbinsäure. *Strahlentherapie*, **120**:315–7.

KUTACEK, M., SPALENY, J. and OPLISTILOVA, K. (1966) Die biosynthetische Inkorporation von externem ^{35}SO$_2$ in Glucobrassicin. *Experientia*, **22**:24–25.

LAUFER, L., GUTCHO, S., CASTRO, T. and GRENNEN, R. (1964) Preparation of radioactive biochemicals by use of yeast. *Biotechnol. Bioengineering*, **6**:127–46.

LAVIK, P. S., MATTHEWS, L. W., BUCKALOO, G. W., LEMM, F. J., SPECTOR, S. and FRIEDELL, H L. (1952) Use of I^{131} labelled proteins in the study of protein digestion and absorption in children with and without cystic fibrosis of the pancreas. *Pediatrics*, 10:667.

LEE, N. D., WISEMAN, R. and TENN, M. (1959) A simplified and exact method for the controlled substitution of proteins with I^{131}. *J. Lab. Clin. Med.*, 54:325.

LEMMON, R. M., TOLBERT, B. M., STOHMEIER, W. and WHITTEMORE, I. W. (1959) Ionizing energy as an aid in exchange tritium labeling. *Science*, 129:1740–1.

LIEBSTER, J., DOBIASOVA, M., KOPOLDOVA, J. and EKL, J. (1961) Préparation par biosynthèse de composés, marqués au radiocarbone. III: Séparation des acides aminés marqués par ^{14}C à partir de l'hydrolysat des albumines de l'algue chlorella vulgaris. *Collect. Czechosl. Chem. Comm.*, 26:1700–7.

LIGHT, A. and SIMPSON, V. (1956) Studies on the biosynthesis of insulin. I: The paper chromatographic isolation of ^{14}C labeled insulin from calf pancreas slices. *Nature, Lond*, 177:225.

LILLY, V. G., BARNETT, H. L., KRAUSE, R. F. and LOTSPEICH, F. J. (1958) A method of obtaining pure radioactive β carotene using phycomyces blakesleeanus. *Mycologia*, 50:862–73.

MAAS, E. A. and JOHNSON, M. J. (1949) Penicillin uptake by bacterial cells. *J. Bacteriol.*, 57:415.

MABRY, C. C., GREENLAW, R. H. and DE VORE, W. D. (1965) Measurement of gastro intestinal loss of plasma albumin: a clinical and laboratory evaluation of ^{51}chromium labelled albumin. *J. Nucl. Med.*, 6:93–108.

MALAMOS, B., MOULOPOULOS, S., KOSTAMIS, P., BALKOURA, M., ANDREOPOULOS, A. and BINOPOULOS, D. (1965) The effect of digitalisation on the disappearance rate of tritiated digoxin from the blood. *Sonderband Strahlentherapie*, 60:310–6.

MANNER, G., BRODA, E. and KELLNER, G. (1957) Untersuchung der Proteinbildung durch Gewebe Kulturen mit Hilfe von Radiokohlenstoff. *Monatshefte Chem. Dtsch.*, 88:896–909.

MARTIN, E., BERKY, J., GODZESKY, C., MILLER, P., TOME, J. and STONE, R. W. (1953) Biosynthesis of penicillin in the presence of C^{14}. *J. Biol. Chem.*, 203:239.

MASOUREDIS, S. P. (1959) Behaviour of intravenously administered ^{131}I diphtheria toxin in the guinea pig. *J. Immunology*, 82:320–27.

MASOUREDIS, S. P. and BEECKMANS, M. L. (1955) Comparative behavior of I^{131} and C^{14} labeled albumin in plasma of man. *Proc. Soc. Exp. Biol. Med.*, 89:398.

MAURER, R., WENZEL, M. and KARLSON, P. (1964) Tritium labelling of natural products. *Nature, Lond.*, 202:896–8.

MAYBERRY, W. E., RALL, J. E., BERMAN, M. and BERTOLI, D. (1965) Kinetics of iodination III: iodination of *N*-acetyl-Tyrosine and *N*-acetyl 3-iodo 1-Tyrosine, studies in a pH-stat system. *Biochem.*, 4:1965–72.

MCAFEE, J. G., STERN, H. S., FUEGER, G. F., BAGGISH, M. S., HOLZMAN, G. B. and ZOLLE, L. (1964) ^{99m}Tc labeled serum albumin for scintillation scanning of the placenta. *J. Nucl. Med.*, 5:936.

MCCALL, M. S. and CAMP, M. F. (1961) A simple technique for prolonging the storage life of I^{131} labeled proteins and polymers. *J. Lab. Clin. Med.*, 58:772–5.

MCCALL, M. S., TIMM, D. L., EISENTRAUT, A. M. and UNGER, R. H. (1962) Preparation of high specific activity glucagon I^{131}. *J. Lab. Clin. Med.*, 59:351.

MCCOMB, A. J. (1964) The preparation of gibberellic acid—^{14}C. *J. Gen. Microbiol.*, 34:401–11.

MCFARLANE, A. S. (1956) Labelling of plasma proteins with radioactive iodine. *Biochem. J.*, 62:135.

MCFARLANE, A. S. (1958) Efficient trace labeling of proteins with iodine. *Nature, Lond.*, 182:53.

MCFARLANE, A. S. (1963a) *In vivo* behaviour of I^{131} fibrinogen. *J. Clin. Invest.*, 42:346–61.

MELICK, R. A., AURBACH, G. D. and POTTS, J. T. (1965) Distribution and half-life of ^{131}I labeled parathyroid hormone in the rat. *Endocrinol.*, **77**:198–202.

MENDENWALD, H. and HABERLAND, G. L. (1957) Synthese von ^{14}C markierter Salicyl-säure ($^{14}CO_2H$), Acetylsalicylsäure ($^{14}CO_2H$) und ($C^{14}COCH_3$), Salicylursäure ($^{14}CO.NH.CH_2.CO_2H$) und gentisinsäure ($^{14}CO_2H$). *Hoppe Zeyler's Z. Physiol. Chem.*, **306**:229–34.

MERCHANT, W. R., MASOUREDIS, S. P. and ELLENBOGEN, E. (1957) The effect of heat and pasteurization on albumin preparation in particular references to radioisotope labeled materials. *J. Clin. Invest.*, **36**:914.

MICHAEL, S. E. (1939) The precipitation of proteins with complex salts. *Biochem. J.*, **33**:924.

MILLER, J. M. (1960) A study of trypsin ^{131}I in rabbits. *Exp. Med. Surg.*, **18**:341–51.

MILLER, W. H., ANDERSON, G. W., MADISON, R. K. and SALLEY, D. J. (1944) Exchange reactions of diiodotyrosine. *Science*, **100**:340.

MISRA, A. L. and WOODS, L. A. (1960) Preparation of radiochemically pure tritium nuclear labelled morphine. *Nature, Lond.*, **185**:304–5.

MOHRING, D., GRAMLICH, F. and WIETHOFF, E. (1960) Zur Markierung von Alkoholdes-hydrogenase mit ^{35}S. *Naturwissenschaften*, **47**:160–5.

MORAVEK, J. and NEJEDLY, Z. (1960) Labelling of 6-mercaptopurine and 6-mercapto-purine riboside by an exchange reaction with elementary sulphur ^{35}S. *Chem. Ind., G.B.*, **19**:530–1.

MOSES, V. and CALVIN, M. (1949) Photosynthesis studied with tritiated water. *Biochem. Biophys. Acta*, **33**:297.

NAISMITH, W. E. F. (1958) The cross-linking of conarachin II with metal salts. *Arch. Biochem. Biophys.*, **73**:255–61.

NOYES, H. E., MCINTURF, C. R. and BLAHUTA, G. J. (1959) Studies on distribution of *Escherichia coli* endotoxin in mice. *Proc. Soc. Exp. Biol. Med.*, **100**:65–8.

NUMEROF, P. (1954) Biosynthesis of streptomycin. I: Studies with C^{14} labeled glycine and acetate. *J. Amer. Chem. Soc.*, **76**:1341.

OBER, R., FUSARI, S. A., COFFEY, G. L., GWYNN, G. W. and GLAZKO, A. J. (1962) Pre-paration of tritium labelled paromomycin (Humatin) by fermentation in a medium containing tritium water. *Nature*, **193**:1289.

ONCLEY, J. L. (1957) Interpretation of data obtained in studies with isotope labeled proteins of biological significance, chemical considerations. *Fed. Proc.* **16**(3), suppl. 1.

PEARSON, J. D. (1959) Preparation of ^{131}I labeled insulin. *Lancet*, **1**:967.

PERMUTT, M. A., PARKER, C. W. and UTIGER, R. D. (1966) Immunochemical studies with lysine-vasopressin. *Endocrinol.*, **78**:809–14.

PETTINGA, C. W. and RICE, C. N. (1952) Insulin fibril formation; application: the iso-lation of ^{35}S labeled insulin. *Fed. Proc.*, **11**:268.

PRESSMAN, D. and EISEN, H. N. (1950) The zone of localization of antibodies. V. *J. Immu-nol.*, **64**:273.

RABINOWITZ, J. L. (1959) The biosynthesis of radioactive 17 β oestradiol. IV: Substrate utilization by testicular homogenates. *Atompraxis*, **5**:98–100.

RACHELE, J. R., KUCHINSKAS, E. L., KNOLL, J. E. and EIDINOFF, M. L. (1959) Hydrogen isotope effects in the *in vivo* utilization of formate. *Arch. Biochem.*, **81**:55.

RAJAM, P. C. and JACKSON, A. L. (1960) Labeling of antibody against the Ehrlich ascites carcinoma with tritium. *J. Lab. Clin. Med.*, **55**:46.

REINER, L., KESTON, A. S. and GREEN, M. (1942) The absorption and distribution of insulin labeled with radioactive iodine. *Science*, **96**:362.

REICHLIN, M. (1966) Antibodies against cytochromes *c* from vertebrates. *J. Biol. Chem.*, **241**:251–3.

RITZ, N. D. and RUBIN, H. (1964) Use of chromium 51 tagged casein for the determination of proteolytic activity. *J. Lab. Clin. Med.*, **63**:344–54.

ROSA, U., PENNISI, F., SCASSELLATI, G., GIAGNONI, F. and GIORDANI, R. (1964) [131]I labeling of fibrinogen by constant current electrolysis. *Biochem. Biophys. Acta*, **86**: 519.

ROSA, U., SCASSELATI, G., PENNISI, F., AMBROSINO, F., LIBERATORI, J., FEDERIGHI, G., DONATO, L. and BIANCHI, R. (1965) Proteins radioiodination by an electrolytic technique. *Sonderband Strahlentherapie*, **60**:258–72.

ROSA, U., PENNISI, F., BIANCHI, R. and DONATO, L. (1967a) Chemical and biological effects of the iodination on human albumin. *Biochem. Biophys. Acta*, **133**:486–98.

ROSA, U., MASSAGLIA, A., PENNISI, G. and ROSSI, C. A. (1967b) Effect of the insulin iodination on the reactivity of the interchain—SS—bonds towards the sulphite. *Biochem. J.*, **103**:407–12.

ROSEN, C. G., EHRENBERG, L. and AHNSTRÖM, G. (1964) Tritium labelling of antibodies. *Nature, Lond.*, **204**:796.

ROWLAND, F. S. and NUMEROF, P. (1957) Radioactive labeling of reserpine by tritium recoil. *Int. J. Appl. Rad. Isotopes.*, **1**:246.

ROWLAND, F. S. and WOLFGANG, A. (1956) Tritium recoil labeling of organic compounds. *Nucleonics*, **14**(8):58.

SACHS, H. (1959) Vasopressin biosynthesis. *Biochem. Biophys. Acta*, **34**:572.

SAWAKI, Y., HUPPERT, M., BAILEY, J. W. and YAGI, Y. (1966) Patterns of human antibody reactions in coccidioidomycosis (demonstrated by radioimmunoelectrophoresis including the use of (I[131]) coccidioidin). *J. Bacteriol.*, **91**:422–7.

SCHMIDT, M. L. and WERNER, G. (1962) Radioaktive Markierung von Tropan–Alkaloïden III. Darstellung von ^{3}H Atropin und ^{3}H Norcocaïn. *Annalen der Chemie*, **656**:149–57.

SCHULTZE, B. (1957) Biological half lives of a single globulin fraction in rabbits. *Biochem. Z.*, **329**:144.

SCHULTZE, B. and HUGHES, W. L. (1965) Untersuchungen über den Abbauort von Eiweiss nach Injection von Cr 51 ribonuclease und Cr 51 Albuminen. *Sonderband Strahlentherapie*, **60**:287–94.

SCOTT, K. G., SMYTH, F. S., PENG, C. T., REILLY, W. A., STEVENSON, E. A. and CASTLE, J. N. (1965). Measurements of the plasma levels of tritiated labelled vitamin–D_3 in control and rachitic, cirrhotic and osteoporotic patients. *Sonderband Strahlentherapie*, **60**:317–24.

SEKIGUCHI, Y. and YOSHIKAWA, T. (1959) Enzymatic synthesis of C^{14} labeled thymidine. *J. Biochem. Jap.*, **46**:1505–11.

SMITH, M. V. and SACHS, H. (1961) Inactivation of arginin-vasopressin by rat kidney slices. *Biochem. J.*, **79**:663.

SONENBERG, M., KESTON, A. S. and MONEY, W. L. (1951a) Studies with labeled anterior pituitary preparations: adrenocorticotropin. *Endocrinology*, **48**:148.

SONENBERG, M., MONEY, W. L., KESTON, A. S., FITZGERALD, P. J. and GODWIN, J. T. (1951b) Localization of radioactivity after administration of labeled prolactine preparation to the female rat. *Endocrinology*, **49**:709.

SONENBERG, M., KESTON, A. S., MONEY, W. L. and RAWSON, R. W. (1952) Radioactive thyroptropic hormones preparations. *J. Clin. Endocrin.*, **12**:1269.

SONENBERG, M., KESTON, A. S. and MONEY, W. L. (1954) The distribution of radioactivity in the tissues of the rat after the administration of radioactive growth hormone preparation. *Endocrinology*, **55**:709.

SONENBERG, M. and MONEY, L. (1955) The fate and metabolism of anterior pituitary hormones. *Rec. Prog. Horm. Res.*, **II**:43.

STADIE, W. C., HAUGAARD, N. and VAUGHAN, M. (1952) Studies of insulin binding with isotopically labeled insulin. *J. Biol. Chem.* **199**:729.

STEINBERG, D., VAUGHAN, C. B., ANFINSEN, C. B. and GORRY, J. (1957) Preparation of tritiated proteins by the Wilzbach method. *Science*, **126**:447.

STEINFELD, J. L., PATON, R. R., FLICK, A. L., MILCH, R. A., BEACH, F. E. and TABERN, D. L. (1958) Distribution and degradation of human serumalbumin labelled with iodine 131 by different techniques. *J. Lab. Clin. Med.*, **51**:756.

STERLING, K. (1951) The turnover rate of serumalbumin in man measured by I¹³¹ tagged albumin. *J. Clin. Invest.*, **30**:1228–37.

STERN, H. S., ZOLLE, I. and McAFEE, J. G. (1965) Preparation of technetium labeled serum albumin (human). *Int. J. Appl. Rad. Isotopes*, **16**:283–8.

STERNLIEB, I., MORELL, A. G., TUCKER, W. D., GREENE, M. W. and SCHEINBERG, I. H. (1961) The incorporation of copper into coeruloplasmin *in vivo*. Studies with copper 64 and copper 67. *J. Clin. Invest.*, **40**:1834.

STRASSMAN, M. (1960). The biosynthesis of the essential aminoacids, arginine, lysine and valine by the yeast *torulopsis utilis*. *Dissert. Abstr.*, **21**:293.

THOMAS, A. W. and NORRIS, E. R. (1925) The "irregular series" in the precipitation of albumin. *J. Amer. Chem. Soc.*, **47**:501.

TSO, T. C. (1965) Biochemical studies on tobacco alkaloïds. VII: Biosynthesis of alkaloïds triply labeled with ¹⁴C, ³H and ¹⁵N. *Phytochemistry*, **5**:278–92.

ULLBERG, S. (1954) Studies on the distribution and fate of S³⁵ labelled benzylpenicillin in the body. *Acta Radiol.*, Suppl. 118.

VANDERHEIDEN, B. S. and BOSZORMENYI–NAGY, I. (1965) Preparation of ³²P labeled nucleotides. *Anal. Biochem.* **13**:496–504.

VAUGHAN, M. and ANFINSEN, C. B. (1954) Non uniform labeling of insulin and ribonuclease synthetized *in vitro*. *J. Biol. Chem.*, **211**:367.

VAUGHAN, M., ANFINSEN, C. B. and GORRY, J. (1957) Preparation of tritiated proteins by the wilzbach method. *Science*, **126**:447.

VOLWILER, W., GOLDSWORTHY, D., McMARTIN, M. P., WOOD, A. P., McKAY, T. R. and FREMONT SMITH, K. (1955) Biosynthetic determination with radioactive sulfur of turnover rates of various plasma proteins in normal and cirrhotic man. *J. Clin. Invest.*, **34**:1126.

VON HOLT, C., VON HOLT, L. and VOELKER, I. (1960) Labeling of insulin with tritium. *Biochem. Biophys. Acta*, **38**:88.

WALDMANN, T. A. (1961) Gastrointestinal protein loss demonstrated by Cr⁵¹-labelled albumin. *Lancet*, **2**:121–3.

WALDSCHANDT, M. (1958) Recherche sur l'albumine ³⁵S dans l'organisme. *Biochem. Z.*, **330**:400–10.

WALTER, H., HAUROWITZ, F., FLEISCHER, S., LIETZE, A., CHENG, H. F., TURNER, J. E. and FRIEDBERG, W. (1957) Metabolic fate of injected homologous serum proteins in rabbits. *J. Biol. Chem.* **224**:107.

WEGELIUS, O. (1960) The localization of radioactivity in the orbit and the thyroid gland after injection of S³⁵ labeled thyrotropin into the carotid artery of guinea-pigs. *Acta Med. Scand.*, **167**:65.

WEYGAND, F., FLOSS, H. G., MOTHES, U., GROGER, D. and MOTHES, K. (1964) Biosynthesis of the ergot alkaloïds: comparison of two possible intermediates. *Z. Naturforsch.*, **19b**:202–10.

WILZBACH, K. E. (1957) Tritium labeling by exposure of organic compounds to tritium gas. *J. Amer. Chem. Soc.*, **79**:1013.

WOODRUFF, N. H. and FOWLER, E. E. (1950) Biological synthesis of radioactive isotopes labeled compounds. *Nucleonics*, **7**:26–41.

WOOL, I. G., SCHARFF, R. and MAGES, N. (1961) *In vitro* synthesis of C¹⁴ corticotropin by isolated rat anterior pituitary. Effect of adrenalectomy. *Amer. J. Physiol.*, **201**:547.

WRIGHT, P. (1959) The effect of insulin antibodies on glucose uptake by the isolated rat diaphragm. *Biochem. J.*, **71**:633.

YALOW, R. S. and BERSON, S. A. (1957) Chemical and biological alterations induced by irradiation of I^{131} labeled human serumalbumin. *J. Clin. Invest.*, **36**:44.
YALOW, R. S. and BERSON, S. A. (1960). Immunoassay of endogenous plasma insulin in man. *J. Clin. Invest.*, **39**:1157.
ZEIG, G., DEVAY, J. E. and COSENS, G. R. (1958). On the biosynthesis of gibberellins by the use of C^{14} labeled substrates. *Plant Physiol.*, **33**, Suppl. 38.

CHAPTER 6

RADIATION DETECTION
AND MEASUREMENT

H. H. Ross

*Analytical Chemistry Division, Oak Ridge National
Laboratory,* Oak Ridge, Tennessee, U.S.A.*

IF RADIOTRACERS are to be used successfully in an experiment, an understanding of the principles and practical aspects of radiation detection is
essential. The proper selection and use of the radiation detector and
detector system may make the difference between a valid experiment or one
which is misleading or in error.

Radiation decay events cannot be detected easily or efficiently with
conventional chemical or physical instrumentation. Thus, over the past
30 years, a special technology has been developed for radiation detection
and measurement. Recently, this field has become quite sophisticated. In
this section are described those radiation-detection systems which are
believed to be the most important for biological investigations. Enough
information about these systems is presented to allow the scientist to select
intelligently the optimum instrument type for a given measurement. For
additional details, the reader is referred to the bibliography at the end of
the section.

It is important to note at the outset that all radiation detectors work on
the principle that a decay event eventually imparts energy to the electrons
in matter. This energy deposition may result from either a primary or
secondary process. In order to fully understand the mechanism of the
detection process, it will be necessary to review briefly the mode of radiation interactions with matter.

* Operated by the Union Carbide Corporation for the U.S. Atomic Energy Commission.

185

1. INTERACTIONS OF RADIATION WITH MATTER

All charged particulate radiation interacts with matter in essentially the same way. This interaction is primarily between the charged particles themselves and the electrons in the atoms of the absorbing matter. These interactions can raise the electrons in the absorbing material to excited states or completely ionize the absorber atoms thus creating primary ion pairs. Since charged-particle interactions are primarily with orbital electrons in the absorbing medium, the specific ionization (ion pairs/unit path length) of a charged particle is greater in high atomic number materials. Thus, lead is a better absorber than aluminum per unit thickness. In many cases of β^- absorption (electrons), the following equation is valid over a large portion of the absorption curve:

$$a_d = a_0 \, e^{-\mu d}, \tag{1}$$

where a_0 = measured activity of source without absorber; a_d = measured activity of source with absorber; μ = absorption coefficient of absorber material (cm^{-1}); and d = thickness of absorber material (cm).

Positrons, like β^-, are charged particles and react with orbital electrons in a similar manner. However, positrons participate in a somewhat unusual secondary interaction not associated with β^- interactions.

As a positron moves through an absorber losing energy in electron interactions, its energy becomes so small that it cannot escape an attracting electron. At this point an electron and positron combine and annihilate each other. Their combined mass is transformed into energy, and momentum is conserved by the emission of two photons in opposite directions, each of which has an energy of 0.511 MeV ($E_\gamma = 1/2 m_e c^2$).

The primary modes of interaction of photons with matter are quite different from that of particulate radiation; however, the ultimate secondary effects are usually the same. The three main modes of photon interaction are photoelectric interaction, Compton interaction, and pair production.

In the photoelectric effect, the photon is considered as interacting with the entire atom with the result that an orbital electron (usually from the K-shell) is ejected with an energy equal to that of the photon less the binding energy of the electron. The photoelectric effect is the major mode of interaction by photons of about 0.5 MeV or less in elements of high atomic weight. This is illustrated by the strong absorption of X-rays by lead. In elements of low atomic number the photoelectric effect is not significant.

The Compton effect is essentially an elastic collision between a free electron and a gamma photon. Energy and momentum are conserved and the incident photon gives up part of its energy to the electron which recoils at an angle to the direction of the original photon. The degraded photon undergoes further similar interactions and usually ends in a photoelectric event. The energy of the photon after a Compton interaction is determined by the angle between the incident and scattered photons and can be calculated by use of the equation:

$$hv' = \frac{hv}{1 + (hv/M_e c^2)\,(1 - \cos\theta)}, \tag{2}$$

where hv' = energy of the scattered photon; hv = energy of the incident photon; $M_e c^2$ = rest energy of the Compton electron; and θ = angle between incident and scattered photons.

Pair production occurs as a result of interaction between an incoming photon and the coulomb field surrounding the nucleus. In this process the photon energy is converted into a $\beta^- - \beta^+$ pair and thus requires an incident photon with at least 1.02 MeV of energy ($2\,M_e c^2$). However, more than this minimum amount of energy is usually required for the observation of significant pair production. Energy, momentum, and charge are conserved by the electron–positron pair and the nucleus in the encounter. Once the pair is formed, the electron and positron continue to interact as described under particulate radiation.

The absorption of photon radiation is almost exactly described by the equation

$$a = a_e\, c^{-\mu d}. \tag{3}$$

where the terms have the same meaning as those of Eq. (1). The numerical values of μ for many materials can be found in various compilations of nuclear data.

It is apparent from the above discussion that although decay energy may appear in a variety of ways, the end result is the formation of ion pairs in matter. The collection and utilization of these ion pairs is the basis for all radiation detection systems.

2. RADIATION DETECTORS

It is difficult to classify radiation detectors into a simple scheme because each has characteristics that may be modified by the manner in which it is used. Adjustment of operating parameters can often be used to achieve some specific mode of response. In the following discussions, detectors will be broadly grouped as gas, solid, liquid, or semiconductor detectors. The basic operating parameters are presented along with the advantages and disadvantages of the system. Typical experimental problems are used as examples.

2.1. GAS-FILLED DETECTORS

One of the oldest and most versatile class of radiation detectors is the gas-filled variety. It has the advantages of high sensitivity, simplicity, and stability. Also, the associated electronics for these detectors can often be austere and inexpensive. Gas-filled detectors can be used to detect virtually any type of decay product when properly designed.

Gas-filled detectors are generally intended to operate in one of three electrical modes. The particular operating mode selected depends on the

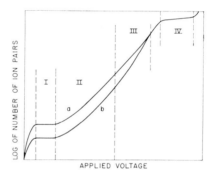

FIG. 1. Number of ion pairs collected versus applied voltage.

information required, the type of sample being investigated, the radiation involved, and physical requirements of the detection system. The criteria for selecting a particular operating mode will become obvious in the following discussion. Like all detectors, gas-filled units depend on the formation of ion-pairs in the bulk of the gas volume caused by the passage of ionizing radiation. Consider an enclosed gas-filled chamber containing two electrodes. A source of variable potential is connected to the electrodes in series with a fixed resistor. If a radioactive source is used to inject a constant number of charged particles into the gas volume, ionization of the gas will occur and the number of ion pairs collected can be measured as a function of the d.c. potential applied to the electrodes. In Fig. 1, data from such measurements are shown. Curves for two types of particles, *a* and *b*, with different specific ionization are presented. Because the ionizing ability of a charged particle depends on its charge density and energy, *a* and *b* may either represent different particle types or identical particles with different kinetic energies.

The important feature to note in Fig. 1 is that the slope of the curves changes a number of times. These slope changes, indicated as regions I—IV, reflect differences in the ion collection mechanisms operating as a function of applied potential. The operation of a gas-filled detector in one of the indicated regions determines the type of response that will be obtained.

2.2. IONIZATION CHAMBER

As the potential is increased from zero on a gas-filled detector, a point is soon reached where no increase in current is observed (region I). This region, the saturation region, defines a gas-filled detector operating as an ionization chamber. The range of voltage over which saturation occurs is dependent upon the spacing and geometry of the electrodes, the pressure and type of filling gas, and the characteristics of the ionization process in the gas.

The construction of ionization chambers (except for choice of insulator material) is not very critical. Almost any nonconducting filling gas can be used; ordinary dry air is quite suitable. Approximately 30 eV are necessary to produce an ion pair in a gas. This value is essentially independent of the energy and type of charged particle. The number of ion pairs generated at saturation will be equal to $NE/30$, where N is the number of charged particles in the chamber and E is the average energy lost by the particles. Thus, in general, for two particles a and b, different saturation values will be observed. If the particles from two samples are identical in type and energy, then the ratio of their saturation values will be equivalent to the ratio of the activity levels of the samples.

The saturation region is obtained with most gases with an applied potential of 100–300 V at s.t.p.

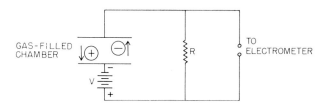

FIG. 2. Schematic diagram of a parallel-plate ionization chamber

However, except for very high radiation fields, the currents produced in ion chambers are quite small and require special measurement methods. The use of an electrometer (Fig. 2) is typical.

As noted above, ion chambers can be used to measure a wide variety of radiation types. The familiar *cutie pie* portable survey meter, which responds to α-, β-, γ-, and X-radiation, is simply an ionization chamber filled with air at atmospheric pressure.

2.3. GAS MULTIPLICATION PROCESSES

If the applied potential on an ionization chamber is increased beyond the saturation level, one observes a rapid increase in the number of ion pairs collected. Since essentially all the ion pairs that are formed in primary interactions are collected at saturation, it is obvious that a new source of ionization appears above the saturation potential. This effect is called multiplication. At high levels of electric field density (between the electrodes), primary ions are accelerated toward the electrodes. In this process they gain sufficient energy to cause secondary ionization of the gas molecules and, hence, the number of ion pairs collected is increased. In region II, the number of pairs collected is proportional to the original ionization; thus the curve for particle *a* maintains a constant value above the curve for particle *b*. Region II is termed the proportional region. A further increase in potential causes the chamber to operate in the region of limited proportionality (III). Finally, in region IV, the Geiger–Mueller (G–M) region, an essentially constant number of ion pairs is collected, regardless of the primary ionization type or energy. The G–M region, characterized by an avalanche process caused by a single ionizing event, represents the highest chamber potential that can be successfully used for radiation detection.

2.4. PROPORTIONAL AND GEIGER–MUELLER COUNTERS

Since the operation of both proportional and G–M counters is based on the production of secondary ionization events in the gas, they will be described together. The following discussion considers the assay of radioactive samples emitting positive or negative electrons or alpha particles.

In counters that utilize a multiplication process, it is necessary to prevent the emission of secondary electrons from the negative electrode caused by bombardment with positive ions of the gas. This secondary emission may initiate new multiplicative processes and give rise to a continuous discharge. The technique to accomplish this is termed quenching. It may be performed by electronic means but is accomplished more usually by the addition of small amounts of a polyatomic gas, such as CH_4 or a halogen, to the counter gas. Collisions of the ions of the counter gas with the polyatomic molecules will cause transfer of the ionic charge to the latter. These will then dissipate most of their energy at the cathode by dissociation. Because of this dissociation, an organic quencher is eventually used up. The operating life of such a counter is approximately 10^9 counts. Halogen atoms tend to recombine after dissociation; halogen quenched tubes have an operating life in excess of 10^{10} counts.

Once the multiplication process has been initiated, the counter is insensitive to new ionizing particles until the discharge has been quenched. The time required for the counter to become sensitive again is called the resolving time τ. During a given measurement, the fraction of time that the counter is insensitive is equal to $R\tau$, where R is the observed counting rate. In G–M counters, where the avalanche is distributed throughout the counter volume, the resolving time is quite long (≈ 300 μsec). For proportional counters, the recovery time is very rapid because the multiplication process is localized to a small volume in the vicinity of the cathode. The resolving time of modern electronic equipment is faster than either the G–M or proportional counter; thus the count-rate limit is a function of the type of counter used for a particular measurement.

The operating range of the proportional counter or G–M counter is determined by observing the rate of change of counting rate with increase in applied voltage. A region, called the plateau, is soon attained in which all of the charged particles produce pulses large enough to be detected. Thus, on the plateau, the counting rate is practically constant. The plateau for a proportional counter has a small slope, $<0.2\%$ per 100 V, over a range of several hundred volts. In contrast to this, the plateaux obtained with G–M tubes have appreciable slopes. For an organically quenched tube, the plateau is about 200–300 V long with a slope of some 1–2$\%$ per 100 V; for a halogen-quenched tube, the plateau is about 100–200 V long, and has a slope of some 3–4$\%$ per 100 V. The obvious advantage of operating on the plateau is that small voltage fluctuations, which are unavoidable, will not affect the counting data.

Because their response is proportional to the energy of the primary ionizing particle, proportional counters may be used for pulse height analysis. In this application, components of different energy are resolved from one another. This differential analysis may be applied to low-energy photons as well as to charged particles. In a proportional counter, 6 cm long and filled with argon at 1 atm, an X-ray of 6 keV will be completely absorbed. The properties of the absorbing gas are important for the detection of photons because the probability of a photoelectric event occurring is proportional to $\sim Z^4$, where Z is the atomic number of the gas. Thus filling the counter with xenon will enable one to detect X-rays of higher energy than is possible in an argon counter. The sensitive dependence of photon detection on the Z of the absorbing gas also is important in the reduction of the background due to X-rays and gamma rays in a counter that is used mainly for detecting β particles. The photon detection efficiency for a typical end-window counter filled with P-10 gas (90% Ar, 10% CH_4) is of the order of 1–2%; changing the filling gas to a mixture of helium and CH_4 effectively reduces photon detection to zero. When increased efficiency is desired, the counter can be filled with gas at greater than atmospheric pressure. In this case, however, special mechanical designs are required.

It should be noted at this point that proportional counters, because of their proportional response to incident radiation, their low resolving time, long life, and approximately horizontal plateaux, offer distinct advantages over G–M counters. However, amplification of the proportional counter output is necessary. Various electronic units, consisting of a preamplifier, a linear amplifier, a scaler with decade scaling strips, a regulated high-voltage supply, a mechanical register, and a timer are commercially available for use with proportional counter tubes.

Both proportional and G–M counters can be fabricated in a number of configurations. The most convenient type to use is one that has a thin window to admit the radiation to be measured (Fig. 3). The window may be made of mica or thin plastic. Usually, for quantitative measurements, a shelf assembly is used to obtain reproducible counting geometries. In some cases, it may be desirable to place the radioactive source directly inside the counting chamber (a windowless counter). This type of counting configuration eliminates the absorption problem of the window when counting "soft" radiation.

As mentioned previously, gas-filled counters have a number of operational and stability advantages. Unfortunately, however, they have a number of disadvantages to biological investigators.

A cursory review of the literature shows that perhaps 75% of the biological investigations carried out with radiotracers utilize the isotopes ^{14}C and ^3H. Both of these isotopes are soft beta emitters. When using gas-filled counters with ^{14}C or ^3H, particular attention must be paid to absorption of the emitted radiation by counter windows or the sample itself. Also, reproducible counting geometries are often difficult to attain. It is only under certain conditions that these difficulties can be overcome. Thus for routine biological assays, gas-filled counters are limited to the measurement of hard beta emitters (^{32}P) or semi-quantitative survey applications.

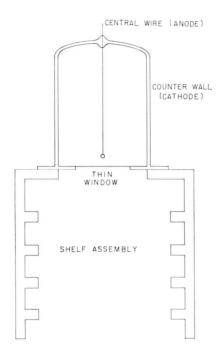

CENTRAL WIRE (ANODE)

COUNTER WALL (CATHODE)

THIN WINDOW

SHELF ASSEMBLY

FIG. 3. G–M counter and shelf assembly

3. LIQUID SCINTILLATION COUNTING

In order to meet the demands of an efficient and sensitive counting method for soft beta radiation, suitable for precise, routine measurements, the technique of liquid scintillation counting was developed. This technique circumvents many of the problems associated with gas-filled detectors and is considered by many to be the method of choice for ^{14}C and ^{3}H assays. The liquid scintillation process has also been used effectively for α, β^+, X-ray, and low energy gamma determinations.

Both the physical basis of the liquid scintillation process and its arts and recipes are much too complex to discuss in great detail in this article.

However, an attempt will be made to present the basic information required to understand the method and permit the reader to consult more extensive discussions for advanced details or specific applications.

3.1. MECHANISM OF THE LIQUID SCINTILLATION PROCESS

The exact mechanism of the liquid scintillation process is still not generally agreed upon by experts in spite of the fact that the phenomenon has been known and used for over 20 years. It is possible, however, to present a reaction scheme that is probably close to correct in its gross aspect. This scheme is important, not only to get a general feeling for the complexity of a liquid scintillator system, but also serves to indicate some of the problems associated with the technique.

A typical liquid scintillator consists of three components: a solvent (L), a primary solute (S_1), and a secondary solute (S_2). The primary solute is sometimes called the primary fluor; the secondary solute the secondary fluor or wave shifter. If a small amount of ^{14}C is introduced *into* the scintillation mixture, a complex series of energy transfer reaction occurs.

$$^{14}C \rightarrow {}^{14}N + \beta^-. \tag{A}$$

Reaction (A) shows the standard decay mode for ^{14}C. Since the decay occurs directly in solution, the released β^- particle is surrounded by an "atmosphere" of solvent molecules.

$$\beta^- + L_1 \rightarrow L_1^*. \tag{B}$$

The particle interacts with a solvent molecule and raises it to an excited state.

$$L_1^* + Ln \rightarrow L_1 + Ln^*. \tag{C}$$

The excitation energy of L_1 can be transferred to other solvent molecules. Reaction (C) may occur several times, each time a solvent molecule is raised to an excited state. However, it is not necessary for reaction (C) to occur at all; L_1^* may proceed directly to (D).

$$Ln^* + S_1 \rightarrow Ln + S_1^*. \tag{D}$$

Eventually an excited solvent molecule reacts with S_1 and raises it to an excited state.

$$S_1^* \rightarrow S_1 + \text{photon (1)}. \tag{E}$$

S_1^* decays to the ground state with the emission of photon (1). Photons emitted by primary solutes are often in the ultraviolet, a spectral region that is sometimes difficult to observe efficiently.

$$\text{photon (1)} + S_2 \rightarrow S_2^*. \tag{F}$$
$$S_2^* \rightarrow S_2 + \text{photon (2).} \tag{G}$$

A secondary solute is used as a wave shifter. The lower energy photon (2), emitted in the visible region, is detected and counted.

For a single given β^- particle, usually more than one product photon is observed. That is, a photon burst occurs for each decay event. The actual number of photons produced is a function of the overall conversion efficiency of scintillator system and the incident beta energy. For all practical

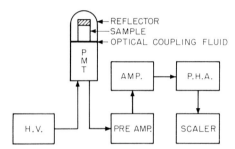

FIG. 4. A basic liquid scintillation counter.

purposes, the conversion efficiency is constant. Thus, the higher the energy of an incident particle the larger is the resulting photon burst; a liquid scintillator system exhibits proportional response.

Although the scintillating mechanism is complex, the time observed from the emission of the β^- particle to the final photon emission is extremely fast. The resolving time for liquid systems is more a function of the electronics used for detection rather than the liquid system itself.

3.2. INSTRUMENTATION FOR LIQUID SCINTILLATION COUNTING

The photon burst that results from the scintillation process is quite feeble, even when caused by an energetic particle. This problem is even more acute when measurements are made with the very soft emitter, ^3H. Therefore, efficient detection of the scintillation process necessitates a sensitive and stable electronic system.

The basic instrumentation for a simple liquid scintillation counter is shown in Fig. 4. The sample to be assayed is dissolved in the liquid scintillator. This container is optically coupled to the face of a photo-multiplier tube (PMT) using a material such as silicone fluid. A reflector is placed over the sample that also can act as a light shield. Light pulses emitted by the sample are converted to electrical pulses by the PMT. These signals are increased by the pre-amplifier and main amplifier. The amplifier output is fed to a pulse-height analyzer (PHA) and then to a scaler. Of course, to determine count rates, a timer is used.

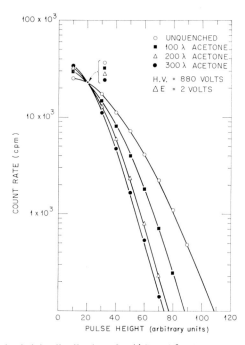

Fɪɢ. 5. Pulse-height distributions for ^{14}C and ^{3}H in a liquid scintillator.

The PHA is usually adjusted to have a fairly large "window", in order to maximize the counting efficiency. The lower discriminator is placed just above the majority of electronic and PMT background noise. The upper discriminator may be adjusted in a variety of ways. Oftentimes, it is not necessary to use an upper discriminator at all; the system is allowed to count all pulses above the threshold setting of the lower level. The typical response for ^{14}C in a liquid scintillator is shown in Fig. 5 as the curve of open circles. At small pulse heights the count-rate is high. As the pulse height increases, a steady decrease in count-rate is observed. Electronic and

PMT background noise in the example is probably excessive below a pulse height of 10 or 15. This, then, is where the lower discriminator would be set. The upper discriminator level might be placed at 120 to increase the counting efficiency.

Since liquid scintillation spectrometry is a proportional counting technique, it is possible to assay two or more isotopes in the same sample. Tritium (^{3}H) has a maximum beta energy of 18 keV while that for ^{14}C is 155 keV. The relative pulse-height distributions of these two isotopes is shown in Fig. 6. If the lower discriminator is set as indicated in the figure, and the upper level is set at infinity, approximately 60% of the ^{14}C can be counted without interference from ^{3}H. Next, the upper and lower discriminator levels are adjusted to bracket the tritium distribution. In this case, the lower pulse-height contribution of ^{14}C will interfere with the

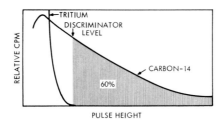

FIG. 6. Relative pulse heights for C^{14} and H^3 in a liquid scintillator.

tritium measurement. It is possible to correct for this interference, however, and obtain a useful value for tritium activity.

The elementary electronic system shown in Fig. 4 is seldom used in modern liquid scintillation counters. It suffers from having high backgrounds, significant drift rates, relatively poor figure of merit, and no immunity to phosphorescense effects occurring in the sample. A more advanced system is illustrated in Fig. 7. This design, introduced in 1954, enjoyed a wide popularity and was probably responsible for the rapid acceptance of the liquid scintillation technique by biological investigators.

In this system, two photomultiplier tubes are used to observe the sample simultaneously. One tube is used for pulse-height analysis; the second is used as a coincidence gate. Random noise pulses occurring in each arm oɩ the system will not be recorded on the scaler unless they happened to occur in coincidence. Thus, a significant reduction in background is realized. Of course, a light pulse occurring in the sample is seen by both tubes in coincidence and the analyzer tube output is routed to the scalers. The preamplifiers, phototubes, and sample are housed in a refrigerated compartment ($\approx 0°$), to reduce thermal noise effects to a practical minimum. In addition to reduced backgrounds, increased figure of merit and freedom from phosphorescence effects are advantages of the system.

The past 5 years have seen the development of even more elaborate electronic systems. Their description is beyond the scope of this discussion and readers are referred to the manufacturers' literature in this field.

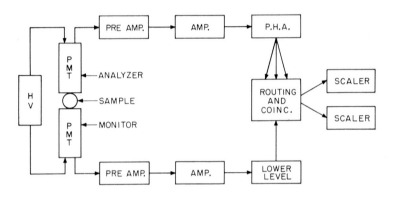

FIG. 7. Coincidence electronics for liquid scintillation counting.

3.3. LIQUID SCINTILLATOR SOLVENTS

It is usually not difficult to select a solvent system for liquid scintillation counting, since the choice is quite limited. Most important is that the solvent transfer energy efficiently from the location of beta ray emission to a scintillator molecule. Other important criteria for solvent selection are:

(1) It must transmit the emitted photons to the detector without degradation (optical transparency).
(2) It must not freeze at the working temperature of the system.
(3) It is desirable to be able to dissolve the sample in the solvent itself or with the help of solubilizing agents.

A large number of solvent systems have been examined; however, aromatic hydrocarbons have been found to be the most successful. Toluene is the most widely used solvent and it is usually considered the standard to which other solvent systems are compared. Other aromatic compounds have been used with equal success but offer no significant advantages and they are not usually available in a sufficiently pure grade. Toluene is an ideal solvent for lipids, steroids, fatty acids, and hydrocarbons. The usefulness of toluene has been extended, by using additives which facilitate solution of such materials as tissue homogenates, amino acids, proteins, body fluids, and $^{14}CO_2$.

Probably the main disadvantage of the toluene system is the inability to dissolve any significant amount of water. To overcome this important objection, mixtures of other solvents with toluene or completely different solvent systems are used. Many exotic recipes are available for specific applications. However, only four or five of these modifications are in widespread use. Table 1 shows the relative counting efficiencies of various pure solvent systems. The limited listing testifies to the short supply of useful solvents.

TABLE 1. RELATIVE COUNTING EFFICIENCY OF VARIOUS SOLVENTS TESTED WITH 0.3% DIPHENYLOXAZOLE AS PHOSPHOR

Compound	Freezing point	Relative efficiency
Toluene	$-95°$	100
Methoxybenzene (anisole)	$-37°$	100
Xylene (reagent, mixed isomers)	$-20°$	97
1,3-dimethoxybenzene	$-52°$	81
N-heptane	$-90°$	70
1,4-dioxane	$+12°$	70
1,2-dimethoxyethane (ethylene glycol dimethyl ether)	$-71°$	60
Benzyl alcohol	$-15°$	38
Diethyleneglycol diethyl ether (Diethyl Carbitol)	$-44°$	32
Acetone	$-94°$	12
Tetrahydropyran	$-81°$	6
Ethyl ether	$-116°$	4
1,1-diethoxyethane	$-100°$	3
Tetrahydrofuran	$-65°$	2
1,3-dioxolane	$-10°$	0
Ethyl alcohol	$-114°$	0
Diethylene glycol monoethyl ether	$-10°$	0
Ethylene glycol monomethyl ether	$-85°$	0
Diethylene glycol	$-8°$	0
Ethylene glycol	$-13°$	0
2,5-diethoxytetrahydrofuran	$-27°$	0
N,N-dimethylformamide	$-61°$	0
Diethyl amine	$-49°$	0
N-methyl morpholine	$-66°$	0
2-ethylhexanoic acid	$-117°$	0

3.4. PRIMARY SCINTILLATORS

The choice of scintillators for liquid counting is even less than that for solvents. The characteristics of a good scintillator are:

(1) It should produce light efficiently when acted upon by beta or alpha radiation. The light output should have a wave length to which the photomultiplier is responsive.

(2) A good scintillator should be sufficiently soluble at the working temperature of the system to permit incorporation of an adequate quantity.

(3) It should be chemically stable for reasonable time periods.

(4) It should be economical at the required concentration.

Although many scintillators have been described since liquid scintillation counting became practical in the early 1950's, few are important today. The first significant scintillator was *p*-terphenyl. It performs well and is inexpensive and stable. Unfortunately, it has limited solubility at the reduced temperatures employed in most counters. The emission maximum of *p*-terphenyl (3406 Å) has a shorter wavelength than the response maximum (4200–4400 Å) of most glass-faced photomultiplier tubes used commercially. However, if quartz-faced photomultipliers are employed, *p*-terphenyl is more closely matched to their response maxima (about 3600 Å).

Under ideal conditions, a good liquid scintillator emits about 7 photons per keV of β-ray energy absorbed in the scintillator. Therefore, for a low-energy beta emitter such as tritium, the most energetic β-rays cause emission of perhaps 130 photons while about half of the events produce less than 45 photons. This light output is distributed over the fluorescence emission spectrum of the scintillator. When *p*-terphenyl is used to measure energetic beta emitters such as ^{14}C, enough photons are produced at the longer wavelengths so that adequate counting results are obtained even though the scintillator is not well matched to the photomultiplier response. However, when measuring a low-energy β-ray emitter such as tritium, where total light output is considerably less, *p*-terphenyl is not an adequate scintillator by itself.

In routine liquid scintillation counting of biological samples, *p*-terphenyl has not been used because of solubility limitations.

The next important scintillator, 2,5-diphenyloxazole (PPO), is still the most widely used type. This efficient photon emitter is quite soluble in all solvents of interest, even at temperatures below 0°. It is stable and relatively inexpensive; the fluorescence maximum is 3800 Å. Therefore, it is better than *p*-terphenyl for matching to photomultiplier response. While PPO is a poorer light emitter than *p*-terphenyl, its performance is almost identical because of its fluorescence maximum at longer wavelengths. By itself, PPO is very adequate for ^{14}C and the more energetic betas.

For ^3H counting, it is advantageous to add a secondary scintillator in order to produce a fluorescence spectrum having an emission maximum of longer wavelength. However, this has been true largely because of the response characteristics of the glass-faced photomultiplier tubes in common use. Now that most commercial liquid scintillation counters contain quartz-faced photomultipliers which have a peak response at short wavelengths, PPO, by itself, should be quite adequate for routine ^3H determination.

Attempts have been made to prepare scintillators more effective than *p*-terphenyl and PPO, but no other material has come into widespread use. 2-phenyl-5-biphenyl-oxadiazole (PBD) is among the best ever described and is superior to PPO. However, for optimum performance, it is used at twice the concentration of PPO.

Since the price of PBD is rather more than that of PPO, its application has been somewhat restricted.

3.5. SECONDARY SCINTILLATORS

The two most important secondary scintillators are 1,4-bis-2-(5-phenyloxazolyl)-benzene (POPOP) and 1,4-bis-2-(4-methyl-5-phenyloxazolyl)-benzene (dimethyl POPOP). These are similar in cost and show little difference in performance. Since Dimethyl POPOP is more soluble, it is preferred in applications where it may be advantageous to use relatively larger quantities than are considered normal. The only other prominent secondary scintillator has been α-naphthyl-phenyloxazole (α-NPO), but this material has been abandoned in general because of inferior performance.

Table 2 is a list of typical liquid scintillator counting solutions. The table is representative but certainly not exhaustive. Mixtures 1, 7, and 8 are particularly recommended.

3.6. SAMPLE PREPARATION

Once the liquid scintillation mixture has been prepared, the last remaining problem is that of introducing the radioactive sample. The most satisfactory and trivial answer to the problem is simply to dissolve the sample

TABLE 2. TYPICAL LIQUID SCINTILLATION COUNTING SOLUTIONS

Solvent		Solute		Figure of merit
Principal	Intermediate	Primary (g/l)	Secondary (mg/l)	
Toluene		PPO(3–5)	POPOP (50–100) Dimethyl POPOP (100–200)	
Toluene		p-Terphenyl(5)	Dimethyl POPOP(500)	
Toluene + Ethanol		PPO	POPOP	4.6–16.2
Xylene (5 parts) + Dioxane (5 parts) Ethanol (3 parts)	Naphthalene (80 g/l)	PPO(5)	α-NPO(50)	32.3
Xylene (1 part) + Dioxane (3 parts) Cellosolve (3 parts)	Naphthalene (80 g/l)	PPO(10)	POPOP(500)	∼60
Dioxane		p-Terphenyl(5)		11.4
Dioxane	Naphthalene (20–120 g/l)	PPO(4–10)	POPOP(50–300)	100–200
Dioxane + Methanol, Ethylene Glycol	Naphthalene (60 g/l)	PPO(4)	POPOP(200)	100
Dioxane (6 parts) + 1,2-Dimethoxy-ethane (1 part)	Anisole (1 part)	PPO(12)	POPOP(50)	50–80
1,2-Dimethoxy-ethane	Naphthalene (100 g/l)	PPO(7)	POPOP(300)	40–45
Dioxane (2 parts) + 1,2-Dimethoxy-ethane (1 part)	Naphthalene (100 g/l)	PPO(7)	POPOP(300)	75–80

directly in the scintillation mixture. As noted, toluene is an ideal solvent for many types of samples. A wide variety of nonpolar solids, liquids, and under certain conditions, gases, can be examined directly in toluene. For aqueous samples, dioxane-naphthalene mixtures are popular.

The liquid scintillation method would be severely limited if it were restricted only to substances soluble in toluene or one of the other solvent mixtures indicated in Table 2. Indeed, many samples of interest are completely insoluble in conventional liquid counting mixtures. Fortunately, many methods are available which either permit the dissolution of normally insoluble materials or provide an efficient means of counting insoluble substances.

The most widely used solubilizing agent is the hydroxide of Hyamine 10-X (Registered Trademark of Rohm & Haas, Inc.) referred to as Hyamine for convenience. This material gained prominence when it was shown to form a toluene-soluble carbonate, permitting simplified $^{14}CO_2$ determinations. Further work with Hyamine has greatly extended its range of application. Samples of amino acids and proteins in Hyamine count efficiently and reproducibly, for example. The highly alkaline nature of the material makes it useful in a host of digestion processes including samples of whole blood, and muscle, bone, liver, brain, and kidney tissues. Residual color from biological samples is sometimes eliminated by the addition of a trace of hydrogen peroxide.

Small quantities of Hyamine have also been advantageous in preventing precipitation of biological materials from aqueous solution when such solution is added to a dioxane-naphthalene solvent mixture. Solubility of many materials such as amino acids, pyrimidines, carbohydrates, and phosphate esters is facilitated. Counting efficiencies for comparable quantities of aqueous solutions of tritiated compounds are as high in this solvent mixture as in toluene–PPO–POPOP when similar quantities of Hyamine are used to effect solution.

Hyamine, though convenient to use, is a severe quenching agent. Use the minimum quantity which will achieve the degree of solubilization and avoid any excess above this amount.

There are many other techniques available for solubilizing samples for liquid scintillation counting. Among these are other reagents such as ethyl alcohol, 2-phenylethylamine, monoethylamine, and alcoholic and aqueous potassium hydroxide. Also, combustion and oxidation methods can be applied. The reader should consult the bibliography for details on these applications.

For insoluble samples, the technique of suspension counting is used. Here, the sample is mechanically dispersed in the liquid scintillation mixture, with or without the aid of a suspending medium. Paper strips or discs, thin-layer chromatography substrates, and a wide variety of other insoluble solids can be counted. For immiscible liquids, emulsions with the liquid scintillator can be formed.

The most popular suspension agent is Cab-O-Sil, an aerated silica with an average particle size of 15 μ and a surface area of 200 m^2/g. Cab-O-Sil suspensions are fluid enough to pour easily but viscous enough to hold a stable suspension. A sample is prepared merely by shaking the insoluble material with a scintillating mixture containing about 4% by weight of Cab-O-Sil in a vial. Such a suspension can hold up to 2 g of sample in a 20 ml volume.

3.7. QUENCHING

Quenching is a term used to describe a reduced conversion or collection efficiency of the scintillator system. One remembers that the mechanism of the scintillation process is complex, requiring a number of energy transfer steps. Any effect that interferes with these transfer steps will reduce light output and hence, quench the system. Quenching occurs primarily in two ways. That which arises from processes not involving photon transfer is termed fluorescence quenching. For example, aldehydes and ketones will compete with solutes for the excitation energy of the solvent and reduce the number of excited solute molecules in the system; alternatively, strong acids often affect the chemical state of the solutes and induce a radiationless transition from the excited state. In both of these cases, the number of photons generated by a given particle is reduced; a shift in the pulse height spectrum is observed. Figure 5 shows the fluorescence quenching effect of acetone in a toluene solvent system.

The second effect, color quenching, is an interference of the photon transmission properties of the liquid. Photons are produced in both the ultraviolet and visible spectral regions. Any sample that absorbs strongly in these regions will interfere with reaction F or with the collection of the secondary photons by the PMT. Thus, quinones that absorb in the near ultraviolet, or biological pigments, that absorb in the visible, are strong color quenchers.

A recognition of the quenching properties of samples is one of the most important facets of liquid scintillation technology. The basic rule of sample preparation is to use the most convenient method that will introduce the minimum amount of quenching.

No matter how carefully one prepares liquid scintillation samples, some degree of quenching occurs in all but ideal systems. Quantitative results can be obtained with virtually any sample, however, by using one of the many available techniques for quench correction. The most generally accepted "standard" technique for correction is the internal standard. Here, the count-rate of a sample to be assayed is compared to the count-rate of a standard added together with the sample. The technique is best illustrated by an example.

The disintegration rate of ^{14}C is to be determined in a sample of liver tissue. The sample is first solubilized in Hyamine and the resulting solution is added to a liquid scintillator. The final counting mixture has a slight residual color due to bio-pigments from the liver tissue. Quenching effects can be expected from both the color and the presence of Hyamine in the system. The sample is placed in a liquid scintillation spectrometer and counted for one minute. The observed count-rate of the sample (R_X) is 754 cpm, using predetermined instrument settings. However, because of the unknown degree of quenching, the 754 cpm has little quantitative meaning.

A sample of ^{14}C labeled toluene having a known disintegration rate $(D_S = 50,000$ dpm) is used as a standard. It is assumed that the addition of a small amount of this standard to the sample will not introduce additional quenching into the system (an assumption known to be valid). A 0.10 ml aliquot of the standard is added directly to the sample; this corresponds to $0.10 \times 50,000$ or 5000 dpm of ^{14}C (D'_S). The sample is recounted giving an observed count rate (R_{XS}) of 2624 cpm. The additional observed counts due to the added standard equals:

$$R_{XS} - R_X = 2624 - 754 = 1870 \text{ cpm}.$$

The counting efficiency of the standard and, thus, the whole sample is:

$$(R_{XS} - R_X)/D_S'; \frac{1870}{5000} = 0.374.$$

The disintegration rate of the sample is therefore:

$$\frac{R_X}{(R_{XS} - R_X)/D'_S}; \frac{754}{0.374} = 2016 \text{ dpm}. \tag{4}$$

where R_X = count-rate of sample; R_{XS} = count-rate of sample plus standard; and D'_S = disintegration rate of standard in sample.

The internal standard method corrects for both color and fluorescence quenching. Of course, the standard must match the sample type; if a tritium sample is to be assayed, a tritium internal standard must be used.

Many commercial instruments use a variation of the internal standard technique for quench correction. This method, the external standard, lends itself to automatic programmed operation. It substitutes for the internal standard a gamma or X-ray emitting source that is brought in close proximity to the sample for the second count. A correction procedure similar to the internal standard is used. This technique yields very acceptable results but is not considered as accurate as the internal standard. It is, however, much more convenient, faster, and avoids radioactive contamination of the original sample. Other quenching correction procedures include the channel ratios method, the balanced quenching technique, and extrapolation procedures.

4. SOLID RADIATION DETECTORS

The radiation detectors discussed in the previous sections have been concerned mainly with the detection of charged particulate radiation. Nonetheless, many isotopes of interest in biological and pharmacological investigations are photon emitters. Efficient and sensitive detection of photon emission is best achieved using solid radiation detectors. The most widely used solid detector is the scintillation crystal. This component, combined with a photomultiplier tube and associated electronics, forms the basis of a complete X or γ-ray detection system.

4.1. THE SCINTILLATION PROCESS

Scintillations produced in fluorescent materials by impinging radiation is one of the oldest methods of detecting radioactive decay. The spinthariscope, used for detecting alpha particles on a ZnS(Ag) fluorescent screen, is now a familiar science toy for children. Decay events are observed as tiny flashes of visible light on the screen.

In modern instrumentation, sodium iodide crystals activated with thallium (NaI(Tl)) are the most versatile scintillators for photon detection. The luminescence of NaI is primarily due to the presence of the thallium activator at a concentration of about 1%. A photon interacts with the crystal by means of all three of the interaction mechanisms: photoelectric absorption, Compton scattering, and pair production. Each of these processes results in the production of high-energy electrons. It is these electrons that cause the luminescence. The electrons in slowing down lose their energy principally to electrons in the crystal lattice. This results in crystal excitation and ionization. The energy deposited in the crystal then migrates to an activator or luminescent center; transition to the ground state occurs by the emission of a light photon or by a nonradiative transition that causes thermal de-excitation of the crystal.

When the scintillation process is used for determining the amount of energy given up by the radiation, each step must transfer a proportional amount of the original radiation energy and must have a constant conversion efficiency for all radiation energies. For a given type of exciting radiation, this efficiency is practically constant. Thus, the light output from a NaI(Tl) detector is essentially a linear function of the exciting energy over a wide range (a proportional detector). The nonlinearity is negligible for all but a few specialized cases in which an energy calibration curve should be established.

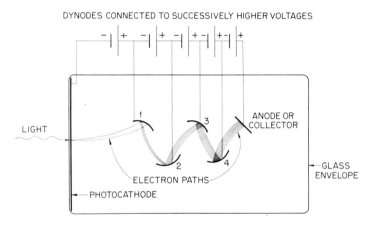

FIG. 8. A simplified representation of a photomultiplier tube.

Other crystal detectors include lithium iodide activated with europium used for neutron spectrometry and cesium iodide, when it is advantageous to use small detectors for photon analysis. Solid organic crystals and scintillating plastics have also been utilized.

The visible light emitted by the crystal is usually detected by a photomultiplier tube. This device consists of a photocathode, several metal plates called dynodes, and a collector plate called the anode. Incoming light flashes interact with the photocathode and eject electrons from the photocathode surface. This is shown in Fig. 8.

These electrons are drawn to the first dynode (labeled 1 in the diagram), where they strike hard enough to knock out two or more electrons. This multiplication process continues down the entire string of dynodes (as many as ten or more) so that a very large resultant shower of electrons appears at the anode. The voltage pulses derived from the PMT are feeble, but an electronic amplifier boosts these voltage pulses up to a level that will trigger a scaling circuit. The photocathode and dynode voltages in the photomultiplier are obtained from a precision high-voltage supply. The spectral sensitivity of conventional PMTs is well matched to the emission of NaI(Tl). The mechanism presented here is the same as that utilized for PMTs used in liquid scintillation counting.

Gain shift phenomena that occur during the course of measurements offer serious limitations to the application of instrumental techniques in gamma spectral resolution. Though these shifts may arise from several sources, the most usual cause is change in the photomultiplier tube. Such shifts occur as a consequence of high counting rates, and in a given detector might involve photopeak drifts of many channels. These gain changes show a hysteresis effect, so that the gain does not immediately return to its normal value when the high activity sample is replaced with a low one. Detectors with guaranteed stability to counting rate effects are now available commercially. Several gain shift correction devices have been proposed.

4.2. COUNTERS

The exponential nature of the attenuation of gamma rays by matter indicates that a portion of the gamma photons from a monoenergetic source reaching the detector will pass completely through the crystal. Others will transfer only part of their energy to the crystal and still others will be completely absorbed. Thus, although the photon beam incident on the crystal is monoenergetic, the output from the crystal-PMT combination exhibits a broad intensity distribution of output pulses. A typical pulse-height distribution (gamma-ray spectrum) of ^{137}Cs, obtained with a NaI(Tl) crystal, is shown in Fig. 9. The major peak at 662 keV is due to the total or photoelectric absorption of the gamma ray and is called the *photopeak*. The remainder of the pulse-height distribution is due to incomplete absorption of the total gamma-ray energy and is called the *Compton distribution*. Obviously, the gamma rays that pass through the crystal with no interaction cause no pulse-height distribution. The spread of pulses within the photopeak, which approximates a Gaussian distribution, stems from several sources. Among these are the process of conversion of energy of ionizing radiation into photons in the scintillator, electron emission from the photocathode, and electron multiplication at the dynodes. A term called resolution has been used to describe the quality of a scintillation detector. Resolution is defined as the photopeak full width at one-half maximum height (X in Fig. 9) divided by the pulse height (or energy) at the photopeak center (Y in Fig. 9). Thus

$$\text{resolution (in } \%) = \frac{X}{Y} \times 100. \qquad (5)$$

NaI(Tl) detectors are limited to an intrinsic crystal resolution that is approximately 6% for the 0.662-MeV gamma ray of [137]Cs. Carefully selected tube-crystal combinations have given resolutions for ^{137}Cs as low

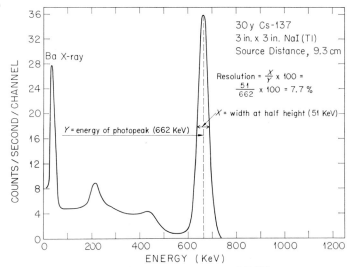

FIG. 9. Gamma-ray spectrum of Cs[137].

as 6.4%. Detector resolution varies approximately inversely as the square root of the gamma-ray energy. A convenient rule-of-thumb is that detector resolution $= kE^{-1/2}$. A typical 3-in. by 3-in. detector with a 7.7% resolution for ^{137}Cs gamma rays might show resolutions of 16% for 0.081 MeV and 5.5% for 1.85 MeV gamma rays. Crystal size *per se* has little correlation with resolution.

Scintillation detectors of 3-in. by 3-in. size are commercially available with 7.5% or better resolution for ^{137}Cs gamma rays, and with guaranteed stability of $<1\%$ drift per day at 1000 cps.

A NaI scintillation counting system may be operated in several modes. One of the most common modes has been described as Geiger-tube substitute scintillation counting. Figure 10 shows a block diagram of this type of counter. These counters are used in applications where the gross gamma counting rate from a sample is all the information that is required. An example of this type of counter is the *well*-type scintillation counter used for most tracer experiments with gamma-emitting nuclides. A typical system will have the high-voltage supply, amplifier, and scaler in one chassis. Auxiliary lead shielding is usually required around the nominal 2 in. shield supplied with most systems to get background counting rates down to 200 cpm. High-energy betas have a relatively high efficiency in these well detectors, therefore it is usually desirable to have an aluminum liner inserted in the well detector to reduce the beta contribution. Radioactive samples in test tubes are then placed in the aluminum liner. The

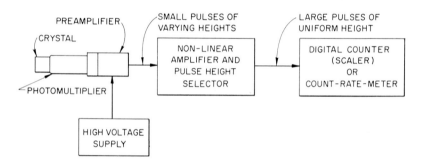

FIG. 10. Geiger-tube-substitute scintillation counter.

amplifier is usually set at the factory to a level just above the noise level of the photomultiplier. To check day-to-day variations in the overall system, it is necessary to count a long-lived standard prepared so as to give reproducible geometry in the well detector. Standards are usually made of natural uranium or other long-lived radionuclides. Natural uranium is a useful standard because of the wide range of energies of gamma rays in the spectrum of the aged uranium.

5. SPECTROMETERS

A scintillation spectrometer differs from the Geiger-substitute counter in that a linear amplifier is used and additional discriminatory circuits are added. The output pulses from the photomultiplier, which are proportional to the energy of the incident gamma ray, are feeble pulses and must be amplified before they will cause the other circuits to function properly. These are amplified with a linear amplifier. Hence, there is linearity in the entire system from the crystal interaction through the preamplifier and linear amplifier. The electronic components of a scintillation spectrometer are termed pulse-height analyzers or kick-sorters. The energy increments into which a pulse-height distribution is divided are called channels.

5.1. SINGLE-CHANNEL ANALYZERS

The simplest pulse-height analyzer consists of a single channel, whereas those more sophisticated may have thousands of channels. Single-channel analyzers have a linear amplifier, two pulse-height selectors, and an anti-coincidence network, as shown in Fig. 11.

As stated previously, pulse-height analyzer may be used to examine pulses from a scintillation detector and sort these voltage pulses into groups corresponding to the original gamma-ray distribution reaching the detector. By setting the proper high-voltage value on the photomultiplier tube and a suitable gain on the amplifier, a single-channel analyzer can be adjusted so that the entire gamma-ray spectrum will fall within the usual 1000 divisions on the pulse-height dial (lower pulse-height selector). The window opening (ΔE) covers that portion of the spectrum between the lower and upper pulse-height selectors. Voltage pulses smaller than those selected by the lower pulse-height selector will be rejected by this discriminator. Pulses large enough to exceed both the lower and upper pulse-height selectors are rejected by the anticoincidence circuit. Therefore, only those voltage pulses that occur *between* the values given by the lower and upper pulse-height selectors will reach the scaler or rate meter. By varying the position of the window opening in relation to a lower pulse height just above electronic noise, the entire pulse-height distribution from a scintillation detector can be determined.

The major limitation of the single-channel analyzer is the long time required to determine the one hundred or so data points necessary to define a gamma-ray spectrum. Single-channel analyzers with a motorized pulse-height selector are available that greatly facilitate the collection of data from a gamma-ray distribution. The output from such an analyzer is fed to a rate meter and then to a strip-chart recorder where a permanent record of the gamma spectrum is obtained. A motorized or scanning single-channel analyzer requires a counting period of approximately 15 min to cover an entire spectrum from a moderately intense source of radioactivity with correspondingly greater times required for weaker sources.

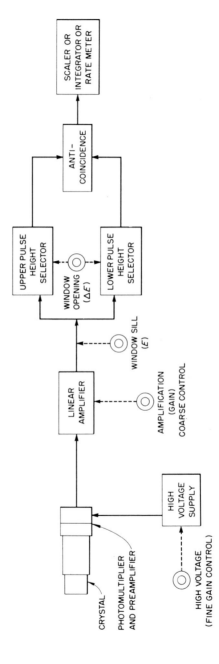

FIG. 11. Diagram of typical single-channel analyzer.

Solid state versions of the single-channel analyzer are available, and are to be preferred over vacuum tube types.

For the smaller laboratory, this equipment is recommended over a gross counting system. If the size of the program is large enough, then a multichannel spectrometer system should be considered.

5.2. MULTICHANNEL ANALYZERS

To reduce the time necessary to accumulate gamma-ray spectrum data, analyzers with a greater number of channels were perfected. There is not only a great increase in speed and convenience when all the data points for a spectrum are accumulated in a single counting interval, but there is improvement in precision of data due to minimization of instrumental drifts. A 20-channel analyzer built up on the principle of 20 single-channel analyzers stacked together was an early successful version of a multi-channel instrument. The major disadvantage of this instrument was the slow read-out and relatively small number of channels. Each of the 20 channels had a scaler and mechanical register or glow-tube register that had to be read out and recorded manually.

Utilizing digital computer techniques for data storage and an analog-to-digital converter, which converts pulse heights to a train of pulses, electronic engineers developed a new type of multichannel analyzer which has revolutionized the fields of gamma-ray spectrometry. The original vacuum-tube designs have now given way to completely transistorized versions with large numbers of channels and many read-out modes.

6. SEMICONDUCTOR DETECTORS

A semiconductor is a material that exhibits electrical properties between those of an insulator and those of a conductor. The conductivity of a typical semiconducting material at room temperature is about 10^3–10^{-6} mho-cm; for insulators, the value is about 10^{-12} mho-cm, whereas for a conductor, it is about 10^6 mho-cm. Because of the intrinsic conduction phenomenon, a semi-conductor has the property that its conductivity increases as the temperature is raised. A conductor displays just the opposite behavior; its conductivity decreases with increasing temperature.

In addition to the intrinsic mode of conduction, a semiconductor exhibits impurity conduction, caused by the presence of impurity atoms in the crystal lattice. Thus, in a semiconductor made of quadrivalent germanium or silicon, pentavalent impurity atoms such as phosphorus, arsenic, or antimony act as electron donors. The material is an *n*-type or electron excess semiconductor, because the extra valence electrons are the carriers of charge. If, instead, trivalent impurity atoms such as aluminum, gallium, or indium are introduced into the crystal lattice, the material will be a *p*-type or electron defect semiconductor.

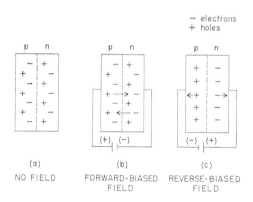

FIG. 12. A semiconductor *p–n* junction.

A semiconductor crystal of *p*-type material, into which a small amount of electron donor has been diffused, contains a *p–n*-junction. As is seen in Fig. 12(a), the electrons and holes diffuse in the material so that the *p*-type region carries a net negative charge, and the *n*-type region, a net positive charge. In the vicinity of the *p–n*-junction, the diffusion of electrons from the *n*-region has filled all the acceptor sites and left the donor sites empty; a depletion layer has been formed. If an electric field is applied to the semiconductor, such that the *p*-type region is at a positive potential with respect to the *n*-region, as in Fig. 12(b), electrons and holes will flow across the junction; electrons toward the anode and holes toward the cathode. If the electric field is reversed, as in Fig. 12(c), so that the *p*-region is at a negative potential with respect to the *n*-region, the flow of current will stop. That is, since the *p*-type region does not contain excess electrons, there will not be a flow of electrons toward the *n*-region; therefore the semiconductor acts as a rectifier. The reverse-biased field then just serves to increase the extent of the depletion layer.

A high electric-field intensity can thus be established in the depletion layer of the semiconductor. This layer acts analogously to a gas-filled ionization chamber in the detection of charged particles. A charged particle passing through the depletion layer produces ion pairs (electrons and holes) that are rapidly collected at the electrodes because of the high-electric field intensity. Moreover, the solid semiconductor radiation

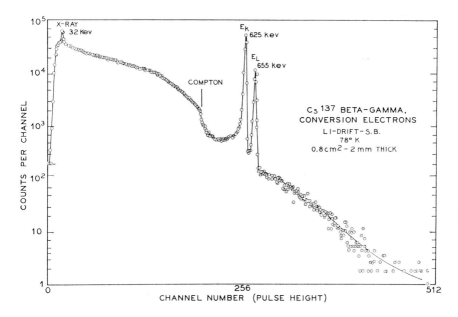

Fig. 13. Gamma-ray spectrum of Cs^{137} taken with a semiconductor detector.

detector possesses several advantages with respect to a gas-filled counter: (1) its higher stopping power makes possible the fabrication of very small detectors, (2) a lower input voltage is required than for gas-filled counting tubes, and (3) the energy necessary to produce an ion pair is much lower, 3.5 eV in silicon as compared to ~ 30 eV in a gas. Thus, for a particle at a given energy, many more ion pairs are formed and collected in the semi-conductor, which results in much higher resolution. It should be noted that depletion layers have also been produced in ion-drifted and surface barrier detectors.

The spectrum of ^{137}Cs obtained with a lithium-drifted semiconductor detector is shown in Fig. 13. Here, the K- and L-conversion electrons from the 0.662 MeV gamma ray are resolved from the continuous spectra of the

216 *Radionuclides in Pharmacology*

0.51 MeV and 1.18 MeV beta particles. In addition to beta-particle detection, semiconductor detectors have been used successfully in the counting of X-rays, alpha particles, and fission fragments.

The resolution of ^{137}Cs in Fig. 12 should be compared with that of Fig. 9. The obviously higher resolution using the semiconductor detector can be an important advantage in some applications.

The semiconductor radiation detector is relatively new and has not yet had appreciable application to biological tracer experiments. However, it is likely that they will supersede other detectors in certain applications for both charged particle and photon counting.

REFERENCES

(A) BOOKS, REVIEWS AND MONOGRAPHS

BELL, C. G. and HAYES, F. N. (eds.). (1958) *Liquid Scintillation Counting.* Pergamon Press, New York, U.S.A.
BIRKS, J. B. (1964) *The Theory and Practice of Scintillation Counting.* Pergamon Press, New York, U.S.A.
CROUTHAMEL, C. E. (ed.). (1960) *Applied Gamma-ray Spectrometry.* Pergamon Press, New York, U.S.A.
DEARNALEY, G. and NORTHROP, D. C. (1964) *Semiconductor Counters for Nuclear Radiations.* John Wiley, New York, U.S.A.
PRICE, W. J. (1958) *Nuclear Radiation Detection.* McGraw-Hill, New York, U.S.A.
STEINBERG, E. P. (1961) Counting methods for the assay of radioactive samples, in *Nuclear Instrumentation and Methods.* John Wiley, New York, U.S.A., pp. 306–66.

(B) ORIGINAL PAPERS

BERNSTEIN, W. and BALLENTINE, R. (1950) Gas phase counting of low energy beta-emitters. *Rev. Sci. Instr.,* 21:158–62.
BLAU, M. and DREYFUS, B. (1945) Multiplier photo-tube in radioactive measurements. *Rev. Sci. Instr.,* 16:245–8.
BORKOWSKI, C. J. (1949) Instruments for measuring radioactivity. *Anal. Chem.,* 21:348–52.
BOUSQUET, A. G. (1949) Counting rate meters versus scalers. *Nucleonics,* 4(2): 67–76.
BROWN, S. C. (1948a, b, c) Theory and operation of Geiger-Muller counters. I: The discharge mechanisms. *Nucleonics,* 2(2): 10–22. II: Counters for specific purposes, *ibid.,* 3:50–64. III: The circuits, *ibid.,* 3(6): 46–61.
EIDINOFF, M. L. (1950) Measurement of radiocarbon as carbon dioxide inside Geiger-Muller counters. *Anal. Chem.,* 22:529–34.
HARDWICK, E. R. and MCMILLAN, W. G. (1957) Study of the scintillation process. *J. Chem. Phys.,* 26:1463–70.
HAYES, F. N., ROGERS, B. S. and LANGHAM, W. H. (1956) Counting suspensions in liquid scintillators. *Nucleonics,* 14(3): 48–51.
JORDAN, W. H. and BELL, P. R. (1949) Scintillation counters. *Nucleonics,* 5(4): 30–41.
LIBBY, W. F. (1947) Measurement of radioactive tracers, particularly C^{14}, S^{35}, T, and other long-lived low-energy activities. *Anal. Chem.,* 19:2–6.

LOEVINGER, R. and BERMAN, M. (1951) Efficiency criteria in radioactivity counting. *Nucleonics*, **9** (1): 26–39.

SANGSTER, R. C. and IRVINE, JR., J. W. (1956) Study of organic scintillators. *J. Chem. Phys.*, **24**:670–715.

SWANK, R. K. (1954) Recent advances in theory of scintillation phosphors. *Nucleonics*, **12** (3): 14–19.

SWANK, R. K. (1954) Nuclear particle detection (Characteristics of scintillators). *Ann. Rev. Nucl. Sci.*, **4**:111–40.

WILLIAMS, D. L., HAYES, F. N., KANDEL, R. J. and ROGERS, W. H. (1956) Preparation of C^{14} standard for liquid scintillation counter. *Nucleonics*, **14** (1): 62–4.

Subsection II

POLYVALENT RADIOPHARMACOLOGICAL METHODS

CHAPTER 7

AUTORADIOGRAPHY IN PHARMACOLOGY

Sven Ullberg, Lars Hammarström, and Lars-Erik Appelgren

Department of Pharmacology, Royal Veterinary College,
Stockholm, Sweden

MOST pharmacological methods aim at recording the effects of drugs on the organs or their interference with biochemical reactions. But important information concerning the mechanism of drug action and toxicity may also be obtained by following the drug itself by studying its distribution and fate in the body.

The procedure which has been used most in studies of the distribution of drugs and other substances of pharmacological interest is taking of samples of body liquids or organs and determining the concentration by some chemical, physical, or biological assay method. The use of radio-isotope techniques in such investigations is gradually increasing. Labeled substances are injected and the concentration in removed samples is measured by liquid scintillation or Geiger counting, for example.

The most obvious advantage of autoradiography compared with a technique based on the quantitative assay of removed organ pieces is that it allows a more precise localization of the drugs in the tissue.

Many investigators therefore start by selecting a number of tissue pieces which they believe to be of special interest and use autoradiography to reveal the distribution pattern within these tissue specimens.

A serious limitation of a technique based on preselection of certain tissue pieces is that it does not favor the making of unexpected findings, e.g. an unforeseen specific localization which may give a new idea of the mode of action of the investigated substance.

If instead a distribution study is begun with whole-body autoradiography (Ullberg, 1954, 1958), a general view of the distribution of practically all tissues of the body can be obtained and the information gleaned is also rather detailed.

Certain tissues which seem to be of special interest according to the whole-body autoradiograms can then be chosen for more detailed localization on the cellular and subcellular level.

In whole-body autoradiography the most common procedure is for a series of mice to be injected intravenously with a labeled compound. Each animal receives a single dose. After various intervals the mice are rapidly deep-frozen and sagittal microtome sections are taken on different levels through the whole frozen bodies. The sections are freeze-dried and pressed against a photographic film. After exposure, the section and film are separated and the pattern of the drug distribution will appear on the developed film. The sections may be stained and mounted under cover glass, or they may be used in their unstained state as references for the interpretation of the autoradiograms.

If about 20 sections are taken on different levels, most tissues and fluids of the body can be studied, including endocrine organs, the different tissues of the eye, teeth and paradental tissues, skin, bone marrow, and joints. The labeled compound in tissue fluids is studied *in situ*. On an autoradiogram of a pregnant female the isotope concentration can be compared in the maternal and fetal tissues.

In the whole-body autoradiograms a labeled substance is usually found to specifically localize in certain sites. Specimens from such areas, or other ones that seem to be of special interest, can be selected for more detailed localization in the light microscope. In some cases it is also possible to combine autoradiography and electron microscopy for still more accurate intracellular localization.

In light microscopy autoradiography the section and photographic emulsion are permanently combined before the exposure. The developed grains in the emulsions are then related to the morphological details of the section.

In electron microscopy autoradiography the principle is the same, with the exception that an ultrathin section is used and this is covered with an emulsion containing only a monolayer of silver bromide grains. After exposure and development, the silver grains appear as electron-dense short spirals in the electron microscope.

1. THE SOLUBILITY OF DRUGS

A technical problem with autoradiography in pharmacology is that most drugs are in a soluble state in the tissues. They are therefore easily dissolved out or dislocated if one uses customary histological techniques: chemical fixation, decalcification, stretching of sections on water, and so on.

In the whole-body autoradiographic technique developed in our laboratory all contact of the tissues with chemicals is avoided, as the animals are frozen before sectioning, and the microtome knife cuts directly through the frozen body. The rapid freezing of the animal also permits short interval studies, e.g. 1 min after intravenous injection.

In light microscopy autoradiography, migration of the labeled compound during tissue preparation and sectioning is prevented either by having the tissue specimen cryostat sectioned, or freeze-dried and embedded in paraffin wax (provided the paraffin wax does not dissolve the labeled substance). The dry sections are then permanently attached to a nuclear plate, which may be made adhesive by pretreatment with a glycerol–ethanol solution. In this way contact with water is avoided while the section is combined with the photographic emulsion.

In electron microscopy autoradiography some of the obstacles relating to work with soluble substances are surmounted, but the method is still generally restricted to investigations of substances that are firmly bound in the tissues.

2. ISOTOPES AND LABELED COMPOUNDS

The main radioisotopes used in autoradiography with drugs are ^{14}C and ^3H (tritium), since most compounds of pharmacological interest are organic and can therefore be labeled with either ^{14}C or ^3H or both. Tritium has the advantage that it gives better resolution owing to the very weak radiation energy of the emitted beta-particles (with consequent short range in the section and photographic emulsion, and relatively small spread of the autoradiographic image). Another advantage of tritium is that it is easier to get tritiated than ^{14}C labeled substances of high specific activity and tritiated compounds are generally less expensive. (The half-life of tritium is 12.3 years compared to 5700 years for ^{14}C.)

On the other hand tritiated compounds are sometimes less reliable with respect to radiochemical purity, and the risk of exchange reactions of the label. Isotope effects have also been observed with tritiated substances. Another disadvantage of tritiated compounds is the low sensitivity in whole-body autoradiography, which is due to the small penetration depth in section and emulsion. (The energy of ^3H is 18 keV compared to 155 keV for ^{14}C: its mean track length in a nuclear emulsion is about 2.5 μ, and for ^{14}C about 100 μ (Rogers, 1967).) For sections in the 20 μ range, a dose (in μci) about 50–100 times larger is needed for work with ^3H than for ^{14}C. With increased section thickness this difference is still more accentuated.

Another problem in whole-body autoradiography with tritium is that the contrast is low in the autoradiographic picture. These inconveniences of ^{3}H decrease with thinner specimens and emulsions; and in electron microscopy autoradiography tritium is also to be preferred to ^{14}C from the sensitivity viewpoint. In our laboratory we prefer to use both a ^{14}C-labeled and a tritiated preparation of a substance, and then predominantly to use the ^{14}C-labeled preparation in whole-body autoradiography, and the ^{3}H-labeled one in microautoradiography.

Another radioisotope that is very suitable for autoradiography is ^{35}S, which is similar to ^{14}C as far as radiation properties are concerned, except for its shorter half-life (87 days). In work with ^{35}S-labeled substances one is not restricted by expense to the use of small experimental animals to the same extent as with ^{14}C investigations.

A radioisotope that from the economical viewpoint can be used still more unrestrictedly is ^{131}I. In work with radioiodine, however, ^{125}I is often to be preferred, because it has a longer half-life and gives better resolution. ^{125}I has thus proved to be well suited for electron microscopy autoradiography, where its very short-ranged extranuclear electrons give good resolution (see Fig. 21, Appelgren *et al.*, 1963; Forberg *et al.*, 1964).

Other isotopes of interest in biological autoradiography are calcium-45, iron-59, iron-55, phosphorus-32 (and phosphorus-33, which is in progress), sodium 22, cobalts-57, -58, and -60, and chlorine-36.

It may be mentioned that it has proved possible to work with isotopes as short-lived as ^{18}F (half-life < 2 hr), both in whole-body and in light microscopy autoradiography (Ericsson and Ullberg, 1958; Ericsson *et al.*, 1960).

The position in the molecule of the radioactive atom(s) is of importance in investigating substances that are split in the body. In such investigations it may be an advantage to have access to two differently labeled preparations of the same substance with the radioactive atom in different sites in the molecule. An example of such a case is given in the application part of the present paper (see Fig. 15).

3. SOME PROBLEMS IN AUTORADIOGRAPHY

It may sometimes be difficult or expensive to get a labeled compound with the desired properties. However, the situation is rapidly improving with regard to access to radioactive isotopes and intermediate components for synthesis of the final products, and in progress in labeling technique.

For pharmacologists it is also important that drug companies are to an increasing extent synthesizing labeled drugs.

It should be remembered that in autoradiography it is just the radioactive atom in the molecule that is registered. This may be regarded as a disadvantage in that metabolized drugs are also registered although they may be biologically inactive. Conjugated substances and labeled fragments of the molecule also show up on the autoradiograms together with the unchanged drug.

But by combining different radioisotope techniques it may be possible to carry out very detailed drug metabolism studies. For example, autoradiography may be combined with a microseparation method (e.g. thin-layer chromatography), and the radioactive spots may be located by using a photographic film or a pulse counter, preferably a scanning device. Whole-body autoradiograms are of great help in selecting the proper tissue pieces for the separation work; these may actually be cut out from thick whole-body sections.

It is also possible to treat some whole-body sections with a solvent before the autoradiographic exposure. This may be done if either the unchanged drug or a major metabolite is selectively soluble in a specific solvent. Neighboring sections can be used, and some of them can be treated with solvents and others left alone. The identity of the substance that is dissolved out can be checked by radiochromatography.

However, the problem caused in autoradiography by the presence of metabolites in the tissues should not be exaggerated. There is generally much less labeled metabolites in the tissues where the substance acts than in the excretory organs.

In whole-body autoradiography a specific localization is often obtained while the metabolization is negligible (e.g. 5 min after intravenous injection), and in some cases the radioactive substance is bound for a long time to its target sites, and remains there when it has left the rest of the body.

4. AUTORADIOGRAPHIC TECHNIQUES

An extensive monography on autoradiographic techniques has been recently presented by Rogers (1967). We shall discuss autoradiographic techniques for use in pharmacology under three main headings:

(1) Whole-body autoradiography.
(2) Light microscopy autoradiography.
(3) Electron microscopy autoradiography.

R.I.P.—I

4.1. WHOLE-BODY AUTORADIOGRAPHY

As experimental animals, adult mice are most frequently used. Each substance to be investigated is mostly injected into a number of mice which are killed after various intervals, the first one 1–5 min after injection, and the last one after 4 or more days. If the placental transfer and fetal distribution is of interest, a series of pregnant mice may be used together with a series of adult male mice.

Other animals that have been sectioned with good results are rats, young cats and monkeys, and newborn dogs and pigs.

The most common route of administration is intravenous injection. Our arrangement for intravenous injection of mice can be seen in Fig. 1(a). The labeled compound is administered in a tail vein. The amount of liquid injected is generally 0.2 ml. Substances that are not water soluble may be dissolved in other solvents, e.g. ethanol, polyethylene glycol, or dimethyl-sulfoxide. For toxicity reasons only small amounts of these solvents can be injected.

The amount of radioactive substance that is used for ^{14}C-labeled compounds is generally 5–10 mcCi per mouse. For tritiated compounds a dose about 100 times larger is required.

After various intervals the animals are anesthetized and rapidly frozen. In connection with being frozen the animals are mounted on large specially made microtome stages (Fig. 1(b), (c)). A metal frame is placed around the stage. The bottom of the basin thus formed is covered with a semiliquid mixture of carboxy-methyl cellulose (CMC) and water. The mouse is placed on this layer and additional CMC-mixture is poured until the mouse is covered.

The entire unit of stage, frame, mouse, and CMC-mixture is then im-

FIG. 1. (a) Injection of a labeled substance into a tail vein of a mouse. The mouse is kept in a transparent plastic cage which allows observation during injection. There is a polyethylene tubing between the syringe and needle. (b) Equipment for embedding. The anesthetized mouse is placed on a large microtome stage where it will be covered with a semiliquid mixture of water and carboxymethyl cellulose (CMC), which after freezing firmly fixes the mouse on the stage. In order to keep the CMC in position before and during freezing the stage is equipped with a frame which is removed after freezing. (c) Freezing of the CMC embedded mouse in hexane cooled with dry ice ($-75°$). (d) The frozen specimen mounted on the microtome after removal of the frame. Some sagittal sections have been taken. (e) "Tape sectioning" of the frozen specimen. A piece of Scotch tape is applied to the upper surface of the block. When cutting, the section comes off attached to the tape. (f) The sections are put on plastic frames and freeze-dried, after which they are brought to room temperature and labeled with radioactive india ink. (g) During the autoradiographic exposure the tape carrying the section is pressed against an X-ray film between two paper clips. To even the pressure soft paper is used as an intervening layer. (h) After exposure the sections are removed from the X-ray films and the films are developed.

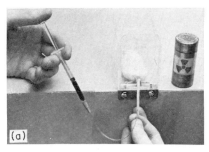

(a)

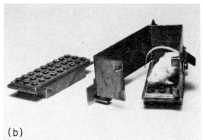

(b)

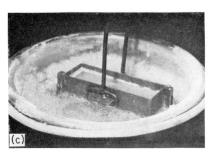

(c)

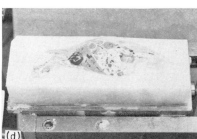

(d)

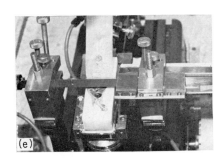

(e)

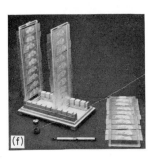

(f)

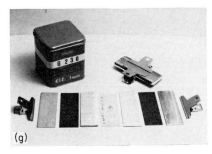

(g)

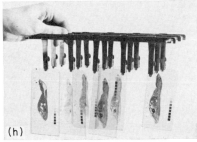

(h)

mersed into hexane saturated with solid carbon-dioxide (temperature about $-75°$). After about 10 min the stage is withdrawn from the cold hexane and the frame is removed. The mouse is now firmly mounted on the stage in a square block of CMC-reinforced ice. To add to the stability of the block the surface of the stage is supplied with a large number of screws (Fig. 1(b)).

The microtome used for sectioning the whole frozen animal is placed in a large freezer kept at $-20°$. A large sledge microtome is used, e.g. Leitz 1300 or Jung type K. The microtome sledge can for convenience be driven by a motor or maneuvered with a pedal.

The microtome knife cuts sagittally through the frozen tissues, including bone and teeth. The sections are discarded until a level is reached where interesting tissues appear on the surface of the block.

In order to get intact sections "Scotch" tape (Minnesota Mining and Manufacturing Co., No. 810) is then applied to the surface of the block with a brush before a final section is taken. The knife cuts under the tape and the section is thus from the beginning attached to the tape.

The section thickness is generally kept at 20 μ. Whole 5 μ sections and occasionally 2 μ sections can also be obtained. Some thicker (e.g. 100 μ) sections are generally also taken; these can be used to get some less detailed autoradiograms with short exposure time (for isotopes except ^3H).

The sections are dried in the freezer, or preferably in a freeze room, and brought to room temperature. Data such as the name of injected substance, time between injection and killing of the animal, and section thickness, are marked on each tape carrying a section with "radioactive india ink" (Fig. 1(f)).

The dried sections are pressed against film in simple presses which are put in light-tight boxes (Fig. 1(g)). The exposure can be made in room temperature, but the section quality is better preserved if the boxes are placed in a cold room or a freeze room.

The films used are roentgen films, for all isotopes except ^3H. For tritium we use nuclear plates, e.g. Ilford G 5.

A common exposure time with 20 μ sections is 3–4 weeks.

After exposure the film and section are separated and the film is developed, fixed, and rinsed.

To facilitate examination a comparison with a stained section is often helpful. The sections can be stained and mounted under cover glass without being removed from the tape. If Canada balsam or the ethanol-soluble mounting medium Euparal® is present on both sides of the tape plus section, no disturbing light refraction from the tape will appear.

Quantitative data concerning the activity in different tissues can be obtained either by impulse counting of punched pieces from the "tape sections" or by densitometry of the autoradiograms. A good reference for the densitometric readings is a stepwedge containing the particular isotope in uniform concentration steps, put beside the section during the auto-radiographic exposure (Berlin and Ullberg, 1963).

Two other methods for whole-body autoradiography which also allow the study of water-soluble substances have been published.

In one of these (Pellerin, 1957), frozen mice are milled with a cutler down to a level at which interesting organs appear. The film is then pressed against the flat surface of the hemi-sectioned mouse for exposure, which is performed in a Dewar flask containing liquid nitrogen. Additional auto-radiograms can be made by milling away more material.

In the second method (Kalberer, 1966) the distribution in rats of an injected substance is studied by sawing sections 2 mm thick through the frozen animals, and then pressing the sections against film in a cold box.

4.2. LIGHT MICROSCOPY AUTORADIOGRAPHY

The most common methods for light microscopy autoradiography are based on a permanent combination of the histological section and the photographic emulsion. After the exposure the section and emulsion are passed together through photographic processing and staining. They are then mounted under cover glass and finally examined together in the microscope, when the developed silver grains in the emulsion are related to the morphological details of the section.

However, most methods that have been described for permanently com-bining section and emulsion do not pay regard to the risk of dislocating water-soluble substances. Such methods are, for example, dipping a section in liquid emulsion (Joftes and Warren, 1955; Kopriwa and Leblond, 1962), or the application of a wet stripping film (Doniach and Pelc, 1950). In autoradiography with soluble substances the contact with water or other solvents has to be avoided in all the different preparation steps until exposure is completed.

4.2.1. *Histologic procedure*

The most common way to avoid relocation during tissue preservation is to freeze the tissue specimen in isopentane or propane cooled with liquid nitrogen.

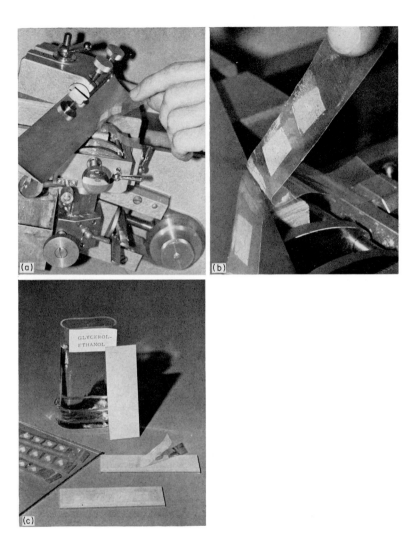

FIG. 2. (a) The sectioning of a freeze dried paraffin-embedded tissue with the aid of a tape, which is pressed onto the surface of the paraffin-block. When cutting the sections come off adhering to the tape. (b) Detail showing the sections on the tape. The sections are flat and the usual stretching on water of paraffin sections can thus be avoided. (c) Dry-mounting. In the dark room the tape with the adhering sections is gently pressed against a glycerol-treated nuclear plate. The glycerol is applied to the emulsion by dipping the nuclear emulsion plate in an ethanol solution of glycerol. After dipping, the plate is left in a vertical position for some minutes to let the ethanol evaporate. The glycerol is absorbed by the gelatin of the emulsion, which makes the surface sticky.

There are then two main alternative methods. One is to mount the freshly frozen tissue on a microtome placed in a cryostat, and take sections at a temperature of $-20°$ to $-70°$; the other is to freeze-dry and embed the tissue in some embedding medium, and then section at room temperature.

Cryostat sectioning is the most reliable of these methods because embedding media are avoided. However, freeze-drying and embedding generally give a better morphology and offer the advantage that an embedded block can be stored. In our experience substances that are not fat-soluble are not dislocated if treated by freeze-drying and subsequent embedding in paraffin wax. In work with fat-soluble substances a water-soluble embedding medium may be used.

Since the stretching of sections on a liquid medium has to be avoided, we have in our laboratory been using tape at the sectioning, as in whole-body autoradiography (Fig. 2(a), (b)).

The tape supports the section, which makes it easier to get whole sections; and it facilitates handling in the subsequent mounting on a photographic plate.

4.2.2. *Autoradiographic procedure*

Sections show some tendency to adhere directly to the gelatin of a photographic emulsion, but in our experience this adherence has not proved sufficiently reliable to prevent some sections from getting loose in large scale work. However, the adhesiveness of the emulsion increases considerably with the addition of a proper amount of glycerol (Hammarström *et al.*, 1965). Photographic slides can be pretreated by being immersed in an ethanol solution of glycerol. The ethanol is allowed to evaporate before the application of the sections (Fig. 2(c)).

During exposure a light pressure is put on the back of the tape. After exposure the tape is removed by xylene. Sections from paraffin-embedded blocks are then simultaneously freed from the paraffin.

The photographic plate carrying the sections is then passed through decreasing concentrations of ethanol, developed, fixed, and rinsed. The sections, still on the photographic plate, are generally weakly stained, passed up the ethanol series, transferred to xylene, and mounted under a cover glass with Canada balsam, and studied by the light microscope with magnification at 400–1000 times.

4.2.3. *Photographic emulsions*

The dry sections can be mounted on nuclear plates, e.g. the Ilford plates. The most sensitive of these is G 5. It is also the most coarse-grained one (mean crystal diameter: 0.27 μ) and has the highest background. G 5-autoradiograms give the best contrast in low-power magnification. The Ilford K-emulsions have a smaller grain size (diameter 0.20 μ) and build up background more slowly. The L-emulsion grains (diameter 0.14 μ) can be observed in the light microscope only in high power magnification.

A thinner emulsion than that of the nuclear plates can be obtained by floating a stripping film (e.g. AR 10, Kodak, England) on a water surface and catching it, emulsion side up, on a glass slide. After it has dried this can be used as an autoradiographic plate.

4.2.4. *Alternative methods*

Cryostat sections can be mounted immediately when sectioned onto an autoradiographic plate. The sections are thus not allowed to dry before exposure. This requires dark-room (safe-light) facilities during sectioning. The exposure has to be carried out well below freezing point. After exposure the sections are thawed, which makes them stick better to the emulsion of the photographic plates (Appleton, 1964).

Stumpf and Roth (1966) have tried cryostat sectioning at very low temperature (down to $-80°$). They have with this arrangement succeeded in getting thin (0.5–1 μ) sections. The sections are immediately freeze-dried. The morphology has allowed the observation of mitochondriae, for example. The good morphology obtained by low-temperature sectioning may be promising with regard to the possibility of obtaining acceptable cryostat sections for electron microscopy autoradiography.

4.3. ELECTRON MICROSCOPY AUTORADIOGRAPHY

The combination of electron microscopy and autoradiography is a relatively new and promising method which, when further improvements have been made, may help us to solve many intricate pharmacological and physiological problems.

4.3.1. *Histologic procedure*

In working with labeled substances that are firmly bound in the tissues, the histological preparation can be carried out with consideration only to morphology using customary electron microscopy techniques.

Attempts have been made to overcome the technical difficulties in regard to water soluble substances but several problems still remain. Some of the critical steps will be considered here.

Fixation fluids have to be avoided if a water soluble isotope is to be localized properly. In spite of the difficulties in obtaining optimal morphology, freeze-drying, or preferably cryostat sectioning seem to be the only reliable ways of starting the tissue preservation without risk of

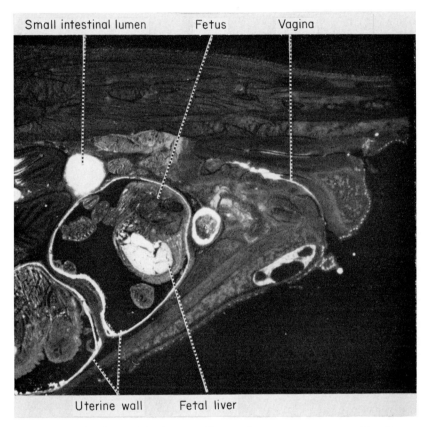

Small intestinal lumen   Fetus   Vagina

Uterine wall   Fetal liver

FIG. 3. Detail of a whole-body autoradiogram from a pregnant mouse 4 hr after subcutaneous injection of ^{14}C-diethylstilbestrol. Note high radioactivity (light areas) in uterine wall, vaginal mucosa and fetal liver. (Bengtsson and Ullberg, 1963.)

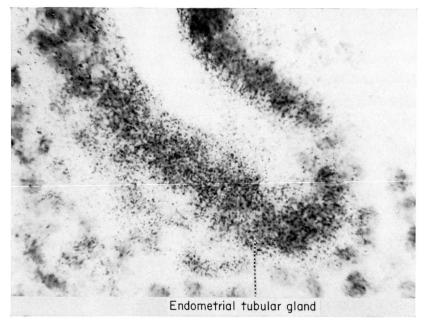

Endometrial tubular gland

FIG. 4. Microautoradiogram from uterus of a mouse 4 hr after subcutaneous injection of ³H-estradiol. Note high uptake (accumulation of silver grains) in endometrial cells. The radioactivity is located mainly in the nuclei of the cells. (Ullberg and Bengtsson, 1963.)

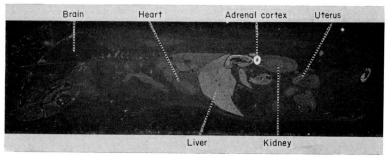

FIG. 5. Autoradiogram of a female mouse 24 hr after an intramuscular injection of ¹⁴C-4-cholesterol. Note the high uptake (light areas) in the adrenal cortex. (Appelgren, 1967.)

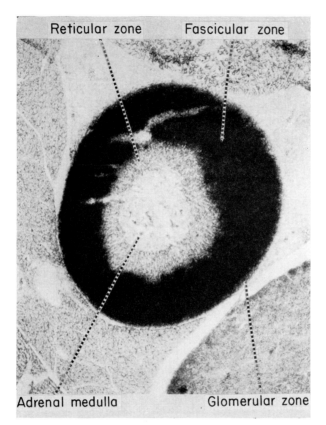

FIG. 6. Microautoradiogram of an adrenal from a mouse 4 days after an intravenous injection of ^{14}C-4-cholesterol. Note the high and specific uptake of ^{14}C in zona fasciculata. The medulla and reticular zone are void of radioactivity. (Appelgren, 1967.)

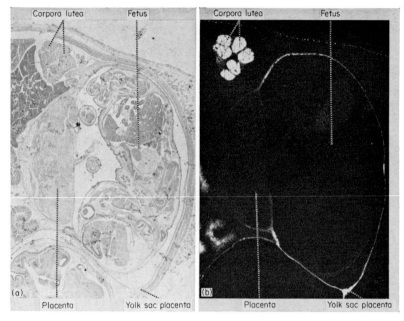

FIG. 7. Detail of whole-body autoradiogram (b) showing the distribution of ^{14}C-4-pregnenolone in a pregnant mouse. Selective accumulation in corpora lutea and yolk sac placenta. (a) is the corresponding section. (Appelgren, 1967.)

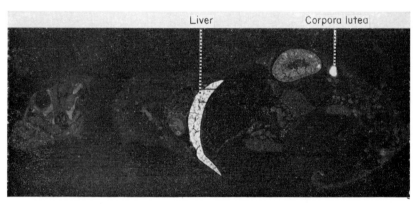

FIG. 9. Distribution of ^{14}C-F6066 in a pregnant mouse. Selective accumulation in ovary and liver. (Hanngren *et al.*, 1965.)

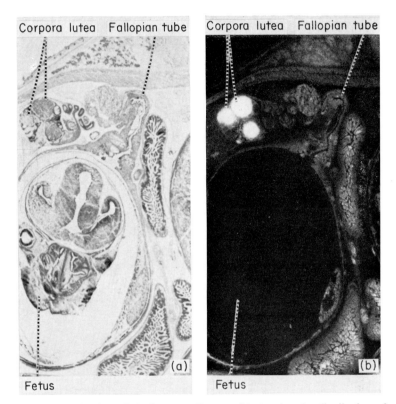

Fig. 10. Detail of whole-body autoradiogram (b) showing the distribution of ^{14}C-F6066 in pregnant mouse. Selective accumulation in corpora lutea. Low concentration in rest of ovary, fallopian tube and uterine wall. No fetal uptake. (a) is the corresponding section. (Hanngren *et al.*, 1965.)

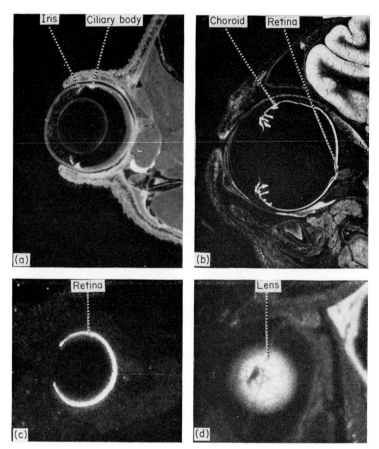

FIG. 11. Autoradiograms showing specific localization in the eye region after intravenous injection of : (a) ³H atropine, localized in the ciliary body and iris (Albanus *et al.*, 1968); (b) ³⁵S-chlorpromazine, localized in the uvea (Cassano *et al.*, 1965); (c) ¹⁴C-labeled vitamin A, localized in the retina (Ullberg, S., Appelgren, L.-E., Hammarström, L. and Hellberg, B., to be published); (d) ¹⁴C-labeled DMSO, localized in the lens (Hellberg, B. and Ullberg, S., to be published).

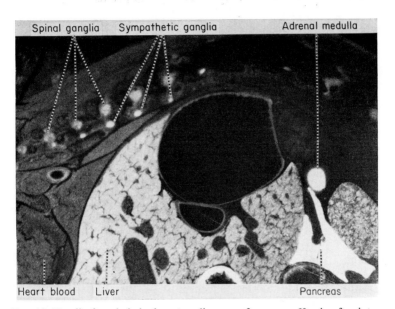

FIG. 12. Detail of a whole-body autoradiogram of a mouse 60 min after intravenous injection of dopa-2-^{14}C. Note marked uptake (light areas) in pancreas,
adrenal medulla and sympathetic ganglia. The concentration in the spinal ganglia
is higher than in the blood. (Hammarström, L., Ritzén, M. and Ullberg, S.,
to be published.)

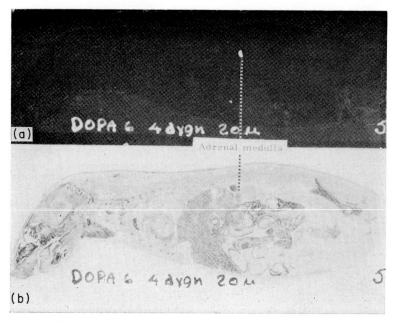

FIG. 13. Whole-body autoradiogram (a) and corresponding section (b) 4 days after injection of dopa-2-^{14}C. Radioactivity, mainly representing adrenaline, exclusively in adrenal medulla. (Rosell *et al.*, 1963.)

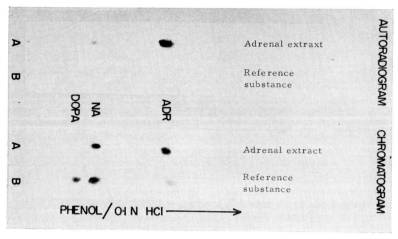

FIG. 14. Chromatographic separation of radioactive components of adrenal 4 days after injection of dopa-2-^{14}C. (Rosell *et al.*, 1963.)

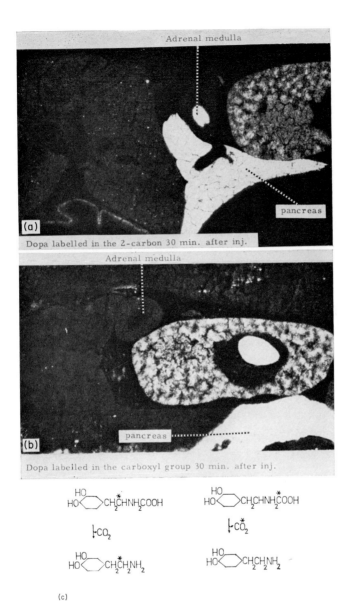

Fig. 15. Details of whole-body autoradiograms from mice 30 min after injection of dopa-2-^{14}C (a) and dopa labeled in the carboxyl group (b). No accumulation of radioactivity in adrenal medulla after injection of carboxyl-labeled dopa. At the conversion of dopa to dopamine the carboxyl group is split off (c). (Ullberg, S., to be published.)

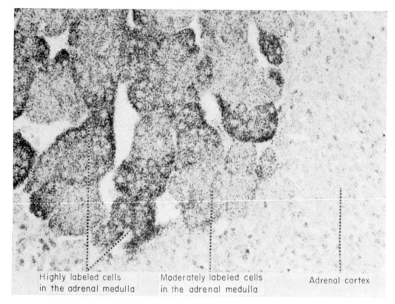

Highly labeled cells
in the adrenal medulla

Moderately labeled cells
in the adrenal medulla

Adrenal cortex

Fig. 16. Microautoradiogram of adrenal from a mouse 5 min after intravenous injection of dopa-2-^{14}C. Some medullary cells show a higher concentration than the others. (Hammarström, L., Ritzén, M. and Ullberg, S., to be published.)

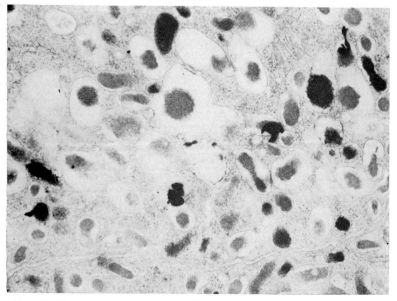

Fig. 17. Electron miscroscopy autoradiogram showing part of cell in adrenal medulla from mouse 4 hr after injection of ^{3}H-dopa. Silver grains over sparsely occurring chromaffin granules. ×46,000. (Elfvin et al., 1966.)

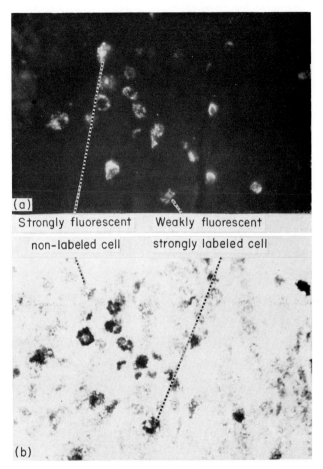

FIG. 18. Fluorescence microphotograph (a) and a microautoradiogram (b) of a part of the gastric mucosa of a mouse which 4 hr before sacrifice was intravenously injected with 5-hydroxytryptophan-³H. Most of the cells show both 5-HT fluorescence and radioactivity, but some strongly fluorescent cells have not accumulated radioactivity and some strongly labeled cells show only weak fluorescence. ×430. (Hammarström *et al.*, 1966.)

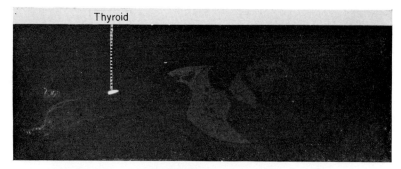

FIG. 19. Whole-body autoradiogram of a mouse 24 hr after intravenous injection of ^{14}C-thiouracil. Note the specific localization in the thyroid. (Hammarström, L. and Ullberg, S., to be published.)

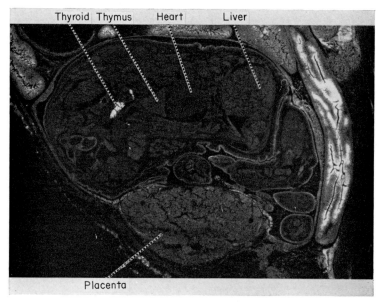

FIG. 20. Detail of a whole-body autoradiogram showing the distribution in the fetus which 4 hr before sacrifice was intravenously injected with ^{14}C-thiourea. Note the specific localization in the fetal thyroid. (Hammarström, L. and Ullberg, S. to be published.)

redistribution.* After freeze-drying, 'a chemical fixation may be obtained by exposing the dried tissue to osmium or aldehyde vapours.

During the embedding, difficulties will arise in cases where the labeled substance is soluble in the embedding agent.

The next technical problem is to take sections without floating them on aqueous media. One may try to collect sections on other liquids that are inert to the labeled substance, or to catch sections with some mechanical device. Koller (1965) has developed a method of collecting dry sections with the aid of an electrostatic field.

Because of the potential risk of isotope loss, contrast staining of the specimen should be postponed until photographic processing is completed.

4.3.2. *Autoradiographic procedure*

Most methods for the application of photographic emulsion to the biological specimen involve the use of liquid emulsion, and are therefore not satisfactory in work with water-soluble substances. They involve such procedures as: (1) dipping the grid in liquid emulsion (Liquier-Milward, 1956; Caro and Palade, 1961; Hay and Revel, 1963; Salpeter and Bachmann, 1964); (2) applying the emulsion with a pipette or a brush (O'Brien and George, 1959; Caro, 1961; Harford and Hamlin, 1961; Pelc *et al.*, 1961; Przybylski, 1961; Clementi and Fumagalli, 1962; Granboulan *et al.*, 1962; Granboulan, 1963); (3) immersing a wire loop into the emulsion, and applying the resulting film onto the grid (George and Vogt, 1959; George, 1961; Hampton and Quastler, 1961; Revel and Hay, 1961; van Tubergen, 1961; Caro and van Tubergen, 1962; Kayes *et al.*, 1962; Meek and Moses, 1963); and (4) centrifugation of the bromide crystals onto the sections (Dohlman *et al.*, 1964).

In the case of water soluble agents Dohlman (personal communication) has obtained good contact between ultrathin sections and emulsions using one of the following methods: one procedure involves centrifuging a monolayer of emulsion onto a Formvar film, and combining it with the section after the emulsion is dried; the other method uses a wire loop to form an emulsion membrane, which is dried before it is applied onto the sections on the grid. The addition of a plasticizer, such as glycerol, to the emulsion improves the uniformity of the emulsion layers.

The emulsion-covered specimens are left in the dark for autoradiographic exposure.

---

*Since the submission of the present paper for publication Appleton and Christensen have described the preparation of freeze sections for electron microscopy in *Autoradiography of diffusible substances* (1969), Eds. L. J. Roth and W. E. Stumpf, Academic Press, New York and London, pp. 301–19, 349–62.

After the photographic development, the obscuring effect of the emulsion might be diminished by enzymatic or chemical digestion of the gelatin (Przybylski, 1961; Revel and Hay, 1961). However, this involves the risk of dislocating some silver grains. The obscuring effect of the emulsion can also be counteracted by contrast staining.

4.3.3. *Resolution*

Compared with light microscopy autoradiography, electron microscopy autoradiography can lead to more detailed and precise observations in two respects: (1) because of the thinness of specimen and the film layer the distance between radiation source and silver grains is diminished, which gives higher autoradiographic resolution; (2) the more detailed morphology observed with the electron microscope makes it possible to relate the silver grains to cell structures that are not satisfactorily recognized in the light microscope.

In light microscopy autoradiography, the resolution depends mainly upon the combined thickness of specimen and film. In electron microscopy autoradiography, the thickness of the specimen is very small compared with the grain size. Therefore the dominating factor which determines the resolution is the size and distribution of the silver halide grains. The most commonly used emulsion, Ilford L 4, has a mean crystal diameter of 0.14μ (1400 Å). When it is combined with 400 Å thick sections the relation of grain diameter to section thickness will be about $3:1$.

In order to relate the silver grains to many interesting structures that are resolvable in the electron microscope, much smaller grains would be desirable.

In 1963 Granboulan reported the use of an emulsion with an average grain size of 700 Å (Gevaert, Scientia NUC 3 07). The Kodak Co. (Rochester) has marketed an emulsion with the grain size of 450 Å. Data on this emulsion are supplied by Salpeter and Bachmann (1963).

4.3.4. *Efficiency*

A serious drawback in work with electron microscopy autoradiography is the long exposure times normally required, which is due to the thinness of the specimen and emulsion layer. Conditions must be chosen in such a way that the exposure time is kept within reasonable limits. It may thus often be wise to work with sections thicker than those that would have given the best morphological details.

A factor which is of great significance for both resolution and sensitivity is the radiation properties of the labeled substance.

Among the radioisotopes of more general biologic interest, tritium has the most favorable properties. The low radiation energy is an advantage from the resolution viewpoint, and it also favors the sensitivity, since the ionization per unit path length is stronger at low particle rate.

Besides tritium, those isotopes which emit extranuclear electrons deserve attention (Forberg *et al.*, 1964). This type of radiation is generally very short-ranged. Among these isotopes the following may be mentioned: ^{125}I, ^{55}Fe, ^{57}Co, and ^{85}Sr.

In our group we have had very good results with the resolution which can be obtained with ^{125}I (Kayes *et al.*, 1962; Dohlman *et al.*, 1964), and it appears probable that this is mainly due to the monoenergetic 3 keV electrons emitted together with more long-ranged radiation.

5. APPLICATIONS

The varying distribution patterns that are observed with different techniques and in using different substances are illustrated by a number of autoradiograms from investigations made in our laboratory.

First a sequence of illustrations will be presented concerning sex hormones and adrenal cortical hormones. The autoradiographic pattern of the synthetic estrogen diethylstilbestrol is very similar to that of the natural estrogens, estradiol and estrone (Bengtsson and Ullberg, 1963). Figure 3 shows how diethylstilbestrol accumulates in the vaginal mucosa and the uterine wall. The distribution picture is thus related to the action of these substances. The non-estrogen steroid compound cortisone showed a very differing pattern (Hanngren *et al.*, 1964).

Within the uterine wall the highest concentration of ^3H-estradiol was found in the endometrial cells (Fig. 4) (Ullberg and Bengtsson, 1963). The accumulation was stronger in the nuclei than in the cytoplasm, which may indicate that the cell proliferating and carcinogenic effect of the estrogen is a direct one on the cell nuclei.

The sites of synthesis of steroid hormones are indicated by the very specific localization of steroid hormone precursors (Appelgren, 1967). Figure 5 illustrates how cholesterol is selectively accumulated in the adrenal cortex. Figure 6 shows that it is mainly the fascicular zone in the adrenal cortex that accumulates the radioactivity, while the inner reticular zone is free of ^{14}C-cholesterol. This picture (Fig. 6) is part of a "whole body microautoradiogram". A 10 μ thick whole body section was permanently attached to an Ilford G 5 nuclear plate.

Cholesterol is also selectively taken up in the ovary, and the immediate precursor of progesterone, pregnenolone, is rapidly and rather exclusively concentrated in the corpora lutea of pregnant mice (Fig. 7).

In this connection a non-steroid compound (F6066) of diphenylethene type (Fig. 8), which shows promise as a contraceptive agent, will be mentioned. It has very weak estrogenic properties and was planned by Ferrosan Ltd., Malmö, the manufacturer of the product, for use against cancer of the genital organs. In whole body autoradiography it was shown to localize very specifically in corpora lutea of pregnant mice (Figs. 9 and 10). This indicated that it might act as a false precursor of progesterone and interfere with the progesterone formation. An antigestagenic effect was also demonstrated in rat experiments (Hanngren *et al.*, 1965). In contrast to stilbestrol, F6066 did not localize specifically in the uterine wall, and it penetrated poorly to the fetus (Fig. 10).

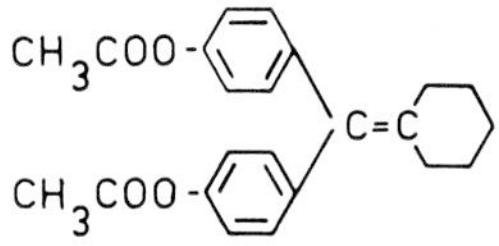

$$CH_3COO- \diagup\!\!\!\diagdown \quad C=C \diagup\!\!\!\diagdown$$
$$CH_3COO- \diagup\!\!\!\diagdown$$

F 6066

Bis(p-acetoxyphenyl)cyclohexylidenemethane

FIG. 8. Structure of the antigestagenic substance "F6066" (Ferrosan Ltd., Malmö, Sweden).

The idea that F6066 interferes with the endogenous production of progesterone is supported by recent findings that the transformation of ^{14}C-pregnenolone to progesterone by ovarian homogenates is blocked (Larsson and Stensson, 1967) and by Appelgren's whole body histochemical finding (1967) that it inhibits the enzyme, 3β-hydroxysteroid dehydrogenase, which effects this transformation.

The very varying pattern which is obtained with different substances is illustrated in Fig. 11, where the localization of four different compounds in the eye can be compared. One autoradiogram shows that tritiated atropine is localized where it is known to interfere with cholinergic mechanisms; in the iris and the ciliary body (Albanus *et al.*, 1968). Another one shows the very selective accumulation of ^{14}C labeled vitamin A in the retina which indicates a rapid turnover of vitamin A in the rhodopsin metabolism (Ullberg, S., Appelgren, L.-E., Hammarström, L., and Hellberg, B., to be published). A third one shows the localization of chlorpromazine-^{35}S (Cassano *et al.*, 1965) in the whole uvea and the outer retina layer, probably due to a pigment affinity, which may be associated with the side effects of light sensitization of chlorpromazine. The fourth eye autoradiogram shows a specific uptake in the lens of the interesting and controversial solvent and drug dimethylsulphoxide-^{14}C (DMSO) which was for some time withdrawn from clinical use because of its lens toxicity (Hellberg, B. and Ullberg, S., to be published).

A sequence of pictures illustrates the fate in the body of the catecholamine precursor dihydroxyphenylalanine (dopa). Labeled dopa is originally taken up in many organs. It is found in especially high concentration in the adrenal medulla and the sympathetic ganglia (Fig. 12) (Hammarström, L., Ritzén, M. and Ullberg, S., to be published). There is also a slight accumulation in the spinal ganglia. The pancreas shows a rather strong but transient accumulation (probably because dopa is initially treated as a protein-forming substance).

The radioactivity from injected dopa rapidly leaves most organs, but is retained for many days in the adrenal medulla (Fig. 13) (Rosell *et al.*, 1963).

The injected dopa is rapidly transformed into catecholamines. Radiochromatography (Fig. 14) shows that 4 days after injection the radioactivity of the adrenal represents mainly adrenaline and to a small extent noradrenaline (NA).

Figure 15 illustrates the possibility of using differently labeled preparations of the same substance where the radioactive atom is in different position in the molecule (Ullberg, S., to be published). If a preparation of dopa is used which is labeled with ^{14}C in the carboxyl group, the catecholamines produced will be non-labeled, and the radioactive CO^2, which is split off when the dopa is decarboxylated, leaves the body with the expired air. In Fig. 15(b) is shown an autoradiogram obtained with carboxyl labeled dopa. No accumulation is seen in the adrenal medulla. This indicates that the decarboxylation of dopa in the adrenal medulla and the disappearance from this site of the split off CO_2 is a very rapid process.

Light microscopy autoradiography shows that the radioactivity after injection of ^{14}C-2-dopa is taken up in higher concentration in some adrenal medullary cells than in others (Fig. 16) (Hammarström, L., Ritzén, M. and Ullberg, S., to be published). Differential staining has indicated that the accumulation is stronger in the adrenaline-forming cells than in noradrenaline forming ones (Elfvin *et al.*, 1966).

An electron microscopy autoradiogram (Fig. 17) of tritiated dopa in an adrenal medullary cell shows that 4 hr after injection most of the radioactive substance is localized in the chromaffin granules (Elfvin *et al.*, 1966).

Figure 18 illustrates the technical possibility of combining autoradiography and fluorescence microscopy of biogenic monoamines using the same section (Hammarström *et al.*, 1966). The two methods seem to give good complementary information; the fluorescence intensity mainly indicating storage size and the autoradiographic accumulation of silver grains the rate of turnover of monoamines, which can thus be compared in different sites under varying conditions.

The selective localization of a drug in its target organ is illustrated by Fig. 19, which shows the high concentration of thiouracil-^{14}C in the thyroid of a mouse 24 hr after injection, when the radioactivity is in the process of leaving the rest of the body (Hammarström, L. and Ullberg, S., to be published). The fetal thyroid also accumulates thiourea preparations. A detail from an autoradiogram of a pregnant mouse (Fig. 20) shows an accumulation in the fetal thyroid after injection of the mother with thiourea-^{14}C (Hammarström, L. and Ullberg, S., to be published). The thyroidal accumulation in the fetus is still more selective than in the adult mouse, as the fetus does not show any significant accumulation in the excretory organs. The fetal thyroid accumulation may explain the fetal hypothyroidism that has frequently been observed after thiourea medication during pregnancy.

Another problem that concerns thyroid metabolism is whether incorporation of iodine into the iodinated thyroid hormones takes place in the cell or in the colloid. It has been discussed whether the accumulation of organically bound radioiodine, which has been observed in light microscopy autoradiography, has been present in the inner cell layer or in the outer colloid region. Electron microscopy autoradiography, with the improved resolution it offers, clearly shows (Fig. 21) that 30 min after injection the radioiodine is totally on the colloid side (Dohlman *et al.*,1964). This may favor the theory that the incorporation of iodine into the organic molecules during the formation of thyroxin and triiodothyronin takes place in the colloid. The very weak monoenergetic extranuclear electrons emitted from ^{125}I give significantly better resolution than the ^{131}I-betas.

Figure 22 shows the distribution of ascorbic acid-1-^{14}C in a pregnant mouse 3 days after an intravenous injection. Ascorbic acid has been accumulated in both maternal and fetal brains, eyes, spinal cords, and adrenals. It has also been taken up in the sympathetic ganglia, thyroid, parathyroid, and pancreatic islets of the mother. Ascorbic acid has been shown to take part in the synthesis of catecholamines, and it is interesting to note that it is accumulated in tissues where this synthesis probably occurs, e.g. the

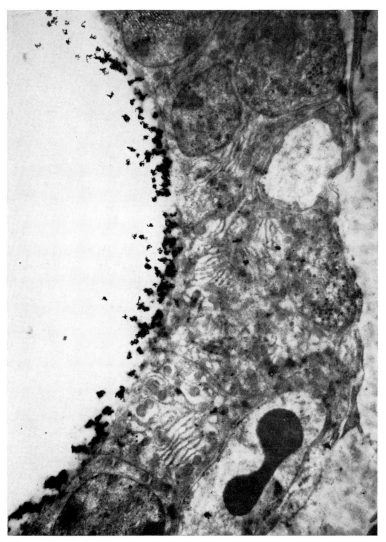

FIG. 21. Electron microscopy autoradiogram of a mouse thyroid, showing the distribution of ^{125}I 1 hr after injection. The radioactivity is confined to the colloid, just outside the thyroid cells. ×7,400. (Dohlman *et al.*, 1964.)

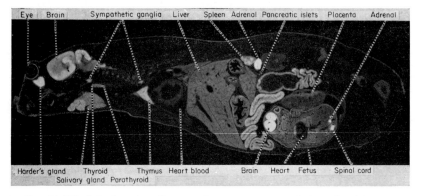

FIG. 22. Whole-body autoradiogram of a pregnant mouse 3 days after intravenous injection of ascorbic acid-1-^{14}C. Note the accumulation in both the maternal and fetal brains, eyes and adrenals. There is also a persistent uptake in the sympathetic ganglia, thyroid, parathyroid and pancreatic islets. No radioactivity is visible in the maternal and fetal blood. (Hammarström, 1966.)

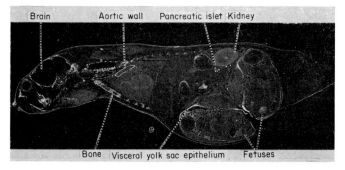

FIG. 23. Autoradiogram of a pregnant mouse 4 hr after an intravenous injection of ^{14}C-2-alloxan. Note accumulation of the pancreatic islets, aortic wall, bone and visceral yolk sac epithelium. (Hammarström and Ullberg, 1966.)

nervous system, adrenal medulla, thyroid, parathyroid, and pancreatic islets (Hammarström, 1966).

Most theories used to explain the diabetogenic action of alloxan are based upon its nonselective distribution. However, whole-body autoradiography has shown that after an intravenous injection of alloxan-2-^{14}C the concentration in the pancreatic islets far exceeded that of any other tissue (Fig. 23). This finding indicates that the morphological changes in the β-cells, observed after administration of alloxan, are preceded by an accumulation of alloxan in these cells (Hammarström and Ullberg, 1966).

REFERENCES

(A) BOOKS, REVIEWS AND MONOGRAPHS

ROGERS, A. W. (1967) *Techniques of Autoradiography*. Elsevier Publishing Co., Amsterdam, London, New York.
ULLBERG, S. (1958) Autoradiographic studies on the distribution of labelled drugs in the body. *Second U.N. Int. Conf. Peaceful Uses of Atomic Energy*, **24**: 248–54.

(B) ORIGINAL PAPERS

ALBANUS, L., HAMMARSTRÖM, L., SUNDWALL, A., ULLBERG, S. and VANGBO, B. (1968) Distribution and metabolism of T-atropin in mice. *Acta Physiol. Scand.* **73**:447-56.
APPELGREN, L.-E. (1967) Sites of steroid hormone formation. Autoradiographic studies using labelled precursors. *Acta Physiol. Scand.*, Suppl., **301**:1–108.
APPELGREN, L.-E., SÖREMARK, R. and ULLBERG, S. (1963) Improved resolution in autoradiography with radioiodine using the extranuclear electron radiation from ^{125}I. *Biochim. Biophys. Acta*, **66**:144–9.
APPLETON, T. C. (1964) Autoradiography of soluble labelled compounds. *J. Roy. Microscop. Soc.*, **83**:277–81.
BENGTSSON, G. and ULLBERG, S. (1963) The autoradiographic distribution pattern after administration of diethylstilboestrol compared with that of natural oestrogens. *Acta Endocr., Copenh.*, **43**:561–70.
BERLIN, M. and ULLBERG, S. (1963) Accumulation and retention of mercury in the mouse. *Archs. Envir. Hlth.*, **6**: 589–601.
CARO, L. G. (1961) Electron microscopic radioautography of thin sections: The Golgi zone as a site of protein concentration in pancreatic acinar cells. *J. Biophys. Biochem. Cytol.*, **10**:37–45.
CARO, L. G. and PALADE, G. E. (1961). Le rôle de l'appareil de Golgi dans le processus sécrétoire. Etude autoradiographique. *C. R. Séanc. Soc. Biol.*, **155**:1750–62.
CARO, L. G. and VAN TUBERGEN, R. P. (1962) High resolution autoradiography. I: Methods. *J. Cell Biol.* **15**:173–88.
CASSANO, G. B., SJÖSTRAND, S. E. and HANSSON, E. (1965) Distribution of ^{35}S-chlorpromazine in cat brain. *Arch. Int. Pharmac. Thér.* **156**:48–58.
CLEMENTI, F. and FUMAGALLI, R. (1962) Intracellular localization in the liver of exogenous 3H-cholesterol: autoradiographic and radiochemical assay. *Expl. Cell Res.*, **28**:604–8.

DOHLMAN, G. F., MAUNSBACH, A. B., HAMMARSTRÖM, L. and APPELGREN, L.-E. (1964) Electron microscopic autoradiography. A method for producing uniform monolayers of silver halide crystals using centrifuge sedimentation. *J. Ultrastruct. Res.*, **10**:293–303.

DONIACH, I. and PELC, S. R. (1950) Autoradiograph technique. *Brit. J. Radiol.*, **23**:184–92.

ELFVIN, L. G., APPELGREN, L.-E. and ULLBERG, S. (1966) High resolution autoradiography of the adrenal medulla after injection of tritiated dihydroxyphenylalanine (DOPA). *J. Ultrastruct. Res.*, **14**:277–93.

ERICSSON, Y. and ULLBERG, S. (1958) Autoradiographic investigations of the distribution of F^{18} in mice and rats. *Acta Odont. Scand.*, **16**:363–74.

ERICSSON, Y., ULLBERG, S. and APPELGREN, L.-E. (1960) Autoradiographic localization of radioactive fluorine (F^{18}) in developing teeth and bones. *Acta Odont. Scand.*, **18**:253–61.

FORBERG, S., ODEBLAD, E., SÖREMARK, R. and ULLBERG, S. (1964) Autoradiography with isotopes emitting internal conversion electrons and auger electrons. *Acta Radiol.*, **2**:241–62.

GEORGE, L. A. II. (1961) Electron microscopy and autoradiography. *Science*, **133**:1423–4.

GEORGE, L. A. II and VOGT, G. S. (1959) Electron microscopy of autoradiographed radioactive particles. *Nature, Lond.*, **184**:1474–5.

GRANBOULAN, P. (1963) Resolving power and sensitivity of a new emulsion in electron microscope autoradiography. *J. Roy. Microscop. Soc.*, **81**:165–71.

GRANBOULAN, P., GRANBOULAN, N. and BERNHARD, W. (1962) Application de l'autoradiographie à la microscopie électronique. *J. Microscopie*, **1**:75–80.

HAMMARSTRÖM, L. (1966) Autoradiographic studies on the distribution of C^{14}-labelled ascorbic acid and dehydroascorbic acid. *Acta Physiol. Scand.*, **70**, suppl. 289, 1–84.

HAMMARSTRÖM, L. APPELGREN, L.-E., and ULLBERG, S. (1965) Improved method for light microscopy autoradiography with isotopes in water-soluble form. *Expl. Cell Res.*, **37**:608–13.

HAMMARSTRÖM, L., RITZÉN, M. and ULLBERG, S. (1966) Combined autoradiography and fluorescence microscopy. Localization of labelled 5-hydroxytryptophan in relation to endogenous 5-hydroxytryptamine in the gastrointestinal tract. *Experientia*, **22**:213–15.

HAMMARSTRÖM, L. and ULLBERG, S. (1966) Specific uptake of labelled alloxan in the pancreatic islets. *Nature, Lond.*, **212**:708–9.

HAMPTON, J. C. and QUASTLER, H. (1961) Combined autoradiography and electron microscopy of thin sections of intestinal epithelial cells of the mouse labelled with H3-thymidine. *J. Biophys. Biochem. Cytol.*, **10**:140–4.

HANNGREN, Å., HANSSON, E., SJÖSTRAND, S. E. and ULLBERG, S. (1964) Autoradiographic distribution studies with ^{14}C-cortisone and ^{14}C-cortisol. *Acta Endocrin.*, *Copenh.*, **47**:95–104.

HANNGREN, Å., EINER-JENSEN, N., and ULLBERG, S. (1965) Specific uptake in corpora lutea of a non-steroid substance with anti-gestagenic properties. *Nature, Lond.*, **208**:461–2.

HARFORD, C. G. and HAMLIN, A. (1961) Electron microscopic autoradiography in a magnetic field. *Nature, Lond.*, **189**:505–6.

HAY, E. D. and REVEL, J. P. (1963) The fine structure of the DNP component of the nucleus. An electron microscopic study utilizing autoradiography to localize DNA synthesis. *J. Cell Biol.*, **16**:29–51.

JOFTES, D. L. and WARREN, S. (1955) Simplified liquid emulsion radioautography. *J. Biol. Phot. Assoc.*, **23**:145–50.

KALBERER, F. (1966) A new method of macro-autoradiography. *Atomlight*, No. 51, 1–7.

KAYES, J., MAUNSBACH, A. B. and ULLBERG, S. (1962) Electron microscopic autoradiography of radioiodine in the thyroid using the extranuclear electrons of I^{125}. *J. Ultrastruct. Res.*, **7**:339–45.

KOLLER, T. (1965) Mounting of ultrathin sections with the aid of an electrostatic field. *J. Cell Biol.*, **27**:441–5.

KOPRIWA, B. M. and LEBLOND, C. P. (1962) Improvements in the coating technique of radioautography. *J. Histochem. Cytochem.*, **10**:269–84.

LARSSON, H. and STENSSON, M. (1967) Effect of bis(*p*-hydroxyphenyl)-cyclohexylidene-methane (F6060) on the conversion of pregnenolone to Δ^4-3-ketosteroids *in vitro*. *Acta Endocr., Copenh.*, **55**:673–84.

LIQUIER-MILWARD, J. (1956) Electron microscopy and radioautography as coupled techniques in tracer experiments. *Nature, Lond.*, **177**:619.

MEEK, G. A. and MOSES, M. J. (1963) Localization of tritiated thymidine in HeLa cells by electron autoradiography. *J. Roy. Microscop. Soc.*, **81**:187–97.

O'BRIEN, R. T. and GEORGE, L. A. (1959) Preparation of autoradiograms for electron microscopy. *Nature, Lond.*, **183**:1461–2.

PELC, S. R., COMBES, J. D. and BUDD, G. C. (1961) On the adaptation of autoradiographic techniques for use with the electron microscope. *Expl. Cell Res.*, **24**:192–5.

PELLERIN, P. (1957) Technique d'autoradiographie à très basse température. *C. R. Acad. Sci.*, **244**:1555–8.

PRZYBYLSKI, R. J. (1961) Electron microscope autoradiography. *Expl. Cell Res.*, **24**:181–4.

REVEL, J. P. and HAY, E. D. (1961) Autoradiographic localization of DNA synthesis in a specific ultrastructural component of the interphase nucleus. *Expl. Cell Res.*, **25**:474–80.

ROSELL, S., SEDVALL, G. and ULLBERG, S. (1963) Distribution and fate of dihydroxy-phenylalanine-2-^{14}C (Dopa) in mice. *Biochem. Pharmac.*, **12**:265–9.

SALPETER, M. M. and BACHMANN, L. J. (1964) Autoradiography with the electron microscope. A procedure for improving resolution, sensitivity and contrast. *J. Cell Biol.*, **22**:469–77.

STUMPF, W. E. and ROTH, L. J. (1966). High resolution autoradiography with dry mounted freeze-dried frozen sections. Comparative study of six methods using two diffusible compounds, ^{3}H-estradiol and ^{3}H-mesobilirubinogen. *J. Histochem. Cytochem.*, **14**:274–87.

ULLBERG, S. (1954) Studies on the distribution and fate of S^{35}-labelled benzylpenicillin in the body. *Acta Radiol.*, Suppl. **118**, 1–110.

ULLBERG, S. and BENGTSSON, G. (1963) Autoradiographic distribution studies with natural oestrogens. *Acta Endocr., Copenh.*, **43**:75–86.

VAN TUBERGEN, R. P. (1961) The use of radioautography and electron microscopy for the localization of tritium label in bacteria. *J. Biophys. Biochem. Cytol.*, **9**:219–22.

CHAPTER 8

BINDING OF DRUGS TO PLASMA AND TISSUE PROTEINS

Yves Cohen

Faculty of Pharmacy, University of Paris, and
Centre d'Études Nucléaires of Saclay, France

INTRODUCTION

The binding of drugs to the constituents of the living organism, and especially to proteins, is one of the fundamental problems in pharmacology, but at the same time one of the most complex problems and one of the most difficult to grasp. By the beginning of the twentieth century P. Ehrlich (1909) considered that in order to have any effect a drug should have a group capable of binding it at the point of impact in the organism, i.e. at a receptor.

But before reaching a receptor, the drug is transported by the blood and may on this level be bound to blood proteins or, more exactly, to the plasma proteins. Research has progressed further into the binding of drugs to plasma proteins than it has with cellular proteins. In fact, plasma albumin is readily to hand, its molecular structure is better known than that of any other tissue protein, and it may therefore be thought that research into the binding of drugs to this protein would serve as a basis for later studies on binding to tissue receptors of protein type. Pharmacological research in this field is following developments in biochemistry, physiology, and molecular biology. The theoretical aspects of protein–drug binding have largely been treated by Klotz (1953), Steinhardt and Beychock (1964), and Nichol *et al.* (1964). More specifically, since Beutner's research in 1925 and 1926 and the papers quoted by Goldstein (1949), the binding of drugs to proteins has been the subject of recent reports by Thorp (1964), Brodie (1964, 1965, 1966), and Van Os *et al.* (1964). Radionuclides and labeled molecules have contributed greatly to this field by facilitating analysis and permitting research on a phased basis. The use of radioactive tracers is rewarding because their lower limit of detection has been reduced to 10^{-5}–10^{-6} millimoles without the destruction of the matter analyzed, and because phenomena can be studied without disturbing the biological equilibria, since indicators of high specific radioactivity are now available. At the present time the studies on the protein binding of radiolabeled drugs are few in number, but in future they should develop owing to the modern means at our disposal and the valuable results to be obtained. In a recent review Cohen *et al.* (1966) quote several papers treating this subject. In this connection we have compiled a table, and have added references to notes and surveys which have appeared in the last 2 years (Table 1).

TABLE 1. STUDIES OF THE BINDING OF LABELLED DRUGS TO PROTEINS

Drug	Label	Author
Oestrone	^{14}C	Wall and Migeon, 1959
		Sandberg *et al.*, 1959
Triamcinolone	^{3}H	Florini *et al.*, 1961
Hydrocortisone	^{14}C	Florini *et al.*, 1961
Tetracycline	^{3}H	Takesue *et al.*, 1960
Heparin	^{35}S	Eiber and Danishefsky, 1959
Trypsin	^{131}I	Miller *et al.*, 1960a, b
Insulin	^{131}I	Wohltmann and Narahara, 1960
Salicylate	^{14}C	Eberhardt, 1963
Phenytoin	^{14}C	
Thiopental	^{14}C	Barlow *et al.*, 1962
Phenobarbital	^{14}C	
Barbital	^{14}C	
Cholographin	^{131}I	
Hypaque	^{131}I	Rosenbaum and Reich, 1966
Renographin	^{131}I	
Folic acid		Neal and Williams, 1965
Cyanocobal amine	^{60}Co	Beal, 1964
		Hardwicke and Jones, 1966
Growth hormone	^{14}C	Colipp and Kaplan, 1966
Thyroid hormones	^{131}I	Salvatore *et al.*, 1966

A paper collecting the communications to the Paris Symposium on plasma protein transport in 1965 gives many references to the protein binding of radioelements, lipids, thyroid hormones, corticosteroids, insulin, vitamins, "circulating" enzymes, bilirubin, toxic substances, and medical drugs (Desgrez and Traverse, 1966). Many studies in basic and clinical physiology, in medical biology, and in biochemistry have been devoted to hormones, to certain vitamins, and to several protein-bound enzymes. They are outside the scope of the present contribution, and we shall not consider them further.

One should call to mind the present conception of the binding of drug to proteins (Koshland, 1963).

Two types of relations are important in the combination of the drugs with the proteins:

(a)   the interactions of the molecule with active sites of the protein; and
(b)   the interactions with other sites of the proteins molecules.

The latter play some part in maintaining the three-dimensional structure of the "active site" and the flexibility of the protein. The forces operating between the protein chains should be of fundamentally the same nature as those which bind other molecules to protein.

One distinguishes between forces of attraction and forces of repulsion. Among attractive forces, reference should be made to *ionic bonds* in which particles which have opposite charges are attracted to each other, and the resulting ionic forces can considerably affect the binding. *Hydrophobic bonds* come into play when a stronger bond is observed between a protein and a molecule on which lateral alkyl chains have been attached. *Dipole interaction* by electrostatic attraction is possible in aqueous solutions by an appropriate alignment of one dipole with another dipole. Of these types of forces, the *hydrogen bond* is the most important. *London forces*, even though they are not specific, can result in an attraction between two aromatic residues which is far more intense than the attraction between an aromatic residue and an aliphatic residue. *Covalence bonds* play no negligible part in the binding of hormones to proteins.

The forces of repulsion cause the rupture of the protein–drug bond by three mechanisms: the interplay of forces of *ionic repulsion* between two ionic charges of the same sign; *dipole–dipole interaction* where again the orientation causes charges of different sign to be juxtaposed; and *steric hindrance* based on electrostatic repulsion the electrons, and on the rigidity of the bonds in relation to tension, compression, and rotation.

These forces of repulsion and attraction are not all brought into play simultaneously. They can intervene in a varying degree and so orient the binding of the drug on the protein. According to the theory of Fisher (1894), revised in the light of the concepts of modern pharmacology, a foreign molecule and a protein may become settled into relation to one another by the close juxtaposition of attractive forces competing with the interaction of forces of repulsion. In such cases a larger homologue, or a structural analogue, may be unable to fix itself on the same site owing to steric hindrance. The mechanical theory of the "template" appears to lack flexibility, and Koshland has proposed the "induced fit theory", according to which:

(a) receptors are flexible and can be modified by interaction with drugs;

(b) precise alignment of the reactive groups is necessary for activity;

(c) the active molecules lead to modifications in the conformation of the receptor which is not so with molecules that are not adapted to the receptors.

The template theory presupposes that receptors have a certain rigidity. In the induced fit theory, in addition to the affinity for the receptor, one assumes, once the protein–drug bond is established, that there is a certain change of the chemical functions of the protein owing to its flexibility.

However, when the labeled drug has a mineral ion it is difficult to draw a distinction between a labile radioelement–protein bond and the incorporation of the radioelement into the protein molecule. For this reason in this paper we shall only consider binding with the free functions —SH, —OH, —NH$_2$, and —COOH of a protein, bonds which simple variations of the pH can destroy.

Most of the papers concerning drug–protein binding seek to find the physico-chemical factors determining the bond so as to explain the particular pharmacological effects observed. They apply to isolated pure proteins or, more often, to blood plasma from various species of animals.

In reference to drug binding with plasma proteins, a description will be given of the physico-chemical and biological factors involved. We shall also describe the methods for which radioelements and labeled molecules represent a significant step forward. The importance of the pharmacological implications of these methods will be analyzed. Finally, the present state of research into the binding of drugs to tissue proteins is briefly considered.

1. BINDING BY PLASMA PROTEINS

It is generally considered that the binding of drugs to plasma proteins is the first phase of a process of transport of the drug from the site of absorption to the receptor site, and the bond is completed in accordance with the physiological mechanism. However, certain authors since Brodie (1964) believe that protein-bound drugs may equally be circulating stores of drugs, stores which at any instant are supplying a certain quantity of drug to the receptor sites and are slowly being replenished.

In the presence of proteins (serum albumin in particular), or of blood plasma, some of the antibiotics and sulfamides partly lose their antibacterial power.

Some steroids related to adrenocortical hormones are bound to plasma proteins, and the duration of their stay in the blood depends on the number of substituents on their carbon skeletons. Derivatives of phenylbutazone, of coumarin, barbiturates, antibacterial sulfamides, and antibiotics have been extensively studied without involving labeled molecules or radioelements.

We shall now consider the physico-chemical factors which have an influence on the binding of drugs, and afterwards the biological characteristics of proteins which lead to a difference in the reactivity of these substances.

1.1. PHYSICO-CHEMICAL FACTORS IN BINDING

The physico-chemical factors are numerous, but their importance varies in degree. One is concerned with the water–lipid partition coefficients, the molecular structure, the electric charge of polar molecules, the dissociation coefficients, and, at the pH of the plasma, with the degree of ionization, the concentration of the drug in the medium, and the temperature. No evidence has as yet been forthcoming to suggest that there are other factors influencing the rates of binding and of dissociation, these latter processes being immediate, or at least so rapid that no curve can be plotted for the binding or dissociation as a function of time.

Water–lipid partition coefficient

The more soluble a substance is, the less chance one has to observe it bound to plasma proteins. *N*-acylation of sulfamides increases the binding of these agents to proteins, but glycuro-conjugation reduces it (see Rieder, 1963). However, it is difficult to establish a constant correlation between the water–lipid partition coefficient and the percentage of binding of the agent to the protein. Thus, for instance, thiopental, for which the heptane–water partition coefficient is 0.95 at pH 7.4, is 82% bound, whereas barbital, for which the corresponding coefficient is 0.005, is 17% bound. On the other hand, salicylic acid, with a partition coefficient of 0.001, is 70% bound. The binding of various carbamates varies with the W/O ratio

(Douglas *et al.*, 1964), while this is not so with the sulfamides (Anton and Boyle, 1964).

Molecular structure

The chemical structure of the molecules that are susceptible to protein binding is varied. At present it is difficult to evince any evidence for a precise relationship between chemical structure and binding to proteins. However, one may suppose, as a first approximation, that the presence of aromatic ring associated with acidic, carboxylic, sulfonic and other functions will favor fixation on albumin. Increasing the weight of molecules by halogen substitutions, as in the case of contrast media, increases protein binding.

Coefficient of acid-base dissociation

The majority of the substances known to bind to proteins are acids: sulfonic dyes (phenol red), diodone, salicylic acid, probenecid, phenyl-butazone, barbiturates, hydantoins, and antibacterial sulfamides. Some bases display a certain binding capacity, i.e. quinine, amidopyrine, and tolbutamide. Even so, among the acids, while salicylic acid is bound, others (amino-salicylic and *p*-aminobenzoic) bind little or not at all.

Ionization of molecules at the PH of plasma

Certain studies have been undertaken at pH values which are distinctly acidic (below 2 for example), or strongly alkaline (above 11). The degree of ionization of the molecules ought to be referred to the blood pH, i.e. about pH 7.4. At this pH it is found that barbital, thiopenthal, pentobarbital, and amidopyrine are practically not dissociated, while salicylic acid or quinine are. Non-dissociation increases the lipo-solubility and the binding of the drug. The molecules not ionized at pH 7.4 are for the most part bound to proteins. Below pH 5 and above pH 9 the binding of sulfamides and barbiturate is diminished. The bonds of alkaloids (morphine, strychnine, etc.) are destroyed at pH 2 (Kramarenko, 1961).

Concentration of the substance in solution

The quantity of protein-bound substance depends on the concentration of the substance in question and on the concentration of the protein. Given the concentration of the protein, if the fixation is nonspecific, one obtains a type of curve similar to absorption isotherms; but if the fixation is specific, at low concentrations the substance will fix itself selectively on one protein, and then above a certain concentration the fixation may be on some other protein. This has been found to be so for cortisone, which binds to transcortin (a_1 globulin) at concentrations below 20 mcg per 100 ml of plasma, and which at higher concentrations binds to serum albumin. The binding of the drug on the protein obeys the law of mass action, and an equilibrium is established between the concentration of free protein and of agent, on the one hand, and the resultant complex, on the other:

$$P + S \underset{k_2}{\overset{k_1}{\rightleftharpoons}} P\text{---}S. \tag{1}$$

Goldstein (1949) has proposed a formula for calculating the fraction of chemical agent bound to protein taking into account the constants k_1 and k_2 of association and dissociation of the complex, the number of sites of binding per protein molecule, and the concentrations in protein and chemical agent.

The ratio of the constants of association k_1 to that of dissociation k_2 in formula (1) is equal to the equilibrium constant K:

$$K = \frac{k_1}{k_2}.$$

The fraction β of chemical substance bound to protein is

$$\beta = \frac{P\text{---}S}{PS + S} = 1 \Big/ \left(1 + \frac{K}{n P} + \frac{S}{n P}\right),$$

where n = the number of binding sites per protein molecule; P = molar concentration in proteins; S = concentration in nonbound chemical agent; $P\text{---}S$ = concentration in bound chemical agent; $PS + S$ = total concentration in chemical agent; and K = equilibrium constant of reaction (1).

The number of binding sites n and the equilibrium constant K can both be affected by the pH, temperature, ionic force, and dielectric constant of the medium.

Keen (1966a) has analyzed the various equations which apply to the binding of several penicillin derivatives to bovine serum albumin, and has distinguished primary binding sites and secondary binding sites.

We agree with Van Os *et al.* (1964) that for a given quantity of protein the bound-drug content tends to some limiting value with increasing free concentration of the drug. If the total concentration of a drug is increased, the free fraction has a tendency to increase abruptly after saturation of the sites of binding. Scholtan and Schmid (1963) and Rolinson and Sutherland

(1965) have tested benzyl-penicillin and cloxacillin and obtained experimental curves corresponding to the theoretical curves of Van Os *et al.* (1964). This phenomenon appears to be fairly general, for we have also come across it in studying the binding of ^{51}Cr to plasma proteins placed in contact with ^{51}CrCl$_3$ (Cohen *et al.*, 1965).

Temperature

The effect of temperature on the binding of drugs to proteins is controversial. Most writers do not regard temperature as being of great importance. According to Wozniak (1960) there is a slight increase in the proportion of bound tetracycline between 2° and 38°. Beyond this point the denaturation of the proteins by heat tends to counteract the binding of the drugs. Any study of drug–protein binding ought clearly to consider the biological nature of the protein and should be carried out in conditions which are compatible with life.

1.2. Biological types of proteins

We have just been discussing a number of factors that are known to be involved in the binding of drugs to proteins, and so far we have refrained from making any reference to the specificity of the plasma proteins, or to the particular protein fraction (serum albumin, serum globulins α, β, or γ). Research in this field, although it has always been precise as to the origin of the protein being studied, has rarely been interested in revealing the differences between the protein fractions involved. Firstly, we shall consider the variations due to the zoological species, and, secondly, the variations related to the protein fractions.

Variations by species

Quite often the drug–protein binding is of the same order for different species, but differences may also be in evidence. Anton (1960) has shown that the binding of sulfadiazine to plasma proteins is not the same for mice, chicks, and dogs as for man, rat, and guinea pig. Sulfamethoxypyridazine and sulfisoxazole are bound much less by the plasma proteins of chicks than by those of some other species, namely man, dog, rat, and guinea pig. The binding of cloxacillin to human serum proteins is weaker than in the case of horse, sheep, rabbit, and calf serum (Rolinson and Sutherland, 1965). It is therefore not advisable to confine studies to one species of animals but to make a comparative study of other species and a study of the human species in particular.

Variations with the kind of serum protein

Serum albumin is by far the most important protein fraction, and it is on this protein that the chemical substances most often bind. The potential number of binding sites is very great, i.e. 100 ionized acidic groups and 86 ionized basic groups per molecule (Keen, 1966a). These groups are the terminal α-carboxyl groups of the amino acids, the β-carboxyl groups of aspartic and glutamic acids, the hydroxy groups of tyrosine, the amino groups of lysine, the guanidine groups of arginine, the terminal α amino groups, and the imidazole groups of histidine (Table 2).

TABLE 2. IONIZED GROUPS PRESENT IN ALBUMIN MOLECULES AT pH 7.4 (AFTER KEEN, 1966a)

Residue	Group	Number of groups per molecule	pK_a	Number ionized at pH 7.4
		Acidic groups		
C-terminal	α carboxyl	1	3.75	1
Aspartic	β carboxyl	99	3.97	99
Glutamic	γ carboxyl			
Tyrosin	Phenolic	19	10.35	0
		Basic groups		
Histidin	Imidazole	16	6.9	6
N-terminal	α amino	1	7.75	0.8
Lysine	ϵ amino	57	9.8	57
Arginine	Guanidine	22	>12	22

Certain more specific globulins play a part in hormone transport, like transcortin, which is capable of binding to cortisol and synthetic corticoids (Weist *et al.*, 1966). With the following intermediaries the binding, almost zero for triamcinolone, is much higher for prednisolone: triamcinolone < dexamethasone = prednisone < cortisol < prednisolone = 17hydroxy-progesterone. When the binding sites of transcortin are saturated, the corticoids fix on albumin.

Certain lipo-soluble substances are bound to lipoproteins. Schen and Rabinovitz (1966) have shown that tetracycline displays an affinity for the α_1 and α_2 lipoproteins and for the various lipids migrating between the α_2 and β_1 globulines in electrophoretic separations.

The foregoing discussion illustrates the principles of studies on drug–protein binding. Drugs studied have sometimes been administered as radioelements or as labeled molecules. More often there has been the use of chemical methods in the classical sense, or of bacteriological assays. The relevance of tracer methods to these studies will now be discussed.

2. TRACER METHODS IN THE STUDY OF PLASMA PROTEIN BINDING OF DRUGS

In the introduction to this chapter a list of papers relating to the binding of radio-tagged drugs to proteins was given. Although not exhaustive, it was a modest list for, in fact, in comparison with classical research along these lines, studies by tracers are few in number and all of them are recent. The radioelements used are: carbon-14, hydrogen-3, iodine-131, iodine-125, sulfur-35, phosphorus-32, mercury-197, and mercury-203, which label hydrocarbon molecules, organic sulfur, or halogen compounds, or even phosphorus and mercury organic compounds. We shall not dwell on the radioactive properties of these tracers, those presented in subsection I, nor on the methods of detection by ion chambers, or Geiger–Mueller counters and scintillation counters associated with the appropriate recording equipment which is described in Chapter 6.

As to methods for measuring radioactivity, we shall confine ourselves to those arrangements or stages of procedures that are the most delicate, or are little known, so as to relate these techniques to the methods of protein fractionation which are considered in more detail elsewhere.

We shall successively consider the ways of purifying the protein–drug complex, namely, centrifugation–congelation, dialysis, ultrafiltration, dextran gel filtration; then the methods of fractionation of the proteins (electrophoresis and autoradiography); and we shall conclude by a review of some less widely used methods.

2.1. CENTRIFUGATION–CONGELATION

On discovering a drug–protein bond, one requires to separate out the resulting complex. This separation is carried out in two stages; firstly, the sedimentation of the blood cells, and, secondly, the separation of the protein complex from the other soluble elements of the plasma. In the case of radioactive tracers the detection of the labeled drug is greatly facilitated by the use of autoradiography. Blood, taken on heparin, is placed in contact with the drug *in vitro* at 37°, or at ambient temperature, in a closed container for a time varying from 1 min to 1 hr. (Alternatively one can administer the labeled drug to the animal first, and then withdraw the blood on anticoagulant.) The blood is then centrifuged in a tube made of plastic, and congealed by immersion in liquid nitrogen. The congealed mass is separated from the tube and delivered to the congelation microtome in a plane perpendicular to the sedimentation. The micro-sections (20 μ) are dried using the method of Ullberg (1954), or the method of Cohen and Delassue (1959) derived therefrom. A radiographic film is applied to the dried section or to the congelated block using the method described by Cohen and Wepierre (1961). The autoradiographic recordings readily show the location of the drug, whether in the erythrocytes, the leucocytes, or in the plasma. By this method it has been possible to show that an apolar volatile hydrocarbon, fat-soluble *p*-cymene, is distributed 1/3 in the plasma and 2/3 in the red blood cells (Wepierre, 1963). These results can be subsequently confirmed by measuring the radioactivity in the plasma and the cells. The advantage of this method is that the result is obtained very quickly as a guide to further inquiries.

2.2. DIALYSIS

Dialysis of a blood serum against a solution of appropriate composition is a simple method mostly used for separating the free molecule from the protein complex. The dialysis membrane is formed from collodion or cellulose acetate, either as a pouch or a tube stoppered at one end. Anton (1960) uses a special arrangement in which a bacterial culture can be produced in the apparatus for performing the dialysis. At intervals of time the radioactivity is measured on a sample of the dialysis solution rather than of the serum. Static dialysis can be replaced by continuous dialysis, the external solution being constantly changed (Acred *et al.*, 1963). The radioactivity in this solution can either be measured point by point, or it can be continuously recorded in the way to be described for dextran gel filtration.

2.3. ULTRA-FILTRATION

Ultrafiltration at laboratory temperature across Visking tubes and under compressed air pressure at 15 psi has been employed by Rolinson and Sutherland (1965). Keen (1966b) has adopted a comparable method after trying ultrafiltration under negative pressure and at body temperature (Keen, 1965). Approximately 0.5 ml of ultrafiltrate can be obtained from 5 ml of serum.

2.4. DEXTRAN GEL FILTRATION

Since the first paper of Porath and Flodin (1959), dextran gel filtration has been used to estimate the plasma protein binding of many compounds.

Barlow *et al.* (1962) thus studied the binding of phenytoin, thiopental, phenobarbital, and barbital. Scholtan (1964) has compared the results obtained by gel filtration with those of dialysis. The results are similar for the drugs tested, namely benzylpenicillin, propicillin, sulfanilamide, and sulfamethoxy-diazin. He thus confirmed the earlier results of Hardy and Mansford (1962). In 1963 Marshall separated epinephrine and norepine-phrine from human plasma. In 1964 Hanson and Nielson evaluated the

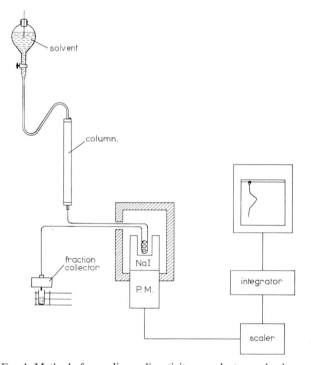

FIG. 1. Method of recording radioactivity on a dextran gel column.

plasma protein binding of Evans blue. We have ourselves used this method to separate pepsin labeled with chromium-51 (Cohen *et al.*, 1967). The principle was simple in that the small molecules are held in a molecular sieve, while large molecules like proteins pass through (Fig. 1). The same solvent (water, citric acid 0.05 M, or the "tris buffer" of Flodin and Killander, 1962) is used both to equilibrate the gel, put to swell in 25 parts of eluate for 72 hr, and to prepare the column and for development. The eluates are collected in samples of 2.4 ml by volume. A spectrophotometric

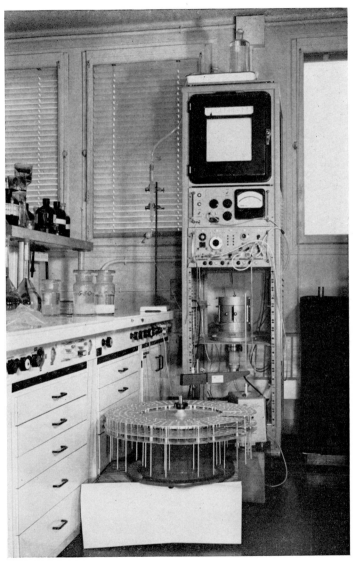

FIG. 2. Apparatus for recording radioactivity on a dextran gel column. (Photograph of Centre d'Etudes Nucleaires de Saclay.)

assay or a biuret reaction (Gornall *et al.*, 1949) detects the proteins; radio-activity can be measured on the labeled substance, either bound to protein, which forms the first radioactive flux, or in the "free" state passing second. In this way Manipol and Spitzy (1962) have been able to separate "free" insulin (labeled with iodine-131) from protein-bound insulin-^{131}I. Ricketts (1966) has fractionated dextran molecules of different molecular weights also labeled with iodine-131.

This technique can be greatly improved by joining on at the end of the sephadex column a polythene catheter which then plunges into the "well" of a sodium iodide crystal of a scintillation counter. The radioactivity is directly recorded as shown in Fig. 2. One of the peaks corresponds to the nonbound tracer and the other to the protein–tracer complex. After passage across the scintillator, the polythene tube is placed above the tubes of a fraction collector. This method can be used along with high-energy γ-ray emitters and β-emitters, which induce bremsstrahlung radiation in the well scintillation counter. The system has not yet been applied to the detection of tracers labeled with carbon-14 or with hydrogen-3, although this may be possible.

The separation of the proteins is effected with gels of sephadex G-75, G-100, and G-200 of increasing porosity (Leach and O'Shea, 1965). A first fractionation can be detected with the sephadex G-100 and G-200 (Porath and Flodin, 1963); however one cannot attain the fine discrimination pro-vided by electrophoretic separation. Figure 3 shows the separation of a mixture of proteins and also of a radioactive tracer (Rousselet, 1967).

2.5. ELECTROPHORESIS AND AUTORADIOGRAPHY

Other methods of protein fractionation are ultracentrifugation, thin-layer chromatography on sephadex (Morris, 1964) and on hydroxy apatite (Kibardin and Lazurkina, 1964), and electrophoresis (Cawley *et al.*, 1965; Fairbanks *et al.*, 1965; Rogers, 1965; Wieme, 1965). Classical electro-phoresis on paper (Block *et al.*, 1955) used largely with unlabeled sub-stances, is also employed with radioactive tracers. Bickel and Bovet, (1962), studied how medicaments deposited in a line are carried on by proteins in their course in the electric field. They observed an interaction between serum albumin and anti-parkinsonian, anti-histaminic, and parasympatholytic substances, and also phenothiazine derivatives. They found no evidence of any interaction with acetylcholine, urea, sympatho-mimetic amines, or curarizing drugs. The interaction with drugs may or may not modify the electrophoretic mobility of the proteins (Murari, 1966).

Morales *et al.* (1966) describe a method whereby one can study the binding of drugs to protein and at the same time check the transport of the drugs and the migration of the protein alone. They applied the method to the protein binding of bilirubin and of aureomycin. The difficulty lies in the detection of the radioactivity. Like Cayen and Anastassiadis (1966), one can cut the paper into strips and immerse them in a scintillating fluid for measuring radioactivity by liquid scintillation; or like Boyd and Mitchell

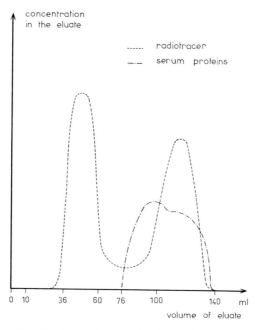

FIG. 3. Separation of a free radiotracer fraction and a protein-bound fraction from blood serum. (Rousselet, 1967.)

(1966) one can replace the water of a polyacrylamide gel (on which the electrophoresis has been performed) by a scintillating solution, and then measure the radioactivity directly; or one can even use the classical method of determining the radioactivity by scanning from end to end of the electrophorogram (Bush, 1963). The resolving power of counters, the windows of which have been collimated, is often insufficient to distinguish the contiguous radioactive peaks corresponding, for instance, to the binding of a radioactive drug to the α_1-globulins or to the α_2-globulins. The two peaks are confusingly recorded as a single large peak. However, since the proportions in albumin, α_1, α_2, β, and γ globulins are given by the degree of optical density of the proteins colored by amido black, there is no difficulty in producing an autoradiogram of the electrophoregram and then measuring the optical density of the dark spots on the radiographic film. This method was first proposed by Murray (1956) and extensively used by Cohen *et al.* (1965). The dried electrophoregram is applied in darkness to a Kodirex radiographic film, and is then left for a period of time which depends on the particular radioelement used, so that the most intense darkening corresponds to a maximal optical density of 0.8. Some experimental results are summarized in Table 3. The exposure time for ^{14}C should be half that used with tritium.

TABLE 3. EXPOSURE TIME OF KODIREX FILM TO SHOW AN 0.002 ml DROP OF ^{51}Cr, ^{198}Au, ^{131}I AND ^{3}H ON PAPER

^{51}Cr (mcC/ml) : time		^{198}Au–^{131}I (mcC/ml):time		^{3}H (mcC/ml):time	
5	2 days	50	min	500	14 days
0.5	8 days	5	6 hr	100	56 days
0.1	1 month	0.5	60 hr	25	150 days

The radiographic film is then developed by standard procedures, and the electrophoresis bands on paper are colored by immersion in a methanol solution saturated with amido black, finally being washed three times in aqueous acetic methanol (Agneray *et al.*, 1959). The paper band, impregnated with a mixture of vaseline oil and α-bromnaphthalene (80/20, V/V), is then placed on a manually operated or automatic densitometer. Optical density is recorded millimeter by millimeter, and displayed on a graph. An identical operation is performed on the autoradiogram. The peaks of optical density are decomposed, and their surface is planimetered. The ratio of each surface area to the total surface area yields the percentage of radioactivity in each fraction. Figure 4 illustrates the improved resolution to be obtained in this way from that obtained in recording the radioactivity by a Geiger–Mueller counter. It is no less necessary to calibrate the optical densitometer in order to be sure of the linearity of its response.

The method has been improved (Cohen *et al.*, 1967) by using a supporting material other than paper, i.e. cellogel or gelatinous cellulose acetate. The bands of cellogel, preserved in a mixture of methanol and water, provide a complete separation of the proteins in $2\frac{1}{2}$ hr, instead of 16–18 hr for paper. The protein spaces are less diffuse than with paper. The phenomenon of labeled molecule tracks is avoided. This supporting material has a disadvantage, in that it has to be dried at 100° after coloration of the proteins before it can be applied to the radiographic film. If the labeled

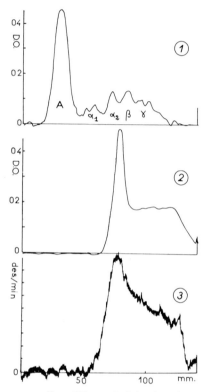

FIG. 4. Simultaneous recording of the optical density of an electrophoregram (1) of the corresponding autoradiogram (2) and of the radioactivity measured on a Geiger counter (3). (Cohen *et al.*, 1965.)

substance is washed out by the coloring reagents, or sublimated by heating to 100°, the autoradiogram will show no binding at all.

One must therefore verify that no loss of radioactivity is involved by these operations.

Figure 5 shows the separation of the albumin–catecholamine-^{14}C complex after mixing of rabbit serum and norepinephrine-^{14}C; the recorded optical density of the electrophorogram and of the autoradiogram is

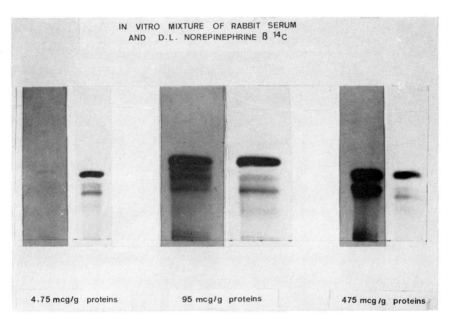

FIG. 5. Electrophoretic separation on cellulose acetate gel of rabbit serum proteins mixed with radioactive norepinephrine.

shown in Fig. 6. We have used this method to study several labeled substances, and we were unable to find any evidence of binding for the following compounds: dimethylbiguanide-^{14}C, paraamino-salicylic acid-^{14}C,

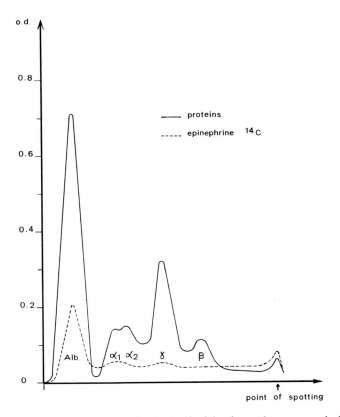

FIG. 6. Recording of the optical density (o.d.) of the electrophoregram and of the
corresponding autoradiogram of a mixture of rabbit serum and radioactive
epinephrine.

ephedrine-^{14}C, chloroquine-^{14}C, and nor-testosterone-^{14}C. The simplicity and ease of this test should ensure its general adoption in studies of
drug metabolism.

Immuno-electrophoresis after Scheidegger (1965), combined with autoradiography, has been employed by Rosenbaum and Reich (1966) to study
the binding of iodized contrast media labeled with iodine-131 in order to
explain the various toxic reactions that are sometimes observed during their

use. By this method one can separate pre-albumin, orosomucoid, albumin, α_1-glycoprotein, haptoglobin, α_2 macroglobulin, ceruloplasmin, transferrin, β_{1c}/β_{1A} globulin, macroglobulin IgM, gamma A (IgA), and gammaglobulin (Igb) in normal man. Iodipamide (Cholographine®) fixes very well on albumin, but not on the other proteins. 3,5, diacetyl amino, 2,4,6-tri-iodo sodium benzoate (Hypaque®), or Renographine® (N-methylglucamine benzoate) do not bind as well to albumin as iodipamide.

Clausen (1966) has observed that a sulfamide labeled with ^{35}S is bound to pre-albumin, albumin, α_1-glycoprotein and to α_2-macroglobulin of human serum all separated and identified by immuno-electrophoresis and autoradiography.

2.6. MISCELLANEOUS

Other methods have been used with varying degrees of success. Ion exchange and precipitation will be considered critically.

Ion exchange

On coming in contact with a well-chosen resin, the free surplus component of a drug can be separated from the component bound to the protein. The resin holds the nonbound tracer.

The resin cannot be separated from the protein solution by decanting or by elution from a column. An appreciable quantity of protein remains adsorbed on the resin, and this will distort the results. Moreover, if the fixing power of the ion-exchange resin is superior to the binding capacity of the protein, the protein-bound labeled derivative is observed to have a constant displacement towards the resin, and in the extreme case the binding, which is governed by the law of mass action, will be zero.

Precipitation

Separation by precipitation, by acids, neutral salts, or by organic solvents, does not seem to be suitable for isolating the radioactive protein–tracer complex: even if the adsorption of the nuclear tracer onto the precipitated particles is not important, one is still faced with the possible destruction of the protein–substance bond. We have ourselves found extreme differences in evaluating serum protein binding of chromium-51, whether the binding was estimated by dialysis or by precipitation of proteins.

3. ADVANTAGES AND DISADVANTAGES OF FRACTIONATION METHODS IN PHARMACOLOGICAL APPLICATIONS

Radioactive tracers permit a finer appreciation of the phenomena observed in the study of drug–protein binding. Their advantages and disadvantages are to be discussed in the following sections.

The advantages are impressive for, in fact, one can bring to light the binding of a protein with a chemical substance, even a paraffinic substance, when the amount of the latter is so small as to be beyond detection by classical chemical and even by biological methods; and this can be done without destroying the protein–drug bond.

Depending on the molecular weight of the protein, or on its electrophoretic mobility, fractionation of the complex permits a precise study of the phenomenon. In conjunction with radioactive measures, automatic recording, autoradiography and evaluation of optical density, fractionation is a method which justifies many more tests and systematic analysis of the saturation of bonds to proteins of different molecular weight. Furthermore, the introduction of radioactive tracers into the cycle of formation or of destruction of the complex permits evaluation of the lifetime of the complex and its recovery from the blood after treatment by methods which have not been mentioned here, but which are considered in detail in Subsection III.

The disadvantages must be brought to light, for they restrict the viability of tracer methods. The main disadvantage is that a global radiation is detected without being sure of the chemical identity of the radioactive molecule. In fact the labeled substance, whether administered to an organism, or mixed with a solution of proteins or blood serum, can be profoundly modified by hydrolysis, oxidation, hydroxylation, conjugation, and methylation. It is therefore necessary to check the identity of the chemical species bound to the protein, and to control constantly by crosschecks the results obtained by means of labeled compounds.

With this proviso, the results are valuable in throwing light upon the physiological and pharmacological significance of protein–drug binding. We shall now consider in turn the role of blood protein storage, the modifications resulting from binding to the blood proteins, the effects produced by the displacement of bound hormones, and finally, the displacement of one drug by another.

3.1. ROLE OF BLOOD PROTEIN STORAGE

It has been found that the binding of drugs to blood proteins protects them against cellular degradation enzymes such as the sulfamide acetylase of pigeon liver (Anton and Boyle, 1964). The bond may stop the drug diffusing beyond the blood compartment so that the concentration of drugs in extracellular fluid, lymph or cerebrospinal fluid will be comparable only to the plasma concentration of the nonbound drug, as found by Verwey and Williams (1962) for penicillin. This implies that the concentration in biological fluids such as milk is dependent upon the nonbound drug concentration in the blood as shown by Rasmussen (1959) for penicillin. It will be useful to study the binding as and when the dosage of new substances becomes established. If the binding keeps the drug away from the receptors, it will be necessary to start the treatment with larger doses and then to reduce them progressively as the binding sites of the serum proteins become saturated. This buffering effect in regard to dosage, may be considered to be of importance in the detoxication of the drugs. On the other hand, the binding may entail an induced fit of the protein molecule, and this will manifest itself in a modification of the electrophoretic mobility of the protein molecule (Murari, 1966), and will accelerate the formation of anti-drugs antibodies.

3.2. DISPLACEMENT OF BOUND HORMONES

Since the number of binding sites is limited, and numerous substances, whether cationic or anionic, may all compete for the same sites, one must expect to observe a displacement of such physiological protein-bound substances as bilirubin, thyroid hormones, or cortico-suprarenal hormones. The death of newborn infants due to jaundice has been attributed to this phenomenon, as also derangement of the thyroid function by radiocontrast media (Lasser *et al.*, 1962) and the intensity of the anti-inflammation properties of certain drugs (Brodie, 1966).

3.3. DISPLACEMENT OF ONE ACTIVE SUBSTANCE BY ANOTHER

Some recent research work has endeavored to explain interaction of drugs in terms of binding to proteins (Kunin, 1964). Thus phenylbutazone displaces from a protein complex the sulfonamides (Anton, 1961), penicillin and its derivatives, phenoxymethyl-penicillin and cloxacillin. Kunin

(1965) and Keen (1966b) have estimated the competitive affinity of several compounds for the binding sites of phenyl-methoxy-penicillin. On human or bovine serum albumin the competitive affinity is in the following decreasing order: salicylate > tolbutamide > sulfinpyrazone > phenyl-butazone > novobiocin > probenecid. It may happen that two antibiotics compete for the same site. Some combinations may therefore result in an attenuation of action, and by no means any enhancement. With anti-coagulants of the coumaro type one finds a danger of bleeding if these are associated with any drug which competes for the same sites on the proteins. The administration of iodized contrast media may likewise prolong the duration of anesthesia after a given dose of pentobarbital.

We have insisted on these few examples of the pharmacological implications of drug binding to blood-plasma proteins in order to emphasize the importance which must be attached to the practical aspect of studies on binding.

4. BINDING BY TISSUE PROTEINS

The binding of drugs by tissue proteins presupposes that the complex formed in the plasma with albumin or globulins has been destroyed. Only the nonbound substances in the lymph or extracellular fluid can combine with tissue proteins. Binding is not proved by the presence of a certain amount of drug in an organ. This may in fact be due to the presence of blood in the vessels of the organ and to the drug remaining in solution in the extracellular fluid of the organ. To produce evidence of binding to a tissue, the tissue must be deprived of blood and careful washing must have removed the original extracellular fluid, so that only molecules bound to the cells remain in the tissue. Autoradiographic detection of a substance in the midst of an organ is not sufficient to prove that this substance has bound with the constituents of the organ. In this case the detection is a first indication of possible binding, but it is necessary to go beyond that. Binding may occur on the level of the cell membrane or within the cell on the nucleus, on cytoplasmic organelles or in the cytoplasmic fluid. It has not been established that the binding may only go on with proteins, since it is known that polypeptides, lipids, and polysaccharides also intervene (Woolley and Gommi, 1966). It therefore becomes necessary to isolate the protein bound to the drug. Furthermore, the protein may be a type of specific "receptor", and be present only in the target organ, or on the other hand, find itself in several tissues, and no longer correspond to the characteristics of a specific pharmacological receptor. This latter protein would constitute a site of loss *vis-à-vis* the drug, and it would act as an "acceptor" with no specificity at all. The term "acceptor" is introduced in order to distinguish binding that is not followed by physiological action from effective binding with the "specific receptor".

For a great many drugs, the protein is an enzyme in relation to which the drugs are substrates. Ariens *et al.* (1964) consider that it is due to labeled molecules that the existence of specific receptors has been directly demonstrated. The research of Waser, reviewed in a recent note (1965), provides proof that curarizing agents are localized on specific receptors, in the motor end plates of the diaphragms of mice. Green (1962) did a survey of the tissue proteins capable of binding with biogenic amines, i.e. histamine, norepinephrine, and 5-hydroxytryptamine. In this immense field of study we shall confine ourselves to considerations affecting methods of study by labeled molecules.

4.1. METHODS OF STUDY

The study of the binding of drugs to tissue proteins can be resolved into the following procedural steps:

(a) production of evidence of binding to a specific tissue;
(b) production of evidence of a cellular bond;
(c) cell fractionation and production of evidence of binding to subcellular fractions;
(d) isolation of the tissue protein, and of the complex with the drug;
(e) demonstration of the specific type of binding and the function of the protein as a "receptor".

Tissue binding

The first phase of research, as mentioned above, is to produce evidence of binding to a specific tissue. Autoradiography on whole animals (Ullberg, 1954), the auto-historadiography of Fischman and Gershon (1964), or as applied by Wohler and Hoffmann (1964) using methyl sulphadiazin-^{35}S, and the methods for measuring radioactivity in homogenized tissue (Petroff *et al.*, 1965), all represent approaches to this problem. The homogenized tissues are mixed with some hyamine to permit the direct measurement of the radioactivity in scintillation fluid. In a recent review this problem has been discussed from a general point of view (Cohen, 1963). McIsaac (1962) has studied the distribution of hexamethonium-^{14}C in the cat, and he found that the quantity of plasma retained in tissues is not negligible: it amounts to 130 mcl of plasma per gram of kidney, 111 mcl per gram of liver, but only 5.3 mcl per gram of skeletal muscle and 9.6 mcl per gram of brain tissue.

By these methods, studies have been made of indomethacin-^{14}C (Hucker *et al.*, 1966), chlortalidone-^{14}C (Beisenherz *et al.*, 1966), serotonin-^{14}C (Gershon and Ross, 1966a and b), mescaline α-^{14}C (Neff *et al.*, 1963), amphetamine-^{14}C (Young and Gordon, 1962), dichloro-isoproterenol-^{3}H (Mayer, 1962), norepinephrine-^{14}C (Kopin *et al.*, 1965), histamine-^{14}C (Snyder *et al.*, 1964; Furano and Green, 1964). This is not the place to give the results in detail, but this list, although incomplete, does show the interest aroused by this method of investigation.

Cellular binding

It is more difficult to produce evidence of cellular binding, since one has to distinguish the drug content of the plasma from that of the extracellular fluids. A measure of tissue plasma by albumin ^{131}I and of extracellular fluid by ^{82}Br is needed (see Robertson, Stoclet, Winbury, and Lamb in subsection III). It is necessary to estimate the radioactive substance concentration of the plasma and of the ultrafiltrate, and then to subtract the calculated quantity from the total quantity found experimentally in the tissue in order to assess the cell content of a drug.

Subcellular binding

After homogenization of a tissue one obtains a pulp consisting of intact cells, broken cells, nuclei, mitochondria, microsomes, and organelles. The homogenates can be extracted directly by the use of different solvents (Wong and Spratt, 1963; Lage and Spratt, 1965), or, alternatively, they can be fractionated by differential sedimentation in a gravitational field following the classical method of Schneider and Hagebom (1950). After having been homogenized in an 0.88 M saccharose solution, the tissue pulp is subjected to low temperature centrifuging at 700 g, 24,000 g, and 105000 g. In each centrifugation one obtains a deposit and a supernatant.

The first deposit P_1 consists of undestroyed cells and nuclei, the second deposit P_2 consists of mitochondria, and the third P_3 of microsomes. The final supernatant contains nonsedimentable elements in solution. The deposit that can readily be obtained by sufficiently long centrifugation with a given field, or on two occasions with the same field, are all measured for radioactivity; but the supernatants are so measured only when no further centrifugation is required. The procedure can be improved by fractionating the P_2 particles into particles A less dense than the solution of saccharose 0.8 M, particles B somewhere between the density of the 0.8 M and 1.2 M solutions of saccharose, and particles C with greater density than that of a saccharose solution of 1.2 M, as proposed by Michaelson and Whittaker (1963).

These operations are schematically represented in Fig. 7. The sub-fractions A, B, and C of P_2 are examined in an electron microscope, and they are composed of myelin, nerve-ending particles (NEP) or synaptosomes, and mitochondria respectively. This method has been used by

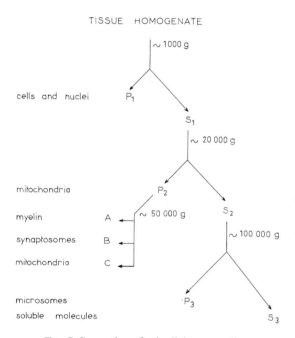

FIG. 7. Separation of subcellular organelles.

Masuoka (1965) and by Glowinski *et al.* (1966) in order to analyze the binding of biogenous amines to varicosities of brain nerve-endings, and by Fisher and Snyder (1965) to detect norepinephrine in the sympathetic ganglia of the cat. Such methods are also becoming increasingly used further afield (Ingrand, 1966; Musacchio *et al.*, 1965) for very different organs (liver and salivary glands). Radioactivity is measured either directly, or after separation of the labeled molecule and its metabolites by a chromatographic process.

Binding to cell protein

It is still necessary to be more precise about the type of the proteic macromolecule to which the pharmacologically active substance is attached. Estimation of nitrogen in the deposit is one element constantly referred to. In the last supernatant, which is supposed to contain only dissolved substances, there are soluble proteins. Talwar *et al.* (1964) fractionated the last supernatant by passage on a column of sephadex G-100. They showed that oestradiol, known to bind to the uterus (De Paepe, 1960; Eisenfeld and Axelrod, 1965), is bound to the first protein fraction to pass the column. It is very difficult to isolate the tissue protein responsible for the binding of the drug in the tissue. In general one comes across a mixture of macromolecules and, on these, dialysis, electrophoresis, and other experiments (Graham, 1960) are carried out using the same methods as those proposed above for plasma proteins.

The task of identifying these tissue proteins is an arduous one. The pharmacologist seeks to find some typical chemical grouping responsible for the capacity for binding, and which might be related to the prosthetic group of an enzyme.

Specific nature of cellular protein

To judge the specificity of the binding, the pharmacologist needs to compare several tissues with each other, e.g. heart and skeletal muscle, intestines or lungs and uterus, liver and brain, etc. Thus, for instance, Talwar *et al.* (1964) observed that a protein fraction which is drawn from the uterus is capable of binding to oestradiol, while the same fraction taken from the lungs does not have this capacity. This uterine fraction acts as a represser of RNA synthesis of *Escherichia coli.* Its binding to oestradiol makes it lose this property. The pulmonary protein is devoid of these effects.

Conscious of this concept of binding to a specific protein regarded as a pharmacological receptor, Ingrand (1966) compared the fixation of ^{51}Cr-labeled cytochrome C to the subcellular organelles of rat liver cells with the binding of ^{51}Cr-labeled heterologous proteins in the same conditions. The cytochrome-*c* presents a bond with the mitochondria which is significantly different to the binding of heterologous proteins. For Wolhtmann and Narahara (1966), besides a "specific accumulation" of insulin ^{131}I in correlation with the biological action of this substance on the permeability of muscle tissue to sugar, there is also a "nonspecific accumulation" independently of hormonal activity which is subject only to the concentration of insulin in the medium. This well illustrates how complicated is the notion of specific binding, since the same tissue may have acceptor sites as well as receptor sites, with no means of differentiating between them other than by kinetic calculation.

4.2. SIGNIFICANCE OF THE METHODS

The methods that have just been described are more often than not very intricate, requiring a long period of time to perform. The results obtained are not entirely lacking in interest, and they advance our knowledge of the distribution of drugs in the organism and in the tissues. But one should not conceal the fact that, beyond descriptive advice, it is still necessary to adduce experimental proof for the hypothesis formulated with regard to specific receptors. Our misgivings stem from the lack of finesse in the methods of fractionation and subcellular analysis, and much less from the tracer methods, although the criticisms we have made previously with regard to plasma proteins may well apply here as well.

In any event we are getting to the heart of living biological matter, since henceforth immunologists are able to follow the binding of a synthetic antigen with certain cells of the reticulo-endothelial system, in order to observe the effects produced by nuclear chromatine antigen interaction and to suggest how antibodies are formed (Roberts, 1966). Research has now proceded beyond the stage of studying the binding of medicinal substances to proteins to explaining the induction of the synthesis of specific proteins, the structure of which is determined by the foreign molecule. We are here touching upon molecular biology. All progress in this field will be exploited in pharmacology.

CONCLUSION

Our knowledge on the binding of drugs to proteins has been advancing slowly over more than half a century. In this chapter we wanted to show how research in this field is rewarding and to show the position of this research in relation to general pharmacology. Certain rules have been evolved, all of which are discussed above. The binding to blood proteins and tissue proteins is influenced by the physico-chemical nature of the particular drug. A better knowledge of the structure of these proteins is necessary for a better understanding of the modalities of the bonds. One has always to wait for biochemists establishing chemical formulae for protein macromolecules before a new step forward can be made in pharmacology.

As regards the theoretical aspect of the problem, the application of such studies to new drugs is not entirely lacking in interest in so far as it leads on to a better knowledge of drugs, and will set dosage on a firm experimental basis.

Radioactive tracer methods have assisted research in association with the well-known techniques of protein separation and fractionation into individualized protein species. Their great merit derives from their convenience to the experimenter, and from the abundance of data which such experiments produce. Experiments can be performed on a much greater scale, and the test parameters (and hence the factors which determine the drug-protein binding) can be systematically analyzed. Moreover, the limits of detection have been pushed beyond all previous expectations, and the precision of these methods once more calls into question some generally accepted theories. On the other hand, the researcher must be on the alert to show a critical spirit; the results have to be confirmed by cross-checking; and, above all, every effort must be made to identify the radioactive molecule detected.

With this condition, one may justifiably speak of some part being played by blood protein storage, one can analyze the mechanism whereby hormones are displaced from their bond to blood macromolecules, and the unwanted effects of an association of drugs can be prevented, and the appearance of specific antibodies of some hormonal medication, for instance, can be anticipated.

In this contribution we have not touched upon the kinetics of protein–drug complexes, or on how long they stay in the blood-stream or on their rates of renewal. Clearly, such research is possible. It is sufficient to apply the methods expounded in Subsection III. Nor have we analyzed the process by which the drug–protein complex becomes dissociated into its two elements. In this respect we know neither the modalities nor the determinism within the living organism. Certainly we shall in future see researchers pay attention to this. If dissociation can appear to be an "accessory question" for blood proteins, it is no less the case for the tissue proteins.

Unfortunately, however, the tissue proteins are less well known than the proteins of blood plasma. The relevant papers are rare, at least in any case those dealing with the binding of drugs. On that account the scientific approach is more prudent: it proceeds stage by stage. Protein in its cytoplasmic medium certainly does not have the same configuration *in vitro* as in solution. The binding has to be studied *in situ* by the methods described in Chapter 7. These methods must have an increasingly large capacity for separation, since the bond has to be detected at the subcellular level, and then the receptive protein molecule needs to be isolated. This molecule may be the "effector" which is to have its equilibrium modified by the drug and so exhibit some mechanical, electric, or chemical change of state; or, on the other hand, the molecule may be an indifferent acceptor, not physiologically involved in the binding.

The tracer method, being nondestructive, seems to us to be the only far-reaching means of analysis of the fundamental mechanisms of the action of drugs. It enables direct evidence of the specific receptor to be obtained, and this has until recently been an abstract concept without objective demonstration.

These concluding remarks which summarize the major lines of research in the field of drug–protein binding, emphasize, if this were necessary, the fundamental contribution of radioactive tracers to this research.

REFERENCES

(a) BOOKS, REVIEWS AND MONOGRAPHS

ARIENS, E. J., SIMONIS, A. M. and VAN ROSSUM, J. M. (1964) Drug receptor interaction: interaction of one or more drugs with one receptor system: II.A.7.3. A direct approach to receptors, in *Molecular Pharmacology*, Vol. 1. Ariens, E. J. (ed.). Academic Press, New York, U.S.A., pp. 267–69.

BLOCK, R., DURRUM, E. and ZWEIG, G. A. (1955) *Manual of Paper Chromatography and Electrophoresis*. Academic Press, New York, U.S.A.

BRODIE, B. B. (1964) Physicochemical factors in drug absorption, in *Absorption and Distribution of Drugs*, Binns, T. B. (ed.). Livingstone, Edinburgh, pp. 16–48.

BRODIE, B. B. (1965) Displacement of one drug by another from carrier or receptor sites. *Proc. Roy. Soc. Med.*, **58**:946–55.

BRODIE, B. B. (1966) Pharmacological and clinical implications of drug transport, in *Transport Function of Plasma Proteins*, Desgrez, P. and De Traverse, P. M. (eds.). Elsevier, Amsterdam, pp. 137–45.

BUSH, I. E. (1963) Advances in direct scanning of paper chromatograms for quantitative estimations, in *Methods of Biochemical Analysis*, Vol. 11. Interscience, New York, U.S.A., pp. 149–209.

COHEN, Y. (1963) Problèmes de pharmacodynamie générale abordés à l'aide de radio-éléments. *Actual. Pharmacol.*, **15**:45–97.

COHEN, Y., WEPIERRE, J. and ROUSSELET, J. P. (1966) Radioactive isotopes in investigating transport phenomena by plasma proteins, in *Transport Function of Plasma Proteins*. Desgrez, P. and De Traverse, P. M. (eds.). Elsevier, Amsterdam, pp. 19–39.

COHEN, Y., WEPIERRE, J. and ROUSSELET, J. P. (1967) Les radio-éléments dans l'étude des phénomènes de transport par les protéines plasmatiques. *Ann. Biol. Clin.*, **25**: 81–106.

DESGREZ, P. and DE TRAVERSE, P. M. (ed.). (1966) *Transport Function of Plasma Proteins*. Elsevier, Amsterdam.

GOLDSTEIN, A. (1949) The interactions of drugs and plasma proteins. *Pharmacol. Rev.*, **1**:102–65.

GREEN, J. P. (1962) Binding of some biogenic amines in tissues, in *Advances in Pharmacology*, Vol. 1. Garattini, S. and Shore, P. A. (eds.). Academic Press, New York, U.S.A., pp. 349–422.

KLOTZ, I. M. (1953) Protein interaction, in *The Proteins, Chemistry, Biological Activity and Methods*. Neurath, H. and Bailey, K. (eds.). Academic Press, New York, U.S.A., 727–806.

KOSHLAND, D. E. (1963) Biological specificity in protein small molecule interactions, in Proc. 1st Int. Pharmacol. Meeting, Vol. 7. Brunings, K. J. (ed.). Pergamon, New York, U.S.A., pp. 161–91.

NICHOL, L. W., BETHUNE, J. L., KEGELES, G. and HESS, E. L. (1964) Interacting protein systems, in *The Proteins, Composition, Structure and Function*. Neurath, H (ed.). Academic Press, New York, U.S.A., pp. 305–403.

SALVATORE, G., ANDREOLI, M. and ROCHE, J. (1966) Thyroid hormones-plasma proteins interactions, in *Transport Function of Plasma Proteins*. Desgrez, P. and De Traverse, P.M. (eds.). Elsevier, Amsterdam, pp. 57–73.

STEINHARDT, J., BEYCHOCK, S. (1964) Interaction of proteins with hydrogen ions and other small ions and molecules, in *The Proteins, Composition, Structure and Function*. Neurath, H. (ed.). Academic Press, New York, U.S.A., pp. 139–304.

THORP, J. M. (1964) The influence of plasma proteins on the action of drugs, in *Absorption and Distribution of Drugs*. Binns, T. B. (ed.). Livingstone, Edinburgh, pp. 64–76.

VAN OS, A. J., ARIENS, E. J. and SIMONIS, A. M. (1964) Drug transference distribution of drugs in the organism, in *Molecular Pharmacology*, Vol. 1. Ariens, E. J. (ed.). Academic Press, New York, U.S.A., pp. 7–52.

WASER, P. G. (1965). Autoradiographic investigation of curarizing and depolarizing drugs in the motor end plate, in *Isotopes in Experimental Pharmacology*. Roth, L. J. (ed.). University of Chicago Press, Chicago, Ill., U.S.A., pp. 99–116.

WIEME, R. J. (1965) *Agar Gel Electrophoresis*, Elsevier, Amsterdam.

(B) ORIGINAL PAPERS

ACRED, P., BROWN, D. M., HARDY, T. L. and MANSFORD, K. R. L. (1963) A new approach to studying the protein-binding properties of penicillines. *Nature, Lond.*, **199**:758–9.

AGNERAY, J., WEPIERRE, J. and PUISIEUX, F. (1959) Décoloration automatique des protéinogrammes sans distillation. Étude des causes d'erreurs. *Ann. Biol. Clin.*, **17**:251–7.

ANTON, A. H. (1960) The relation between the binding of sulfonamides to albumin and their antibacterial efficacy. *J. Pharmacol.*, **129**:282–90.

ANTON, A. H. (1961) A drug induced change in the distribution and renal excretion of sulfonamides. *J. Pharmacol.*, **134**:291–303.

ANTON, A. H. and BOYLE, J. J. (1964) Alteration of the acetylation of sulfonamides by protein binding, sulfinpyrazone and suramin. *Canad. J. Physiol. Pharmacol.*, **42**: 809–17.

BARLOW, C. F., FIREMARK, H. and ROTH, L. J. (1962) Drug plasma binding measured by sephadex. *J. Pharm. Pharmacol.*, **14**:550–5.

BEAL, R. W. (1964) The plasma protein binding of radioactive vitamine B-12. I: Factors influencing *in vitro* binding. *J. Clin. Lab. Med.*, **63**:968–76.

BEISENHERZ, G., KOSS, F. W., KLATT, L. and BINDER, B. (1966) Distribution of radio-activity in the tissues and excretory products of rats and rabbits following administration of C^{14} Hygroton. *Arch. Int. Pharmacodyn.*, **161**:76–93.

BEUTNER, R. (1925) The binding power of serum for drugs tested by a new *in vitro* method. *J. Pharmacol.*, **25**:365–380.

BEUTNER, R. (1926) The reaction between serum and alkaloids. *J. Pharmacol.*, **29**: 95–103.

BICKEL, M. H. and BOVET, D. (1962) Relationship between structure and albumine-binding of amines tested with crossing-paper electrophoresis. *J. Chromatog.*, **8**:466–74.

BOYD, J. B. and MITCHELL, H. K. (1966) Measurement of the radioactivity in carbon 14 and tritium labelled proteins that have been separated by disk electrophoresis. *Analyt. Biochem.*, **14**:441–54.

CAWLEY, L. P., EBERHARDT, L. and SCHNEIDER, D. (1965) Simplified gel electrophoresis. II: Application of immunoelectrophoresis. *J. Lab. Clin. Med.*, **65**:342–54.

CAYEN, M. N. and ANASTASSIADIS, P. A., (1966) A simplified technique for the liquid scintillation measurement of radioactivity on paper chromatograms containing C^{14} and H^3 labeled compounds. *Analyt. Biochem.*, **15**:84–92.

CLAUSEN, J. (1966) Binding of sulfonamides to serum proteins physico chemical and immuno chemical studies. *J. Pharmacol.*, **153**:167–75.

COHEN, Y., BLANCHARD-PELLETIER, O. and BONFILS, S. (1967) Le marquage de la pepsine par le chlorure de chrome ^{51}Cr. Choix des conditions techniques et des contrôles. *C. R. Soc. Biol. Paris* **160**: 2272-7.

COHEN, Y. and DELASSUE, H. (1959) Modification de la méthode d'autoradiographie de S. Ullberg sur coupe de souris entière. *C. R. Soc. Biol. Paris*, **153**:300–4.

COHEN, Y. and WEPIERRE, J. (1961) Méthode d'étude autoradiographique de substances marquées volatiles. 1er Symposium Européen d'Autoradiographie dans les Sciences Med. Rome, Rapport C.E.A. 2071, Centre d'Études Nucléaires de Saclay.

COHEN, Y., WEPIERRE, J. and PONTY, D. (1965) Fixation du chrome 51 sur les fractions protéiques de sérum sanguin, in *Radioaktive Isotope in Klinik und Forschung*, Vol. 6, Fellinger, K. and Höfer, R. (eds.). Urban u. Schwarzenberg, München, pp. 273–86.

COLLIPP, P. J., KAPLAN, S. A. (1966) Interaction of ^{14}C labeled human and bovine growth hormone with serum proteins. *Biochim. Biophys. Acta*, **117**:416–23.

DE PAEPE, J. C. (1960) An autoradiographic study of the distribution in mice of oestrogens labelled with carbon 14 and tritium. *Nature, Lond*, **185**:264–5.

DOUGLAS, J. F., BRADSHAW, W. H., LUDWIG, B. J. and POWERS, D. (1964) Interaction of plasma protein with related 1–3 propanediol dicarbamates. *Biochem. Pharmacol.*, **13**: 537–9.

EBERHARDT, H. (1963) Der Salizylgehalt der Rattenorgane nach parenteraler Verabreichung von radioaktivem Natriumsalizilat. *Arch. Int. Pharmacodyn.*, **143**:205–18.

EHRLICH, P. (1909) Uber den jetzigen Stand der Chemotherapie. *Ber. dtsch. Chem. Ges.* **42**:17–47.

EIBER, H. B. and DANISHEFSKY, I. (1959) Distribution of injected heparin in different blood fractions. *Proc. Soc. Exp. Biol. N.Y.*, **102**:18–20.

EISENFELD, A. J. and AXELROD, J. (1965) Selectivity of oestrogen distribution in tissues. *J. Pharmacol.*, **160**:469–75.

FAIRBANKS, G., LEVINTHAL, C. and REEDER, R. H. (1965) Analysis of C^{14} labeled proteins by disc electrophoresis. *Biochem. Biophys. Res. Commun.*, **20**:393–9.

FISCHER, E. (1894) Einfluss der Configuration auf die Wirkung der Enzyme. *Ber. dtsch. Chem. Ges.*, **27**:2985.

FISCHER, J. E. and SNYDER, S. (1965) Disposition of norepinephrine H^3 in sympathetic ganglia. *J. Pharmacol.*, **150**:190–5.

FISCHMAN, D. A. and GERSHON, M. D. (1964) A method for studying intracellular movement of water soluble isotopes prior to radioautography. *J. Cell Biol.*, **21**:139–43.

FLODIN, P. and KILLANDER, J. (1962) Fractionation of human serum proteins by gel filtration. *Biochim. Biophys. Acta*, **63**:403–10.

FLORINI, J. R., PEETS, E. A. and BUYSKE, D. A. (1961) Plasma half-life, tissue distribution and excretion of triamcinolone ^{3}H. *J. Pharmacol.* **131**:287–93.

FURANO, A. V. and GREEN, J. P. (1964) The uptake of biogenic amines by mast cells of the rat. *J. Physiol. Lond.*, **170**:263–71.

GERSHON, M. D. and ROSS, L. L. (1966a) Radioisotopic studies of the binding, exchange and distribution of 5-hydroxy-tryptamine synthetized from its radioactive precursor. *J. Physiol. Lond.*, **186**:451–76.

GERSHON, M. D. and ROSS, L. L. (1966b) Location of sites of 5 hydroxytryptamine storage and metabolism by radioautography. *J. Physiol. Lond.*, **186**:477–92.

GLOWINSKI, J., SNYDER, S. H. and AXELROD, J. (1966) Subcellullar localization of H³ norepinephrine in the rat brain and the effect of drugs. *J. Pharmacol.*, **152**:282–92.

GORNALL, A. G., BARDOWILL, C. J. and DAVID, M. M. (1949) Determination of serum proteins by means of the biuret reaction. *J. Biol. Chem.*, **177**:751–66.

GRAHAM, J. D. P. (1960) Binding of ¹⁴C.J.11 by isolated tissue. *J. Physiol. Lond.*, **152**:50P–51P.

HANSEN, P. and NIELSEN, C. (1964) The binding of Evans blue to plasma proteins. An evaluation using adsorption onto Sephadex. *Scand. J. Clin. Lab. Invest.*, **16**:491–7.

HARDWICKE, J. and HOWEL JONES, J. (1966) The nature of the vitamine B-12 binding protein in human serum. *Brit. J. Haemat.*, **12**:529–35.

HARDY, T. L. and MANSFORD, K. R. L. (1962) Gel filtration as a method of studying drug-protein binding. *Biochem. J.*, **83**:34P–35P.

HUCKER, H. B., ZACCHEI, A. G., COX, S. V., BRODIE, D. A. and CANTWELL, N. H. R. (1966) Studies on the absorption, distribution and excretion of indomethacin in various species. *J. Pharmacol.*, **153**:237–49.

INGRAND, J. (1966) Le cytochrome C marqué au chrome 51. I: Préparation, analyse et distribution intracellulaire. *Biochem. Pharmacol.*, **15**:1649–53.

KEEN, P. M. (1965) The binding of three penicillins in the plasma of several mammalian species as studied by ultrafiltration at body temperature. *Brit. J. Pharmacol.*, **25**:507–14.

KEEN, P. M. (1966a) The binding of penicillines to bovine serum albumin. *Biochem. Pharmacol.*, **15**:447–63.

KEEN, P. M. (1966b) The displacement of three anionic drugs from binding to bovine serum albumin by various anionic compounds. *Brit. J. Pharmacol.*, **26**:704–12.

KIBARDIN, S. A. and LAZURKINA, V. B. (1965) Thin layer chromatography of proteins on plates coated with hydroxy apatite. *Biochemistry, USSR*, **30**:483–6.

KOPIN, I. J., GORDON, E. K. and HORST, W. D. (1965) Studies of uptake of l norepinephrine ¹⁴C. *Biochem. Pharmacol.*, **14**:753–9.

KRAMARENKO, V. P. (1961) Binding of alkaloids by proteins. *Farmatsevt Zh. Kiev.*, **16**:16–20.

KUNIN, C. M. (1964) Enhancement of antimicrobial activity of penicillins and other antibiotics in human serum by competitive serum binding inhibitors. *Proc. Soc. Exp. Biol. N.Y.*, **117**:69–73.

KUNIN, C. M. (1965) Inhibition of penicillin binding to serum proteins. *J. Lab. Clin. Med.*, **65**:416–31.

LAGE, G. L. and SPRATT, J. L. (1965) H³ digoxin metabolism by adult male rat tissues *in vitro*. *J. Pharmacol.*, **149**:248–56.

LASSER, E. C., FARR, R. S., FUJIMAGARI, T. and TRIPP, W. N. (1962) The significance of protein binding of contrast media in Roentgen diagnosis. *Amer. J. Roentg.*, **87**:338–60.

LEACH, A. A. and O'SHEA, P. C. (1965) The determination of protein molecular weights of up to 225000 by gel filtration on a single column of sephadex G-200 at 25° and 40°. *J. Chromatog.*, **17**:245–51.

MCISAAC, R. J. (1962) The relationship between distribution and pharmacological activity of hexamethonium-N-methyl ¹⁴C. *J. Pharmacol.*, **135**:335–43.

MANIPOL, V. and SPITZY, H. (1962) Separation of I¹³¹ labelled protein-bound insulin from "free" insulin. *Int. J. Appl. Rad. Isotopes.*, **13**:647–8.

MARSHALL, C. S. (1963) The use of sephadex G-25 for the separation of catecholamines from plasma. *Biochim. Biophys. Acta*, **74**:158–9.

MASUOKA, D. (1965) Monoamines in isolated nerve ending particles. *Biochem. Pharmacol.*, **14**:1688–9.

MAYER, S. E. (1962) The physiological disposition of H³ dichloro isoproterenol. *J. Pharmacol.*, **135**, 204–12.

MICHAELSON, I. A. and WHITTAKER, V. P. (1963) The subcellular localization of 5 hydroxy tryptamine in guinea pig brain. *Biochem. Pharmacol.*, **12**:203–11.

MILLER, J. M., ROBINSON, D. R. and WILLIARD, R. F. (1960a) A study of trypsin ¹³¹I in rabbits. *Exp. Med. Surg.*, **18**:341–7.

MILLER, J. M., WILLIARD, R. F. and POLLACHEK, A. A. (1960b) An investigation of trypsin ¹³¹I in patients. *Exp. Med. Surg.*, **18**:352–70.

MORALES-MALVA, J. A., JAPAG-HAGAR, M. and ISRAEL-BUDNICK, S. (1966) A preparatory paper electrophoresis method for the study of the transporting capacity of serum proteins. *Clin. Chim. Acta*, **14**:667–71.

MORRIS, C. T. (1964) Thin layer chromatography of proteins on sephadex G 100 and 200. *J. Chromatogr.*, **16**:167–75.

MURARI, G. (1966) Ricerche sul legame farmaco proteico: influenza del furazolidone e della nitro furantoina sulla mobilita elettroforetica di frazioni seriche bovine. *Arch. Ital. Sci. Farmacol.*, **14**:224–7.

MURRAY, I. M. (1956) Interaction of stabilized radiogold colloid and plasma proteins. *Proc. Soc. Exp. Biol. N.Y.*, **91**:252–5.

MUSACCHIO, J. M., FISCHER, J. E. and KOPIN, I. J. (1965) Effects of chronic sympathetic denervation on subcellular distribution of some sympathomimetic amines. *Biochem. Pharmacol.*, **14**:898–900.

NEAL, G. E. and WILLIAMS, D. C. (1965) The fate of intravenously injected folate in rats. *Biochem. Pharmacol.*, **14**:903–14.

NEFF, N., ROSSI, G. V., CHASE, G. D. and RABINOWITZ, J. L. (1964) Distribution and metabolism of mescaline C¹⁴ in the cat brain. *J. Pharmacol.*, **144**:1–7.

PETROFF, C. P., PATT, H. H. and NAIR, P. P. (1965) A rapid method for dissolving tissue for liquid scintillation counting. *Int. J. Appl. Rad. Isotopes*, **16**:599–601.

PORATH, J. and FLODIN, P. (1959) Gel filtration: A method for desalting and group separation. *Nature, Lond.*, **183**:1657–9.

PORATH, J. and FLODIN, P. (1963) Gel filtration, in *Protides of the Biological Fluids*, Vol. 10. Peeters, H. (ed.). Elsevier, Amsterdam, pp. 290–7.

RASMUSSEN, F. (1959) Mammary excretion of benzylpenicillin, erythromycin and penethamate hydroiodide. *Acta Pharmacol. Kbh.*, **16**:194–200.

RICKETTS, C. R. (1966). Isotopically labelled macromolecules in biological research: Dextran labelled with radioactive iodine. *Nature, London.*, **210**:1113–5.

RIEDER, J. (1963) Physikalisch-chemische und biologische Untersuchungen an Sulfonamiden. *Arzneimittel-Forsch.*, **13**:81–103.

ROBERTS, A. N. (1966) Cellular localization and quantitation of tritiated antigen in mouse lymph nodes during early primary immun response. *Amer. J. Path.*, **49**:889–909.

ROGERS, L. J. (1965) A simple apparatus for disc electrophoresis. *Biochim. Biophys. Acta*, **94**:324–9.

ROLINSON, G. N. and SUTHERLAND, R. (1965) The binding of antibiotics to serum proteins. *Brit. J. Pharmacol.*, **25**:638–50.

ROSENBAUM, E. H. and REICH, S. B. (1966) Binding of radiographic contrast media to serum protein demonstrated by immunoelectrophoresis and radio autography. *Radiology*, **86**:515–9.

ROUSSELET, J. P. (1967) Contribution à l'étude pharmacologique du transport des colloïdes d'or radioactif par le sang et les exsudats séreux, Rapport C.E.A.R. 3064 Centre d'Etudes Nucléaires de Saclay.

SANDBERG, A. A., SLAUNWHITE, W. R. and ANTONIADES, H. N. (1961) Effects of time and steroid concentration on binding of ¹⁴C oestrogens in human plasma. *Proc. Soc. Exp. Biol. N.Y.*, **106**:831–4.

SCHEIDEGGER, J. J. (1955) Une microméthode de l'immunoélectrophorèse. *Int. Arch. Allergy, Basel*, 7:103–10.

SCHEN, A. J. and RABINOVITZ, M. (1966) The affinity of tetracycline for human serum lipoproteins demonstrated by fluor immunoelectrophoresis. *Israel. J. Med. Sci.*, 2:86–7.

SCHNEIDER, W. C. and HAGEBOM, G. H. (1950) Intracellular distribution of enzymes. V: Further studies on the distribution of cytochrome C in rat liver homogenates. *J. Biol. Chem.*, 183:123–8.

SCHOLTAN, W. (1964) Vergleichende quantitative Bestimmung der Eiweissbindung von Chemotherapeutica mittels Sephadex und Dialyse. *Arzneimittel-Forsch*, 14:146–9.

SCHOLTAN, W. and SCHMID, J. (1963) Die Bindung der Antibiotica an die Eiweisskörper des Serums. *Arzneimittel-Forsch.*, 13:288–94.

SNYDER, S. H., AXELROD, J. and BAUER, H. (1964) The fate of C^{14} histamine in animal tissues. *J. Pharmacol.*, 144:373–9.

TAKESUE, E. I., TONELLI, G., ALFANO, L. and BUYSKE, D. A. (1960) A radiometric assay of tritiated tetracycline in serum and plasma of laboratory animals. *Int. J. Appl. Rad. Isotopes*, 8:52–9.

TALWAR, G. P., SEGAL, S. J., EVANS, A. and DAVIDSON, O. W. (1964) The binding of oestradiol in the uterus: A mechanism for derepression of RNA synthesis. *Proc. Nat. Acad. Sci. Wash.*, 52, 1059–66.

ULLBERG, S. (1954) Studies on the distribution and fate of ^{35}S labelled benzylpenicillin in the body. *Acta Radiol.*, Suppl., 118:1-110.

VERWEY, W. F. and WILLIAMS, H. R. (1962) Binding of various penicillins by plasma and peripheral lymph obtained from dogs, *Antimicrobial Agents and Chemotherapy*, pp. 484–91.

WALL, P. E. and MIGEON, C. J. (1959) *In vitro* studies with 16 ^{14}C oestrone: distribution between plasma and red blood cells of man. *J. Clin. Invest.*, 38:611–18.

WEIST, F., ZICHA, L., WOLF, F. and SAUERBREY, C. (1966) Experimentelle Untersuchungen über Eiweissbindung 50 wie Resorption von dexamethason-isonicotinsauer Ester nach Inhalation und rektaler Applikation. *Arzneimittel-Forsch.*, 16:667–70.

WEPIERRE, J. (1963) Contribution à l'étude de la perméabilité cutanée à l'aide d'une substance lipophile, le p-cymène marqué au carbone 14, Science thesis Université de Paris.

WÖHLER, F. and HOFFMANN, G. (1964) Autoradiographische Untersuchungen über das Verhalten eines radioaktiven Sulfonamides (5 methyl Sulfodiazin S^{35}) imgewebe. *Arzneimittel-Forsch.*, 14:1222–5.

WOHLTMANN, H. J. and NARAHARA, H. T. (1966) Binding of insulin ^{131}I by isolated frog sartorius muscles. Relationship to changes in permeability to sugar caused by insulin. *J. Biol. Chem.*, 241:4931–9.

WONG, K. C. and SPRATT, J. L. (1963) Assay of radioactive digoxin in liver tissue. *Biochem. Pharmacol.*, 12, 577–602.

WOOLLEY, D. W. and GOMMI, B. W. (1966) Serotonin receptors. VI. Methods for the direct measurement of isolated receptors. *Arch. Int. Pharmacodyn.*, 159:8–17.

WOZNIAK, L. A. (1960) Studies on binding of tetracyclines by dog and human plasma. *Proc. Soc. Exp. Biol. N.Y.*, 105:430–3.

YOUNG, R. L. and GORDON, M. W. (1962) The disposition of ^{14}C amphetamine in rat brain. *Biochem. Pharmacol.*, 9:161–7.

CHAPTER 9

QUANTITATIVE ISOTOPIC METHODS FOR MEASURING ENZYME ACTIVITIES AND ENDOGENOUS SUBSTRATE LEVELS

R. E. McCaman

Division of Neurosciences, City of Hope Medical Center, Duarte, California, U.S.A.

1. INTRODUCTION

MORE and more, pharmacologists are becoming interested in the study of enzyme reactions. This interest is related to an attempt to understand the effects of drugs at the cellular level. In some instances, the principal effect of a drug may be the direct consequence of its effect on the activity of an enzyme(s). In other instances, metabolism of drugs by enzymes may lead to inactivation or conversion to a more active compound. Pharmacologists have also shown a great interest in studying the enzymes involved in the metabolism of many substances, naturally present in tissues, which have pronounced pharmacologic properties. Such substances would include acetylcholine, 5-hydroxytryptamine, γ-aminobutyric acid, histamine, and various catecholamines. Thus the study of enzyme catalyzed reactions has provided important basic biochemical information as well as an understanding of the mechanism of action of many pharmacologic agents.

The measurement of enzyme activities has involved diverse instrumentation and techniques. The early studies utilized bioassay, manometric, titrimetric, and colorimetric procedures. In recent years fluorometric techniques have gained more widespread use because of their high sensitivity and specificity. A high sensitivity and specificity are also characteristic of isotopic procedures and, with the ever-increasing number of labeled analogs of natural and pharmacologic compounds, these procedures represent another valuable approach to the study of enzyme reactions.

While isotopic compounds have a long history of use in qualitative and semi-quantitative studies, only recently have they been used for the

275

quantitative measurement of enzyme activities. The major objective of this chapter will be to (a) present in some detail several examples of isotopic methods used for the quantitative assay of enzyme-catalyzed reactions; (b) use these examples to illustrate that isotopic techniques have a potential sensitivity, convenience, and reliability equal to or greater than those of other techniques currently used for the quantitation of enzyme-catalyzed reactions; and (c) use such examples to assist the reader in understanding the general principles of these procedures so that he may use them to develop additional methods appropriate for his needs.*

2. METHODS FOR MEASURING ENZYME ACTIVITIES
IN VITRO

In the course of this chapter the general features of established isotopic procedures will be discussed. The discussion of the various methods will be primarily concerned with (a) the peculiar advantages of an isotopic procedure over that of some other established procedure for the study of a particular enzyme reaction; (b) various reasons for selecting a particular chemical compound as a labeled substrate; and (c) the additional physical and chemical factors that play an important (albeit frequently unemphasized) role in the development of successful methodology. No attempt will be made to provide complete experimental detail which can be obtained from the appropriate reference material.

Before considering specific methods, it might be appropriate to emphasize certain characteristics which are desirable in any enzyme assay. Such an assay should be quantitative, sensitive, specific, unaffected by side reactions, and sufficiently convenient to permit a rapid analysis of several samples at one time. The procedure should permit the measure of enzyme activities with crude tissue homogenates as well as with partially purified enzyme preparations. For pharmacologic studies, it would be particularly desirable to have a method which was unaffected by the presence of a drug or antimetabolite.

---

* List of abbreviations used in this chapter: CMP, cytidine monophosphate. AMP, adenosine monophosphate. TMP, thymidine monophosphate. UMP, uridine monophosphate. CDP, cytidine diphosphate. CTP, cytidine triphosphate. CDP glucose, cytidine diphosphoglucose. GDP glucose, guanosine diphosphoglucose. UDP glucose, uridine diphosphoglucose. TPN, TPNH, Triphosphopyridine nucleotide (oxidized and reduced forms, respectively): the more modern nomenclature is $NADP^+$, NADPH ($+ H^+$)-nicotinamide-adenine di-nucleotide phosphate. DPN, DPNH, diphosphopyridine nucleotide (oxidized and reduced forms, respectively): the more modern nomenclature is NAD^+, NADH($+H^+$)-nicotinamide-adenine di-nucleotide.

The significance of the above characteristics might best be illustrated by considering the advantages and deficiencies of several methods for the assay of monoamine oxidase. Monoamine oxidase activity has been measured by several procedures including oxygen consumption, liberation of ammonia, and disappearance of substrate. More recently Green and Haughton (1961) have described a colorimetric method for the enzymatically-generated aldehyde. These investigators specified several disadvantages of the previous methods which were overcome by their procedure. Their criticisms included (a) the lack of sensitivity and considerable variability (or error) due to secondary reactions when oxygen consumption was used as a measure of the reaction; (b) the laborious character inherent in the measure of ammonia liberation which makes it difficult to use in the assay of several samples; and (c) the undesirable aspects of substrate utilization methods for kinetic studies. The subsequent development of a fluorometric procedure for the measure of monoamine oxidase (see Udenfriend, 1962) appears to offer additional sensitivity and convenience, and it is applicable to crude tissue homogenates.

Several other fluorometric techniques have recently come into use (see Udenfriend, 1962). These procedures appear to have many of the desirable characteristics specified above. They are convenient, reliable, and much more sensitive than other techniques currently in use. There are, however, limitations to these techniques since many compounds of biological interest do not exhibit a natural fluorescence and cannot be induced to do so. Further, the use of fluorometric methods to study the effects of various pharmaceutical agents on enzyme reactions is often seriously affected by the fluorogenic character of the pharmaceutical agents, themselves. And, finally, the utilization of fluorometric techniques, not infrequently, requires considerable time and effort on behalf of the investigator to purify the auxiliary chemical and enzymatic reagents in order to reduce their contributions to the fluorescence of the blank.

2.1. SENSITIVITY OF ISOTOPIC METHODS

It may be of interest to compare the inherent sensitivity of isotopic procedures* to that of colorimetric or fluorometric procedures currently in use. For purposes of the present discussion the "limit sensitivity" of a procedure is defined as that amount (moles) of material which will give rise

---

* All of the isotopic procedures discussed in this chapter employ scintillation counting for the measure of radioactivity. Thus, the calculations of sensitivity and various other aspects of discussion will be based on the assumption that scintillation counting is used for measurement of radioactivity.

to a corrected signal (counts, optical density, or fluorescence) which is equal in magnitude to that obtained from the "blank". Suppose, for example, in some fluorometric procedure a reagent blank having 25 units of fluorescence is obtained. If 50 units of fluorescence are obtained from a sample containing, in addition to the basic reagent, 10^{-11} M of some fluorogenic substance, the net fluorescence $(50 - 25 = 25)$ is equal to that of the blank. By definition, then, the "limit sensitivity" of such a method is 10^{-11} M of this sub-

TABLE 1. CALCULATION OF SENSITIVITY OF ISOTOPE PROCEDURE AND COMPARISON
TO THAT OF OTHER METHODS

Physical technique	"Limit sensitivity"
Colorimetric	10^{-8}–10^{-9} M
Fluorimetric	10^{-10}–10^{-11} M
Isotopic	1.3×10^{-11} M[a]

[a] Sample calculation for "limit sensitivity" of isotopic procedure:*

$$10^{-3} \frac{M}{mCi} \times \frac{mCi}{2.2 \times 10^9 \text{ dpm}} \times \frac{dpm}{0.7 \text{ cpm}} = \frac{6.5 \times 10^{-13} \text{ M}}{cpm}$$

if "machine blank" = 20 cpm
then 1.3×10^{-11} M = limit sensitivity.

* The values used for this calculation are (a) the reciprocal of the assumed specific activity, (b) the constant relating dpm to millicuries, and (c) an assumed counting efficiency of 70% for ^{14}C in liquid scintillation counting procedures.

Reaction:

^{14}C-Serotonin $\longrightarrow$ ^{14}C-Aldehyde $\longrightarrow$ (Acid)
^{14}C-Tyramine $\longrightarrow$ ^{14}C-Aldehyde $\longrightarrow$ (Acid)
^{14}C-Dopamine $\longrightarrow$ ^{14}C-Aldehyde $\longrightarrow$ (Acid)

Incubation (10 mcl):	KPO_4 (pH 7.2)	0.1 M/l
	^{14}C Serotonin (1 mCi/mM)	8×10^{-4} M/l
	Tissue	1–40 mcg

Postincubation: 1 mcl 3 N HCl
                      50 mcl ethyl acetate
                      Remove aliquot of organic layer
                      Wash with 0.3 N HCl (30 mcl)
                      Remove organic layer and count

Coefficient of variation: 2–3%
Limit sensitivity: 10^{-11} M

FIG. 1. Outline of procedure for microassay of monoamine oxidase activity.

stance. This rather arbitrary way of expressing sensitivity is derived from experience with fluorometric techniques where the instruments either have no absolute calibration or the calibrations, when present, are used rather arbitrarily. In fluorescence (as well as isotopic) measurements, it is the ratio of the corrected sample reading to that of the blank that determines the sensitivity of the method. It should be obvious that when the "limit sensitivity" is expressed in this fashion, an increase in the reagent blank of a given procedure (due to contaminating fluorescence of the substrates and reagents or inadequate removal of the residual radioactive substrate in the isotopic procedures) results in a decrease of the sensitivity. Conversely, a reduction of the reagent blank (for example, to the level of fluorescence obtained with pure or redistilled water, or to the machine background of scintillation spectrometer) results in the maximum sensitivity obtainable with these techniques.

The theoretical "limit sensitivity" for a ^{14}C-labeled compound may be calculated (Table 1) by assuming a value for the specific activity (i.e., 1 mCi/mM) and the counting efficiency for the scintillation spectrometer (70%). It is also necessary to know the value of the "machine blank" (assumed to be 20 cpm) for a given instrument at a specific high voltage setting. Making these assumptions then, the calculations as shown in Fig. 1 give rise to a value of 1.3×10^{-11} M of labeled material. Using approximately similar calculations, one obtains values of 10^{-10}–10^{-11} M for fluorometric methods and 10^{-8}–10^{-9} M for colorimetric procedures. The values obtained for a colorimetric procedure are based on the assumption that the molar absorbance is in the range of 10^6–10^7 M^{-1} cm^2 and that the samples are read in microcells (50 mcl). If the optical density measurements were obtained in larger reading volumes (i.e. 1 ml or more, cf. fluorometric techniques), the sensitivity of the colorimetric procedures would be proportionately less. The values for the "limit sensitivity" of fluorometric procedures are based on the determination of pyridine nucleotides by the procedure of Lowry *et al.* (1957).

It is apparent from the above considerations that the inherent sensitivity of the isotopic procedures is at least comparable to that of the fluorometric procedures and much greater than that of colorimetric procedures. However, it should be emphasized that the sensitivity of the isotopic procedures could be increased perhaps 10–100-fold by using a radioactive material with a higher specific activity (see later). It should also be noted that the "limit sensitivity" for a ^{3}H-labeled material would be approximately one-third that of a ^{14}C-labeled compound (assuming an equal specific activity) due to the lower counting efficiency of ^{3}H-labeled compounds. This difference is usually offset by the much higher specific activities of ^{3}H-labeled materials.

2.2. ISOTOPIC METHODS IN CURRENT USE

To achieve the maximum level of sensitivity for an isotopic procedure, it is necessary to effect an adequate separation of the labeled enzymatic product from the residual labeled substrate. Usually this must be done under conditions where the amount of labeled product represents only 0.1–5% of the quantity of labeled substrate. Further, the procedure involved should allow essentially quantitative recovery of the labeled product. For practical reasons, the procedure should be sufficiently convenient and rapid so that several samples may be analyzed simultaneously. In the subsequent sections, the general features of a number of isotopic methods will be considered, attempting where possible, to analyze both their advantages and disadvantages and, thus, to establish criteria useful in the development of future methodology.

All of these procedures depend on some physical (or chemical) mode of separation of the enzymatic product from the labeled substrate. Thus the methods will be grouped according to the physical (or chemical) technique used. It should be emphasized that the following citations are not intended to represent a complete list of isotopic methods for quantitation of enzyme activities. Rather, these examples have been selected to illustrate the general utility of isotopic techniques. Frequent emphasis will be placed on the potential and actual use of isotopes in the development of micro-techniques in which the high inherent sensitivity of such procedures is used maximally.

2.2.1. *Solvent extraction*

The first group of isotopic procedures to be discussed depends on a simple single solvent extraction which separates labeled product from labeled substrate very effectively. Typical of such procedures is that for measuring monoamine oxidase activity (McCaman, 1961; McCaman *et al.*, 1965) as outlined in Fig. 1. With this procedure, three different labeled substrates were available for detailed studies: 5-hydroxytryptamine, tyramine, and dihydroxyphenylethylamine (dopamine). The same general principle was used by Wurtman and Axelrod (1963) with ^{14}C-tryptamine as the substrate.

In this reaction the substrate, a primary amine, is oxidatively deaminated to yield the corresponding aldehyde as the initial product. However, in the presence of oxygen and/or an additional enzyme (aldehyde oxidase) some portion of the aldehyde is further oxidized to a secondary product (the corresponding acid). Because of this secondary reaction, quantitation of the initial reaction has been difficult when either oxygen consumption or the appearance of aldehyde served as a measure of the reaction. However, with the use of the isotopic procedure, the secondary reaction is of little to no consequence for the following reasons: (a) the total amount of both the aldehyde and acid is stoichiometrically equivalent to the quantity of amine that is deaminated; (b) and since the ionizable functional groups (carboxyl and phenolic) of both products are undissociated at an acid pH, the solvent extraction results in a quantitative recovery of both products simultaneously (McCaman *et al.*, 1965). The solvent (ethyl acetate), with a specific gravity of less than 1.0, is present as an upper phase. Thus an aliquot of the upper (organic) layer may be conveniently and rapidly removed, washed with another small volume of acid and a final aliquot placed in a scintillation vial for counting. The procedure is simple, rapid (as many as 150–200 samples may be analyzed in one day), and is highly reproducible (coefficient of variation of 2–3%). The sensitivity of this procedure is approximately 10^{-11} M when ^{14}C-serotonin with a specific activity of 1 mCi/mM is used. The "reagent blank" is essentially equal to that of the "machine blank" (background), since labeled serotonin and/or tyramine are not soluble in ethyl acetate at an acid pH. Occasional lots of the ^{14}C-dopamine have presented problems because of trace contaminants which are labeled and which are extracted from acidified aqueous solutions into ethyl acetate.

This procedure serves to illustrate a particularly useful advantage of isotopic substrates, namely that they may be used with considerable ease to study the effects of various antimetabolites or enzyme inhibitors (McCaman *et al.*, 1965). In a study of competitive inhibitors of enzyme activity, it is desirable to conduct certain tests at low substrate concentrations and, therefore, at suboptimal reaction rates. The great sensitivity of the isotopic methods greatly facilitates such studies. Furthermore, the quantitative effect of adding any unlabeled inhibitor is directly reflected in the amount of labeled product formed.* Structurally similar analogs, which often interfere with colorimetric or fluorometric assays, have no influence on the determination of the labeled products. This feature of isotopic procedures makes it possible, for example, to study the effect of added unlabeled serotonin (itself a substrate) on the metabolism of ^{14}C-tyramine by

* The exception would be where the added material in some way interferes with the physical method of recovering the labeled product. Such an effect would seldom be expected but may be readily checked.

TABLE 2. ENZYME REACTIONS WHICH CAN BE MEASURED ISOTOPICALLY BY EMPLOYING SOLVENT EXTRACTION PROCEDURES

Enzymes		Labeled substrate	(Co-substrate)	Labeled product(s) isolated	References
1. Amine oxidase	(a)	^{14}C-5-OH-Tryptamine		5-OH-Indoleacetaldehyde (acid)	McCaman, 1961
	(b)	^{14}C-Tyramine		3-OH-Phenylacetaldehyde (acid)	McCaman et al., 1965
	(c)	^{14}C-Dopamine	(O$_2$)	3,4-Dihydroxyphenylacetaldehyde (acid)	
	(d)	^{14}C-Tryptamine		Indoleacetaldehyde	Wurtman and Axelrod, 1963
2. Methyl transferases	(a)	^{3}H-Adrenaline	(SAMe)[a]	Metanephrine	Axelrod et al., 1959
	(b)	SAMe-^{14}C	(3,4-Dihydroxybenzoate)	3-Methoxy-4-OH-benzoate	McCaman, 1965
	(c)	SAMe-^{14}C	(N-acetylserotonin)	5-O-Methoxy-N-acetyl serotonin	Axelrod et al., 1961
	(d)	SAMe-^{14}C	(Histamine)	N-Methylhistamine	Axelrod et al., 1961
	(e)	SAMe-^{14}C	(Phenylethanolamine)	N-Methylphenylethanolamine	Axelrod, 1962
	(f)	SAMe-^{14}C	(Desmethylimipramine)	N-Methylimipramine	Dingell and Sanders, 1966
3. Hydroxylases		SAMe-^{14}C	(Tyramine) (COMT)[b]	3-Methoxy-4-OH-phenyl-ethylamine	Axelrod et al., 1965
4. Acyl-transferases	(a)	^{14}C-Carnitine	(Acyl CoA)	Acyl (oleyl, palmityl) carnitine	McCaman and McCaman, 1967
	(b)	^{14}C-ethanolamine	(Acyl CoA)	Palmitylethanolamide	Bachur and Udenfriend, 1966
	(c)	^{14}C-α-glycerol-PO$_4$	(Acyl CoA)	Phosphatidic acid	Goldfine, 1966
	(d)	^{14}C-Acyl CoA	(Diglyceride)	Triglyceride	Weiss et al., 1960

5. Miscellan-eous transferases				
(a)	CDP-Choline-^{14}C	(Diglyceride)	Phosphatidylcholine	Weiss *et al.*, 1958
(b)	CDP-Choline-^{14}C	(Ceramide)	Sphingomyelin	Sribney and Kennedy, 1958
(c)	GDP-Mannose-^{14}C	(Diglyceride)	-D-mannosyl-diglyceride	Lennarz and Talamo, 1966
(d)	UDP-galactose-^{14}C	(Sphingosine)	Psychosine	Cleland and Kennedy, 1960
(e)	^{3}H-CTP	(Phosphatidic acid)	CDP-diglyceride	Carter and Kennedy, 1966
(f)	^{14}C-Inositol	(CDP-diglyceride)	Phosphatidylinositol	Paulus and Kennedy, 1960
(g)	^{14}C-α-glycerol-PO$_4$	(CDP-diglyceride)	Phosphatidyl glycerolphosphate	Kiysau *et al*, 1963
(h)	^{14}C-serine	(CDP-diglyceride)	Phosphatidylserine	Borkenhagen *et al.*, 1961

[a] SAMe = S-adenosylmethionine.
[b] COMT = catechol-*O*-methytransferase.

monoamine oxidase. Indeed, it is possible to study the enzymatic deamination of two separate amines simultaneously by using two different labels
(^{3}H and ^{14}C). Much valuable information concerning association and
dissociation constants, the presence of two distinct enzymes, etc., could be
obtained by this technique.

In Table 2 are listed several isotopic methods currently used which
employ solvent extraction to separate the labeled substrate and the labeled
product. These examples demonstrate how certain differences between substrate and product, in this case, solubility, have been used successfully to
devise new or improved enzyme assays.

Axelrod *et al.* (1959) described an assay for catechol-*O*-methyl transferase in which ^{3}H-adrenaline was the labeled substrate (Table 2, 2(a)).
With the development of this method and the studies which have followed,
the important role of *O*-methyl transfer reactions in the intermediary
metabolism of sympathomimetic amines has been more fully appreciated.
The product, ^{3}H-metanephrine, formed in the presence of *S*-adenosyl-
methionine and the enzyme, was extracted from the aqueous incubation
mixture with a toluene-isoamyl alcohol system. This solvent system extracted a significant amount of ^{3}H-adrenaline (i.e. gave a high reagent
blank) and incompletely extracted the ^{3}H-metanephrine (i.e. gave low
product recovery). These two factors resulted in a method whose sensitivity
was considerably less than the theoretical maximum (see above). The
modifications described by McCaman (1965) have resulted in a marked
improvement in the sensitivity of the assay by (1) introducing the label in
the form of ^{14}C-*S*-adenosylmethionine which, because of the highly
charged sulfonium group, has little tendency to be extracted by organic
solvents; (2) choosing a co-substrate (dihydroxybenzoate) which results in
greater enzyme activity; and (3) selecting a solvent (ethyl acetate) which
results in quantitative recovery of the labeled product (Table 2, 2(b)). This
example demonstrates the importance of judicious choices in the selection
of the labeled substrate and the solvent in order to obtain maximum
sensitivity.

Axelrod *et al.* (1961) have also developed a procedure for measuring the
activity of the enzyme which carries out the *O*-methylation of *N*-acetyl-
serotonin (hydroxyindole-*O*-methyltransferase). The labeled substrate in
this case was ^{14}C-*S*-adenosylmethionine and chloroform was used as the
solvent for the selective extraction of the ^{14}C-methoxymelatonin (Table 2,
2(c)). The efficiency of the extraction and the overall convenience of the
methodology appears to be quite good. With this method it has been
possible to study the regional distribution of this enzyme in nervous tissue.

The enzyme appears to be almost exclusively located in the pineal gland, in contrast to the ubiquitous distribution of catechol-*O*-methyl transferase, suggesting that at least two distinct enzymes catalyze *O*-methylation reactions (Axelrod *et al.*, 1961).

A number of *N*-methyl transfer reactions have been studied using [14]C-*S*-adenosylmethionine as the labeled substrate (Table 2, 2(d)–(f)). With the procedure for measuring the enzyme activity of imidazole-*N*-methyl transferase (Table 2, 2(d)), much interesting information concerned with histamine metabolism has been obtained (Axelrod *et al.*, 1961; Snyder and Axelrod, 1965). It should be emphasized that the solvent system (toluene-isoamyl alcohol) utilized in these studies, while convenient for scintillation counting, in this case also does not result in quantitative extraction of the ^{14}C-methylhistamine nor does it completely exclude contamination from the [14]C-*S*-adenosylmethionine. However, this solvent does appear to be useful in several different methods and has been used in the study of *N*-methyl transferases responsible for *N*-methylation of phenylethanol-amine (Axelrod, 1962) and desmethylimipramine (Dingell and Sanders, 1966). Whether or not these are different enzymes or the same enzyme remain to be determined.

The formation of dihydroxy derivatives (catechols) of phenolic amines and indoles is an important step in the intermediary metabolism of these compounds. Axelrod *et al.* (1965) have described a procedure which is broadly applicable to the study of the hydroxylase(s) which catalyze such conversions (Table 2, 3). This procedure utilizes the enzyme, catechol-*O*-methyl transferase, as an analytical reagent. Thus, when monophenols are incubated with a suitable tissue extract in the presence of [14]C-*S*-adenosyl-methionine and added catechol-*O*-methyl transferase, the dihydroxy compound formed is immediately *O*-methylated. Subsequently, the radioactive *O*-methyl derivative is extracted into toluene-isoamyl alcohol (as above for other methylation assays) and serves as the indirect, but proportionate, measure of hydroxylase activity present in the tissue extract. The results of these investigators strongly suggest there are several distinct hydroxylases which have widely different substrate specificities (Axelrod *et al.* 1965). Since continued study of these enzymes would appear to require many structurally different substrates, the wide applicability of the toluene-isoamyl alcohol solvent system may outweigh the disadvantages indicated above. It is also apparent from the above studies that the [14]C-*S*-adenosyl-methionine, which is now commercially available with a high specific activity, is an extremely useful substrate in the study of methyl transferase reactions.

The studies of Feldstein and Wong (1965) supplement the above discussion of the choice of solvent systems for selective extraction of the various metabolic products. These investigators have developed a series of elaborate extraction procedures for the isolation of all the anticipated products resulting from the *in vitro* metabolism of ^{14}C-hydroxytryptophan. These studies would appear to have considerable value in the study of the influence of various drugs on the enzymes involved in these reactions. In addition, the thorough investigation of the differential solubility of these metabolites in different solvent systems might be useful in improving the sensitivity of existing methods or developing future procedures involving solvent extraction.

The remaining reactions (Table 2, 4 and 5) have a common characteristic; they represent metabolic conversions in which at least one of the products has lipid properties (minimum solubility in aqueous solutions, highly soluble in organic solvents). All of these reactions also involve the transfer of a molecule with a low molecular weight (and for the most part highly polar) and with high solubility in aqueous solutions. In these cases solvent extraction affords virtually quantitative separation of product and substrate. For example, the activity of carnitine acyltransferase may be readily determined when ^{14}C-carnitine and palmityl- or oleyl-CoA are the substrates (Table 2, 4(a)). The ^{14}C-acylcarnitine is quantitatively extracted from the incubation mixture by chloroform with little to no contamination from ^{14}C-carnitine (McCaman, M. W. and McCaman, R. E., to be published). Procedures for following the enzymatic formation of palmityl-ethanolamide (Bachur and Udenfriend, 1966) and phosphatidic acid (Goldfine, 1966) involve essentially similar extraction procedures. In the latter example (Table 2, 4(c)), the ^{14}C-α-glycerophosphate is not yet commercially available, but is readily prepared bioenzymatically with high yields. The use of solvent extraction for studying the enzymatic formation of triglycerides (Table 2, 4(d)) is somewhat less efficient, since both the labeled substrate (^{14}C-palmityl CoA) and its hydrolysis product (^{14}C-palmitate) exhibit lipid solubility properties. However, Weiss *et al.* (1960) have observed that, when labeled triglyceride is extracted into carbon tetrachloride and thoroughly washed with strong salt solutions made basic with ammonia, the organic phase (containing triglyceride) is freed of residual labeled palmityl CoA and palmitate. The transferase reactions shown in the final portion of Table 2, (5(a)–(h)), also result in the formation of lipid products having strong hydrophobic characteristics. These labeled products are quantitatively extracted into organic solvents (usually chloroform) which completely excludes contamination by the labeled water-soluble precursors.

Isotopic methods for the quantitative assay of three additional enzyme activities involved in lipid metabolism have also been described. These enzymes catalyze the hydrolysis of labeled lipids (which must be prepared in the laboratory) to yield labeled water-soluble fragments. They provide a measure of the enzymatic hydrolysis of sphingomyelin (Kanfer *et al.*, 1966), ceramides (Gatt, 1966), and cerebrosides (Brady *et al.*, 1965). The essential difference between these procedures and those discussed above is that solvent extraction is used to remove (and recover) the labeled substrate, leaving the water-soluble product in the aqueous phase for counting and determining the enzyme activity. While removal of the substrate can be accomplished with essentially the same efficiency as extraction of the products in the previous examples, it is all the more significant in these last three examples since the substrates are not commercially available and their recovery and reuse makes for a much more efficient use of these valuable chemicals.

The above examples should serve to illustrate the convenience, rapidity, and general utility of solvent extraction for developing isotopic methods. When the product(s) of an enzyme-catalyzed reaction exhibits distinctly different solubility characteristics than that of the substrate(s), solvent extraction might well be considered as the procedure of choice. While the solubility differences are readily apparent in the latter examples (for example, between inositol and phosphatidylinositol), very often simple substitution of methyl groups (as *O*-methoxy or *N*-methyl) produce marked changes in the solubility characteristics of a compound. However, it should be emphasized that many organic solvents cause severe quenching in a given counting medium. If this occurs, it may be necessary to evaporate the solvent before counting or substitute a less troublesome one. As an example, labeled lipid products (Table 2, 4(a)–(h)) are readily soluble in both carbon tetrachloride or chloroform. However, the former causes severe quenching while chloroform has little apparent effect on scintillation counting in a toluene-scintillator system (McCaman and Cook, 1966). Finally, it should be noted that manipulation of the pH or salt content of the aqueous phase may significantly affect the outcome of the procedures employing solvent extraction.

2.2.2. *Diffusion techniques*

Volatilization or sublimation has also been used to effect a separation of labeled product and substrate. Any enzyme catalyzing the production of $^{14}CO_2$ may be readily studied with isotopic procedures if the substrate can be obtained with the label (^{14}C) in the appropriate position. Examples of enzyme-catalyzed reactions utilizing ^{14}C-labeled substrates which give rise to $^{14}CO_2$ are listed in Table 3 (a)–(e). Isotopic methods are described for quantitation of glutamic decarboxylase (Albers and Brady, 1959); 5-hydroxytrytophan decarboxylase (McCaman, 1962a; McCaman *et al.*, 1965); 6-phosphogluconic dehydrogenase (Pastan *et al.*, 1963); histidine decarboxylase (Levine and Watts, 1966) and phosphatidyl serine decarboxylase (Borkenhagen *et al.*, 1961). These studies were greatly facilitated because the appropriate labeled substrates were commercially available (except for the labeled phosphatidylserine (Table 3, 1(e)). The procedure in all examples involved termination of the enzyme reaction by acidification. The gaseous $^{14}CO_2$ which is evolved diffused through a limited space and was "trapped" in Hyamine.* The strongly basic character of Hyamine and the high solubility of Hyamine-carbonate in toluene has encouraged wide use of this compound as a trapping agent for $^{14}CO_2$. While Hyamine does cause quenching in high concentrations (Brown and Badman, 1961), the quantities used in the above procedures do not pose a serious problem in this respect. Suggestions for other trapping agents and techniques for collection of $^{14}CO_2$ may be found in a recent review by Rapkin (1964).

Acetic acid is another compound which is readily volatilized. This factor has permitted the development of methods to study the metabolic conversions of labeled acetate to non-volatile products (Table 3, 2(a), (b)). Utilizing ^{14}C-acetate (along with ATP and CoA), Schuberth (1965) described a convenient procedure for following the enzymatic formation of acetyl CoA (Table 3, 2(a)). This represents another example of removal of the labeled substrate rather than direct isolation of the product. Complete removal of the acetate requires at least two evaporations of the acidified incubation mixture with carrier acetic acid added prior to each evaporation. The isotopic procedure for measuring the activity of choline acetylase involves essentially the same principle (Schuberth, 1963). The procedure for measuring the formation of acetylcholine is much less sensitive and reliable than that for acetyl CoA since the former involves two enzyme reactions and requires some finite quantity of ^{14}C-acetyl CoA being present at all times. The ^{14}C-acetyl CoA, being nonvolatile, results in a high and to some extent variable "blank".

Isotopic procedures have been described which involve the formation of tritiated water (^3HOH) which is collected by sublimation. Hutton *et al.* (1966) prepared a hydroxyproline-deficient protein (substrate) which contains a residue of 3,4-^{3}H-L-proline. Enzyme-catalyzed hydroxylation of the

* Hyamine, *p*-(di-isobutylcresoxethoxyethyl)-dimethylbenzyl-ammonium hydroxide.

TABLE 3. ENZYME REACTIONS WHICH CAN BE MEASURED ISOTOPICALLY BY EMPLOYING DIFFUSION TECHNIQUES

Enzyme		Labeled substrate	(Co-substrate)	Measured product	References
1. Decarboxylases	(a)	Glutamate 1-^{14}C		$^{14}CO_2$	Albers and Brady, 1959
	(b)	5-OH-Tryptophan-3-^{14}C		$^{14}CO_2$	McCaman, 1962(a)
	(c)	1-^{14}C-6 phosphogluconate	(TPN)	$^{14}CO_2$	Pastan *et al.*, 1963
	(d)	^{14}C-Histidine		$^{14}CO_2$	Levine and Watts, 1966
	(e)	^{14}C-Phosphatidylserine		$^{14}CO_2$	Borkenhagen *et al.*, 1961
2. Miscellaneous	(a)	^{14}C-Acetate	(ATP, CoA)	Acetyl CoA	Schuberth, 1965
	(b)	^{14}C-Acetate	(ATP, CoA, choline)	Acetylcholine	Schuberth, 1963
	(c)	^{3}H-Deoxyuridylate	(methylene tetra-hydrofolate)	^3HOH	Lomax and Greenberg, 1966

labeled proline residues results in the concomitant release of a tritium atom which equilibrates with water. Similarly, Lomax and Greenberg (1967) have developed an assay for thymidylate synthetase activity based on the release of tritium (as tritiated water) from deoxyuridylate-5-^{3}H (Table 3, 2(c). The apparatus and procedure described by Hutton *et al.* (1966) for the recovery of tritiated water is reported to be very rapid, allowing many samples to be processed in the same day.

2.2.3. *Secondary chemical reactions*

The term "secondary chemical reaction" is used here to indicate the result of the addition of a chemical agent which reacts with the product of an enzyme reaction to yield still another product. Examples of such reactions might include: (a) precipitation of quaternary compounds (such as choline and carnitine) as insoluble reinecke salts or periodides; (b) formation of hydrazones from aldehydes and keto acids; (c) precipitation of sulfates or phosphates as insoluble barium or silver salts, etc. The purpose of using these secondary reactions, in conjunction with isotopic methods, is to produce a derivative of the labeled enzymatic product or substrate that makes their separation more convenient and efficient.

The procedure for measuring the activity of choline acetylase (McCaman, 1963; McCaman and Hunt, 1965) may be used to demonstrate the effectiveness of such an approach (Fig. 2). The labeled substrate ^{14}C-acetyl CoA (commercially available), in the presence of choline and tissue preparations, gives rise to ^{14}C-acetylcholine. The addition of ammonium reinecke results in the formation of an insoluble reinecke salt of the ^{14}C-acetylcholine (product) and the choline (unlabeled substrate). The latter (present in large excess) serves as a carrier material which insures quantitative precipitation of the ^{14}C-acetylcholine. This aspect of the method is not fortuitous, but rather absolutely essential, since it is known that reinecke salts do not result in quantitative precipitation of acetylcholine in the absence of choline (McCaman, unpublished results). Further, the amount (0.1–20 picoM) of acetylcholine generated in these experiments would result in such a small quantity of precipitate that visualization and subsequent washing, etc., of the precipitate would be virtually impossible. ^{14}C-Acetyl CoA has little tendency to form an insoluble reinecke derivative, but it is generally necessary to wash the ^{14}C-acetylcholine-choline-reinecke precipitate at least once to remove the last traces of labeled substrate physically trapped in the precipitate. If it is desired to use higher concentrations of ^{14}C-Acetyl CoA than that indicated, it may be necessary to include unlabeled acetyl CoA in the washing step to reduce the blank. The reinecke precipitate is completely solubilized by the addition of acetone (or alcohol–acetone mixtures) and a known aliquot may be removed and added to a scintillator toluene solution to determine its radioactivity. In the quantities indicated here, neither the acetone nor the pink coloration of the reinecke solution results in significant quenching. If larger quantities of material are to be counted, the addition of a small quantity (0.5 ml) of Hyamine (1 M/l in methanol) is advisable.

Reaction:
$$^{14}\text{C-acetyl CoA} + \text{choline} \longrightarrow \text{CoA} + {}^{14}\text{C-acetylcholine}$$

Incubation (10 mcl):

K_2HPO_4 (pH 7.4)	1×10^{-1} M/l
Choline	5×10^{-3} M/l
^{14}C-acetyl CoA (S.A. 10)	5×10^{-5} M/l

Postincubation:

1 mcl 3 N TCA–0.2 M/l choline (centrifugation)
10 mcl aliquot
20 mcl 5 mM/l acetyl CoA–0.5 N HCl
7 mcl NH$_4$–reineckate
Centrifuge remove SN, wash with 0.3 N HCl (50 mcl)
Acetone to dissolve ppt. and count.

Coefficient of variation: 3%.
Limit sensitivity: 10^{-12} M.

FIG. 2. Outline of procedure for microassay of cholineacetylase activity.

When the specific activity of ^{14}C-acetyl CoA is approximately 10 mCi/mM, the "limit sensitivity" of this procedure is approximately 10^{-12} M of ^{14}C-acetylcholine. The "reagent" blank is generally only a few cpm greater than the "machine" blank (background). This procedure is convenient and highly reproducible giving a coefficient of variation of less than 3%. With this procedure choline acetylase activity in samples of nervous tissue weighing as little as 0.2–20 mcg has been measured (McCaman and Hunt, 1965).

There are at least two side reactions which could affect the quantitative measure of the activity of this enzyme: (a) the hydrolysis of ^{14}C acetyl-CoA by acetyl-CoA deacylase which would give rise to ^{14}C-acetate and CoA; and (b) hydrolysis of ^{14}C-acetylcholine by choline esterase. The enzyme catalyzing the latter reaction was completely inhibited by the addition of eserine to the incubation mixture.* The presence of acetyl-CoA deacylase

---

* When the sensitivity of this procedure is used maximally, the ^{14}C-acetylcholine can be measured when its concentration in the incubation mixture is only 10^{-6}–10^{-7} M. Such concentrations are so low relative to the substrate constant K_s of cholinesterase (0.5×10^{-3} M/l) that appreciable metabolism does not take place even in the absence of cholinesterase inhibitors.

in tissues was of no consequence as long as the concentration of the ^{14}C-acetyl-CoA was maintained in sufficient quantities to saturate the choline acetylase during the incubation period.

Recently, Fonnum (1966) proposed an alternate procedure for the assay of choline acetylase (Table 4, 2) which differs from the above in two aspects: (a) utilization of ^{14}C-acetate as the labeled substrate and the addition of an acetyl CoA generating system to the incubation mixture (partially purified acetyl CoA synthetase, ATP and CoA); and (b) precipitation of the choline and ^{14}C-acetylcholine with tetraphenylborate (rather than with reinecke salts). The tetraphenylborate precipitation results in quantitative recovery of the acetylcholine. However, the use of a two-stage reaction, in which the synthesis of acetylcholine is dependent on the synthesis of acetyl CoA, would complicate studies of the direct effects of various metabolic (or pharmacologic) agents on choline acetylase activity *per se*.

While choline is quantitatively precipitated as a reinecke salt, the reinecke salts of certain other quaternary compounds containing anionic groups (choline phosphate, betaine and carnitine) are more soluble. However, this effect is, to some extent, pH dependent.* At an acid pH (<2), choline phosphate and betaine can be recovered as an insoluble reinecke salt to the extent of 30–40% (compared to 100% recovery of choline). At an alkaline pH (>10), choline phosphate and betaine will not form insoluble derivatives to any measurable extent (although the recovery of choline is still 100% at this pH). These differences form the basis for isotopic methods for measuring the activities of choline phosphokinase (McCaman and Cook, 1966) and choline oxidase (Goldberg and McCaman, to be published). In the case of choline phosphokinase (Table 4, 3), the ^{14}C-choline phosphate (product) is separated from ^{14}C-choline (substrate) by complete removal of the latter as an insoluble reinecke salt at an alkaline pH. The supernatant solution (containing ^{14}C-choline phosphate and a trace of ^{14}C-choline) is recovered and unlabeled choline (carrier) added, followed by a second precipitation with the reinecke solution. The insoluble reinecke salts are again removed (centrifugation). The supernatant solution now contains all of the enzymatically-formed ^{14}C-choline phosphate (97–101%) and less than 0.01% of the ^{14}C-choline. The reproducibility of the method is such that a coefficient of variation of 3% or less is obtained and the "limit sensitivity" of the procedure is 10^{-11} M when the specific activity of the ^{14}C-choline is approximately 1 mCi/mM. In the choline oxidase assay, the betaine aldehyde is converted to betaine in the

* McCaman, R. E., unpublished results.

TABLE 4. ENZYME REACTIONS WHICH CAN BE MEASURED ISOTOPICALLY BY EMPLOYING SECONDARY CHEMICAL REACTIONS

Enzyme	Labeled substrate	(Co-substrate)	Labeled product isolated	Secondary reactant	References
1. Choline acetylase	^{14}C-Acetyl CoA	(Choline)	Acetylcholine	Reinecke	McCaman and Hunt, 1965
2. Choline acetylase	^{14}C-Acetate	(ATP, CoA, Choline)	Acetylcholine	Tetraphenyl-borate	Fonnum, 1966
3. Choline P-kinase	^{14}C-Choline	(ATP)	Choline-PO_4	Reinecke	McCaman and Cook, 1966
4. Carnitine acetylase	^{14}C-Acetyl CoA	(Carnitine)	Acetylcarnitine	Periodide	McCaman *et al*, 1966
5. *N*-methyl transferase	SAMe-^{14}C	(Norepinephrine)	Epinephrine	Reinecke	Fuller and Hunt, 1965
6. Folic acid reductase	^{14}C-Folic Acid	(TPNH)	Tetrahydro-folate	Zinc	Rothenberg, 1966
7. Serine trans-hydroxymethylase	Serine-3-C^{14}	(Tetrahydrofolate)	"C_1"	Dimedon	Taylor and Weissbach, 1965
8. CMP-sialic acid synthetase	^{14}C-Sialic acid	(CTP)	(CMP Sialic) $^{14}CO_2$	BH_4, hydrolysis, decarboxylation	Kean and Roseman, 1966

presence of a partially purified aldehyde dehydrogenase and DPN and the same procedure as described above is used to remove the residual labeled substrate, choline (Goldberg and McCaman, to be published).

Quaternary compounds containing anionic groups may be quantitatively precipitated as insoluble periodides (Wall *et al.* 1960). Thus ^{14}C-acetyl carnitine, formed as the result of carnitine acetylase activity (Table 4, 4), may be isolated quantitatively as an insoluble periodide (McCaman *et al.*, 1966). The unlabeled carnitine, present in substrate quantities, serves as a carrier during the precipitation of ^{14}C-acetylcarnitine. There is less tendency for the ^{14}C-acetyl CoA to be trapped in the periodide precipitates than in the reinecke precipitates of choline discussed above, thus in this case the blank is equivalent to background even with high concentrations of ^{14}C-acetyl CoA.

Fuller and Hunt (1965) have developed a convenient and sensitive assay for *N*-methyl transferase activity which is also based on the quantitative removal of the labeled substrate (Table 4, 5). They observed that ^{14}C-*S*-adenosylmethionine could be effectively removed as an insoluble reinecke salt (using unlabeled *S*-adenosylmethionine as carrier). Quantitative recovery of the enzymatically-formed ^{14}C-epinephrine was obtained. The "limit sensitivity" of this procedure was many-fold greater than the procedure using solvent extraction (Table 2, 2(e)), since a low recovery of the labeled product and a high blank was obtained with the latter.

The procedure for folic acid reductase, as developed by Rothenberg (1966), utilizes ^{14}C-folic acid and TPNH as the substrates (Table 4, 6). The ^{14}C-tetrahydrofolic acid produced during the course of the enzyme reaction is selectively precipitated with zinc salts. Taylor and Weissbach (1965) developed an isotopic method for the measure of serine transhydroxy-methylase which catalyzes the transfer of a radioactive "C_1" fragment from serine-3-C^{14} to tetrahydrofolate (Table 4, 7). The active one-carbon unit ("C_1") readily forms a complex with dimedon. The radioactive dimedon-"C_1" complex can be separated by solvent extraction from the starting labeled substrate (^{14}C-serine) and measured by scintillation counting.

Kean and Roseman (1966) used a two-stage secondary reaction to measure CMP-sialic acid synthetase (Table 4, 8). At the conclusion of the enzyme incubation, two labeled compounds are present, ^{14}C-sialic acid (substrate) and ^{14}C-CMP-sialic acid (enzymatic product). The ^{14}C-sialic acid is selectively reduced to the dihydro-form by the addition of boro-hydride, while the product, a glycoside, is not reduced. Following destruction of the excess borohydride (with the addition of excess glucose), the ^{14}C-CMP-sialic acid is hydrolyzed to give free ^{14}C-sialic acid. The free acid is decarboxylated (evolving $^{14}CO_2$) under conditions where the dihydro-sialic(reduced substrate) is not. The $^{14}CO_2$ is trapped in a methyl cellosolve-ethanolamine mixture and serves as the indirect measure of ^{14}C-CMP-sialic acid synthesis. In spite of the number of steps involved, this procedure appears to be quite rapid and several samples may be processed at one time. While the release of $^{14}CO_2$ from ^{14}C-sialic acid was not quantitative in the procedure as routinely used by these authors, it was directly pro-portional to ^{14}C-sialic acid concentration (over the range of 0.005–0.10 mсм). By only a slight modification of this procedure, an isotopic pro-cedure for assaying sialyltransferase has been developed (Jourdian *et al.*, 1963).

Wegener *et al.* (1965) described an isotopic procedure to study the enzymatic condensation of ^{14}C-glyoxylate with short-chain fatty acid acyl CoA derivatives. This procedure is based on the ability of glyoxylate (substrate) to form a nitrophenyl-hydrazone, which may be separated from the labeled products of the reaction. The method, as currently used, measures substrate utilization. However, it might become much more sensitive and convenient by slight modifications which would permit the radioactive product(s) to be measured.

The principal objective of using secondary chemical reactions as illu-strated above is to make the separation of the labeled substrate and the labeled product(s) more convenient and more quantitative. Generally, these procedures result in a selective and marked change in the solubility properties of the product (or substrate). There are, of course, many other potentially useful chemical reactions appropriate for the production of a wide variety of secondary products. Many of these could be used effectively in conjunction with the prudent selection of appropriate radioactive sub-strates to produce an array of sensitive and specific assays for enzyme studies.

2.2.4. *Adsorption techniques*

The fourth group of isotopic procedures is based on the principle of selective adsorption to effect a separation between labeled products and substrates (Table 5). While the technique of column chromatography employing ion-exchange resins, charcoal, cellulose, etc. has had wide application in the separation of complex mixtures, this technique is usually much too cumbersome to be used for the study of enzyme-catalyzed reactions, particularly on a micro scale. However, the same sorbants may be used, in a greatly simplified fashion, to resolve a two-component mix-ture (i.e. labeled substrate vs. labeled product). Such simplifications in-volve, for example, the use of these sorbants in a "batch operation". Either

TABLE 5. ENZYME REACTIONS WHICH CAN BE MEASURED ISOTOPICALLY BY EMPLOYING VARIOUS SORBANTS

Enzymes		Labeled substrate	Co-substrate	Labeled product isolated	Sorbant	References
1. Esterases		Acetyl-1-^{14}C-chlorine		Acetate	Resin (CG-120)	Reed *et al.*, 1966
2. Kinases	(a)	^{14}C-choline	(ATP)	Choline-PO$_4$	Resin (AG-1)	McCaman, 1962b
	(b)	^{14}C-glucose	(ATP)	Hexose-PO$_4$	DEAE disc	Sherman, 1963
	(c)	^{14}C-glycerol	(ATP)	Glycerol-PO$_4$	DEAE disc	Robinson and Newsholme 1966
	(d)	XMP (^{3}H or ^{14}C)	(ATP)	XDP, XTP	DEAE disc (P'tase)	Furlong, 1963
	(e)	^{3}H-d UMP-5t	methylenetetra-hydrofolate	^{3}HOH	Charcoal	Roberts, 1966a
3. Hydroxylases	(a)	Tyrosine-3,5-^{3}H		^{3}HOH	Resin (AG-50)	Nagatsu *et al.*, 1964
	(b)	^{14}C-Tryptophan		Serotonin	Resin (CG-50)	Green and Sawyer, 1966
4. Transaminases		^{14}C-α-Ketoglutar-ate	Amino acid	Glutamate	Resin (AG-50)	Albers *et al.*, 1962
		^{14}C-pyruvate		Pyruvate		
5. Transferases	(a)	^{14}C-choline-PO$_4$	(CTP)	CDP choline	Charcoal	Borkenhagen and Kennedy, 1957
	(b)	UDP-galactose-^{14}C	(glucose)	Lactose	Resin (AG-1)	Babad and Hassid, 1966
6. Miscellaneous	(a)	^{3}H-folate	(TPNH)	^{3}HOH	Charcoal	Roberts, 1966
	(b)	^{14}C-N-Acetyl neuraminic		N-acetyl manosamine	Resin (AG-1)	Brunetti *et al.*, 1962
	(c)	^{14}C-glucose-1-PO$_4$	(CTP)	CDP-glucose	Resin (AG-1), (P'tase)	Mayer and Ginsburg, 1966
	(d)	^{14}C-glucose-1-PO$_4$	(GTP)	GDP-glucose	Charcoal	Barber, 1966

the substrate or product may be selectively adsorbed by mixing the sample with a small quantity of sorbant in a test tube. After a brief centrifugation, the radioactivity in an aliquot of the supernatant solution serves as a direct measure of the unadsorbed metabolite and, thus, a measure of the enzyme activity. These sorbants may also be used in small sintered glass funnels. In this case a sample (0.01–1.0 ml) passes rapidly through the column and the effluent from the column (or the eluant after washing), containing the radioactive substrate (or product), is a measure of the reaction. Techniques such as these can be very sensitive and convenient for assaying a hundred or more samples in one day, even though they are based on principles that more conventionally require many hours or a day for the processing of a single (complex) sample.

Reed *et al.* (1966) developed an isotopic procedure for the quantitative assay of cholinesterase (Table 5, 1). This procedure depends on the separation of ^{14}C-acetate (product) from ^{14}C-acetylcholine (substrate) by complete adsorption of the latter on a cation exchange resin. The adsorption of unhydrolyzed ^{14}C-acetylcholine is carried out in a batch operation, with the resin (followed by an addition of ethanol which terminates the enzyme reaction) added directly to the incubation mixture. After centrifugation, the radioactivity in an aliquot of the supernatant liquid is determined and serves as a direct measure of ^{14}C-acetate liberated by acetylcholinesterase. This method permits a rapid and accurate determination of the enzymic hydrolysis of nanomole quantities of acetylcholine and is useful for a variety of incubation conditions including a wide range of substrate concentrations.

An isotopic microprocedure for the assay of choline phosphokinase (Table 5, 2(a)) utilizes a small column (1 × 1 cm) of anion exchange resin in a sintered glass funnel to separate ^{14}C-choline phosphate (product) from ^{14}C-choline (substrate). The rapid flow rate of these microcolumns facilitates the removal of the unadsorbed ^{14}C-choline by a series of washes, and the subsequent elution of the ^{14}C-choline phosphate in a small volume of eluant (McCaman, 1962b). Although this procedure employs a resin in a "column operation", the procedure involves essentially a batch separation in which all of the manipulations (sample application, washing, elution) are carried out so rapidly that fifty or more samples may be processed in a couple of hours. It should also be noted that in our laboratory this procedure has been replaced by the more convenient and sensitive alkaline reinecke precipitation procedure (see Table 4, 3).

Sherman (1963) described a sensitive isotopic procedure for the assay of hexokinase employing discs of anion exchange paper (Table 5, 2(b)). When

an aliquot of an incubation mixture is applied to a small disc of DEAE*
paper, the enzymic product (^{14}C-hexose phosphate) is strongly adsorbed.
The radioactive substrate (^{14}C-hexose) may be rapidly washed from the
disc in a suction funnel apparatus, or several marked discs may be collected
in a beaker and washed *en masse* (batch washing). The radioactivity of the
^{14}C-hexose phosphate is measured while it is still adsorbed to the DEAE-
disc. This technique would appear to be suitable for the assay of almost
any enzyme catalyzing the conversion of a neutral or cationic substrate to
an anionic product. Recently Robinson and Newsholme (1966) have
adopted this technique in an isotopic assay for glycerol kinase (Table 5,
2(c)). After washing the DEAE disc to remove the ^{14}C-glycerol (substrate),
the radioactivity on the disc (^{14}C-glycerophosphate) was determined
directly by scintillation counting.

The procedure of Furlong (1963) for assay of nucleotide kinase activity
embodies the same technique as the above (DEAE adsorption) but uses, in
addition, a partially purified phosphatase as an auxiliary reagent (Table 5,
(d)). In this assay a radioactive mononucleotide (i.e. AMP, CMP, TMP, or
UMP) and ATP serve as the substrates and the enzymatic products are
labeled nucleotide di- and tri-phosphates. Before application to the DEAE
disc the samples are pretreated with the partially purified phosphatase
which results in the selective enzymic hydrolysis of the labeled mononucleotide (substrate) to the corresponding nucleoside. The nucleosides are
not adsorbed on the DEAE. On the other hand, the radioactive nucleotide
di- and tri-phosphates, which are not attacked by the phosphatase, are
quantitatively adsorbed on the disc and provide a direct isotopic measure
of the kinase activity.

Roberts (1966a) described an isotopic assay for thymidylate synthetase
in which the residual substrate (^{3}H-deoxyuridylate) is removed by batch
adsorption onto charcoal. The radioactivity present in the supernatant
fluid (containing the tritiated water) is a direct measure of enzyme activity
(Table 5, 2(e)). This procedure is very similar in principle to that of Lomax
and Greenberg (1967) discussed above. The former would appear to be the
more convenient procedure and is reported to be more sensitive.

The use of specially prepared tritiated substrates has permitted the
development of convenient assays for enzyme-catalyzed hydroxylation
reactions in which the displaced tritium atoms are released in a form that
equilibrates with water (to form ^{3}HOH). Thus, Nagatsu *et al.* (1964) were
able to develop a convenient and sensitive assay for tyrosine hydroxylase

---

* DEAE: anion exchange paper made from diethylaminoethyl cellulose.

utilizing L-tyrosine-3,5-^{3}H as the substrate (Table 5, 3(a)). In this reaction two labeled products are generated:

$$\text{L-Tyrosine-3,5-}^3\text{H} + \text{O}_2 \xrightarrow{\text{Enzyme}} {}^3\text{HOH} + \text{L-DOPA-5-}^3\text{H}.$$

The separation of the labeled dihydroxyphenylalanine (DOPA) from the labeled tyrosine requires techniques too cumbersome to permit the analysis of many samples and would require relatively large quantities of the reactants. However, the ^{3}HOH may be rapidly and conveniently separated from the ^{3}H-tyrosine and ^{3}H-DOPA by adsorbing the latter two compounds either on charcoal (Pomerantz, 1964) or on Dowex-50 (Nagatsu *et al.*, 1964) or by sublimation (see Table 3, 2(c)).

Green and Sawyer (1966) described an assay procedure measuring the conversion of tryptophan to 5-hydroxytryptophan by a hydroxylase present in tissue extracts (Table 5, 3(b)). This assay depends upon the presence of 5-hydroxytryptophan decarboxylase in the tissue extracts to convert the ^{14}C-5-hydroxytryptophan to ^{14}C-5-hydroxytryptamine. The selective adsorption of the latter compound onto a cation exchange resin (GC-50) is the basis for the procedure. It is essential to add a monoamine oxidase inhibitor (tranylcypromine) to the enzyme incubation mixture, since no ^{14}C-5-hydroxytryptamine is observed in its absence. In fact, the result obtained when the monoamine oxidase inhibitor is omitted serves as a "blank" for this assay. The procedure requires the extraction of the radioactive products from the incubation mixture into an organic solvent (butanol) and then re-extraction into an acidified aqueous phase before the sample can be applied to the resin. Recently, an alternative isotopic procedure for tryptophan hydroxylase has been described by Lovenberg *et al.* (1967). In this case the enzymatic product is trapped in a pool of unlabeled 5-hydroxytryptophan (carrier) and is subsequently decarboxylated by L-amino acid oxidase to give ^{14}C-5-hydroxytryptamine. The amine is adsorbed on permutit, washed until free of residual substrate, then eluted with ammonia. It seems possible that both of the above procedures could be greatly simplified by using tryptophan-5-^{3}H and measuring the hydroxylation directly as the formation of tritiated water (cf. procedure of Nagatsu *et al.*, 1964). Charcoal should effectively remove the unmetabolized substrate or any other labeled indole byproducts (such as tryptamine or 5-hydroxytryptamine).

An extremely sensitive and convenient procedure for the isotopic assay of a variety of transaminases has been described by Albers *et al.* (1962). The procedure utilizes a ^{14}C-α-keto acid (pyruvate or α-ketoglutarate) as the labeled substrate in conjunction with an L-amino acid as the amino donor (Table 5, 4). The reaction mixture is transferred directly to a small column (1 × 1.5 cm) of cation exchange resin (Dowex 50), rapidly washed to remove the unmetabolized substrate (^{14}C-keto acid), and the ^{14}C-amino acid (enzymic product) is eluted in a small volume of NH_4OH. The radioactivity in the alkaline eluates serves as the direct measure of the reaction. These investigators obtained evidence in support of the separate identities of several transaminases. An isotopic procedure for the assay of a transaminase acting on γ-aminobutyric acid (Hall and Kravitz, 1967) utilizes essentially similar techniques.

Phosphocholine-cytidyl transferase, which catalyzes the following reversible reaction:

$$\text{phosphocholine} + \text{CTP} \rightleftharpoons \text{CDP-choline} + \text{pyrophosphate},$$

may be measured in several ways by using (a) labeled phosphocholine(^{14}C- or ^{32}P-) and isolating the labeled product (CDP-choline) on charcoal; (b) ^{32}P-pyrophosphate and isolating the labeled product (CTP) on charcoal; and (c) CDP-choline-^{14}C, removing this substrate with charcoal, and measuring the labeled product, ^{14}C-phosphocholine, in the supernatant solution. In terms of the efficiency and convenience of separation of labeled substrate from labeled product, all three procedures are probably equivalent. However, the second of these approaches might be seriously affected by the occurrence of an exchange reaction, while the enzymic hydrolysis of CDP-choline by a pyrophosphatase (to yield phosphocholine) would present serious difficulties with the third approach. The first procedure (Table 5, 5(a)) would appear to be the one of choice and has been described by Borkenhagen and Kennedy (1957). In this procedure charcoal added directly to the incubation mixture adsorbs the ^{14}C-CDP-choline. Then the ^{14}C-choline phosphate is removed by washing, and the labeled product assayed after elution from charcoal with an alcoholic ammonia solution.

The enzymatic formation of ^{14}C-lactose may be conveniently detected after removal of the unmetabolized substrate (UDP-galactose-^{14}C) on a small column of anion exchange resin (Babad and Hassid, 1966; Table 5, 5(b)).

The isotopic procedure for folic acid reductase described by Roberts (1966b) utilizes as the enzymic substrate, folate which is labeled by gaseous exchange with tritium (Table 5, 6(a)). When the folate is reduced by the enzyme (in the presence of TPNH) subsequent chemical oxidation releases one half of the radioactivity at position 7 (in the pteridine ring) as tritiated water. After removal of the residual labeled substrate by adsorption onto charcoal, the tritiated water is measured by liquid scintillation counting. This procedure appears to be several-fold more sensitive and at least as convenient as the zinc precipitation procedure described above (see Table 4, 6).

Brunetti *et al.* (1962) have described an isotopic procedure for the enzyme that cleaves *N*-acylneuraminic acid (Table 5, 6(b)). In this procedure a small column of anion exchange resin (Dowex 1) is used to adsorb the residual labeled substrate, and the labeled product of the reaction (*N*-acyl-mannosamine), collected in the column effluent, is measured by scintillation counting. It should be emphasized again that this procedure (as well as several of those mentioned previously) can be used for the recovery (and reuse) of the unmetabolized substrate. This is a valuable asset when the labeled substrate(s) are not readily available or are expensive to prepare.

The enzymatic formation of ^{14}C-CDP-glucose (Mayer and Ginsberg, 1966) or ^{14}C-GDP-glucose (Barber, 1966) from ^{14}C-glucose-1-phosphate and the respective nucleotide triphosphate are currently measured by column chromatographic techniques (Table 5, 6(c), (d)). It seems likely that these procedures could be greatly simplified by using a phosphatase to form free glucose (Mayer and Ginsberg, 1966). The labeled product (^{14}C-CDP-glucose) might then be conveniently and selectively adsorbed onto either a DEAE-disc or charcoal as described above (cf. Table 5, 2(b), (c), and 5(a)).

Vahouny *et al.* (1963) have reported on a rapid procedure for the effective separation of cholesterol and cholesterol esters. This separation is carried out on microscopic slides coated with silicic acid (thin layer chromatography). The complete separation of labeled sterols and their derivatives, as observed in these studies, indicates that this procedure might provide an extremely sensitive and convenient isotopic assay for sterol esterification and esterases.

In summary, the examples discussed above show that sorbants, such as anion and cation exchange resins, charcoal, and DEAE cellulose, can be used to effect rapid and efficient separations between labeled substrates and products of certain enzyme reactions. In those instances where obvious differences in the net charge of substrate vs. product occur, exchange resins or the DEAE disc have been used. Often charcoal is useful where one of the two constituents to be separated is a nucleotide. In any case, these sorbants, which are more conventionally used to effect elaborate chromatographic separations, can, on occasion, be used in a much simpler fashion to provide a complete separation of only two or three components.

2.2.5. *Miscellaneous procedures*

Finally, a few isotopic procedures for enzyme assays which cannot readily be placed in the above categories should be mentioned. For example, glycogen biosynthesis may be studied by isotopic procedures using ^{14}C-UDP-glucose-(glucose-labeled) as one of the substrates. The selective isolation of the labeled product (glycogen) is accomplished by precipitation with trichloracetic acid in ethanol (Palasi *et al.*, 1966). Turner *et al.* (1966) have described an ultramicromethod for the measurement of pepsin, in which denatured hemoglobin labeled with radioactive iodine (^{131}I) is the substrate. Proteolysis is measured by release of acid-soluble radioactivity. The procedure with only minor modification is reported to be applicable to the assay of many other proteolytic enzymes. There are numerous experiments present in the current literature in which isotopic procedures have been used to follow the incorporation of low molecular weight labeled precursors into macromolecules (i.e. proteins, nucleic acids, polysaccharides, mucopeptides, mucolipids, etc.). In these assays, frequently the high molecular weight labeled polymer which is formed may be precipitated by acid, alcohol, etc., and in this way readily separated from its precursor. Unfortunately, many of these reactions are too complex to be studied step by step, as yet. Further, the labeled precursors or intermediates for many of these reactions are not generally available and require considerable specialized experience and equipment for their preparation. Thus broad pharmacologic investigations (isotopic or otherwise) of these enzyme-catalyzed reactions will generally be limited by our ability to describe and develop methodology for the individual steps of these complex processes.

3. METHODS FOR REACTIONS *IN VIVO*

In the previous sections, the discussion of isotopic methods suitable for quantitative assay of enzyme activities has been limited to examples which involved a well-defined single-step reaction (*in vitro* assay) where such factors as pH, substrate concentration and side reactions can be rigidly controlled. By definition, control of these factors in an *in vivo* assay is virtually impossible. Consequently, it is not possible to categorize or discuss the "quantitative" aspects of isotopic enzyme assays *in vivo* in the same way as was used in the previous sections of this chapter. Even if it is assumed that one had available a reliable and selective method for the isolation of a metabolite arising *in vivo* from a labeled substrate, it would be difficult to be certain whether or not (a) the metabolite arose exclusively as the result of the activity of a single enzyme, much less the designated one; (b) the quantity of the metabolite recovered from a given tissue was directly proportional to the enzyme present in that tissue (*in vitro* assay conditions usually are planned so that this relationship holds); or (c) whether an appreciable quantity of the metabolite had been converted (through subsequent enzyme metabolism) to chemical forms which, for various reasons, were not measured. The effects of such factors* as the route of administration, permeability barriers, and protein binding, to mention but a few, are largely unknown and often beyond the control of the investigator. Thus in the author's opinion any general attempt to obtain even a semi-quantitative value of enzyme activity *in vivo* is precluded. (See also Hanson and Clark, 1962; Sourkes, 1966.)

Notwithstanding the above considerations, there are a few examples in which isotopic methods for studying enzyme-catalyzed reactions *in vivo* have been useful for certain pharmacologic studies. For example, Hanson and Clark (1962) described a procedure for the "quantitative" measure of *inhibition* of dihydroxyphenylalanine decarboxylase *in vivo*. Their assay, based on the measurement of radioactivity in the respiratory CO_2 after injection of ^{14}C-carboxy-labeled dihydroxyphenylalanine, would appear to be a much more rapid and, in some respects, a more direct approach to the measure of decarboxylase activity *in vivo* than was previously available (Clark, 1959). Similarly, Okita (1964) used a continuous monitoring of respiratory $^{14}CO_2$ in studying the effects of drugs on the oxidation of labeled substrates. The relative effects of drugs on catecholamine metabolism *in vivo* has been reported by Rutschmann *et al.* (1964) and Udenfriend *et al.* (1966). In the latter studies, it was necessary to isolate, identify and measure each of the various enzymic products. Axelrod and co-workers carried out a series of studies (both *in vitro* and *in vivo*) to determine the quantitative significance of enzyme-catalyzed *O*-methylation vs. deamination as the major metabolic route for catecholamine inactivation (see Axelrod, 1966).

It should be obvious that in the above examples isotopes were not used for the primary purpose of measuring the activity of an enzyme *per se*. Rather they were concerned with obtaining a relative measure of potency of different drugs or a relative measure of importance of different metabolic pathways.

---

* Many of the factors alluded to here as affecting the interpretation of *in vivo* metabolism of labeled compounds are covered in detail in other chapters of this volume.

4. METHODS FOR MEASURING ENDOGENOUS SUBSTRATES

The measurement of endogenous levels of such compounds as acetylcholine, serotonin, histamine, etc., has been of much interest to pharmacologists. In most cases this is an exceedingly difficult analytical problem because of the minute quantities of these compounds present. Thus procedures for the measurement of endogenous metabolites must, of necessity, have a high level of sensitivity and specificity. For these reasons fluorometric techniques have proven very useful in the study of tissue levels of catecholamines and indoleakylamines (see review of Udenfriend, 1962). Isotopic techniques also have the requisite level of sensitivity and under the appropriate circumstances are suitable for the measurement of endogenous metabolites.

Snyder *et al.* (1966) have described an isotopic procedure for the measurement of tissue histamine (Table 6, 1). In this procedure, a trace quantity of ^{3}H-histamine is added to tissue extracts containing an unknown quantity of histamine. The histamine (both labeled and unlabeled) is converted to ^{14}C-*N*-methyl histamine in the presence of ^{14}C-*S*-adenosyl methionine and the enzyme histamine-*N*-methyl transferase. The doubly labeled methyl-histamine is selectively extracted into an organic solvent and independent measures of the radioactivity due to ^{14}C and ^{3}H are obtained. It has been shown that the ratio of ^{14}C/^{3}H radioactivity is directly proportional to the quantity of histamine present in the tissue extracts. This assay is extremely sensitive (0.002–1.0 mcg of histamine) and specific. The latter characteristic is a consequence of the specificity of the methyl transferase.

Double-label assay techniques, using partially purified enzymes to form secondary derivatives, have been used for the assay of other tissue constituents. These would include assays for tissue levels of S-adenosylmethionine (Baldessarini and Kopin, 1966) and of *N*-acetylserotonin (Baldessarini, unpublished observations). It should be emphasized that the double-label technique does not require complete conversion of the tissue constituent to a secondary product because one label indicates the dilution by the tissue constituent (^{3}H), while the other (^{14}C) indicates the degree of reaction. It should also be noted that these procedures do not require the careful and laborious purification of tissues and reagents characteristic of other (i.e. fluorometric) procedures.

The isotopic procedures for the determination of substrate levels of pyridine nucleotides (Table 6, 3 and 4) use a pair of enzymes which can be

TABLE 6. ENDOGENOUS SUBSTRATES WHICH MAY BE DETERMINED BY EMPLOYING ISOTOPIC PROCEDURES

Substrate	Procedure	Measured product	References
1. Histamine	Add'n: ³H Histamine (trace) ¹⁴C-Me-SAMe Histamine N-Methyl transferase	$^3H/^{14}C$ 1,3-Methylhistamine (solvent extraction)	Synder et al., 1966
2. *S*-Adenosyl methionine	Add'n: ¹⁴C-Me-SAMe (trace) ³H-N-Acetyl Serotonin Hydroxyindole-O-Methyl transferase	$^3H/^{14}C$ *O*-Me-*N*-Acetyl-serotonin (solvent extraction)	Baldessarini and Kopin, 1966
3. TPN, TPNH	1° Add'n: 1-¹⁴C glucose-6-P, NH_4^+, Ketoglutarate, glutamic dehydrogenase, glucose-6-phosphate dehydrogenase 2° Add'n: TPN 6-phosphogluconic dehydrogenase	$^{14}CO_2$	Pastan et al., 1963 Serif et al., 1966
4. DPN, DPNH	Add'n: 1-¹⁴C-ketoglutarate, lactate, glutamic dehydrogenase, lactic dehydrogenase	$^{14}CO_2$ (glutamic decarboxylase)	Serif and Butcher, 1966

related in a metabolic cycle. The principle underlying these procedures is the same as that described by Lowry *et al.* (1961) for the fluorometric deter-

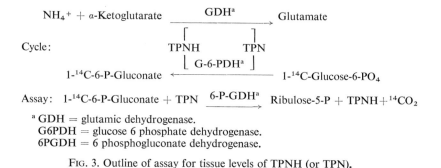

Cycle:

$NH_4^+ + \alpha$-Ketoglutarate $\xrightarrow{\text{GDH}^a}$ Glutamate

1-^{14}C-6-P-Gluconate $\longleftarrow$ 1-^{14}C-Glucose-6-PO$_4$

TPNH   TPN

G-6-PDH^a

Assay: 1-^{14}C-6-P-Gluconate + TPN $\xrightarrow{\text{6-P-GDH}^a}$ Ribulose-5-P + TPNH$+^{14}$CO$_2$

^{a} GDH = glutamic dehydrogenase.
G6PDH = glucose 6 phosphate dehydrogenase.
6PGDH = 6 phosphogluconate dehydrogenase.

Fig. 3. Outline of assay for tissue levels of TPNH (or TPN).

mination of tissue levels of the pyridine nucleotides. These techniques involve a "cycling" phenomenon which is illustrated (Fig. 3) in the assay of TPNH (Pastan *et al.*, 1963). The tissue extract is treated with dilute alkali to destroy the oxidized pyridine nucleotides present. The extract containing TPNH is then added to an incubation mixture containing 1-^{14}C-glucose-6-phosphate, ammonia, α-ketoglutarate and the purified enzymes, glutamic dehydrogenase and glucose-6-phosphate dehydrogenase. The TPNH present in the tissue extract initiates the formation of glutamate and TPN (glutamic dehydrogenase). The latter product, in turn, initiates the production of ^{14}C-6-phosphogluconate and TPNH (glucose-6-phosphate dehydrogenase). This TPNH then "recycles" through the paired enzyme-catalyzed reactions to produce multiples (depending on the number of cycles in a given time of incubation) of glutamate and ^{14}C-6-phosphogluconate. Ultimately (after 50–100 cycles), the reaction is terminated and ^{14}C-6-phosphogluconate formed is converted quantitatively (in presence of TPN and 6-phosphogluconic dehydrogenase) to ^{14}CO$_2$. The radioactivity in the ^{14}CO$_2$ is proportional (but amplified several-fold by cycling) to the level of TPNH originally present in the tissue extracts (cf. Serif *et al.*, 1966).

The specificity of the reaction for TPN vs. TPNH (and DPN vs. DPNH) depends upon the selective destruction of the unwanted nucleotide by base or acid, respectively. The discrimination between TPN vs. DPN (or TPNH vs. DPNH) results from the substrate (nucleotide) specificity of at least one enzyme of the pair used for the cycling reaction. Thus, the isotopic determination for TPN and TPNH (Table 6, 3) differs from that for DPN and DPNH (Table 6, 4) by the pair of enzymes (and substrates) used for the cycling reaction and consequently, the purified enzyme used in the "analytical" step resulting in the evolution of $^{14}CO_2$.

It should be noted that the amount of cycling (and, therefore, the sensitivity) is different for each of the isotopic procedures and is less in both procedures than that obtained by Lowry *et al.* (1961). The lower amplification (cycling) in the isotopic procedures is the result of the incubation conditions (and enzymes) and is not related to the use of isotopes *per se*. If conditions were selected so that the isotopic procedures resulted in cycling factors approximately equal to those obtained in the fluorometric procedures, the former (isotopic) would be expected to be the more sensitive technique (see Table 1).

5. MISCELLANEOUS CONSIDERATIONS
5.1. LIMITS OF SENSITIVITY

A principal factor which determines the ultimate sensitivity of the isotopic methods discussed in this chapter is the specific activity of the measured compound. Obviously, the higher the specific activity, the greater the inherent sensitivity. In an early section of this chapter, the "limit sensitivity" of a ^{14}C-labeled compound with a specific activity of 1 mCi/mM was calculated to be approximately 1.3×10^{-11} M. Suppose this theoretical ^{14}C-labeled compound contained 6 carbon atoms. If each of the carbons were labeled with pure carbon-14 (whose specific activity is 64 mCi/mM) the compound could have a *maximum theoretical* specific activity of 384 mCi/mM (6×64), and would result in a corresponding increase (384-fold) in the sensitivity of measurement of this compound. There are, however, several practical limitations to such a consideration. First, labeled materials having a maximum theoretical specific activity (in terms of carbon content) seldom can be prepared either on a commercial basis or in the laboratory. In fact, as one attempts to produce a given compound with a higher and higher specific activity, there is generally a disproportionate increase in the cost of such an effort; second, the chemical stability of labeled compounds is generally inversely related to its specific activity; the higher the specific activity, the less stable is the material in storage. Finally, the inherent "blank" of a given method for isolating a labeled product may be such that it precludes that an increase in sensitivity will result from the use of materials with a higher specific activity. For example, suppose that, under a given set of conditions for the measure of choline acetylase (Table 4, 1), the sample (containing 10^{-11} M of enzymatically-synthesized ^{14}C-acetylcholine) had a measured radioactivity of 100 cpm while that of the reagent blank was 10 cpm. Let us further assume that both of these counts are corrected for background and that the 10 cpm for the blank represents *unavoidable* contamination by ^{14}C-acetyl CoA. If a ^{14}C-acetyl CoA preparation of 10-fold greater specific activity were used, it may be assumed (all other conditions being equal) that the reagent blank and sample would contain counts of 100 and 1000 cpm respectively. Thus, although the count obtained for the sample would be proportionately higher, the count for the reagent blank also is proportionately higher. Since the "limit sensitivity" was defined as the ratio of radioactivity in the sample (corrected for reagent blank) to that of the reagent blank (*vide supra*), this ratio remains at 9/1 for both of the above examples (90/10 and 900/100). Therefore, under conditions in which the blank is significantly greater than background, it is apparent that the use of a higher specific activity would not result in an increase in sensitivity. If, on the other hand, the radio-activity of the "reagent blank" was undetectable (much less than that of the background or "machine blank"), the use of a substrate with a higher specific activity would be expected to increase the sensitivity of the procedure.

5.2. MICROTECHNIQUES

Frequently it may be necessary to measure enzyme activities of very small tissue samples (a few micrograms or less). In this situation, the use of micropipettes, microtubes, etc., is dictated by the size of tissue sample available. Even when sample size is not limiting, there are several advantages to conducting isotope experiments on a microscale. The reduction in the quantity of isotope used in a given microscale experiment results in a substantial savings in the cost of the experiment as well as increased safety for personnel. Perhaps not so obvious is the reduction of quenching effects in scintillation counting solutions resulting from the use of small volumes (microliters) of aqueous solutions and organic solvents. Frequently experiments carried out on a microscale can be carried out more efficiently and more rapidly with respect to solvent extractions, isolation and washing of precipitates, and diffusion distance, etc. Additional descriptions of the techniques and apparatus appropriate for conducting isotopic assays on microgram and submicrogram quantities of tissue may be found in recent reviews by McCaman (1966, 1968).

5.3. CHOICE OF ISOTOPES

Most of the previous discussion of methods has been restricted to examples in which ^{14}C- or ^{3}H-labeled compounds were utilized. While this is largely the result of the ubiquity of these two elements in nature, it is also related to other factors: (1) more than 90% of the labeled biochemicals commercially available contain one of these two isotopes; (2) both ^{14}C and ^{3}H emit β-radiation of weak to moderate energy and, therefore, pose no serious health hazard in tracer quantities as described herein; and (3) both of these isotopes have a long half-life compared to the very short half-lives of ^{35}S (87 days), ^{32}P (14 days), and ^{131}I (8 days), which obviates the necessity of making frequent corrections for the loss of radioactivity due to short-term decay. Two problems may be encountered when compounds containing ^{32}PO$_4$ or ^{35}SO$_4$ are used to measure enzyme-catalyzed reactions. The first concerns their ability to enter into "exchange" reactions (rather than net synthesis); the second is the ease with which these compounds become strongly adsorbed to glass surfaces. The former of these considerations may markedly influence the interpretation of certain data and must be properly controlled. The latter requires that glassware used for a given experiment be discarded or placed aside until suitable decay has taken place to reduce the contamination to an acceptable level.

When a choice must be made between ^{14}C- vs. ^{3}H-labeled materials, the following general considerations may be helpful. The ^{3}H-labeled compounds are generally cheaper and are available with exceptionally high specific activities. Since ^{3}H is more easily introduced into compounds, a greater variety of ^{3}H-labeled materials may be synthesized (see Wilzbach, 1963). However, several factors may favor the use of ^{14}C-labeled compounds. For example, scintillation counting of ^{14}C is less susceptible to quenching. Further, the ^{14}C-label is stable in contrast to the ^{3}H-label which may frequently be present in a "loose" or "exchangeable" form. Finally, the large atomic weight difference between tritium and hydrogen atoms may produce artifacts (isotope effects) in certain types of enzyme studies. In contrast, the "isotope effects" of ^{14}C may be considered to be relatively unimportant.

5.4. SCINTILLATION COUNTING TECHNIQUES

The specific techniques and composition of scintillator solutions used in scintillation counting are nearly as varied in number as there are scintillation counters. The variety of scintillator-counting fluid recipes is just as frequently based on the subjective experiences of the investigator as on the restrictive demands of a particular procedure. The recent review (Rapkin, 1964) of various aspects of scintillation counting techniques may be helpful in deciding among the available alternatives.

9. RESUME

The underlying theme for this chapter has been a discussion of the general principles which have contributed to an efficient use of isotopes for the quantitative assay of enzyme activities. The examples cited have focused primarily on the use of ^{14}C-labeled substrates in assays of single-step enzyme-catalyzed reactions *in vitro*.

The following points have been emphasized: (a) that a commercially available labeled substrate was used; (b) that the labeled substrate constituted no particular health hazard nor presented problems due to chemical instability; (c) that the overall procedure was relatively simple and did not require highly specialized apparatus; and (d) that certain aspects of the technique contributed to the formulation of general principles which would aid in the development of future methodology.

Various methods currently in use have illustrated that supporting techniques, such as solvent extraction, adsorption and desorption, secondary chemical reactions, etc., are crucial to the development of isotopic methods. An intimate knowledge of the purity and stability of the isotopic substrate as well as its general chemical and physical properties is also essential. A careful selection of the labeled substrate will often minimize the consequences of side reactions and allow full advantage to be taken of the physical or chemical technique used for the isolation of the labeled metabolic product.

Isotopic procedures for the assay of enzyme activities will be found to offer many methodologic advantages. Their intrinsic sensitivity is equal to or greater than that of other procedures (fluorescence, absorption, titration) currently used for biochemical studies. They may be used for the quantitative assay of a variety of enzymatic activities and endogenous levels of metabolic intermediates. In some cases the isotopic methods may represent the only way that a convenient and reliable chemical measure of an enzyme activity or tissue constituent may be obtained. Often the conditions of an isotopic procedure may be manipulated so that the consequences of secondary (or unanticipated) metabolic reactions, which would lead to gross errors with other types of procedures, are negligible. Frequently the necessity of using highly purified chemicals (solvents) or enzymes as auxiliary reagents as required by other forms of analysis (especially fluorescence), is avoided. Finally, a particular advantage of these techniques is the ease with which they may be used to study the effects of antimetabolites or inhibitors of enzyme activities.

REFERENCES

(A) BOOKS, REVIEWS AND MONOGRAPHS

AXELROD, J. (1966) Methylation reactions in the formation and metabolism of catecholamines and other biogenic amines. *Pharmacol. Rev.*, **18**:95–113.

McCAMAN, R. E. (1968) Application of tracers in quantitative histo- and cytochemical studies, in *Advances in Tracer Methodology* Rothchild, S. (ed.). Plenum Press, New York, U.S.A., pp. 87–202.

RAPKIN, E. (1964) Liquid scintillation counting 1957–1963. A review. *Int. J. appl. Rad. Isotopes*, **15**:69–87.

UDENFRIEND, S. (1962) *Fluorescence Assay in Biology and Medicine.* Academic Press, New York, U.S.A.

(B) ORIGINAL PAPERS

ALBERS, R. W. and BRADY, R. O. (1959) The distribution of glutamic decarboxylase in the nervous system of the rhesus monkey. *J. Biol. Chem.*, **234**:926–8.

ALBERS, R. W., KOVAL, G. J. and JAKOBY, W. B. (1962) Transamination reactions of rat brain. *Exp. Neurol.*, **6**:85–89.

AXELROD, J. (1962) Purification and properties of phenylethanolamine-*N*-methyl transferase. *J. Biol. Chem.*, **237**:1657–60.

AXELROD, J., ALBERS, W. and CLEMENTE, C. D. (1959) Distribution of catechol-*O*-methyl transferase in the nervous system and other tissues. *J. Neurochem.*, **5**:68–72.

AXELROD, J., INSCOE, J. K. and DALY, J. (1965) Enzymatic formation of *O*-methylated dihydroxy derivatives from phenolic amines and indoles. *J. Pharmacol. Exp. Therap.*, **149**:16–22.

AXELROD, J., MacLEAN, P. D., ALBERS, R. W. and WEISSBACH, H. (1961) Regional distribution of methyl transferase enzymes in the nervous system and glandular tissues, in *Regional neurochemistry*, Kety, S. S. and Elkes, J. (eds.). Pergamon Press, New York, U.S.A., pp. 307–11.

BABAD, H. and HASSID, W. Z. (1966) Soluble uridine diphosphate D-galactose: D-Glucose β-4-D-galactosyltransferase from bovine milk. *J. Biol. Chem.*, **241**:2672–8.

BACHUR, N. R. and UDENFRIEND, S. (1966) Microsomal synthesis of fatty acid amides. *J. Biol. Chem.*, **241**:1308–13.

BARBER, G. A. (1966) GDP-glucose pyrophosphorylase from peas, in *Methods in Enzymology*, Vol. 8, Colowick, S. P. and Kaplan, N. O. (eds.). Academic Press, New York, U.S.A., pp. 266–8.

BALDESSARINI, R. J. and KOPIN, I. J. (1966) *S*-adenosylmethionine in brain and other tissues. *J. Neurochem.*, **13**:769–77.

BORKENHAGEN, L. F. and KENNEDY, E. P. (1957) The enzymatic synthesis of cytidine diphosphate choline. *J. Biol. Chem.*, **227**:951–62.

BORKENHAGEN, L. F., KENNEDY, E. P. and FIELDING, L. (1961) Enzymatic formation and decarboxylation of phosphatidylserine. *J. Biol. Chem.*, **236**:PC28–30.

BRADY, R. O., KANFER, J., and SHAPIRO, D. (1965) The metabolism of glucocerebrosides. I: purification and properties of a glucocerebroside-cleaving enzyme from spleen tissue. *J. Biol. Chem.*, **240**:39–43.

BROWN, W. O. and BADMAN, H. G. (1961) Liquid-scintillation counting of ^{14}C-labelled animal tissues at high efficiency. *Biochem. J.*, **78**:571–8.

BRUNETTI, P., JOURDIAN, G. W. and ROSEMAN, S. (1962) The sialic acids. III: distribution and properties of animal *N*-acetylneuraminic aldolase. *J. Biol. Chem.*, **237**:2447–53.

CARTER, J. R. and KENNEDY, E. P. (1966) Enzymatic synthesis of cytidine diphosphate diglyceride. *J. Lipid Res.*, **7**:678–83.

CLARK, W. G. (1959) Studies on inhibition of L-DOPA decarboxylase *in vitro* and *in vivo*. *Pharmacol. Rev.*, **11**:330–49.

CLELAND, W. W. and KENNEDY, E. P. (1960) The enzymatic synthesis of psychosine. *J. Biol. Chem.*, **235**:45–51.

DINGELL, J. V. and SANDERS, E. (1966) Methylation of desmethylimipramine by rabbit lung *in vitro*. *Biochem. Pharmacol.*, **15**:599–605.

FELDSTEIN, A. and WONG, K. K. (1965) Analysis of 5-HTP-^{14}C and its metabolites. *Anal. Biochem.*, **11**:467–72.

FONNUM, F. (1966) A radiochemical method for the estimation of choline acetyltransferase. *Biochem. J.*, **100**:479–84.

FULLER, R. W. and HUNT, J. M. (1966) A micromethod for the assay of phenethanolamine *N*-methyl transferase. *Anal. Biochem.*, **16**:349–54.

FURLONG, N. B. (1963) A rapid assay for nucleotide kinases using ^{14}C- or ^{3}H-labeled nucleotides. *Anal. Biochem.*, **5**:515–22.

GATT, S. (1966) Enzymatic hydrolysis of sphingolipids. I: Hydrolysis and synthesis of ceramides by an enzyme from rat brain. *J. Biol. Chem.*, **241**:3724–30.

GOLDFINE, H. (1966) Acylation of glycerol-3-phosphate in bacterial extracts. Stimulation by acyl carrier protein. *J. Biol. Chem.*, **241**:3864–6.

GREEN, A. L. and HAUGHTON, T. M. (1961) A colorimetric method for the estimation of monoamine oxidase. *Biochem. J.*, **78**:172–5.

GREEN, H. and SAWYER, J. L. (1966) Demonstration, characterization, and assay procedure of tryptophan hydroxlyase in rat brain. *Anal. Biochem.* **15**:53–64.

HANSSON, E. and CLARK, W. G. (1962) Studies on DOPA decarboxylase inhibitors *in vivo* by use of ^{14}C-carboxyl-labeled DOPA. *Proc. Soc. Exp. Biol. Med.* **111**:793–8.

HALL, Z. W. and KRAVITZ, E. A. (1967) The Metabolism of γ-Aminobutyric Acid (GABA in the Lobster Nervous System—I. GABA-glutamate transaminase., *J. Neurochem.*, **14**:45–54.

HUTTON, J. J., JR., TAPPEL, A. L. and UDENFRIEND, S. (1966) A rapid assay for collagen proline hydroxylase. *Anal. Biochem.*, **16**:384–94.

JOURDIAN, G. W., CARLSON, D. M. and ROSEMAN, S. (1963) The enzymatic synthesis of sialyl-Lactose. *Biochem. Biophys. Res. Com.*, **10**:352–8.

KANFER, J. N., YOUNG, O. M., SHAPIRO, D. and BRADY, R. O. (1966) The metabolism of sphingomyelin. I: Purification and properties of a sphingomyelin-cleaving enzyme from rat liver tissue, *J. Biol. Chem.*, **241**:1081–4.

KEAN, E. L. and ROSEMAN, S. (1966) CMP-sialic acid synthetase. (cytidine-5′-monophospho-sialic acid synthetase), pp. 208–15. In *Methods in Enzymology*, Vol. 8, Colowick, S. P. and Kaplan, N. O. (eds.). Academic Press, New York, pp. 208–15.

KIYASU, J. Y., PIERINGER, R. A., PAULUS, H. and KENNEDY, E. P. (1963) The biosynthesis of phosphatidylglycerol. *J. Biol. Chem.*, **238**:2293–8.

LENNARZ, W. J. and TALAMO, B. (1966) The chemical characterization and enzymatic synthesis of mannolipids in *Micrococcus lysodeikticus*. *J. Biol. Chem.*, **241**:2707–19.

LEVINE, R. J. and WATTS, D. (1966) A sensitive and specific assay for histidine decarboxylase activity. *Biochem. Pharmacol.*, **15**:841–9.

LOMAX, M. I. S. and GREENBERG, G. R. (1967) A new assay of thymidylate synthetase activity based on the release of tritium from deoxyuridylate-5-^{3}H. *J. Biol. Chem.*, **242**:109–13.

LOVENBERG, W., JEQUIER, E. and SJOERDSMA, A. (1967) Tryptophan hydroxylation: measurement in pineal gland, brainstem, and carcinoid tumor. *Science*, **155**:217–19.

LOWRY, O. H., PASSONNEAU, J. V., SCHULZ, D. W. and ROCK, M. K. (1961) The measurement of pyridine nucleotides by enzymatic cycling. *J. Biol. Chem.*, **236**:2746–55.

LOWRY, O. H., ROBERTS, N. R. and KAPPHAHN, J. I. (1957) The fluorometric measurement of pyridine nucleotides. *J. Biol. Chem.*, **224**:1047–64.

MAYER, R. M. and GINSBURG, V. (1966) CDP-glucose pyrophosphorylase from *Salmon-*

ella paratyphi, in *Methods in enzymology*, Vol. 8, Colowick, S. P. and Kaplan, N. O. (eds.). Academic Press, New York, U.S.A., pp. 256–8.

McCaman, R. E. (1961) A new micromethod for monoamine oxidase. *Fed. Proc.*, **20**:344.

McCaman, R. E. (1962a) A microradiometric method for 5-hydroxytryptophan decarboxylase. *Fed. Proc.*, **21**:365.

McCaman, R. E. (1962b) Intermediary metabolism of phospholipids in brain tissue: microdetermination of choline phosphokinase. *J. Biol. Chem.*, **237**:672–6

McCaman, R. E. (1963) Microdetermination of choline acetylase and its distribution in nervous tissue. *Fed. Proc.*, **22**:170.

McCaman, R. E. (1965) Microdetermination of catechol-*O*-methyl transferase in brain. *Life Sci.*, **4**:2353–9.

McCaman, R. E. (1966) Isotopic method for determining enzyme activity in microgram and submicrogram quantities of tissue. *Isotop. Radiat. Technol.*, **3**:328–34.

McCaman, R. E. and Cook, K. (1966) Intermediary metabolism of phospholipids in brain tissue. III: Phosphocholine-glyceride transferase. *J. Biol. Chem.*, **241**: 3390–4.

McCaman, R. E. and Hunt, J. M. (1965) Microdetermination of choline acetylase in nervous tissue. *J. Neurochem.*, **12**:253–9.

McCaman, R. E., McCaman, M. W., Hunt, J. M. and Smith, M. S. (1965) Microdetermination of monoamine oxidase and 5-hydroxytryptophan decarboxylase activities in nervous tissues. *J. Neurochem.*, **12**:15–23.

McCaman, R. E., McCaman, M. W. and Stafford, M. L. (1966) Carnitine acetyltransferase in nervous tissue. *J. Biol. Chem.*, **241**:930–4.

Nagatsu, T., Levitt, M. and Udenfriend, S. (1964) A rapid and simple radioassay for tyrosine hydroxylase activity. *Anal. Biochem.*, **9**:122–6.

Okita, G. T. (1964) *In vivo* oxidation of ^{14}C-labeled intermediates and of drugs as measured by a continuous $^{14}CO_2$ monitor, In *Isotopes in Experimental Pharmacology*. Roth, L. J. (ed.). University of Chicago Press, chap. XVI, pp. 191–203.

Palasi, C. V.-, Rosell-Perez, M., Hizukuri, S., Huijing, F. and Larner, J. (1966) Muscle and liver UDP-glucose: α-1,4-Glucan α-4-glucosyltransferase (glycogen synthetase), In *Methods in Enzymology*, Vol. 8, Colowick, S. P. and Kaplan, N. O. (eds.). Academic Press, New York, U.S.A., pp. 374–84.

Pastan, I., Wills, V., Herring, B. and Field, J. B. (1963) Pyridine nucleotides in the thyroid. I: A method for the measurement of oxidized and reduced triphosphopyridine nucleotides with the use of 6-phosphoglucomate-1-^{14}C. *J. Biol. Chem.*, **238**:3362–5.

Paulus, H. and Kennedy, E. P. (1960) The enzymatic synthesis of inositol monophosphatide. *J. Biol. Chem.*, **235**:1303–11.

Pomerantz, S. H. (1964) Tyrosine hydroxylation catalyzed by mammalian tyrosinase: An improved method of assay. *Biochem. Biophys. Res. Comm.*, **16**:188–94.

Reed, D. J., Goto, K. and Wang, C. H. (1966) A direct radioisotopic assay for acetylcholinesterase. *Anal. Biochem.*, **16**:59–64.

Robinson, J. and Newsholme, E. A. (1966) A radiochemical enzymic activity assay for glycerol kinase. *Biochem. J.*, **101**:41P.

Roberts, D. (1966a). An isotopic assay for thymidylate synthetase. *Biochem. J.*, **5**:3546–48.

Roberts, D. (1966b) An isotopic assay for dihydrofolate reductase. *Biochem. J.*, **5**:3549–51.

Rothenberg, S. P. (1966) A rapid radioassay for folic acid reductase and amethopterin. *Anal. Biochem.*, **16**:176–9.

Rutschmann, J., Pacha, W., Kalberer, F. and Schreier, E. (1964) A method for the study of drug influence on catecholamine metabolism using L-DOPA (2,5,6-^{3}H),

In *Isotopes in Experimental Pharmacology.* Roth, L. J. (ed.). University of Chicago Press, pp. 295–306.

SCHUBERTH, J. (1963) Radiochemical determination of choline acetyltransferase. *Acta Chemica Scand.* 17:S233–S237.

SCHUBERTH, J. (1965) On the biosynthesis of acetyl coenzyme A in the brain. I: The enzymic formation of acetyl coenzyme A from acetate, adenosine triphosphate and coenzyme A. *Biochim. biophys. Acta*, 98:1–7.

SERIF, G. S. and BUTCHER, F. R. (1966) Pyridine nucleotides. I: Radiometric determination of minute quantities of diphosphopyridine nucleotides. *Anal. Biochem.*, 15:278–86.

SERIF, G. S., SCHMOTZER, L. and BUTCHER, F. R. (1966) Pyridine nucleotides. II. Radiometric determination of minute quantities of triphosphopyridine nucleotides. *Anal. Biochem.*, 17:125–34.

SHERMAN, J. R. (1963) Rapid enzyme assay technique utilizing radioactive substrate, ion exchange paper and liquid scintillation counting. *Anal. Biochem.*, 5:548–54.

SNYDER, S. H., BALDESSARINI, R. J. and AXELROD, J. (1966) A sensitive and specific enzymatic isotopic assay for tissue histamine. *J. Pharmacol. Exp. Therap.*, 153:544–549.

SNYDER, S. H. and AXELROD, J. (1965) Sex differences and hormonal control of histamine methyltransferase activity. *Biochim. Biophys. Acta.* 111:416–21.

SOURKES, T. L. (1966) DOPA decarboxylase: substrates, coenzyme, inhibitors. *Pharmacol. Rev.*, 18:53–60.

SRIBNEY, M. and KENNEDY, E. P. (1958) The enzymatic synthesis of sphingomyelin. *J. Biol. Chem.*, 233:1315–22.

TAYLOR, R. T. and WEISSBACH, H. (1965) Radioactive assay for serine transhydroxymethylase. *Anal. Biochem.*, 13:80–4.

TURNER, M. D., TUXILL, J. L., MILLER, L. L. and SEGAL, H. L. (1966) An ultramicro method for the measurement of pepsin. *Anal. Biochem.*, 16:487–99.

UDENFRIEND, S., ZALTZMAN-NIRENBERG, P., GORDON, R. and SPECTOR, S. (1966) Evaluation of the biochemical effects produced *in vivo* by inhibitors of the three enzymes involved in norepinephrine biosynthesis. *Mol. Pharmacol.*, 2:95–105.

VAHOUNY, G. V., BORJA, C. R. and WEERSING, S. (1963) Radioactive and analytical determination of free and esterified cholesterol following micro thin-layer silicic acid chromatography. *Anal. Biochem.*, 6:555–9.

WALL, J. S., CHRISTIANSON, D. D., DIMLER, R. J. and SENTI, F. R. (1960) Spectrophotometric determination of betaines and other quaternary nitrogen compounds as their periodides. *Anal. Chem.*, 32:870–4.

WEGENER, W. S., REEVES, H. C. and AJL, S. J. (1965) An isotopic method for assaying the condensation of glyoxylate with acetyl-CoA and other short-chain fatty acid acyl-CoA derivatives. *Anal. Biochem.*, 11:111–20.

WEISS, S. B., SMITH, S. W. and KENNEDY, E. P. (1958) The enzymatic formation of lecithin from cytidine diphosphate choline and D-1,2-diglyceride. *J. Biol. Chem.*, 231:53–64.

WEISS, S. B., KENNEDY, E. P. and KIYASU, J. Y. (1960) The enzymatic synthesis of triglycerides. *J. Biol. Chem.*, 235:40–4.

WILZBACH, K. E. (1963). The gas exposure technique for tritium labeling, In *Advances in Tracer Methodology*, Vol. I, Rothchild, S. (ed.). Plenum Press, New York, U.S.A., pp. 4–11 and 28–31.

WURTMAN, R. J. and AXELROD, J. (1963) A sensitive and specific assay for the estimation of monoamine oxidase. *Biochem. Pharmacol.*, 12:1439–41.

Subsection III

RADIOISOTOPE COMPARTMENTAL
ANALYSIS IN PHARMACOLOGY

CHAPTER 10

THEORETICAL ASPECTS OF COMPARTMENTAL ANALYSIS*

James S. Robertson

Medical Physics Division, Medical Research Center, Brookhaven National Laboratory, Upton, N.Y.

1. INTRODUCTION

THE tracer concept may be illustrated by an example. Consider the use of leaves floating on the surface of a river as markers for the rate of flow of the water. Differences in rates and direction of flow for the various parts of the stream become much more obvious than they would be without the markers. The leaves, however, are not useful as tracers for vertical components of the flow, for subsurface flow rates, or for details involving dimensions smaller than a few leaf diameters. The basic reason for this deficiency is, of course, that leaves are different from water. For some purposes the differences are not important, while for others they are limiting factors.

Like the leaves, other tracers also serve as indicators for the movements of labeled substances, and show components of such movement that in general are not apparent in direct observation of the unlabeled material. And, in further analogy to the leaves, any tracer's reliability is limited by the extent to which its properties duplicate those of the substance being traced. At the atomic level minor differences in chemical and physical properties may be important, and isotopes of the element being traced make the most nearly perfect tracers, whereas when large molecules are to be traced, even replacement of an atom of one element by one of a different element may give a satisfactory tracer. At each level of complexity there are limitations on the amount of information that can be obtained from an analysis of tracer data.

* Research supported by the U.S. Atomic Energy Commission.

The purpose of this article is to examine some of the fundamental relationships between the kinetics of tracers and the things traced, particularly as these are applicable to studies using labeled pharmaceutical materials in mammalian systems, and with further emphasis on the interpretation of the kinetics of tracer behavior in terms of compartmented systems.

Although the terminology will be kept as general as possible, at some times it will be most convenient to assume that the tracer is a radioactive nuclide. However, to the extent that the basic assumptions, such as identity of behavior at the unit level of interaction (which depends upon the nature of the labeled substance) and nonperturbation of the system by the tracer, hold, the principles are applicable to all tracers, and the terminology can be translated into that appropriate to the method actually used. Some drugs, by virtue of their being dyes, of being fluorescent, or having other identifying characteristics are self-labeled and can be traced by physical methods without requiring specific chemical analyses. In these cases the units used for intensity or concentration may usually be substituted directly for activity concentration.

Contributions to the theory of tracer kinetics in general, and analysis by the compartmental method in particular, are dispersed widely throughout the literature. Some of the most important articles are in physical and chemical journals; others are in pharmacological, physiological, biophysical, biochemical, and other bio-medical journals. The references given have been selected largely on the basis of giving key or general references (books and reviews) to the older literature, with direct references to the recent literature only, the dividing line being about 1960.

2. DEFINITIONS AND DISCUSSION OF TERMINOLOGY

Several of the terms used in the preceding introduction have special or restricted meanings when used in discussions of tracer kinetics. However, there has not been universal agreement as to the exact meanings of certain words, the best word to express certain concepts, or the symbolic notation to be used. In this article the recommendations of the International Committee for Radiological Units (ICRU) Task Group on Tracer Kinetics (Brownell *et al.*, 1968) will be adopted. The following terms, in particular, are defined.

System. An assemblage of interrelated objects, into which a tracer can be introduced and either its exit from or concentration within the system or its components can be determined.

In the present discussion a system may be the entire body or some portion of the body. The term "system" will be used to denote the largest entity under consideration.

Label. A marker, tag or indicator distinguishable by the observer but (at least in principle) not by the system, and used to identify a population (molecules, cell, etc.) being traced.

Tracer. Labeled particles or members of a population. An ideal tracer is indistinguishable by the system from the unlabeled population.

Tracee. The material that is traced. This term is proposed by the Task Group on Tracer Kinetics (Brownell *et al.*, 1968) to represent unambiguously what has previously been referred to as unlabeled substance, mother substance, etc. in tracer kinetics articles. Unless indicated otherwise, the term "tracee" will include unlabeled plus labeled substance.

Specific activity. The concentration of the label relative to the tracee. This broad definition is consistent with usage in tracer studies, and permits a fairly wide range of units such as mCi/g, mCi/mEq or counting rate per gram to be used. The basic concept of the relative number of radioactive to nonradioactive atoms is preserved, but it is not necessary to reduce all numerical values to these units explicitly.

Compartment. An anatomical, physiological, chemical, or physical subdivision of a system throughout which the ratio of concentration of the tracer to that of the tracee is uniform at any given time.

This definition implies the assumption of rapid mixing of the tracer with its unlabeled counterpart within a given compartment, so the same transfer probabilities can be assigned to tracer and tracee. Uniform concentration of the tracee in the compartment is not an essential assumption; uniform specific activity is.

The relationships among a system and its compartments, tracer and tracee are illustrated in Fig. 1. Figure 2 shows some different ways of representing compartmented systems.

Steady state. In tracer kinetics a system is regarded as being in the steady state if the amounts and concentrations of the tracee remain constant in each compartment for the duration of the experiment.

When steady state systems are under consideration, the additional assumption that tracee inflow and outflow rates are constant is also usually made, but this is an independent constraint on the system.

Rate constant. The question of whether the term "turnover rate" should have dimensions of quantity per time or fraction per time has been debated

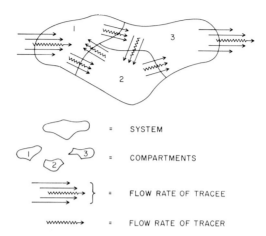

FIG. 1. Schematic representation of a *system* comprising three *compartments*. The transfer rate of the *tracer* is indicated by the wavy-shafted arrow, while that of the *tracee* is represented by the cluster of straight and wavy arrows.

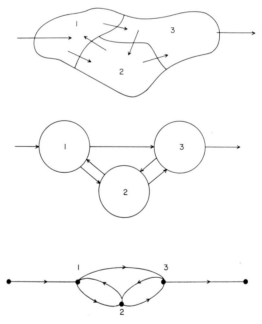

FIG. 2. Reduction of diagram of a *compartmented system* from the style used in Fig. 1, through the commonly used mode of separated areas to the more abstract representation of the compartments as nodes in a network. The latter method is used by Rescigno and Segre (1966).

in the literature. In the present article "rate" will imply quantity per time, and "rate constant" or "transfer constant" will be used to denote a fraction per time.

More extensive discussions of the above and other terms are available in the tracer kinetics task group report cited above, and in a number of books and reviews, particularly those by Sheppard (1962), Bergner (1961, 1966), Rescigno and Segre (1966), and Robertson (1957, 1962).

2.1. SYMBOLS

A confusing aspect of the tracer kinetics literature has been the tendency for individual investigators to invent their own notation systems. In an effort to promote some uniformity in this respect, the ICRU Task Group on Tracer Kinetics recommends the notation system presented in Table 1, which will be used here. In this notation upper-case letters are used for system parameters and lower-case letters for the corresponding tracer variables, where applicable. Usually a parameter or variable is represented by the first letter of its name, the exceptions being k for the rate constant, in conformance with widespread usage, and a for specific activity, with s being reserved for designating Laplace transform functions.

It should be noted that R_{ij} is used to mean the rate of transport into compartment i from compartment j, in contrast to the reverse notation (R_{ij} = from i into j) which some authors use. The recommended notation conforms to the rows, column subscripting notation of matrix algebra. The diagonal entries R_{ii} are used for the total of the outflow rates for the ith compartments. The latter convention is permissible because, under the assumption of uniform specific activity within a given compartment, all tracee outflows from that compartment have the same specific activity at a given time. The specific activities in the inflows, however, depend on those in their source compartments, so the inflow rates must be treated individually. Another consideration is that outflow, *per se*, does not change the specific activity of the source compartment, but the inflow does, if its specific activity is different from that in the compartment. Similarly, the rows, column matrix notation is used for the subscripts of the coefficients in the solution equations, with A_{jk} being the kth element in the jth row of the [A] matrix.

The k_{ij} are defined as fractional outflows, $k_{ij} = R_{ij}/Q_j$. Their subscripts also conform to the row, column matrix convention when the equations are in terms of tracer quantity. For equations in specific activity or concentration units it is sometimes more convenient to define the k's as inflow

TABLE 1. SYMBOLS

	Tracer (1)	Tracee (2)	Medium volume (3)	Specific activity (1)/(2)	Tracer concentration (1)/(3)
Quantity in compartment j	q_j	Q_j	V_j	$a_j = \dfrac{q_j}{Q_j}$	$c_j = \dfrac{q_j}{V_j}$
Transport rate constant into compartment i from j	k_{ij}	k_{ij}	k_{ij}		
Transport into compartment i from j	$r_{ij} = k_{ij}q_j$	$R_{ij} = k_{ij}Q_j$	$F_{ij} = k_{ij}V_j$		
Transport into system at compartment i	r_{i0}	R_{i0}	F_{i0}		
Exponential description of quantity in compartment j	$\sum_n q_{jn}e^{-\lambda_n t}$			$\sum_n a_{jn}e^{-\lambda_n t}$	$\sum_n c_{jn}e^{-\lambda_n t}$

fractions (Robertson, 1962) but only k's defined in terms of outflows are used here. Flow into the system from the outside is described by $R_{io}a_0$, with Q_0, and hence k_{io}, not being defined. For ideal tracers, the k's defined in terms of the system parameters are applicable to the tracer:

$$k_{ij} = \frac{R_{ij}}{Q_j} = \frac{r_{ij}}{q_j}.$$

For mathematical purposes, this relationship will be assumed to hold.

Except to indicate values at particular times, functions of time, $f(t)$, are written without the (t). Thus q implies $q(t)$, and $q(0)$ is the value of q at time zero.

The term $f(s)$ is defined as the Laplace transform of $f(t)$, with

$$f(s) = \int_0^\infty f(t)\, e^{-st}\, dt.$$

These transforms are useful in solving differential equations in t by reducing them to algebraic equations in s. Since st is dimensionless, s has the

TABLE 2. SELECTED LAPLACE TRANSFORMS (WEAST *et al.*, 1964)

$f(t)$	$f(s)$
$\dfrac{df(t)}{dt}$	$sf(s) - f(0)$

INVERSE TRANSFORMS

$f(s)$	$f(t)$
$\dfrac{1}{s}$	1
$\dfrac{1}{s-a}$	e^{at}
$\dfrac{1}{(s-a)(s-b)}$	$\dfrac{1}{a-b}\,(e^{at} - be^{bt})$
$\dfrac{s}{(s-a)(s-b)}$	$\dfrac{1}{a-b}\,(ae^{at} - be^{bt})$
$\dfrac{1}{(s-a)(s-b)(s-c)}$	$-\dfrac{(b-c)e^{at} + (c-a)e^{bt} + (a-b)e^{ct}}{(a-b)(b-c)(c-a)}$

dimension t^{-1}, and the transform space is sometimes referred to as the frequency domain. Tables of Laplace transforms are now widely available in collections of mathematical tables. Table 2, abstracted from the *Handbook of Mathematical Tables* (Weast, Selby & Hodgman, 1964), gives the transformations used in the examples below.

3. THE ROLE OF TRACERS IN PHARMACOLOGY

Although closely related, the uses of tracers in pharmacology and in physiology have some important differences.

In physiological studies the tracee is normally present in the system, often in a steady state, and the usual problem is to determine, through the use of the tracer, the distribution of the tracee in the system and the rates of its transfer between subdivisions of the system. Thus what is observed is the rate of penetration of the tracer into the domain of the unlabeled tracee (interfusion, Sheppard, 1962), with concepts such as "apparent volume of distribution" and "total exchangeable mass" being based on the ratio of the concentrations of tracer and tracee at some particular time after injection of the tracer. Similarly, many biochemical, metabolic and diagnostic studies involve following the tracer through paths regarded as being characteristic of those of the unlabeled tracee. In these studies the behavior of the tracer is not of intrinsic interest; the tracer is a tool for obtaining information about the kinetics of the tracee. Robertson (1964) has reviewed the role of the tracer method in developing concepts of kinetics in physiology. Studies of transfer rates in steady state systems were largely out of reach before the advent of isotopic tracers.

In pharmacological studies, however, the tracer is more typically a labeled drug that is foreign to the system and is not represented by an unlabeled counterpart normally present within the unperturbed system. The drug itself and its degradation products may be the objects of interest. Numerous studies using labeled drugs are discussed in recent publications by Roth (1965) and by Andrews *et al.* (1966).

A question may arise, when a foreign substance is being traced, as to the meaning of the concentrations and rates that are found, in terms of the parameters of the system. Since the kinetics of their distribution are not determined by those of a preexisting tracee, what does govern the kinetics of such substances? The answer to this depends on the physical and chemical nature of the substance in relation to the system—whether it remains in the circulation, becomes distributed in the total body water or localizes in specific tissues, whether it is catabolized or remains intact, etc.

Also, almost by definition, drugs produce biochemical and physiological changes in the system, and these changes may in turn affect the kinetics of the drug. To a large extent, however, the rates of distribution of a drug are determined by system parameters. For example, the kinetics of colloidal preparations that are selectively removed from the circulation by the reticulo-endothelial system will depend on, and in turn may be used to measure, the blood flow rate to the spleen and liver.

The tendency of the tetracyclines to be retained in mineralized tissues has been discussed by Ibsen and Urist (1964). This aspect of their metabolism is similar to that of calcium, and studies of one substance supplement those of the other.

To the extent that the dependency on system parameters is rate determining, the drug's kinetics may be used to measure properties of the system, or the latter may be used to predict the rate of distribution of the drug. Thus, while in a sense in the case of a labeled drug, the tracer and tracee are one and the same, for some purposes the drug may be regarded as a tracer for a normal component of the system.

3.1. COMPARTMENTAL MODELS

The mammalian organism is far too complex to analyze in complete detail in any one experiment, but for most purposes complete detail is as unnecessary as it is impossible to attain.

Model building is the art of selecting and representing those features of the system under study that both are of interest and are susceptible to analysis.

For example, suppose that the rates of uptake of several substances by the thyroid gland are to be compared. For this purpose the thyroid may be regarded as a single entity, or compartment. However, for a study of the path of iodine in the synthesis of the thyroid hormone, it is necessary to consider several compartments, or chemical phases, within the gland. Even so, for the latter study the individual cells are not considered separately, although minor differences in the reaction rates may be expected on a cell-by-cell basis. For determining the drug dose rate required to maintain a given concentration level in the blood, the entire body may be regarded as a single compartment. Thus the degree of subdivision used is often dictated by the objectives of the experiment.

Alternatively, the data may set limits on the degree of subdivision that it makes sense to consider. For example, suppose that the retention of a tracer in the body as measured by whole-body counting or from the analysis of excretory products can accurately be described by a single component exponential equation: $q = q(0)\, e^{-\lambda t}$. This result is consistent with a one-compartment open-system model. That is, an equation that can be fitted to the data can be derived from a mathematical description of this model.

Such a result does not prove, and should not be interpreted as meaning, that the tracer is uniformly distributed in the body or that the body "really" consists of a single compartment, although both of these assumptions may have been used in analyzing the model. All that can be said in this case is that with respect to the tracer used, the body behaves *as if* it were a single compartment with the rate constant indicated by the λ in the equation. Actually the same data could result from a complicated interplay of diverse rates which happen to interact together to produce the observed result. There is, however, no way to extract additional rate information from the data given, and analysis in terms of a more complicated system would give indeterminate results.

When several exponential components are needed to describe the data, the use of more complicated compartmental models is justified. In general, however, and as will be shown below, there is not a $1:1$ correspondence between the turnover rate constants for the compartments of the model and the exponential components of the curve. Also, it may not be possible, or correct, to identify a given compartment in the model with an anatomical or chemical subdivision of the biological system.

Thus a model is a simplified representation of the biological system that retains certain features of the system and is compatible with the data available. A physical model may be a drawing or other abstract representation of the system. Either the equations that describe the physical model, or the solution equations, those which describe the data, may be regarded as a mathematical model. Of course it is also possible to go directly to the mathematical representation without consciously constructing a physical model.

In practice, it often happens that either the model derived from the system does not lead to a satisfactory description of the data, or a model that is found to give a good fit to the data is inconsistent with the constraints imposed by one's knowledge of the biological system. The reconciliation of these conflicting concepts by modification of the model, obtaining additional data, and reexamining the quality of the fit is part of the process of model building. Both mathematics and intuition, both science and art are involved in the process. In favorable cases this may lead to insight into the processes under study.

In the analysis of compartmental systems, differential equations are most often used, although equivalent results may be obtained through stochastic approaches (Marsaglia, 1963; Pavoni *et al.*, 1964), and for some problems integral equations may be more appropriate (Berkowitz, Sherman and Hart, 1963; Branson, 1946; Stephenson, 1960a, b; Zierler, 1962, 1962, 1964). Because of its general applicability the differential equation method will be emphasized in the analysis that follows.

3.2. LITERATURE SURVEY

It is of special interest to note at this point that some of the basic principles of this method of analysis were established by Teorell (1937) in studies of drug kinetics. The mathematical methods have subsequently been developed by many authors, notably Sheppard and Householder (1951), Hart (1955–66), Berman and Schoenfeld (1956, 1960), Bergner (1960, 1965), Stephenson (1960), Sheppard (1962), Yudilevich *et al.* (1962), Hart (1963), Hart and Weller (1963), Nicolescou-Zinka (1964), Myhill *et al.* (1965), and Rescigno and Segre (1966).

Bio-medically oriented introductions to the mathematical methods used in compartmental analysis are available in the books by Defares and Sneddon (1960) and Searle (1966).

Explicit formulas for the analysis of two- and three-compartment systems have been obtained in a variety of forms. These include Gurpide *et al.* (1964), Leitner (1965), Patten (1966), Potter *et al.* (1963), Robertson *et al.* (1957), Sharney *et al.* (1965), Shore (1961), Skinner *et al.* (1959), and Solomon (1960).

Recent applications that are pertinent to the theory of compartmental analysis include Bauer (1965), Belcher and Jones (1960), Bergner (1964), Brownell *et al.* (1960), Hart (1965), Koch (1962), Lushbaugh *et al.* (1966), Pollycove and Mortimer (1961), Threefoot (1962), and Worsley (1962).

4. DIFFERENTIAL EQUATION METHODS

Given the assumption of a model system in the steady state, with constant transfer rates and with well mixed compartments, tracer kinetics can be described by a set of ordinary first-order linear differential equations with constant coefficients. For an n compartment open system there are n equations of the form

$$\frac{dq_i}{dt} = -R_{ii}\,a_i + \sum_{\substack{j=0 \\ j \neq i}}^{n} R_{ij}\,a_j \quad (i = 1, 2, \ldots, n). \tag{1}$$

By substituting $a_j = \dfrac{q_j}{Q_j}$ and $k_{ij} = \dfrac{R_{ij}}{Q_j}$, we obtain:

$$\frac{dq_i}{dt} = k_{ii}\,q_i + \sum_{\substack{j=1 \\ j \neq i}}^{n} k_{ij}\,q_j + \sum R_{i0}\,a_0 \quad (i = 1, 2, \ldots, n). \tag{2}$$

In the descriptions of these equations, by "ordinary" is meant that there is only one independent variable, in this case time t. "First order" indicates that no derivative higher than the first is used. "Linear" means that the coefficients are constants or functions of the independent variable and are not functions of any of the dependent variables.

The third term in the right-hand member of Eq. (2) appears only with open systems with labeled inflow from outside of the system.

This type of equation is also used to describe first-order chemical reactions, and sometimes confusion arises on the point of whether its use in compartmental analysis implies the assumption that only first-order chemical reactions are involved in determining transfer rates. Such is not the case. In steady-state systems with constant transfer rates first-order equations may be used independently of the actual order of any chemical reactions that may be involved. This simplification is admissible because, with both the amount Q_i present and the exit transfer rates R_{ii} for a given compartment being constant, the exit transfer rate is a constant fraction k_{ii} of the amount present, and the actual reaction order is irrelevant. Conversely, a tracer experiment in a steady-state system is not useful in determining the reaction order.

For any system or compartment that does not meet the assumptions used above, linear equations may not be appropriate, and nonlinear methods are needed (Hart, 1957; Jeffay, 1963; Sheppard, 1962; and Resigno and Segre, 1966).

As may be shown by several methods, the solutions of Eq. (2) have the general form:

$$q_i = \sum_{j=1}^{n} A_{ij}\,e^{-\lambda_j t} \quad (i = 1, 2, \ldots, n). \tag{3}$$

Methods for obtaining explicit expressions or numerical values for the A_{ij}'s and the λ_j's of Eq. (3) in terms of the constants of Eq. (2) are given below. The solution equations may thus be used to predict the behavior of a tracer in a system for which the compartment sizes and transfer rates of the tracee are known or to describe experimental data. Solving the inverse problem of deducing the system parameters from the experimental data is the more common goal, but techniques for solving the forward problem are also essential in model analysis.

Equations (2) and (3) have q as the independent variable. For compatibility with experimental data it may be desirable to use equations in concentration or specific activity. Or, for analysis by analog computer methods, specific activity may be more convenient, because the tracer behaves as if differences in specific activity were the driving forces, and at the final equilibrium the specific activities will be equal. In an open system the final specific activity is that of the inflow, which may be zero.

The units of quantity, concentration and specific activity are interrelated as follows

$$a = q/Q = Vc/Q = c/C; \tag{4}$$

$$c = q/V = Qa/V = Ca. \tag{5}$$

For example, for the two-compartment closed system $1 \rightleftarrows 2$, with $R_{12} = R_{21} = R$, the differential equations in the three different units, q, a, and c, are

Quantity	Specific activity
$\dfrac{dq_1}{dt} = -\dfrac{R}{Q_1} q_1 + \dfrac{R}{Q_2} q_2$	$\dfrac{da_1}{dt} = -\dfrac{R}{Q_1} a_1 + \dfrac{R}{Q_1} a_2$

$$\tag{6}$$

Concentration
$\dfrac{dc_1}{dt} = -\dfrac{R}{Q_1} c_1 + \dfrac{R}{Q_1}\dfrac{C_1}{C_2} c_2$

Quantity	Specific activity
$\dfrac{dq_2}{dt} = \dfrac{R}{Q_1} q_1 - \dfrac{R}{Q_2} q_2$	$\dfrac{da_2}{dt} = \dfrac{R}{Q_2} a_1 - \dfrac{R}{Q_2} a_2$

$$\tag{7}$$

Concentration
$\dfrac{dc_2}{dt} = \dfrac{R}{Q_1}\dfrac{C_2}{C_1} c_1 - \dfrac{R}{Q_2} c_2$

Inspection of Eqs. (6) and (7) show that the matrix of coefficients for specific activity is the transpose (rows exchanged for columns) of that for quantity, and that for concentration is like that for specific activity but also includes the C_i/C_j factors. When $R_{ij} = R_{ji}$ for all ij's, these relationships apply to n-compartment systems as well. For equations in specific activity and concentration units the R_{ij}'s in row i are divided by Q_i; with quantity units, the R_{ij}'s in column j are divided by Q_j.

4.1. SOLUTIONS

Assuming the inflow specific activity a_0 to be constant, the Laplace transforms of Eq. (2) have the form

$$sq_1(s) - q_1(0) = - k_{ii} q_k(s) + \sum_{\substack{j=i \\ j \neq i}}^{n} k_{ij} q_j(s) + R_{i0} a_0/s. \qquad (8)$$

Equation (8) may be solved for $q_i(s)$ as a set of linear algebraic equations. Rearranging gives

$$(s + k_{11}) q_1(s) - k_{12} q_2(s) \ldots - k_{1n} q_n(s) = q_1(0) + R_{10} a_0/s$$

$$- k_{21} q_1(s) + (s + k_{22}) q_2(s) \ldots - k_{2n} q_n(s) = q_2(0) + R_{20} a_0/s$$

$$\cdot \qquad \cdot \qquad \cdot \qquad \cdot$$

$$\cdot \qquad \cdot \qquad \cdot \qquad \cdot$$

$$- k_{n1} q_1(s) - k_{n2} q_2(s) \ldots + (s + k_{nn}) q_n(s) = q_n(0) + R_{n0} a_0/s. \qquad (9)$$

The λ's of Eq. (3) are obtained from Eq. (9) by substituting $-\lambda_j$ for s in the coefficients of the left member of Eq. (9) and extracting the n roots of the polynomial obtained as the determinant of the coefficients.

$$
\begin{vmatrix}
(-\lambda_j + k_{11}) - k_{12} \ldots & & -k_{1n} \\
-k_{21} & +(-\lambda_j + k_{22}) \ldots -k_{2n} & \\
\cdot & \cdot & \cdot \\
\cdot & \cdot & \cdot \\
\cdot & \cdot & \cdot \\
-k_{n1} & -k_{n2} & +(-\lambda_j + k_{nn})
\end{vmatrix} = 0.
$$

$$(10)$$

The roots of λ may be expressed as

$$(\lambda_j - \lambda_1)(\lambda_j - \lambda_2) \ldots (\lambda_j - \lambda_n) = 0. \tag{11}$$

It is assumed that the λ_j's are distinct. The problem of multiple roots requires special consideration (Searle, 1966).

For closed systems, one of the λ_j's is zero, and one of the terms in Eq. (3) is a constant.

The same set of n λ's appears in the solution equation for each compartment in the system. The λ's are independent of the starting boundary conditions and of a_0, and can be expressed in terms of the k's only. For these reasons, the λ's are among the invariants of the system (Berman and Schoenfeld, 1956). The values for the A_{kj}'s, however, do depend on the initial conditions of the experiment and upon a_0 as well as upon the system parameters. The general expression for the A_{kj}'s derived by Berman and Schoenfeld (1956) for an n-compartment system with unlabeled inflow is, in the present notation,

$$A_{kj} = \sum_{i=1}^{n} \left(\frac{\Delta_{ik(\lambda)}}{\Delta(\lambda)} q_i(0) \right) (\lambda_i - \lambda_j), \tag{12}$$

where $\Delta_{ik}(\lambda)$ is the cofactor for the ith row and kth column of the matrix in Eq. (10), and $\Delta(\lambda)$ is the polynomial on the left in Eq. (11).

Perhaps the method of handling open systems that is simplest to express in general terms is to regard an n compartment open system as a form of an $(n + 1)$ compartment closed system. However, when all of the inputs are constants it may be simpler to evaluate the A's by using Eq. (12) with $[q_i(0) - R_{i0}a_0/\lambda_i]$ substituted for $q_i(0)$. The input a_0's do not have to be equal, but do have to be constant for this to be applicable.

4.2. CALCULATION OF SYSTEM PARAMETERS FROM EXPERIMENTAL DATA

For the inverse problem, the A_{ij}'s and λ_j's are obtained experimentally by fitting Eq. (3) to the data (Perl, 1960), and the problem is to use this information to calculate the system (or model) parameters. This may be done by substituting the right-hand members of Eq. (3) for the q_i's in Eq. (2), equating corresponding terms in the result and the derivative of Eq. (3), and solving for the k_{ij}'s. From the k_{ij}'s and the boundary conditions, explicit solutions for the R's and Q's are obtained.

R.I.P.—N

Substitution in Eq. (2) gives:

$$\frac{dq_i}{dt} = - k_{ii} A_{i1} e^{-\lambda_1 t} - k_{ii} A_{i2} e^{-\lambda_2 t} \cdots$$

$$+ k_{ij} A_{ji} e^{-\lambda_1 t} + k_{ij} A_{j2} e^{-\lambda_2 t} + \ldots + \ldots, \text{ etc.}$$

(13)

Differentiation of Eq. (3) gives:

$$\frac{dq_i}{dt} = - A_{i1} \lambda_i e^{-\lambda_1 t} - A_{i2} \lambda_2 e^{-\lambda_2 t} - \ldots, \text{ etc.} \qquad (14)$$

For the right-hand members of Eqs. (13) and (14) to be equal, the co-efficients of corresponding exponential terms have to be equal. These equations may be expressed concisely as:

$$[k] [A] = [A][\lambda], \qquad (15)$$

where $[k]$ is the matrix in Eq. (10), without the λ's, $[A]$ is the array of A_{ij}'s in Eq. (3) and $[\lambda]$ is the diagonal matrix having the $-\lambda_j$'s along the diagonal and zeros elsewhere.

$[A]^{-1}$ is defined as the inverse of the $[A]$ matrix, with the property that the matrix product $[A][A]^{-1} = [I]$, the unit matrix, with 1's on the principal diagonal, and zeros elsewhere. Since $[k][I] = [k]$, Eq. (15) may be solved for $[k]$ by post multiplication of both members by $[A]^{-1}$:

$$[k] = [A] [\lambda] [A]^{-1}. \qquad (16)$$

The procedure of translation of the k's into the Q's and R s depends on the model being used. If q_i and a_i are both available for the same instant of time, these establish Q_i by the relationship $q_i = Q_i a_i$, then $R_{ji} = Q_i k_{ji}$, etc. The chain of relationships is greatly simplified if $R_{ij} = R_{ji}$.

Equation (16) implies that all of the A's and λ's have to be known for solutions of $[k]$ to be possible. Constraints on the model in the form of absence of transfers between certain compartments, however, serve to reduce the items of data needed. The three-compartment closed system can be solved completely from data in the initially labeled compartment only (Robertson *et al.*, 1957). When the data available are inadequate to fully determine the parameters of a model, a certain range of values are possible. The computer program developed by Berman *et al.* (1962, 1963) accepts incomplete data and produces solutions within the compatible ranges.

4.3. EXAMPLES

One-, two-, three-, and some four-compartment systems are sufficiently simple that the appropriate equations may be solved by desk calculations. In principle the more complicated systems could be solved also, but in practice the terms encountered rapidly become discouragingly unwieldy.

4.3.1. *The one-compartment open system and the two-compartment closed system*

Analysis in terms of the one-compartment open system, $\rightarrow 1 \rightarrow$, or the two-compartment closed system $1 \rightleftarrows 2$ is suggested if the tracer data can accurately be described by an equation consisting of a constant and a single exponential term

$$q = E + (A - E)\, e^{-\lambda t}. \tag{17}$$

The analyses of these two models are not difficult, but the methods used in their solution serve well as prototypes for the more complicated problems.

For the one-compartment system, equating the rate of change to the difference between inflow and outflow of the tracer gives:

$$\frac{dq_1}{dt} = \frac{dq_1\, a_1}{dt} = R_{10}\, a_0 - R_{01}\, a_1. \tag{18}$$

For the steady state, $R_{10} = R_{01} = R$:

$$\frac{dq_1}{dt} = Q_1 \frac{da_1}{dt} = Ra_0 - Ra_1. \tag{19}$$

If the inflow specific activity a_0 is an undefined function of t, it is not possible to solve Eq. (19) for q_1 or a_1. Alternatively, the equation may be used to solve for R directly:

$$R = \frac{dq_1/dt}{a_0 - a_1}. \tag{20}$$

Thus if experimental values for dq_1/dt or da_1/dt, a_0 and a_1 are obtained for the same time, t, R (or R/Q_1) is determined. This method may be used in cases where only a certain organ is of interest and the data necessary to satisfy Eq. (20) can be obtained, but where, because of the complexity of the rest of the system, a_0 is a correspondingly complicated function of time and is not defined by the data available, or is nonintegrable.

Equation (19) can also be solved for q_1 or a_1 if a_0 is exponential or some other integrable function. In particular, if a_0 is zero or a constant, the method of solution outlined above is applicable.

For specific activity, using the definition $k_{01} = R/Q$, the Laplace transform applied to Eq. (19) gives

$$sa_1(s) - a_1(0) = k_{01} a_0/s - k_{01} a_1(s), \tag{21}$$

$$sa_1(s) + k_{01} a_1(s) = k_{01} a_0/s + a_1(0). \tag{22}$$

Solving Eq. (21) with Laplace transforms

$$a_1(s) = \frac{k_{01} a_0}{s[s + k_{01}]} + \frac{a_1(0)}{[s + k_{01}]}. \tag{23}$$

By the inverse transform

$$a_1 = a_0 + [a_1(0) - a_0]\, e^{-k_{01}t}. \tag{24}$$

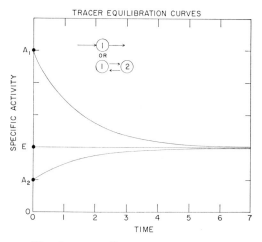

TRACER EQUILIBRATION CURVES

FIG. 3. Tracer equilibration curves for one-compartment open or two-compartment closed systems. Each of the exponential curves shown approaches the equilibrium level with a half-time of one time unit on the abscissa ($\lambda = 0.69315$).

If $a_1(0) < a_0$, the result will be a growth curve characterized by the factor $(1 - e^{-\lambda t})$ and approaching a_0 asymptotically from below, as shown in Fig. 3. If $a_1(0) > a_0$, the result will be an exponential decay curve, again approaching a_0 asymptotically, but from above, also shown in Fig. 3.

Relating Eq. (24) to Eq. (17), we have

$$E = a_0, \tag{25}$$

$$A = a_1(0), \tag{26}$$

$$\lambda = k_{01}. \tag{27}$$

From these, the size of the compartment and the rate of flow of the tracee may be calculated:

$$Q_1 = q_1(0)/a_1(0), \tag{28}$$

$$R = k_{01} Q_1. \tag{29}$$

If $a(0) = 0$, Eq. (28) is not applicable. In this case simultaneous values for q and a obtained at some other time T may be used:

$$Q_1 = q_1(T)/a(T). \tag{30}$$

By a similar line of reasoning, the equations for specific activity in a two-compartment steady-state closed system are, with $k_{11} = k_{21}$ and $k_{22} = k_{12}$:

$$\frac{da_1}{dt} = -k_{21} a_1 + k_{21} a_2, \tag{31}$$

$$\frac{da_2}{dt} = k_{12} a_1 - k_{12} a_2. \tag{32}$$

The corresponding Laplace transforms are

$$sa_1(s) - a_1(0) = -k_{21} a_1(s) + k_{21} a_2(s), \tag{33}$$

$$sa_2(s) - a_2(0) = k_{12} a_1(s) + k_{12} a_2(s), \tag{34}$$

and the solutions in transform space are

$$a_1(s) = \frac{a_1(0)}{s + k_{21} + k_{12}} + \frac{k_{12} a_1(0) + k_{21} a_2(0)}{s[s + k_{21} + k_{12}]}, \tag{35}$$

$$a_2(s) = \frac{a_2(0)}{s + k_{21} + k_{12}} + \frac{k_{12} a_1(0) + k_{21} a_2(0)}{s[s + k_{21} + k_{12}]}, \tag{36}$$

$$\text{Let } C = \frac{k_{12} a_1(0) + k_{21} a_2(0)}{k_{21} + k_{12}}. \tag{37}$$

It is readily shown that $C = E$, the equilibrium specific activity, defined as

$$E = \frac{Q_1 a_1(0) + Q_2 a_2(0)}{Q_1 + Q_2}. \tag{38}$$

With this substitution, the inverse transforms of Eqs. 35 and 36 are

$$a_1 = E + (a_1(0) - E)\, e^{-(k_{21} + k_{12})t}, \tag{39}$$

$$a_2 = E + (a_2(0) - E)\, e^{-(k_{21} + k_{12})t}. \tag{40}$$

From the definition of E, Eq. (38), it is apparent that if $a_1(0) \neq a_2(0)$, E will have a value intermediate to the two initial specific activities. Therefore, considering a_1 and a_2, one will approach E from above and the other from below (Fig. 3). For equations in q, the equilibrium levels for the two compartments are different.

The two-compartment data may also be fitted by Eq. (17). The relationships of the constants in Eq. (17) to the parameters of the system are somewhat different, however, than in the one-compartment case. For two compartments:

$$\lambda = k_{21} + k_{12}, \tag{41}$$

$$A_{12} = (A - E)_1 = a_1(0) - E, \tag{42}$$

$$A_{22} = (A - E)_2 = a_2(0) - E. \tag{43}$$

From Equation 16:

$$k_{21} = \frac{\lambda A_1}{a_1(0) - a_2(0)} = \frac{\lambda A_{12}}{A_{12} - A_{22}}, \tag{44}$$

$$k_{12} = \frac{\lambda A_2}{a_2(0) - a_1(0)} = \frac{\lambda A_{22}}{A_{22} - A_{12}}. \tag{45}$$

If $a_1(0) \neq 0$ and $a_2(0) \neq 0$:

$$Q_1 = \frac{q_1(0)}{a_1(0)}, \quad Q_2 \frac{q_2(0)}{a_2(0)}, \tag{46}$$

$$R = k_{21} Q_1 = k_{12} Q_2. \tag{47}$$

Or, if $a_1(0) \neq$ and $a_2(0) \neq 0$

$$Q_2 = \left[\frac{q_1(0)}{E} - Q_1 \right]. \tag{48}$$

At this point it is apparent that the curves fitted to the data are the same for the one-compartment open and for the two-compartment closed systems, but the interpretations are different. The selection of the model to use, therefore, is dictated by considerations other than the data-fitting curves. In more complicated systems ambiguities of this sort are more prominent and there may be a number of models that give equally good fits for the data. Additional experiments may be needed to distinguish among the possibilities. In the three-compartment closed system which follows, the solution equations have the same form when the tracer is initially in an end compartment as when it is initially in the middle compartment, but of course the interpretations are different.

4.3.2. *The three-compartment closed system*

Analysis of the three-compartment closed system is illustrated by a numerical example, using the system serving as the basis for Fig. 4, $1 \rightleftarrows 2 \rightleftarrows 3$. With $Q_1 = 8$, $Q_2 = 10$, $Q_3 = 15$, $R_{12} = R_{21} = 40$, $R_{23} = R_{32} = 30$, $q_1(0) = 264$, and $q_2(0) = 0$, we have $k_{21} = 5$, $k_{12} = 4$, $k_{32} = 3$, and $k_{23} = 2$. Equation (2) becomes

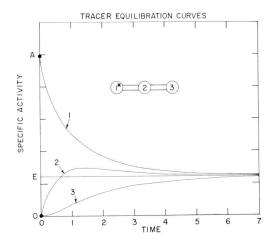

FIG. 4. Tracer equilibration curves for specific activity in a three-compartment steady-state, closed system with $Q_1 = 8$, $Q_2 = 10$, $Q_3 = 15$, $R_{12} = R_{21} = 40$, $R_{23} = R_{32} = 30$, and with all of the tracer initially in compartment 1. Each of the three curves is the resultant of two exponential components, with $\lambda_1 = 11$ and $\lambda_2 = 3$.

$$\frac{dq_1}{dt} = -5q_1 + 4q_2 + 0,$$

$$\frac{dq_2}{dt} = 5q_1 - 7q_2 + 2q_3,$$

$$\frac{dq_3}{dt} = 0 + 3q_2 - 2q_3, \tag{49}$$

and Eq. (10), with all signs reversed is

$$\begin{vmatrix} \lambda - 5 & 4 & 0 \\ 5 & \lambda - 7 & 2 \\ 0 & 3 & \lambda - 2 \end{vmatrix} = 0. \tag{50}$$

Solving Eq. (50) for λ

$$(\lambda - 11)(\lambda - 3)(\lambda - 0) = 0, \tag{51}$$

$$\lambda_1 = 11, \lambda_2 = 3, \lambda_3 = 0. \tag{52}$$

For each of the three values of λ, the corresponding matrices in Eq. (50) are

$$\lambda = 11 \qquad\qquad \lambda = 3 \qquad\qquad \lambda = 0$$

$$\begin{bmatrix} 6 & 4 & 0 \\ 5 & 4 & 2 \\ 0 & 3 & 9 \end{bmatrix}, \begin{bmatrix} -2 & 4 & 0 \\ 5 & -4 & 2 \\ 0 & 3 & 1 \end{bmatrix}, \begin{bmatrix} -5 & 4 & 0 \\ 5 & -7 & 2 \\ 0 & 3 & -2 \end{bmatrix}, \tag{53}$$

and the corresponding minors, or cofactors, k'_{ij}, are, with k'_{ij} substituted for the corresponding k_{ij},

$$\begin{bmatrix} 30 & -45 & 15 \\ -36 & 54 & -18 \\ 8 & 12 & 4 \end{bmatrix}, \begin{bmatrix} -10 & -5 & 15 \\ -4 & -2 & 6 \\ 8 & 4 & 12 \end{bmatrix}, \begin{bmatrix} 8 & 10 & 15 \\ 8 & 10 & 15 \\ 8 & 10 & 15 \end{bmatrix}. \tag{54}$$

Applying Eq. (12) by substituting values from the above matrices of cofactors, the left member of Eq. (51), and q_1 (0) for the appropriate variables generates the coefficients for the solution equation:

$$A_{11} = \frac{30}{(11 - 3)(11 - 0)}(264) = 90, \tag{55}$$

$$\cdot$$
$$\cdot$$
$$\cdot$$

$$A_{33} = \frac{15}{(0 - 11)(0 - 3)}(264) = 120, \tag{56}$$

with the answers:

$$q_1 = 90\,e^{-11t} + 110\,e^{-3t} + 64, \tag{57}$$

$$q_2 = -135\,e^{-11t} + 55\,e^{-3t} + 80, \tag{58}$$

$$q_3 = 45\,e^{-11t} - 165\,e^{-3t} + 120. \tag{59}$$

The curves shown in Fig. 4 are directly related to this result, but are for specific activities instead of quantities.

Because initially only q_1 (0) has a nonzero value, only the upper rows of the cofactors in Eq. (54) are used in Eqs. (55) and (56). The second and third rows would be involved with positive q_2 (0) and q_3 (0), respectively.

For the inverse problem, with $[\lambda]$ and $[A]$ known,

$$[A]^{-1} = \begin{bmatrix} 90 & +\ 110 & +\ 64 \\ -135 & 55 & 80 \\ 45 & -165 & 120 \end{bmatrix}^{-1} = \begin{bmatrix} \dfrac{1}{264} & \dfrac{-1}{220} & \dfrac{1}{990} \\[2mm] \dfrac{1}{264} & \dfrac{1}{660} & \dfrac{-1}{330} \\[2mm] \dfrac{1}{264} & \dfrac{1}{264} & \dfrac{1}{264} \end{bmatrix} \tag{60}$$

(For a method of obtaining $[A]^{-1}$ from $[A]$, see Searle (1966).)

Applying Eq. (16):

$$[A]\,[\lambda]\,[A]^{-1} = [k]$$

$$\begin{bmatrix} 90 & 110 & 64 \\ -135 & 55 & 80 \\ 45 & -164 & 120 \end{bmatrix} \begin{bmatrix} -11 & 0 & 0 \\ 0 & -3 & 0 \\ 0 & 0 & 0 \end{bmatrix} \begin{bmatrix} \dfrac{1}{264} & \dfrac{-1}{220} & \dfrac{1}{990} \\[2mm] \dfrac{1}{264} & \dfrac{1}{660} & \dfrac{-1}{330} \\[2mm] \dfrac{1}{264} & \dfrac{1}{264} & \dfrac{1}{264} \end{bmatrix},$$

$$= \begin{bmatrix} -5 & 4 & 0 \\ 5 & -7 & 2 \\ 0 & 3 & -2 \end{bmatrix}, \tag{61}$$

which agrees with the original $[k]$ in Eq. (49). Thus this example illustrates the major steps in generating the A's and λ's from the k's and $q(0)$'s, and of solving the inverse problem of calculating the k's from the A's and λ's.

5. TRANSFER FUNCTIONS

In some problems interest may be limited to describing the time course of the tracer in one compartment as a function of that in another compartment without direct concern for the rest of the system. The techniques for reducing complicated linear systems to the elements essential for such an analysis have been developed by Rescigno and Segre (1966), and the following discussion is based largely on their presentation. Network diagrams of the type illustrated in Fig. 2 are used in these analyses, with the compartments being represented as nodes, and the flow between compartments is represented as arms, or directed line segments. The tracer function for a given node is determined by the products of the nodes contributing flow to it times their respective arms. Four rules for simplifying the network are given (Rescigno and Segre, 1966). In the present notation, to obtain $q_b(s)$ terms of $q_a(s)$:

"1. Those nodes which receive no contribution from q_a and those nodes which do not contribute to q_b and the nodes that leave them, can be eliminated.

"2. Two arms in series can be substituted with an arm equal to their product, and their intermediate node can be suppressed.

"3. Two arms in parallel can be substituted by an arm equal to their sum.

"4. All the arms entering a node can be substituted by arms entering all immediately successive nodes; each new arm is equal to the product of the suppressed arm times the arm that connects the terminal node of the suppressed arm with the terminal node of the new arm."

Application of these rules is straightforward in the absence of loops, or recycling, which lead to "closed arms" with values denoted by T_{ii}, and introduce $(1 - T_{ii})$ terms in the denominator for every arm entering node i.

Eventually, under application of the above rules, a transfer function $g(s)$ with

$$g(s) = \frac{q_b(s)}{q_a(s)} \tag{62}$$

or

$$q_b(s) = q_a(s)\, g(s) \tag{63}$$

is obtained. The antitransform of $g(s)$, $G(t)$, is known as the weighting function. The antitransform of Eq. (63) is

$$q_b(t) = \int_0^t q_a(\theta)\, G(t - \theta)\, d\theta = \int_0^t q_a(t - \theta)\, G(\theta)\, d\theta \qquad (64)$$

in which the integral is called the convolution integral relating the function $q_b(t)$ to $q_a(t)$. Like the λ's discussed above, the $G(t)$'s are invariants of the system, being determined by the Q's and R's independently of the initial distribution of the tracer. For a unit "spike" function, in which the tracer is present in compartment n only momentarily,

$$q_n(t) = G(t). \qquad (65)$$

A continuous function such as $q_a(t)$ may be regarded as an integral of a series of unit functions with $d\tau$ as the increment of time and $q_a(\tau)\, d\tau$ as the element of quantity, giving

$$q_b(t) = \int_0^t q_a(\tau)\, G(t - \tau)\, d\tau. \qquad (66)$$

Several numerical methods for calculating the weighting functions and transfer functions are reviewed by Rescigno and Segre (1966).

In the analysis of a compartmental system, if the transfer function between two compartments is known, certain deductions may be made about the system, and if several transfer functions are known, the system can be determined to a corresponding degree. The operations involved are closely related to those described in the preceding section.

When the transfer rates in opposite directions between all pairs of compartments in a chain are equal, there is reciprocity between the transfer functions operating in opposite directions. In this case the specific activity curve in compartment i following an initial injection in compartment j is the same as the curve in compartment j following injection of the same quantity of tracer into compartment i (Robertson, 1957). The quantities of tracer transported in these two experiments are different, of course, but the amounts of tracee represented are equal.

6. COMPUTER METHODS

6.1. ANALOG

General purpose electronic analog computers are useful in compartmental analysis as differential equation solvers. In this method, combinations of operational amplifiers are used to differentiate and integrate as well as to perform the ordinary arithmetic operations. Sizes of compartments (Q) may be represented as capacitances, the tracer variable as a voltage, and flow rates by currents. Each individual term in a system may thus be represented, and the entire problem becomes a system of interconnections and feedback loops.

Another analog method, that does not require the use of differential equations, and that may also be achieved with hydrodynamic and other analog devices involves direct representation of the system. In the electrical direct analogs, again the representation is in terms of capacitance, voltage, and current. The flow between two compartments is simulated by connecting the two capacitors through a resistor. In its pure form this method may be used only in systems having equal tracee flow rates in opposite directions between two compartments. Operational amplifier methods may, however, be used as one-way pumps to supplement the resistor-capacitor circuits and a wide variety of steady-state systems can be represented satisfactorily.

Particularly for simple systems, the analog methods are useful in providing inexpensive solutions of compartmental problems. Since the curve-fitting is usually done by eye, however, the objectivity and accuracy of the digital methods are difficult to match. Analog methods are particularly useful in the model-building stages to establish the degree of complexity needed. Among recent applications of analog methods in tracer studies are publications by Schepers and Winkler (1963) and Silverman and Burgen (1961).

6.2. DIGITAL

The digital computer methods used in compartmental analysis typically use the matrix algebra techniques discussed above. With unit cycle times in the modern computers being less than a microsecond, operations involving matrix inversion and matrix multiplication that would hardly be practical by slower methods are achieved with great speed and precision. Being free from the physical constraints inherent in the analog methods, the digital methods have a correspondingly greater flexibility. By the same token, more care is required in programming to conform to realistic operations.

One difficulty with the matrix method is that in principle a complete set of A's and λ's is needed for all compartments of the system. The program developed by Berman *et al.* (1962) and Berman (1963) handles this by introducing arbitrary values for the missing information. The degrees of freedom correspond to the number of arbitrary values needed. Calculated values for the tracer variable are compared with the observed values, and through an iterative process the estimates are revised until either a satisfactory fit is achieved or a preset arbitrary number of iterations permitted is exceeded. The method can also be used to determine the limits of the parameters within which lie all solutions giving satisfactory fits to the available data. The program was developed for execution by a 32 K memory IBM-7094 computer, but has subsequently been adapted to other computers.

Data may be supplied to digital computers in the form of punched cards or punched tape or on magnetic tape. Data acquisition devices can often be designed to produce large parts of the input data directly in the form needed.

7. DISCUSSION

Objections to the methods of compartmental analysis are sometimes expressed. These take various forms, including objecting to the initial assumptions, preferring other methods, and challenging the validity of all tracer methods. Mixtures of well-taken points and simple misunderstandings are involved. These will be considered in order of increasing complexity of the system.

In a few special cases isotopic effects do occur, and in a chain of reactions in which an isotope effect occurs at a key stage, the effect may be multiplied so that a small error at the key stage becomes a large one in the overall function (Bigeleisen, 1963). However, given an ideal tracer, the probability of its transfer from a given location or state to another is the same as that for its unlabeled counterpart in the same original state. This is practically by definition of the ideal tracer, and disagreement at this level amounts to asserting that no two molecules or particles can exhibit the same behavior, if they have the slightest difference in structure. When large molecules or particles are labeled, the requirements for an ideal tracer are met by isotopic labels within any reasonable standard of precision.

The macroscopically observable behavior of the tracer and tracee, however, may be quite different, particularly in the study of steady-state systems. In editorializing on this, Reizenstein (1966) expresses the concept as "Tracers do trace in the sense that there is a mathematically defineable relation between the behavior of a tracer and that of its unlabeled equivalent." However, the next question is "How should the mathematical relationships be formulated?"

In problems like determining the average time of passage in studies of flow through a capillary network, a method that does not require assumptions concerning the structure of the system may be desirable, and non-compartmental methods are useful. By the same token, these methods do not yield any information about the internal structure.

The compartmental method is one of wide applicability, but it is not completely general and does have definite limitations that must be recognized. If there is a continuous gradient of specific activity between two locations, any finite compartmentalization of the intervening path is obviously artificial, and can yield only approximations to the exact answers. In a review of the validity of tracer kinetic methods Bergner (1962) does not find the compartmental method useful in studies of metabolic turnover.

Alternatively, there are defineable subdivisions of the body such as the circulation, the extracellular fluid and the intracellular fluid, that are separated by definite structural boundaries and which may also be associated with definite discontinuities of concentration. In problems exemplified by the transfer of calcium from blood to bone, mixing in the blood is fast, relative to the transfer processes involved. For substances for which the efficiency of uptake can be established, the rate of uptake of a tracer by a tissue may be used to measure the rate of blood flow to that tissue. On the other hand, in general the rate of transfer of an electrolyte between blood and extravascular fluid across capillary membranes cannot be deduced from the rate of tracer disappearance from the blood, because the rate of blood flow, rather than the rate of transfer, is the rate-limiting process and will be what is measured.

Thus an element of caution has to be introduced into any analysis by the compartmental method. The criterion of curve-fitting, while essential, is not sufficient unless a purely phenomenological interpretation is all that is desired. Those situations in which definite anatomical subdivisions of the system can be assigned to the compartments deduced from tracer analysis must be regarded as unusual. Even so, the method does provide a way to assign upper and lower limits on the quantities and transfer rates involved. When the assumptions required for compartmental analysis can be accepted, the method provides a powerful tool for interpreting the behavior of tracers. When the basic assumptions cannot be accepted, the use of the method is at best questionable. Like any tool, the compartmental method of analysis should only be used for the intended purpose. The extensive literature on the subject indicates that there are many practical applications of the compartmental method, and the growing availability of computers can be expected to accelerate the rate of growth of these applications.

REFERENCES

(A) BOOKS, REVIEWS AND MONOGRAPHS

ANDREWS, G. A., KNISELY, R. M. and WAGNER, H. N. (1966) *Radioactive Pharmaceuticals*. U.S. Atomic Energy Commission, Division of Technical Information, CONF-651111, Oak Ridge., Tenn., U.S.A.

BAUER, G. C. H. (1965) Tracer techniques for the study of bone metabolism in man, in *Advances in Biological and Medical Physics*, vol. 10. Lawrence, J. H. and Gofman, J. W. (eds.). Academic Press, New York, U.S.A. pp. 227–75.

BIGELEISEN, J. (1963) *Chemistry of Isotopes*, BNL 828 (T-323).

DEFARES, J. G. and SNEDDON, I. N. (1960) *The Mathematics of Medicine and Biology*. North-Holland Pub. Co., Amsterdam.

JEFFAY, H. (1963) Measuring turnover rates in the nonsteady state, in *Advances In Tracer Methodology*, vol. 1, Proceedings of the Fifth Annual Symposium on Tracer Methodology, October 20, 1961 (Rothchild, S. (ed.).) Plenum Press, New York, U.S.A., pp. 217–21.

LUSHBAUGH, C. C., BERGNER, P.-E. E. and TAUXE, W. N. (1966) (eds.). *Compartments, Pools and Spaces in Medical Physiology*. Oak Ridge Inst. of Nuclear Studies Conf 661010 Oak Ridge, Tenn., U.S.A.

RESCIGNO, A. and SEGRE, G. (1966) *Drug and Tracer Kinetics*. Blaisdell Pub. Co., Waltham, Mass. (Italian edition, Editore Boringhieri Societa per azioni, Torino, 1961.)

ROBERTSON, J. S. (1962) Mathematical treatment of uptake and release of indicate substances in relation to flow analysis in tissues and organs, in *Handbook of Physiology*, Section 2. Circulation v. I., Washington. American Physiology Society, pp. 617–44.

ROBERTSON, J. S. (1964) *The Impact of Isotopic Tracers on Physiological Concepts*. Brookhaven Natl. Lab., BNL 857 (T 341).

ROTH, L. J. (ed.) (1965) *Isotopes in Experimental Pharmacology*. University of Chicago Press, Chicago, Ill., U.S.A.

SEARLE, S. R. (1966) *Matrix Algebra for the Biological Sciences*. John Wiley, New York, U.S.A.

SHEPPARD, C. W. (1962) *Basic Principles of the Tracer Method*. John Wiley, New York, U.S.A.

SOLOMON, A. K. (1960) Compartmental methods of kinetic analysis, in *Mineral Metabolism*, Vol. 1, Pt. A (Comar, C. L.) and Bronner, F. (eds.). Academic Press, New York, U.S.A., pp. 119–67.

STEPHENSON, J. L. (1960b) Integral equation description of transport phenomena in biological system, *Proceedings Fourth Berkeley Symposium on Mathematical Statistics and Probability*, University of Calif. Press, Berkeley, Calif., U.S.A., p. 335.

WEAST, R. C., SELBY, S. M. and HODGMAN, C. D. (1964) *Handbook of Mathematical Tables*. Chemical Rubber Co., Cleveland, Ohio, U.S.A.

YUDILEVICH, D., MARTIN, P. and BUSTOS, S. (1962) A method to process information from multiple tracer experiments, in 4th Inter-American Symposium on the Peaceful Application of Nuclear Energy, Mexico City, April. Washington, Pan Amer. Union, 1962, vol. 2, pp. 77–83 (in Spanish).

ZIERLER, K. L. (1964) Basic aspects of kinetic theory as applied to tracer-distribution studies, in *Dynamic Clinical Studies with Radioisotopes*. Knisely, R. M. and Tauxe, W. N. (eds.). U.S. Dept. Commerce TID-7678, pp. 55–79.

(B) ORIGINAL PAPERS

BELCHER, E. H. and JONES, N. C. (1960) The mathematical analysis of ^{51}Cr deposition in organs following the injection of ^{51}Cr-labelled red cells. *Clin. Sci.* 19:657–63.

BERGNER, P.-E. E. (1960) On the solution of the compartmentalized tracer system. *Expl. Cell Res.*, 20:579–80.

BERGNER, P.-E. E. (1961) Tracer dynamics. I: A tentative approach and definition of fundamental concepts. II: The limiting properties of the tracer system. *J. Theoret. Biol.*, 1:120–40, 359–81.

BERGNER, P.-E. E. (1962) The significance of certain tracer kinetical methods especially with respect to the tracer dynamic definition of metabolic turnover. *Acta Radiologica*, Suppl., Stockholm, 210.

BERGNER, P.-E. E. (1964) Tracer dynamics and the determination of pool-sizes and turnover factors in metabolic systems. *J. Theoret. Biol.*, 6, 137–58.

BERGNER, P.-E. E. (1965) Exchangeable mass: Determination without assumption of isotopic equilibrium. *Science*, 150:1048–50.

BERGNER, P.-E. E. (1966) Tracer theory: A review. *Isotopes Radiat. Technol.* 3,245–62.

BERKOWITZ, J. M., SHERMAN, J. L. and HART, H. E. (1963) The rate of decarboxylation of mevalonic acid-1-C^{14} in man. *Ann. N.Y. Acad. Sci.*, 108:250–8.

BERMAN, M. and SCHOENFELD, R. (1956) Invariants in experimental data on linear kinetics and the formulation of models. *J. Appl. Physics.*, 27:1361–70.

BERMAN, M. and SCHOENFELD, R. L. (1960) A note on unique models in tracer kinetics. *Expl. Cell Res.*, 20: 574–8.

BERMAN, M., WEISS, M. F. and SHAHN, E. (1962) Some formal approaches to the analysis of kinetic data in terms of linear compartmental systems. *Biophys. J.*, 2:290–310.

BERMAN, M. (1963) The formulation and testing of models. *Ann. N.Y. Acad. Sci.* 108: 250–8.

BRANSON, H. (1946) A mathematical description of metabolizing systems. I. *Bull. Math. Biophys.*, 8:159–65.

BROWNELL, G. L., GREENFIELD, E. and BRENTANI, P. (1960) Mathematical analysis of tracer data in Ca and Sr studies. *Strahlentherapie Sonderbände*, 45:1–11.

BROWNELL, G. L., BERMAN, M. and ROBERTSON, J. S. (1968) Nomenclature for tracer kinetics. *Int. J. Appl. Rad. Isotopes* 19: 249–62.

GURPIDE, E., MANN, J. and SANDBERG, E. (1964) Determination of kinetic parameters in a two-pool system by administration of one or more tracers. *Biochemistry*, 3: 1250–5.

HART, H. E. (1955–66) Analysis of tracer experiments. I: Non-conservative steady-state systems. II: Non-conservative non-steady-state systems. III: Homeostatic mechanisms of fluid flow systems. IV: The kinetics of general N compartment systems. V: Integral equations of perturbation-tracer analysis. VI: Determination of partitioned initial entry functions. VII: General multi-compartment systems imbedded in non-homogeneous inaccesible media. *Bull. Math. Biophys.*, 17:87–94 (1955); 19:61–72 (1957); 20:281–7 (1958); 22:41–52 (1960); 27:417–29 (1965); 27:Suppl. 1, 329–32 (1965); 28:261–82 (1966).

HART, H. E. (1963) (ed.) Multicompartment analysis of tracer experiments. *Ann. N.Y. Acad. Sci.*, 108:1–338.

HART, H. E. (1965) Determination of equilibrium constants and maximum binding capacities in complex *in vitro*. *Bull. Math. Biophys.* 27:87:98.

HART, H. E. and WELLER, C. A. (1963) Recent developments in multicompartment tracer analysis. *Trans. N.Y. Acad. Sci.*, 26:64–74.

IBSEN, K. H. and URIST, M. R. (1964) The biochemistry and the physiology of the tetracyclines. *Clin. Orthopaedics*, 32:143–69.

Koch, A. L. (1962) The evaluation of the rates of biological processes from tracer kinetic data. I: The influence of labile metabolic pools. *J. Theoret. Biol.*, 3:283–303.

Leitner, F. (1965) The use of two radiotracers for transfer-rate determination in closed two compartment systems. *Bull. Math. Biophys.*, 27:431–4.

Marsaglia, G. (1963) *Stochastic Analysis of Multicompartment Systems.* Report D1-82-0280, Boeing Scientific Laboratory.

Myhill, J., Wadsworth, G. P. and Brownell, G. L. (1965) Investigations of an operator method in the analysis of biological tracer data. *Biophys. J.*, 5:89–107.

Nicolescou-Zinca, D. (1964) Measurement of metabolic pools by a new method, that of dynamic isotope dilution. *Minerva Nucl.*, 8:312–13.

Patten, B. C. (1966) Equilibrium specific activity relationships in two-compartment exchange systems. *Health Phys.*, 12:521–4.

Pavoni, P., Vitali, O. and Pieraccini, L. (1964) Multi-compartment models and statistical methods for the study of biological processes by means of tracer substances. *Panminerva Med.*, 6:457–64.

Perl, W. (1960) A method for curve-fitting by exponential functions. *Int. J. Appl. Radiat. Isotopes*, 8:211–22.

Pollycove, M. and Mortimer, R. (1961) The quantitative determination of iron kinetics and hemoglobin synthesis in human subjects. *J. Clin. Inv.*, 40:753–82.

Potter, C. S., Rosevear, J. W. and Ackerman, E. (1963) The kinetic analysis of transport between two constant-volume compartments in a closed system under non-steady-state conditions. *Phys. Med. Biol.*, 7:473–80.

Reizenstein, P. (1966) Do tracers trace? (Editorial) *Blood*, 27:744–7.

Robertson, J. S. (1957) Theory and use of tracers in determining transfer rates in biological systems. *Physiol. Rev.*, 37:133–54.

Robertson, J. S., Tosteson, D. C. and Gamble, J. L. (1957) The determination of exchange rates in three-compartment steady-state systems through the use of tracers. *J. Lab. Clin. Med.*, 49:497–503.

Schepers, H. and Winkler, C. (1963) Investigations on radioiodine kinetics, especially the initial iodide phase in the thyroid gland using an electronic simulator. *Strahlentherapie Sonderbände*, 53:19–26.

Sharney, L., Wasserman, L. R., Gevirtz, N. R., Schwartz, L. and Tendler, D. (1965a) Multiple-pool analysis in tracer studies of metabolic kinetics. I: General considerations and solutions of simpler systems (one and two pools). II: Three-pool models and partial systems. *J. Mt. Sinai Hosp.*, 32:201–61.

Sharney, L. *et al.* (1965b) Significance of the time lag in "tracer" movement: Representation of unidirectionally-connected pool sequences by time lag. *Amer. J. Med. Electron.*, 4:95–9.

Sheppard, C. W. and Householder, A. S. (1951) The mathematical basis of the interpretation of tracer experiments in closed steady state systems. *J. Appl. Phys.* 22:510–20.

Shore, M. L. (1961) Biological applications of kinetic analysis of a two-compartment open system. *J. Appl. Physiol.*, 16:771–82.

Silverman, M. and Burgen, A. S. (1961) Application of analogue computer to measurement of intestinal absorption rates with tracers. *J. Appl. Physiol.*, 16:911–13.

Skinner, S. M., Clark, R. E., Baker, N. and Shipley, R. A. (1959) Complete solution of the three compartment model in steady state after single injection of radioactive tracer. *Amer. J. Physiol.*, 196:238–44.

Stephenson, J. L. (1960a) Theory of transport in linear biological systems. I. Fundamental integral equation. II: Multiflux problems. *Bull. Math. Biophys.* 22:1–17; 113–38.

Teorell, T. (1937) Kinetics of distribution of substances administered to the body. I: The extravascular modes of administration. *Arch. Intern. Pharmacodyn.* 57:205–55.

THREEFOOT, S. A. (1962) Some factors influencing interpretation of studies of body water and electrolytes with isotopic tracers. *Progr. Cardiovascular Diseases*, **5**:32–54.

WORSLEY, B. H. (1962) Selection of a numerical technique for analyzing experimental data of the decay type with special reference to the use of tracers in biological systems. *Biochim. Biophys. Acta.* **59**:1–24.

ZIERLER, K. L. (1962) Circulation times and the theory of indicator-dilution methods for determining blood flow and volume. In *Handbook of Physiology*, Section 2, Circulation, vol. 1, Hamilton, W. F. and Dow, P. (eds.). Amer. Physiol. Soc., Washington, pp. 585–615.

ZIERLER, K. L. (1963) Theory of use of indicators to measure blood flow and extracellular volume and calculation of transcapillary movement of tracers. *Circulation Res.* **12**:464–71.

CHAPTER 11

METHODS OF BODY COMPARTMENTS ANALYSIS: APPLICATIONS IN PHARMACOLOGY

J. C. Stoclet

Pharmacodynamics Laboratory, Faculty of Pharmacy, University of Strasbourg, France

INTRODUCTION

THE term compartment here signifies a fraction of a living organism within which a tracer is continuously and uniformly distributed or a subdivision of a model to analyze the diffusion of the tracer within the organism. The compartments thus defined have limits of very different types—anatomical, physiological, chemical, or physical; and only rarely do they correspond to structural or functional units of the human body. Nevertheless, this method of describing organisms has proved to be of great use in physiology and, more recently, in pharmacology as well, since it makes possible *in vivo* studies of body composition and its variations under the influence of drugs in the organism.

The concept of body compartments has developed considerably over the past century. In 1866 Claude Bernard defined an interior liquid medium, which is today called the extracellular fluid, and he drew a clear distinction between the chemical composition of the extracellular and intracellular fluids. Later it became possible to consider the quantitative aspect of the problem by using the methods of tracer dilution. Thus Grehant and Quinquaud (1882) measured the red cell volume by combination with a known quantity of carbon monoxide. The volume-dilution of markers dissolved in injectable solutions, used for the first time for urea by Marshall and Davis (1914), made it successively possible to determine plasma volume by using dyes (Keith *et al.*, 1915; Dawson *et al.*, 1920), extracellular fluid with sodium thiocyanate, and total body water with deuterium oxide (Hevesy and Hofer, 1934).

These studies on liquid volumes of the organism show that certain

349

tracers are stopped by physiological membranes. For instance, dyes bound to plasma proteins do not diffuse through the capillary wall nor does the thiocyanate ion penetrate into cells. Thus the concept of body compartment progressively evolved towards the notion of a dilution space for tracer substances. Only with the advent of a wide range of artificial radio-elements was it developed by Moore (1946): radioisotopes enabled not only liquid volumes to be measured *in vivo* but also various inorganic or organic masses in which dilution takes place by a series of exchanges or transfers; only a slightly modified technique was required for the latter purpose, whatever labeled mineral or organic substance entered the body composition. In addition to this, nuclear indicators allowed the evaluation of the rate or degree of the renewal processes to which the various body compartments are subject. These measurements of electrolyte or organic compartments constituted an effective isotopic dissection of the organism.

Tracers introduced into the circulation diffuse at different rates according to the organ under consideration and the state of circulation. Local circulation may therefore be studied by the use of appropriate indicators as considered in Chapter 12. We confine ourselves here to studying the compartments of the whole living organism regarded as a "system" (see Chapter 10).

A compartment will include extracellular or cellular, mineral, or organic portions, which in reality are distributed in different quantities or concentrations in different tissues. The compartmental study of tracer dilution in organisms first requires an analysis of the temporal variations of tracer concentration in blood plasma, since blood plasma is the only homogeneous body fluid that can be sampled without difficulty. But the physiological interpretation of the results very often requires complementary data obtained by analysis of heterogeneous tissues and simultaneous measurement of several compartments with different tracers.

The task of the pharmacologist is still further complicated by the disturbances that a drug often causes in the renewal and size of the compartments being studied. Two possibilities are open to him: either the effect of the drug on the compartments or the drug distribution within the organism can be studied. The particular problems that arise will be discussed with some examples. But first we shall explain the principle used in the dilution of radioactive tracers and the various techniques which enable the method to be applied to the measurement of body compartments in pharmacology, restricting ourselves to results obtained in studying the principal compartments of the living organism.

1. GENERAL METHODS OF STUDY

All measurements of body or tissue compartments *in vivo* are based on studying the dilution of tracer substances introduced into the blood circulation.

Very many different substances can be used as tracers, but radioactive tracers are by far the most common since they are the simplest to measure in very low concentration. Tracers that are not naturally occurring constituents of the organism, e.g. radioiodinated albumin or labeled drugs, enable dilution volumes to be measured while labeled forms of naturally occurring constituents further permit a measurement of the mass of substance in which they are diluted, so long as one no longer studies the plasma concentration of the tracer but the changes in its specific activity, i.e. the ratio of the quantity of tracer or its concentration in the medium to the total quantity or total concentration of substance both labeled and unlabeled. In this connection it should be mentioned that isotope effects rarely feature in body compartment studies.

The methods of measuring radioactivity are studied in Chapter 6. In the following pages we disregard the physical decay of the radioactive tracers. The effect of such decay has been studied by Perrault *et al.* (1967).

1.1. ISOTOPE-DILUTION METHOD AND ISOTOPIC EQUILIBRIUM

It is necessary for the indicator to be introduced into the organism in a sufficiently small quantity for it to be regarded as negligible so that no change in the observed compartments will take place as a result and so that the indicator will undergo no change within the organism, i.e. it should neither be formed nor destroyed. However, it is possible to use metabolizable organic molecules if they can be separated from their metabolites, and if such metabolism is borne in mind in analyzing the results. The attributes required in a tracer are treated in greater detail by Robertson in Chapter 10. It should be added that the liquid volume in which the tracer is administered should itself be small enough not to alter the steady state appreciably.

The case of labeled nor-adrenaline can be quoted as an example of the precautions to be taken when tracers are used. It is generally known that upon introduction into an organism this drug quickly disappears from the blood and accumulates in nerve endings, more particularly in the heart (Brodie and Beaven, 1963). In the course of their first experiments these authors found two compartments of cardiac nor-adrenaline. On using a tracer of higher specific radioactivity, or labeling the cardiac nor-adrenaline by injection of a labeled precursor (^{3}H-dopa), it was noticed that one of the two compartments was in fact formed by the nor-adrenaline injected into the animal. A dose of nor-adrenaline-^{3}H as low as 1 mcg per kg of body weight seemed *a priori* to be a tracer dose, but in reality it was not, for it is no longer negligible once it has become concentrated in the nerve endings. A dose as low as 0.1 mcg of nor-adrenaline-^{3}H per kg of body weight has to be reached before it constitutes a real tracer dose (Costa *et al.*, 1966).

The dilution method uses the principle that if an indicating substance is introduced into a system where it spreads uniformly, the total volume V of the system is given by the ratio of the quantity R of indicator retained by the system at the moment of time t to the concentration $[Rt]$ of the indicator in the system at the same instant:

$$V = \frac{R}{[Rt]}. \tag{1}$$

By substituting into this formula the specific activity RSt of the tracer in the system at the instant t in place of the concentration, we obtain the mass M of the observed substance present in the system

$$M = \frac{R}{RSt}. \tag{2}$$

This definition implies that the indicator is distributed uniformly in a system formed by one homogeneous compartment and achieves an equilibrium, i.e. the concentration or specific radioactivity becomes constant after a period of "equilibration". Equations (1) and (2) only apply at equilibrium, that is to say the time measured from the moment of administration must be greater than the period of time required for equilibration of the tracer.

The majority of substances present in the organism are not localized in a single homogeneous compartment but are distributed between different compartments where they are subject to more or less rapid turnover phenomena and into which the tracer soon penetrates by transfer or metabolism (if a precursor is used as tracer). In addition to this, excretion processes continually reduce the quantity of indicator retained by the organism. Therefore an actual isotopic equilibrium will hardly ever occur after a single administration of tracer. However, it is to be observed that excretion of many substances proceeds slowly in relation to diffusion of these substances within the organism, while the various renewal processes sometimes proceed at such different rates that under some experimental conditions the slowest are negligible compared with the fastest. Accordingly, the concentration of tracer can become stable in the most accessible compartment long enough for one to talk of "apparent" equilibrium. The volume V given by Eq. (1) is then called the "apparent diffusion space", and the mass M from Eq. (2) the "apparent exchangeable mass". If the apparent exchangeable mass of the observed substance is less than the total quantity contained in the organism, the difference is said to be "nonexchangeable". However, this does not imply that the nonexchangeable mass is subject to no turnover process; it only means that the exchanges which originate from this mass are too slow to influence in any appreciable way the isotopic equilibrium under the conditions of the experiment. Thus only a small fraction of the calcium contained in the skeleton is exchangeable (Neuman and Neuman, 1953, 1958). This fraction can itself be broken down into several subfractions for which the exchanges are more or less rapid (Bauer *et al.*, 1955a, b).

In the absence of apparent equilibrium, the study of body compartments consists of following the temporal change in the specific radioactivity of the labeled molecule or of its metabolic derivatives after administering a single dose of indicator. These kinetic studies involve more or less complex calculations which are treated in Chapter 10. Another experimental procedure sometimes used consists of realizing an actual isotopic equilibrium by maintaining constant the specific radioactivity of the observed substance by a continuous introduction of tracer. Either approach, with the aid of nuclear indicators, will enable the determination of the functional characteristics of renewal. Their application in pharmacology will be discussed after we have explained the methods of measuring dilution spaces and exchangeable mass following a standard period of equilibration.

These different methods apply to an organism in the steady state, i.e. to an organism whose bodily composition does not vary appreciably during the experiment. This equilibrium state of the constituent parts of the body is entirely independent of the isotopic equilibrium, which may or may not arise after the introduction of the tracer: even though the composition of each compartment may remain unchanged, this in no way implies that the specific radioactivity of this part will undergo no change in the course of time because of turnover phenomena. It will be seen later that many drugs upset the steady state, and so add a further complication to the interpretation of the results. For the present we shall assume that the steady state is respected.

(a) *Measurement of diffusion space and exchangeable mass*

In this method the nuclear indicator is injected into the blood (generally intravenously), and the plasma or blood radioactivity is then measured after a standard period of equilibration. The values experimentally found in the blood plasma refer in fact to the accessible compartment as a whole; this may be the whole of the organism or a part.

Knowing the radioactivity of the tracer administered at the beginning of the experiment, the diffusion space or exchangeable mass can then be

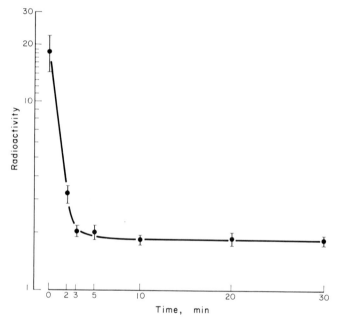

FIG. 1. Temporal variation of radioactivity (% of administered dose) per milliliter of plasma after intravenous injection of Na ^{82}Br in rats of 200 g. Mean values of experimental determinations with fiducial limit $P = 0.05$.

obtained from Eqs. (1) or (2) without difficulty. A variant of this method consists of measuring the specific urinary radioactivity that is at any instant equal to the specific plasma radioactivity.

Equilibrium is reached relatively quickly depending on the type of tracer and the animal species. For the diffusible ions Cl^-, Na^+, and Br^-, equilibrium is established very quickly where it occurs. In the rat ^{82}Br diffuses spatially within minutes (Fig. 1), whereas in man equilibrium is reached more slowly (Nicholson and Zilva, 1957), the process taking several hours. Equilibrium can be much more delayed for larger molecules such as insulin, which diffuse only slowly in the water of the connective tissue (Cotlove, 1954). On the other hand, ^{42}K disappears very quickly from the circulation (Sheppard *et al.*, 1953; Walker and Wilds, 1952).

In the special case of ^{82}Br in the rat, we have been able to regard the excretion as negligible throughout the diffusion period (Stoclet, 1966); but generally the quantity excreted between the injection of the tracer and the time when the sample is taken has to be considered, even when the elimination is sufficiently slow to speak of apparent equilibrium. In this case the radioactivity R appearing in Eqs. (1) and (2) becomes the difference between the administered quantity R_0 of indicator and the fraction R_e which is excreted during the equilibration period:

$$V = \frac{R_0 - R_e}{R\,t}. \tag{3}$$

However, Eq. (3) does not apply in two special cases where a dilution space can still be measured.

In the first case, if the tracer undergoes rapid excretion to an indeterminate extent, the blood concentration will decrease according to a function which contains two exponential terms. The curve for the variation of plasma concentration with time then shows, using semi-logarithmic coordinates, a fast and a slow component. By extrapolating the slow component to zero time, the dilution space can be calculated provided that diffusion is much more rapid than excretion. In practice it suffices to take 3 or 4 samples after the diffusion period and calculate the concentration at zero time by extrapolation on semi-logarithmic paper. Everything behaves as though the diffusion were instantaneous, and it is sufficient to use Eqs. (1) or (2). This method has been applied by Cachera and Barbier (1941a, b) to the measurement of the diffusion space of sodium thiocyanate.

In the case where equilibrium is reached slowly while excretion is rapid, an analysis of the curve showing the variation of concentration with time after a single injection does not permit a distinction between elimination and diffusion to be made. Nevertheless, an experimental design described by Gauding and Levitt (1949) for inulin does enable the dilution space to be measured. A continuous perfusion of the tracer substance is arranged so as to compensate for its excretion throughout the diffusion period. The total quantity of tracer retained by the organism and the plasma concentration are then measured.

The two variants on the measurement of diffusion space that have just been described are kinetic methods applied to a particularly simple case (a single compartment). The first is applied during the transition to equilibrium and the other at equilibrium. These kinetic methods also enable us to measure the degree or rate of renewal processes, as will be seen below.

(b) *Kinetics of transition to isotopic equilibrium*

The kinetic study of the distribution within organisms of a nuclear indicator injected in a single dose (generally intravenously), consists of analyzing the temporal variation of specific radioactivity in the blood plasma and possibly in different tissues or organs and in the excreta.

The results of the study can be interpreted by means of a model in which the organism is represented by a set of compartments between which transfers occur and in which phenomena of metabolism and excretion may take place. The theory of compartmental analysis and the associated mathematical interpretation are treated at length in Chapter 10. Detailed reviews have also been published on this subject (Robertson, 1957, 1962; Solomon, 1953, 1960; Sheppard, 1962; Segre, 1965). Without returning to the theory of the method, we confine ourselves to presenting some of the problems raised in applying it in practice.

The main difficulty arises from the practical impossibility of measuring the specific radioactivity in each compartment. Except for the blood plasma and the red cells, all the organs or tissues have different extracellular and intracellular structures in which the observed substance is renewed at different rates and therefore occurs in various compartments. The following operations have therefore to be performed in sequence:

(1) From data drawn directly from the experiment, find the relation which describes the decrease of specific radioactivity with time in the blood plasma.

(2) In the light of the foregoing relation, select one or more models to describe the distribution of the observed substance and its movements within the organism.

(3) From the selected model, or each model retained, calculate the size and renewal rate for each compartment and the relations which describe the variation of specific radioactivity with time in each compartment.

(4) Finally, verify the model by comparing the values calculated from the model with the values measured experimentally (excretion, specific radioactivity in the tissues); this last operation may make it

possible to choose between the various models that have been considered up to this point.

We must first emphasize the limitations of the conclusions to be drawn from any kinetic study of tracer distribution in the transition to isotopic equilibrium. We will then illustrate how the method is put into practice by taking a definite example, and consider the various experimental approaches in which the method can be used.

Each phenomenon of absorption, excretion, exchange, synthesis, or degradation of the substance being studied has repercussions on the distribution of the tracer in the organism, and *theoretically* can be measured by using the relation which describes the variation of the specific radioactivity in the blood plasma with time, *provided* the existence of each of these phenomena is known in advance and a practical means of identifying the values calculated for the phenomena is available. *In practice* the method only enables phenomena of very different degree to be distinguished (by a factor of at least 10 according to most authors), and so it only provides more or less approximate values.

The specific plasma radioactivity decreases with time in accordance with a relation that contains n exponential additive terms when the organism may be associated with a closed system of $(n + 1)$ compartments, or with an open system of n compartments. In the latter and more general case the organism is related to the external medium by the phenomena of absorption and excretion, the rates of which are equal to one another during the test period if the steady state is maintained. Since the number of compartments concerned is not known in advance in the majority of studies, this number is found by the analysis of the curve for the decrease of specific plasma radioactivity with time.

The graphical, numerical, and analog methods for this analysis are treated in Chapter 10. None of them enable the required function to be obtained unambiguously except in the simplest cases where the system comprises two or, at the very most, three compartments which are very different in their renewal rate and size.

In fact the transport of a substance very often has circumstances which are qualitatively or quantitatively different for each organ and tissue and even for each cell. In the extreme case the system should be divided into as many compartments as there are extra- and subcellular fractions. Fortunately, certain tissues and fluids make up a very substantial part of the organism (extracellular fluid, striated muscular fibres, neurones, and bone for instance), and in these the functional characteristics of renewal of the observed substance are approximately similar. The analysis of the decrease of specific plasma radioactivity RS as a function of time t is therefore often (but not always) possible.

In this case we have a relation of the type

$$RS = \sum_{i=0}^{n} A_i\, e^{-S_i t}, \tag{4}$$

which contains n additive exponential terms where the constants A_i and S_i are complex functions of the real size and rate of renewal of the n compartments (for an open system with one input and one output). This relation is correspondingly more easily established for a smaller number of exponential terms n, and for constants A_i and S_i which differ appreciably from one another, i.e. for fewer compartments with greater differences in size and renewal rate. Several functions, sometimes corresponding to different numbers n, can describe the phenomenon with an approximately close probability, i.e. their calculated values coincide with the test values allowing for experimental approximation. But the body can reasonably be described as a system of n compartments for Eq. (4) in which the constants A_i and S_i differ by a factor of at least 10 between one exponential term and another. Otherwise complementary experimental data are required in order to select Eq. (4).

In all cases, study of the variations of concentration of tracer in the blood plasma enables only a hypothesis to be formed as to the number of body compartments into which the tracer spreads, while the size and renewal rate of these compartments can only be calculated later once the relationships between these compartments and their respective positions are known; that is to say a model is needed. The choice of model therefore calls for further data or hypotheses since it is essential for later calculations.

By way of example, the problems posed by kinetic studies and the conclusions to be drawn can be illustrated by referring to studies of calcium transport in the living rat (Stoclet, 1958, 1960a, b, 1964a, b, 1966). After injection of a tracer dose of ^{45}Ca the specific plasma radioactivity RS_1 decreases for 48 hr in accordance with an equation which contains five additive exponential terms. The constants A_i and S_i of each of these terms can be determined graphically since they are very different from one term to another. Thus for a female rat of 200 g in diestrus, we have, for instance, the equation

$$RS_1 = 137\, e^{-120t} + 17\, e^{-15t} + 11\, e^{-1.2t} + 4.9\, e^{-0.17t} + 1.4\, e^{-0.02t} \tag{5}$$

where time t is measured in hours (Fig. 2).

The foregoing equation corresponds to a model with five compartments having one input and one output. Since the calcium content of the blood plasma and of the organs varies only within very narrow limits, the system can be deemed to be in the steady state, i.e. the instantaneous loss of calcium to the external medium by the system is compensated by the incoming gain. The homeostatic control of blood calcium level and skeletal

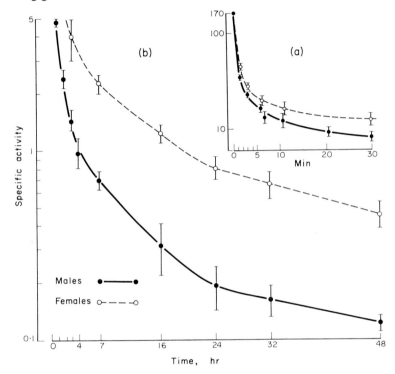

FIG. 2. Decrease of specific radioactivity (% of injected dose per mg of Ca) in blood plasma of male and female rats of 200 g for 30 min (a), and 48 hr (b) after intravenous injection of $^{45}Ca\ Cl_2$. Calculated curves and mean values of experimental determinations with fiducial limit $P = 0.05$.

calcium transport have been the subject of research which, together with the study of body composition, has enabled a model (Fig. 3) to be selected which appears to correspond to Eq. (5).

The skeleton contains the major part of the calcium in vertebrates, about 99% in the rat (Hammett, 1925a, b). Owing to the phenomena of physico-chemical transfer (Neuman and Neuman, 1953) and physiological formation of new bone, the greater part of the ^{45}Ca injected into the animal becomes fixed in bone. The transfer reactions, owing to their degree, would mask all the other phenomena if these reactions affected the whole of the bone calcium; but in fact they are restricted to a very small fraction of it (Neuman and Neuman, 1958). So it can be accepted that calcium fixed in bone by osteogenesis has the same specific radioactivity as that of blood plasma at the instant when the calcium left it, while the calcium liberated

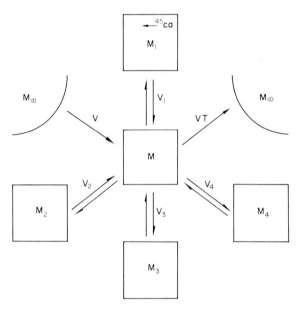

FIG. 3. Open mamillary model with five compartments representing the distribution of calcium transport in the rat organism. M_∞, external medium; M_i, calcium masses of each compartment; V_i flow rates.

in the plasma by osteolysis has no radioactivity since this calcium comes from bone that was formed before the injection of the tracer (Bauer *et al.*, 1955a, b). In other words, a labeled calcium atom which is trapped by the skeleton remains irreversibly fixed throughout the duration of the experiment (48 hr) without feedback. Such an atom can be regarded as lost to the system just as if it were excreted from the organism. The model in Fig. 3 illustrates the position by apportioning the nonexchangeable bone calcium to the calcium of the external medium which is of infinite mass and has therefore zero specific radioactivity. The steady state is maintained since the rate of input V of calcium due to osteolysis and absorption is equal to the rate of output V_t from the system by osteogenesis and excretion. The calcium content of the blood plasma is therefore held constant, despite varying absorption of calcium, by regulation of the excretion, osteogenesis, and osteolysis, which have been studied by Aubert *et al.* (1961, 1963).

It is known that intravascular mixing of an ion that is intravenously injected into the organism takes a few seconds (Zierler, 1962); while diffusion through the capillary barrier is slower. It seems reasonable to represent the organism by a mammillary model where one central compartment M, representing the interstitial spaces, is the origin of calcium transfers to four peripheral compartments M_1, M_2, M_3, and M_4, which are characterized by their respective calcium exchange rates V_1, V_2, V_3, and V_4. It has already been seen that one of these compartments (M_1 in Fig. 3) can represent the blood plasma into which the tracer is introduced, whilst the other three compartments M_2–M_4 would represent cellular media and the exchangeable bone fraction. This mammillary arrangement is considered to be the most realistic one for the majority of applications of compartmental analysis to the living organism. All the same, it presupposes the existence of an interstitial sector of homogeneous composition despite its dispersion in very different tissues; this hypothesis will be discussed later in the present paper. In this particular case it is assumed that the calcium of each of the peripheral compartments of the model is in exchange only with the calcium of the central compartment. This hypothesis is partly justified because it is unlikely that the exchangeable bone calcium could be exchanged with the calcium of some other tissue without passing through the intermediary interstitial fluid; but we cannot exclude the possibility of two compartments existing in series and representing calcium within the cellular medium (which is certainly not homogeneous).

The validity of a model can be tested by comparing the calculations from the model with other experimental data. In the example under consideration, each compartment can in fact be associated with a sector of the organism where the quantity of calcium corresponds to the model and into which ^{45}Ca penetrates in accordance with the kinetics predicted by the model and Eq. (5). The measured parameters (mass, rate) thus assume a physiological significance.

It was assumed above that compartment M_1 represents blood plasma. The mass of calcium in blood plasma is estimated to be 0.6 mg by the kinetic method. The same figure is obtained from measurements of the volume (5.5 ml on average) of blood plasma and its calcium content (107 mcg/ml) using similar animals. From another aspect the homogeneity of the plasma calcium, considered as a body compartment, has been demonstrated by dialysis experiments, i.e. the specific radioactivity of the various fractions of plasma calcium (ionized, nonionized ultrafiltrable, protein bound nonultrafiltrable) is the same even immediately after administration of the ^{45}Ca (1 min).

It is less easy to verify the hypotheses in regard to the other compartments of the model. An indirect approach is to analyze the variation of the specific radioactivity in the organs. It is known in fact that the internal medium of each organ comprises several nondissociable structures between which the calcium is distributed, e.g. residual blood plasma in the capillaries, interstitial fluids, connective tissue, and muscle fibres. The state of the calcium in each of these organs can be regarded as a compartmental subdivision whether corresponding or not to one of the various phases of the internal medium.

At each instant t the radioactivity r^t_x of some organ x is the sum total of the radioactivities of each of the forms of calcium which this organ contains. In this case

$$r^t_x = \sum_{i=0}^{n} RS^t_i\, m_i, \qquad (6)$$

where terms m_i represent the mass of calcium of each compartment contained in the organ, and RS^t_i is the specific radioactivity of the respective compartments at time t.

The variation with time of the specific radioactivity in each of the compartments of the model can be calculated from Eq. (5). It is therefore possible to apply Eq. (6) at different instants t as often as may be necessary to calculate each fraction m_i by a set of x equations with x unknowns. The calculated values of m_i can be verified in the following manner: their sum total should be equal to the quantity m_x of the observed substance (total calcium in this context) present in the organ and determined experimentally; also Eq. (6) should be satisfied at any time t. In the latter respect the temporal variation of the specific radioactivity RS_x of the calcium of the organ is calculated by the equation

$$RS_x = \frac{RS_i \cdot m_i}{m_x}, \qquad (7)$$

where RS_x and RS_i are time functions, while m_i and m_x are constants. One then verifies that the calculated curve for RS_x as a function of time corresponds at any instant to the experimentally determined specific radioactivity of the calcium of the organ. This check clearly has no significance at times for which Eq. (6) is applied, since the values of m_i have been calculated from data (RS_x) obtained at these determined times. On the other hand, the check does show that the same values of m_i would be found at whatever time was chosen for the calculations.

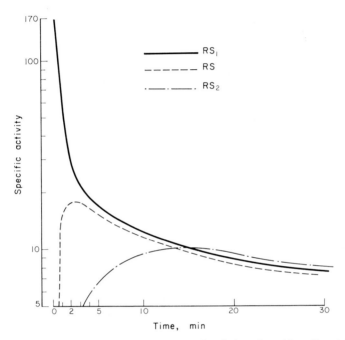

FIG. 4. Calculated curves representing temporal variation of specific radioactivity RS_i (% of injected dose per mg of Ca) as a function of time in the central compartment M (RS) and in the peripheral compartments of the model (Fig. 3): plasma (RS_1) and compartment M_2 (RS_2) for 30 min after injection of ^{45}Ca Cl$_2$ in the male rat of 200 g.

The variation with time of the specific radioactivity of the calcium of the different compartments is illustrated in Figs. 4 and 5 for the example under consideration. It will be seen from Fig. 4 that the specific radioactivity of the calcium of the central compartment M, which is assumed to represent the interstitial fluids, tends asymptotically to the radioactivity of the plasma calcium, so that after about 5 min the difference has become negligible (i.e. the difference is less than the experimental error in measurement). The specific radioactivity of the calcium of the other peripheral compartments increases and even exceeds that of the central compartment before decreasing to the same level as the central compartment (Fig. 5). If our model is sound, in each tissue or organ we should find that the specific radioactivity increases rapidly after injection of tracer to reach maximum in about 2 min (the time required for ^{45}Ca to invade the extracellular media), and then decreases to remain continually somewhere between the specific radioactivity of the extracellular calcium (in practice the plasma

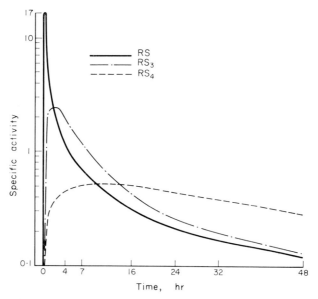

Fig. 5. Calculated curves representing temporal variation of specific radioactivity RS_i (% of injected dose per mg of Ca) as a function of time in the central compartment M (RS) and the peripheral compartments M_3 (RS_3) and M_4 (RS_4) of the model (Fig. 3) for 48 hr after injection of ^{45}Ca Cl$_2$ in the male rat of 200 g.

specific radioactivity) and that of the calcium of the cellular compartments represented in the observed tissues. This was actually found to be the case in all the organs analyzed.

Before proceeding further with an analysis of the results obtained at the tissue level, we will consider the central compartment M, which is assumed to represent the "interstitial" medium. This medium contains all the extracellular fluids of the organ, excluding blood plasma; and its composition is generally considered to be identical to that of a plasma ultrafiltrate (Manery, 1954). We have measured its volume (the dilution volume of ^{82}Br minus the plasma volume), and on average it was found to be 45 ml for rats of 200 g; also, according to our calculations, the calcium content is 2.6 mg. The concentration of calcium in the interstitial medium should thus be about 58 mcg/ml, which is less than the concentration of a plasma ultrafiltrate. In fact the interstitial medium is not homogeneous; it contains not only interstitial fluids but also the fundamental matter of the connective tissue where the calcium concentration is not uniform (Bozler, 1963).

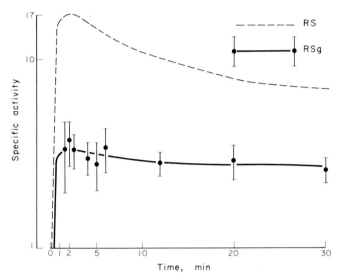

FIG. 6. Temporal variation of specific radioactivity (% of dose injected per mg of Ca) in gastrocnemius muscle (RS_g) and in the extracellular compartment (RS) for 30 min after intravenous injection of ^{45}Ca Cl_2 in the male rat of 200 g. Calculated curves and mean values of experimental determinations with fiducial limit $P = 0.05$.

However, considering experiments that have been performed on actual tissues, it does seem that the specific radioactivity of the whole of the interstitial calcium may well be regarded as homogeneous, and little different from that of blood plasma 2 or 3 min after injection of tracer.

By autoradiographs of ^{45}Ca in frog skeletal muscles, Cosmos and Van Kien (1961) showed that the interstitial calcium is labile and easily eliminated by washing the muscles in a Ringer solution lacking calcium. On the other hand, calcium of muscle fibres remains bound under the same conditions. In Figs. 6 and 7 the variation with time of the specific radioactivity of the calcium of rat gastrocnemius muscle is compared with the variation of the specific radioactivity of the calcium of different compartments. At the start of the experiment there is a sudden large increase of the specific radioactivity of muscle calcium (Fig. 6), representing rapid invasion of the extracellular fluids by the tracer. Thereupon (Fig. 7) the specific radioactivity of the gastrocnemius rejoins that of the plasma in about 2 hr, and

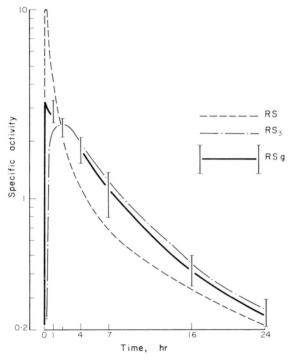

FIG. 7. Temporal variation of specific radioactivity (% of dose injected per mg of Ca) in gastrocnemius muscle (RS_g) and in the extracellular (RS) and "bound" cellular (RS_3) compartments for 24 hr after intravenous injection of $^{45}Ca\ Cl_2$ in the male rat of 200 g. Calculated curves and experimental determinations with fiducial limit $P = 0.05$.

then exceeds it, to remain constant between the specific radioactivity of the extracellular medium and that of compartment M_3, which is intended to represent bound cellular calcium. By using Eqs. (6) and (7), the total calcium (60 mcg/g) of the muscle can be divided between extracellular calcium (11 mcg/g) and bound cellular calcium (49 mcg/g), and the renewal rate of each of these fractions can be measured (ten times greater for extracellular than for bound cellular calcium). Satisfactory agreement is found between these calculations and the experimental results (Figs. 6 and 7).

The extracellular volume of the gastrocnemius (^{82}Br space) has been measured in experiments on rats, and on the average it was evaluated at 126 mcl/g. This volume corresponds to the interstitial space because the rats were bled when sacrificed, and it was verified that the tissue samples contained only negligible quantities of blood (Cohen and Stoclet, 1963). The calcium content of the interstitial spaces of the gastrocnemius should therefore be about 87 mcg/ml. This is distinctly higher than the figure of 58 mcg/ml quoted above for the whole of the interstitial spaces of the organism, but it can be assumed that the extracellular calcium of muscle is to a large extent localized in the connective tissue, the heterogeneity of which as regards calcium content, was mentioned above.

Striated muscle fibers form a sufficiently large proportion of the organism for the renewal of calcium there to be an appreciable factor in the decrease of the specific plasma radioactivity after injection of ^{45}Ca, hence these fibers form the major part of one of the compartments. An approximate calculation shows that the calcium contained in the whole of the striated fibers of a rat of 200 g must be between 3 and 4 mg, while the bound cellular calcium in the female rat of this weight is found to be 5.6 mg. Compartment M_3, which is referred to as "bound cellular calcium" (Fig. 3), contains principally calcium of the striated fibres but it includes also calcium contained in other tissues and organs (e.g. the large intestine where we have found it).

The argument which has just been developed in reference to bound cellular and interstitial calcium has been applied to the other compartments of the model (Fig. 3), using data collected from a large number of organs where we have analyzed the variation of specific radioactivity and measured the extracellular volume. All this research and the work done by other authors on calcium excretion and transport in bone tissue (Aubert and Milhaud, 1960), warrants the physiological interpretation illustrated by Fig. 8.

It should be stressed that this physiological interpretation has only been possible because of the considerable data obtained quite independently of the kinetic study alone of ^{45}Ca in plasma and organs. In itself the kinetic study only enables the observed substance to be apportioned between compartments with very different renewal rates. The example of calcium further illustrates this point. If the foregoing study is carried out with male rats of the same weight (200 g) as the females previously used, it is found that the specific radioactivity decreases much more rapidly after injection of ^{45}Ca into males than into females. The model for the analysis, however, has exactly the same number of compartments, and each male compartment has a rate of renewal similar to that for the corresponding one in the female (Stoclet, 1966a, 1966; Stoclet and Cohen, 1963), but the size of these compartments is considerably larger in the male rat. Under these conditions the mass of calcium contained in the central compartment and in compartments M_2 and M_3 (the interstitial, diffusible cellular and bound cellular calcium respectively) amounts to 23 mg, and it can be no longer localized in the soft tissue, i.e. it corresponds partly to the exchangeable

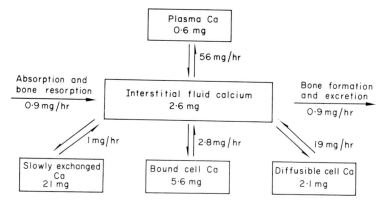

Fig. 8. Calcium distribution and transport in the organism of the female rat of 200 g.

calcium of the skeleton. For one and the same weight, 200 g, male rats are in a period of rapid growth, whereas females at this weight are older and will barely grow any more; bone calcium exchange is much greater in the young rat than in the older animal. In the males, different proportions of exchangeable bone calcium (Bauer *et al.*, 1955a, b) appear to increase the mass of the calcium compartments of the soft tissues, for they are renewed at the same rate. The kinetic study does not enable a distinction to be drawn between phenomena of closely similar degree but of very different nature.

From all these facts it follows that the compartments of a model for kinetic studies on the distribution of tracers in the organism are seldom entirely homogeneous. There are grouped together, in one compartment, parts where the tracer is distributed *approximately* homogeneously, that is to say where the specific radioactivity is roughly uniform. In fact these compartments are "pools", in which the tracer is rapidly distributed compared with the rate at which it leaves the pool.

The error introduced by grouping several compartments in a single pool can become very considerable if the pool is very heterogeneous since the specific radioactivity of the various compartments is then very different whatever the time owing to the absence of real isotopic equilibrium. This is the case, in particular, in a simplified method used by a number of authors to avoid the calculations and hypotheses necessary for compartmental analysis. The method consists in measuring only the last part of the curve for the decrease of specific radioactivity of the plasma or tissue. In this case the relation between specific radioactivity RS and time t is a simple exponential which is represented by a straight line on a semilogarithmic plot. The tracer is assumed to be distributed in a single pool of which the size P and renewal rate V are easily calculated from the relation

$$RS = \frac{R_0}{P} e^{-V/Pt}, \tag{8}$$

where R_0 is the total radioactivity of tracer introduced into the organism at the start of the experiment.

The results obtained by the use of this simplified method are affected by errors which have been evaluated for the case of calcium (Aubert and Milhaud, 1960; Aubert *et al.*, 1958, 1963; Aubert, 1965). Referring solely to the linear part of the curve of decrease of specific plasma radioactivity (semilogarithmic coordinates), one is assuming that the calcium of the organism is contained in a single pool from which it leaves by processes of ossification and excretion. In this case the error in measuring the rate of departure from the pool is relatively less than the error in measuring the mass of the pool. These two errors are greater for a pool of larger mass. So when the pool is very large, as in cases of bone hyperactivity, an error up to 100% can be made in measuring the mass of calcium and up to 40% in measuring the rate.

Likewise, Montanari *et al.* (1963) were able to demonstrate a 50% error in measuring the rate of renewal of tissue nor-adrenaline with labeled nor-adrenaline, when both compartments of tissue nor-adrenaline are combined in a single pool.

Despite the importance of these errors, it does not seem that simplified methods should always be rejected in pharmacology. In effect they permit comparison of the results obtained when a single factor is varied; for example, the presence or absence of a drug. But measurements of renewal rates are only exact in reference to compartments which are homogeneous in content. Since the model is never more than an arbitrary simplification, a systematic error arises which is difficult to assess, and this always adds to the margin of uncertainty due to the approximation of experimental measurements.

From the experimental point of view, there are two techniques for studying the variation of plasma radioactivity with time. Either successive blood samples can be taken, or, alternatively, radioactivity can be measured continuously by an extracorporal circulation tube or tap.

When successive blood samples are taken, one must be sure that the amount of sample is negligible in relation to total blood volume so as not to disturb the physiological state of the animal. Furthermore, since the samples should be taken quite quickly one after the other to enable the curve for the variation of the radioactivity with time to be analyzed, the technique in question is not always applicable to the study of quickly changing phenomena, particularly as the radioactivity should be assumed to be almost constant during the time necessary for the sampling.

However, the use of efficient counting methods (especially by scintillation) and of permanent catheters in most cases enables small quantities to be sampled quite frequently without appreciably altering the steady state.

The other technique of continuously recording the variations of blood radioactivity by an extracorporal circulation avoids the disadvantages inherent in the sampling method, but it runs into other difficulties which limit its use. The animal is anesthetized and the blood which is removed at the cardiac extremity of a severed artery (e.g. the carotid), runs through a circuit with a counting facility before being reintroduced into the peripheral end of the artery or into a vein. The experimental details are described by several authors (Morel, 1950; Kimbel, 1965; Chivot, 1966). It is only pointed out here that the apparatus should include an integrator, analog, or preferably digital, the time constant of which should be adjusted to the kinetics of the phenomenon being studied. Furthermore, precautions must be taken to avoid excessive cardiac fatigue due to the diversion. This method is particularly suited to the study of quickly changing phenomena because the experiment is limited to a few hours anyway in view of the operating conditions. It offers the great advantage of avoiding extrapolation from point to point since the radioactivity is known at each instant; but it has the disadvantage of only being applicable for short periods to gamma-ray emitters (at least with apparatus currently available), and of only measuring radioactivity, not specific radioactivity. All the same, this latter drawback can to some extent be reduced by measuring the concentration of tracer at the start of the experiment and at the end. A modification of this technique has been proposed for a beta-emitter, ^{14}C, by Bonet-Maury *et al.* (1954), who collimated a counter under a mouse ear. This avoids the disadvantages of extracorporal circulation, but the method is less accurate and measurements are confined to a less general range.

Whenever specific radioactivity is measured in other tissues and organs at the same time as in the plasma, one very often has to sacrifice animals by groups at varying times after injection of the tracer. In this case the body compartments are measured much less precisely than in the methods outlined above, and the statistical study of the results becomes very difficult. The calculations are made upon average values which have a margin of uncertainty owing to individual variation. On the other hand, in the kinetic study on the plasma of each animal, the mass and the renewal rate of each compartment are calculated before proceeding to statistical calculations (variance, etc.) to compare the results obtained on different batches of animals (e.g. either treated with a drug or not treated).

Some authors adopt a different procedure based on the identity of the specific radioactivity in the plasma and urine at the instant it is voided. Except for very prolonged studies where the specific radioactivity varies only slowly, catheters appear to be required to avoid the dead space represented by the urine paths and especially the problems of stagnation and mixing in the bladder.

With natural molecules of endogenous origin, e.g. steroid hormones, the rate of production in the organism can be calculated by analyzing the development of the specific radioactivity of a urine metabolite after injection of labeled hormone (Pearlman, 1957; Petersen, 1965).

Total body radioactivity can also be measured instantaneously by finding the difference between the quantity of tracer injected and the quantity of tracer or its metabolites excreted.

In conclusion, kinetic studies in the transition to isotopic equilibrium are relatively simple to perform, but interpretation of the results is complicated. The latter involves calculations which often necessitate the use of an analog or digital computer and often requires supplementary data, especially measurement of the various fluid volumes in the organism.

(c) *Isotopic equilibrium*

Isotopic equilibrium is achieved when the specific radioactivity of the tracer has become constant in the organism. This method permits a simple interpretation of the rate at which the tracer, or a metabolite, appears in a compartment (Zilversmit *et al.*, 1943; Buchanan, 1961).

Whenever the labeled molecule is a substance foreign to the organism, the isotopic equilibrium is achieved automatically. This is the case for a large number of drugs.

If the drug is not metabolized, the variation of plasma or tissue radioactivity after administering a single dose of tracer can be studied to analyze the distribution and excretion of the drug by a procedure analogous to that proposed above for the kinetics of the transition to equilibrium: it is no longer specific radioactivity which varies, but the concentration of the drug. The only real point in labeling the drug is to create analytical techniques which generally are much more sensitive and much simpler than administering a dose of the drug itself. Very small doses can be given in this way which will possibly have no significant pharmacological action; one could not in this case speak of a steady state as far as the concentration of the observed substance in the tissues and fluids is concerned, but it is necessary to have regard as much as possible to the steady state of other constituents of the organism.

However, if the drug is metabolized in the organism, even though it may form no part of the normal constituents of the organism, the measurement of total radioactivity no longer has any significance; the drug and its various metabolites need to be separated beforehand. The results in respect of blood plasma are then interpreted by means of a model and the calculations described above. The kinetic study of the specific radioactivity of the various metabolites, each of which can be regarded as one compartment, will then enable the rate of every catabolic reaction to be measured. In this way the various modes of breakdown and excretion of the drug can be quantitatively determined by analysis of the excreta.

In the case where the substance being studied is a molecule which is naturally present in the organism, either of endogenous (metabolism) or exogenous (absorption) origin, isotopic equilibrium is never achieved after a single dose of tracer for the reasons explained above. However, the specific radioactivity of the observed substance can be kept constant by continual administration of tracer. The results obtained by this method can be interpreted without complicated calculations, but the experiment is very difficult to perform. The problems arising here have been discussed by Chevallier (1963). If the renewal time of the observed substance is short, the tracer is administered by perfusion. Conversely, if the renewal time is long, the tracer is ingested for several weeks by a constant regime.

For substances that are exclusively exogenous in origin, the specific radioactivity, after sufficient time has elapsed for adaptation, remains unchanged even if variations of concentration occur in the plasma or in an organ. With substances of endogenous or hybrid origin, however, it may be a different situation if the rate of synthesis of the substance by the organism varies during the experiment. It is therefore essential to determine the precise amplitude of the variations of specific radioactivity throughout one "circadian cycle". Generally speaking, equilibrium cannot be achieved unless the interval of time between two consecutive administrations of labeled compound is less than the average renewal time. It is therefore worthwhile splitting the dose and arranging a continuous recording of the specific radioactivity.

One elegant method consists in the continuous measurement of the specific radioactivity of exhaled $^{14}CO_2$ after administration of a tracer labeled with ^{14}C. Since very many drugs and constituents of the organism contain carbon and are degraded by respiratory oxidation to CO_2, this particular method has an immense field of application. Le Roy *et al.* (1960) have described a device for continuous recording of expiratory $^{14}CO_2$ in man. For laboratory animals, Chevallier *et al.* (1962) have described a closely similar method for studying isotopic equilibrium after administration of cholesterol labeled with ^{14}C; Okita (1965) used an analogous apparatus to study respiratory oxidation of glucose under the influence of different drugs. A current of air circulates through an air-tight circuit which includes the cage in which the animal breathes. The exhaled $^{14}CO_2$ is led into a system containing an apparatus for measuring radioactivity (flow counter or ionization chamber) and one for measuring total CO_2.

The constituents of exclusively endogenous origin are derivatives of their precursors. An isotopic equilibrium can be achieved in this case by administering a precursor, the radioactivity of which is maintained constant. With compounds of hybrid origin (endogenous and exogenous), isotopic equilibrium can be achieved in the organism by introducing the labeled compound or a precursor itself into the food.

Once isotopic equilibrium has been achieved and verified, there is no difficulty in determining the size and distribution of transfer spaces, these here being defined in terms of the collection of molecules susceptible to transfer from the organs into the plasma and vice versa. If the specific radioactivity in an organ is equal to that found in the plasma, this implies that all the substance contained in the organ is entirely renewed. If, however, the specific radioactivity is less than that in the plasma, only some of the molecules are renewed; the renewal is in proportion to the ratio of the specific radioactivities in the organ and plasma. Knowing the specific radioactivity of the substance in each organ and the quantities of substance present there, the mass renewed in each organ is calculated. On the other hand, rates of transfer can only be determined by a kinetic study of the renewal process during the period of time preceding equilibrium (lag period), or during the period which succeeds it (after stopping the administration of the tracer).

For a compound of hybrid origin (endogenous and exogenous), the method of isotopic equilibrium further enables the rate of endogenous formation to be measured, and excretion to be distinguished from secretion, as shown by Chevallier (1963) with cholesterol.

If the specific radioactivity in the plasma is less than that of the administered compound, it is implied that, independently of the quantity of labeled compound appearing each day in the plasma, a further quantity of the same compound (synthesized or absorbed as the case may be) is being discharged which dilutes the specific radioactivity. Thus the correlation between absorption and synthesis can be studied by varying the concentration of the observed substance under the same conditions.

In other respects it is generally known that the specific radioactivity of excreted molecules is equal to that of plasma molecules since, by definition, excretion is the transfer of plasma molecules into the external medium. If a specific radioactivity less than that of the plasma molecules is found in the excreta (at isotopic equilibrium), it is implied that a secretion of unlabeled substance (synthesized by the cells of the intestinal wall, for example) has been added to the excretion (provided, of course, that the tracer is administered parenterally, and that the observed substance of alimentary origin and nonabsorbed is negligible in the fecal matter).

1.2. PRESENTATION OF RESULTS

The majority of authors refer the results obtained by compartmental analysis to the body weight. Although this method of reference may be sufficient for the pharmacologist, it should be pointed out that other methods of reference can be adopted, especially the "lean body" and the "body cellular" mass.

It has been argued by Ljungren et al. (1957), Moore et al. (1963), and Miller and Weil (1963), that the form of presentation in which results are *referred* to body weight is a very imperfect method, which ought rigorously to be replaced by analysis *as a function* of the body weight. Since there is not always a linear relationship between the body constituents and the body weight, in most cases an expression of the type $y = ax + b$ (where y

is the observed constituent, x is the weight, and a and b are constants) can be regarded as a good approximation for analyzing a limited group of values. When the results are simply referred to the body weight (the ratio y/x), the constant b is neglected, i.e. the ratio y/x can differ significantly between two groups where x is different, even if the relation between y and x can be expressed in terms of the same regression equation. In practice, significant differences between ratios of one bodily constituent to the weight of groups of different weight can become insignificant if they are expressed in a more physiological way as a function of the weight, and vice versa.

An example is given by Haxhe (1964). The comparison of many results in respect of men and women shows that total water and some cellular components (red cell volume and intracellular fluid) are significantly higher in men when referred to body weight, whereas the extracellular constituents show no significant difference at all in this system of reference. On the other hand, as a function of the weight, all the constituents, including those of the extracellular sphere (except plasma space), are higher in men than in women.

The phrase "as a function of body weight" can itself be somewhat misleading in certain cases. For instance, in the same example reported by Haxhe (1964), the presence of a different quantity of fat in the two sexes calls for a form of presentation which would exclude the variable introduced by the fatty surface area. Hence Haxhe was obliged to express his results as a function of the "lean body" mass and the "body cellular" mass.

The concept of lean-body mass becomes indispensable in cases where a comparison is made between groups of individuals or animals whose nutritional state may be very different. It is generally known that adipose tissue consumes very little oxygen, whereas lean tissue, which includes the active cellular mass, is the principal consumer of oxygen and contains almost all the elements of the hydroelectrolyte structure. In expressing the results per unit weight of lean-body mass, Haxhe (1964) no longer found any difference between the body composition of men and women, even though the same experimental results were significantly different in reference to body weight or as a function of this weight.

The lean-body mass, used as a system of reference, enables different groups to be compared, while excluding fat as an individual variable. But the relative proportion of cellular and extracellular constituents in the lean-body mass can vary. Hence Moore *et al.* (1963), and Moore and Boyden (1963), suggested that results in respect of cellular functions or constituents should be referred to the *body cellular mass*.

In the following section it will be seen that isotopic methods enable the lean-body mass and the body cellular mass to be determined.

2. PRINCIPAL BODY COMPARTMENTS

At the present time a number of body compartments are measured by pharmacologists in order to study drug distribution within organisms, or to analyze the modes of action of drugs. The majority of kinetic studies of the distribution of tracers in organisms can be interpreted only if the principal extracellular and cellular fluid volumes are known. Their measurement entails determining the dilution space of appropriate tracers, the choice of tracers here depending on the functional characteristics of the sectors of the organism being studied, and also on the need to measure several compartments *simultaneously*, a situation in which pharmacologists often find themselves. This calls for a veritable isotopic dissection of the organism, which will be considered after studying the measurement of compartments individually.

The various tracer-dilution methods for the determination of body compartments in organisms are equally applicable to the measurement of compartments in organs or tissues. It is sufficient to relate the concentration of tracer in the organ to its concentration in the plasma to obtain the space occupied by the tracer in the organ. Within a tissue the mass of substance exchanged since the start of the experiment is equal to the ratio of the concentration of tracer in the tissue to the specific radioactivity in the plasma. Any exchangeable mass or diffusion space in an organ or tissue must be measured at equilibrium (or at least at apparent equilibrium), as in the case of the organism as a whole.

The plasma volume and interstitial volume of an organ are frequently measured in order to analyze the distribution of a substance (by difference) between the extracellular and cellular media.

2.1. PLASMA VOLUME

In order to measure plasma volume, tracers should be stopped by the capillary barrier, should not appreciably penetrate into red cells, should quickly and uniformly mix with the blood plasma, and should be eliminated (by excretion or metabolism) only slowly so that the plasma concentration is stable for a sufficiently long time.

No tracer perfectly satisfies all these requirements, but several produce satisfactory results. Very often proteins are used, labeled *in vivo* or *in vitro*.

For labeling *in vivo*, use is made of a dye (e.g. Evans blue) that attaches itself to the albumin molecule (Rawson *et al.*, 1959). *In vitro*, some plasma proteins are labeled with radioiodine, viz. human serum albumin (Fine and Seligman, 1944; Crispell *et al.*, 1950; McFarlane, 1958), and gamma-globulins or fibrinogen (Baker, 1963a, b). At present three isotopes of iodine with different half-lives (iodine-125, iodine-131, and iodine-132) are available, permitting a judicious choice to be made in experiments with multiple tracers (see Chapter 5).

These various tracers spread uniformly throughout the plasma volume in the course of a few minutes in man and still more quickly in laboratory animals. The stability of labeled molecules is good, and they leave the vascular network slowly. All the same, for precise measurements it is prudent to take several blood samples and to apply extrapolation (Noble and Gregersen, 1946; Pritchard *et al.*, 1955). Furthermore, results obtained with the various proteins labeled with iodine tend to differ slightly from one another. Thus fibrinogen does not mix with the whole of the plasma (Polosa and Hamilton, 1963), whilst serum albumin and dyes produce slightly too high values owing to the diffusion of these substances into the extravascular spaces (Baker, 1963a, b).

The values obtained by the tracers mentioned above are generally closely similar to one another when employed in the usual way. Other methods are not unanimously accepted. In particular, plasma volume would seem to be overestimated when ^{51}Cr chromium chloride is used as the tracer.

2.2. RED CELL VOLUME

Red cells labeled with radioisotopes enable the red cell volume to be measured simply and accurately. The labeled cells are distributed within minutes throughout the total volume, and loss during the mixing period is small.

In vivo red cells can be labeled with radioactive iron-55 or iron-59 (Hahn *et al.*, 1941; Bonfils *et al.*, 1963), and *in vitro* with potassium-42 (Yalow and Berson, 1951), phosphorus-32 (Reeve and Veall, 1949), or preferably with chromium-51, which leaves the cells less quickly (Mollisson and Veall, 1955) and simplifies the labeling (Sterling and Gray, 1950).

The experimental details in the measurement of red cell volume in man and animals are very similar (Cohen and Ingrand, 1960; Cohen and Stoclet, 1960). In this respect the subject's own red cells are labeled by contact with a solution of $Na_2{}^{51}CrO_4$ and then injected.

2.3. BLOOD VOLUME AND HEMATOCRIT

Blood volume may be evaluated by adding the simultaneously measured red cell and plasma volumes or from consideration of either of these volumes and the hematocrit.

The red cell and plasma volumes have been measured simultaneously in the animal (Everett *et al.*, 1956; Tala *et al.*, 1956; Bonfils *et al.*, 1963), using red cells labeled with iron-59 and human serum albumin labeled with iodine-131. All these authors found hematocrit differences according to the vascular area being considered, as would have been foreseen by microscopical examination of the vessels (Chaplin and Mollison, 1953). For instance, in the rat the hematocrit, which is 36% in blood from the heart cavity, or from the vena cava, is only 32% in the vessels of the striated muscles.

Generally speaking, the hematocrit measured on a sample of venous blood is greater than the hematocrit of whole blood. Therefore blood volume as calculated from measurements of red cell volume and the venous hematocrit (the only one accessible for direct measurement) (see Cohen and Stoclet, 1960), will have a systematic error. All the same, the error should only be about 3% for the total blood volume (Baker, 1963a). But in order to evaluate the volume of blood contained in an organ correctly, it is necessary to measure red cell volume and plasma volume at the same time.

2.4. EXTRACELLULAR AND INTERSTITIAL WATER

The ambiguity of the term "extracellular fluid" shows the difficulty that very often arises in identifying a body compartment with any anatomical section of the organism. The term "extracellular fluid" has been given as many meanings as there have been indicators proposed for measuring it.

It is now generally agreed that the extracellular fluid should be defined physiologically to include that part of the total water and of the dissolved substances which is not contained in the cell. The extracellular water includes plasma water, interstitial water, water of the connective tissue, water contained in the bones and cartilages, and "transcellular" water—a term applied by Edelman *et al.* (1952) to fluids which have traversed the cells or have been produced by them (cerebrospinal fluid, water of the digestive tract, bile, serous fluids, and so on).

The term "interstitial fluid" is also given several different meanings. From a structural point of view it is defined as the liquid filling the lacunar spaces between the cells. No indicator can measure the volume of this liquid exclusively. On the other hand, it is possible to measure the extracellular fluid that is not contained in the vascular layer. This fraction is sometimes referred to as the interstitial fluid. It is equal to the difference between the extracellular and plasma volumes; it thus includes the water and dissolved materials of the fundamental substance of the connective, bony and cartilaginous tissues, and of the transcellular fluids as well as the properly so-called interstitial fluid.

Extracellular water cannot be measured directly (no more than plasma water), since labeled water becomes diffused in the total water of the organism. An indicator is therefore required which will quickly diffuse throughout the extracellular fluids, without appreciable loss during diffusion, and without penetrating into the cells or becoming attached to their membrane.

Numerous substances have been proposed as indicators for measuring extracellular volume. None corresponds perfectly to the requirements that have just been stated.

Large molecules, like inulin and saccharose, easily cross the capillary barrier and are stopped completely by cell membranes. No difficulty arises in measuring their concentration in the fluids of the organism because they can be labeled with carbon-14 or even with radioiodine (Brooks *et al.*, 1960). Unfortunately, however, they diffuse only slowly and partially into the connective tissue of muscles and tendons, and this represents a large part of the extracellular fluid (Cotlove, 1954; Elkington and Danowski, 1955). The slowness of diffusion can be a very serious inconvenience for pharmacologists wishing to analyze the action of drugs on body or tissue compartments: a technique of constant-flow perfusion is then necessary (Schwartz *et al.*, 1949).

Mannitol, thiocyanate, and thiosulphate ions have also been proposed, but must apparently be rejected, perhaps because of excessive or irregular renal or extrarenal clearance (Swan *et al.*, 1954); or, in the case of thiocyanate, because of penetration into the intracellular sector. The same applies to ^{24}Na which is, in addition, concentrated in the bone (Edelman *et al.*, 1954a, b).

Two indicators seem to be left, namely a beta emitter radio-sulphate ^{35}S and a gamma emitter $^{82}Br^-$. Both of these indicators are rapidly diffusing ions, which are particularly suited to pharmacological studies.

The cellular penetration of $^{35}SO_4$ can be regarded as negligible during the time of experimentation; it is not converted into organic sulfate and it diffuses into the major part of the extracellular fluids (Walser *et al.*, 1953). Nevertheless, an elective fixation to cartilaginous tissue can be pointed out

(Cohen and Delassue, 1959). This indicator can now be employed without great difficulty by the use of resin chromatography and liquid scintillation measuring techniques (Savoie and Jungers, 1965).

However, the indicator most used for the sake of convenience is still ^{82}Br, which is diluted in a space identical to that of chlorine (Brodie *et al.*, 1939), and is easier to handle than the chlorine isotopes. Many papers have shown that chlorine is almost entirely found outside cells (Manery, 1954, 1961; Cotlove and Hoghen, 1962), except red cells, where the chlorine content is not negligible, although a correction can be made for this. But the dilution space of ^{82}Br, even corrected for its content in red cells, slightly overestimates the extracellular fluid space (by about 8% according to Cheek, 1961) owing to the very low quantity of chlorine present in the cells and its greater concentration in the connective tissue (Mannery and Hastings, 1939). As we have seen already (Fig. 1), a uniform distribution of ^{82}Br is achieved very rapidly, and numerous authors have described the details of its employment (Haxhe, 1964). It should be noted, however, that in certain cases chlorine, and hence bromine too, may be able to penetrate cells, and so lead to an overestimation of the extracellular fluid, e.g. in suprarenalectomized animals or in animals undergoing a form of treatment which leads to a suprarenal deficiency (Nicholson and Zilva, 1960).

Study of the renewal of dissolved substances entering into the composition of the extracellular fluid becomes a special case for each substance. In every case, however, the speed of "capillary transfer" is such that continuous recording of radioactivity is necessary. This topic is discussed in the paper of Morel (1950) on ^{24}Na.

2.5. TOTAL BODY WATER

The total quantity of water may be measured by means of water labeled with one of the isotopes of hydrogen, deuterium, or tritium. After the first experiments of Hevesy and Hofer (1934), measurement of total water by deuterium oxide remained out of favor owing to difficulties of measurement until methods were developed for determining heavy water in biological fluids by densitometry (Schloerb *et al.*, 1950) and mass spectrometry (Solomon *et al.*, 1950). Water labeled with tritium (tritiated water) was proposed by Pace *et al.* (1947), but this came into common use only after the work of Prentice *et al.* (1952) and the development of liquid scintillation counting (Langham *et al.*, 1956). The dilution space of deuterium oxide is almost identical to that of tritiated water (Anbar and Lewitus, 1958; Gaebler and Choitz, 1964).

Other tracers have been proposed, but all produce less precise results than the foregoing. This applies in particular to urea (Dalton, 1964), or to antipyrine or its derivatives, *N*-acetyl-4-amino-antipyrine, and 4-iodo-antipyrine labeled with iodine-131 (Talso *et al.*, 1955). It seems that iodo-antipyrine should be discarded because a part of the iodine is lost by the molecule and excreted (Flora *et al.*, 1962). Also, antipyrine itself is rapidly excreted, which calls for several blood samples (extrapolation) or measurement of the excreted fraction. Finally, antipyrine does not always reach a uniform concentration in the organism in cases of oedema (Faller *et al.*, 1955).

Water labeled with an isotope of hydrogen therefore seems to be the indicator to be preferred for measuring total body water. Hansard (1964) stressed that tritiated water is particularly convenient and advantageous in that it quickly reaches equilibrium with the body water, it binds very little to proteins, and it is not metabolized. Seitchik *et al.* (1963) have reported that with D_2O equilibrium is reached much more slowly during the period of gestation than outside this period.

2.6. LEAN-BODY MASS AND MASS OF FAT

Measuring the *mass of fat* is an important consideration in studying the composition of the body. On the other hand, *lean-body mass* is an interesting index to which the measurements of particular body compartments can be referred. Both may be measured directly or indirectly, and for either the method of tracer dilution offers interesting possibilities.

Until the dilution method was used, the mass of fat had to be measured by methods which were either inaccurate or else were restricted to specialized laboratories. These procedures, very often based on measuring body density, have been reviewed by Lim (1963). It used to be the practice, with variable results, to measure the fatty mass by dilution of very fat-soluble gases such as cyclopropane (Lesser *et al.*, 1952 and 1960), radiokrypton (Davidson *et al.*, 1956), or both gases at the same time in order to improve accuracy (Lesser and Zak, 1963). But by 1945 Pace and Rathbun had shown that the mass of fat can be measured indirectly as the difference between total weight and lean weight, the lean weight itself being an estimate obtained from the total body water which forms a constant fraction. Since then it has been proposed to estimate lean-body mass by measuring total potassium (Forbes and Hursh, 1961). Such measurements are based on the assumption that the lean mass, as evaluated from one of its constituents, remains constant. According to Kyle *et al.* (1963), changes of weight of body fat can reasonably be calculated by subtracting from the changes of body weight the sum total of the changes of body water and of body proteins.

2.7. CELLULAR MASS OF THE BODY

The cellular mass of the body can be estimated by measuring cellular potassium or cellular water. But since cellular water can be estimated only in terms of the difference between total body water and extracellular water, it is a less precise index of cellular mass than is potassium (owing to the uncertainties associated with the estimation of the extracellular fluid).

The exchangeable potassium was proposed as a criterion of the body composition by Talso *et al.* (1960), for all cells contain potassium at a concentration of approximately 150 mEq/l, while the quantity of extra-cellular and bone potassium is low. It is sufficient to multiply the exchange-able potassium (as measured by dilution of ^{42}K) by a constant coefficient in order to calculate the cellular mass (Moore and Boyden, 1963; Moore *et al.*, 1963), provided that a check is made to verify that no deficiency of cellular potassium has arisen due to the particular substances being studied. Also a correction can be introduced for the active cellular mass by measuring the urinary excretion of creatinine (which provided an estimate of the mass of muscle).

2.8. SIMULTANEOUS MEASUREMENTS

Simultaneous measurements of several bodily compartments are particu-larly interesting to the pharmacologist who is analyzing the distribution of a labeled drug in the organism, or the effect of a drug on several different compartments. In either case it is generally necessary to measure plasma volume and the volumes of the cellular and extracellular water. In this latter respect the composition of the cellular and extracellular parts should also be analyzed.

Simultaneity of the measurements is particularly important whenever the organism is not in its steady state under the influence of the drug; but this poses the practical problem of measuring the concentration of several tracers in the same sample. This calls for a judicious choice of tracers.

As already seen, the simultaneous measurement of plasma and red cell volumes involves using red cells labeled with ^{59}Fe rather than with ^{51}Cr so as to allow counting in the presence of ^{131}I. The problems of counting obviously become increasingly complicated for a larger number of tracers.

The first truly isotopic dissection of the organism was proposed by Moore (1946), who measured simultaneously blood plasma volume, extracellular fluid volume, total body water, and the exchangeable masses of sodium and potassium. Other techniques have since been proposed, the results of which are reported in monographs published by Moore *et al.* (1963) and by Haxhe (1964). Special reference may be made, for example, to the solutions proposed by Belcher *et al.* (1960), Haxhe (1963) and Fernandez *et al.* (1966).

These multiple-tracer methods not only permit simultaneous measurement of the volume or mass of several body compartments, but also enable the distribution of water and the concentration of substances dissolved in the cellular, extracellular, and plasma media to be deduced by appropriate subtractions. By repeating the measurements on the same animal, the physiological variations of the body composition can be evaluated (Haxhe, 1963) and then, possibly their modifications under the influence of drugs.

3. EFFECT OF DRUGS ON THE SIZE AND RENEWAL OF COMPARTMENTS

The study of how body compartments are influenced by drugs is obviously one way of analyzing the mode of action of these drugs. But such studies are also of interest in research into new drugs by providing relatively simple and specific tests in certain cases.

Before illustrating these various possibilities, it must be stressed that the introduction of a drug into the organism is always liable to induce changes of composition and thus disrupt the steady state of the body. So one must always be sure that a new steady state has been reached under the influence of the drug, or bear in mind the transient conditions in the interpretation of the results. In either case, the methods that allow the test animal to be used as its own control are particularly advantageous. Very often it is possible to find experimental conditions in which variations of size or renewal rate of the body compartments under the influence of the drug are slight for the duration of the experiments.

Thus Garrett *et al.* (1962, 1963) performed an analog computer study of a steroid hormone, 6-α-methylprednisolone and its effect on the kinetics of ^{47}Ca in the dog. They studied the kinetics of ^{47}Ca in the blood and the excreta for four or five consecutive test periods—prior to treatment, twice during treatment by daily oral administration of steroid, and once or twice after cessation of treatment. They were thus able to show that modifications of calcium transport in the organism occur not only under the influence of the treatment, but also when the treatment is stopped (compensation effect).

The open mamillary model with four compartments, considered above, enables excellent agreement to be obtained between the calculations and test results, as far as excretion is concerned. Unfortunately, the most interesting point suggested by the results, i.e. modification of the fixation of calcium on to bone and of its resorption under the influence of 6-α-methylprednisolone, could not be verified by the method employed. The authors tried performing bone biopsies during each kinetic study of ^{47}Ca so as to measure the specific radioactivity of the bone, but the results were too variable to be capable of interpretation, probably owing to the heterogeneity of the skeleton. In order to confirm the hypothesis permitted by the analog computation, they would have had to analyze the skeleton as a whole, as was done by Aubert and Milhaud (1960), although, obviously, this would have entailed sacrificing the animal and thus losing the benefit of repeated experiments on the same animal.

In other similar cases, it could be of interest to verify that the selected model truly corresponds to physiological reality before the analog computer is used to analyze the results of numerous kinetic studies which have been repeated on the same animal under different conditions. Very often such verification requires experiments to be performed specially for the purpose as suggested above in regard to the kinetics of equilibration.

The action of a drug may have an effect on the size or the renewal rate of the various body compartments or it may influence the absorption or excretion rates of some substance, or even affect all these phenomena together. The results are then interpreted using the same model for the treated as for the control animal; only the parameters of the model are altered. But in other cases the model itself may be modified by adding or removing a compartment or a metabolic pathway for instance. Thus, as we have seen above, transfers of bone calcium are added to the calcium renewal of the soft tissues in animals which grow rapidly.

On the other hand, in the case of body compartments of some organic substance, compartmental analysis in the presence of a drug assumes significance only in the light of supplementary metabolic studies. Thus, for instance, the tissue reserves of nor-adrenaline are depleted by reserpine or amphetamine, but for each case the metabolic pathway is different (see the review by Costa *et al.*, 1966).

To close this section we illustrate by examples the possibilities open to the pharmacologist of studying the effect of drugs on body compartments.

Many papers are concerned with the action of drugs on the transport of water and electrolytes. In the first instance the action of hormones (and their derivatives) which are responsible for homeostatic regulation of the composition and volume of the fluids of the organism has been reviewed by Gomirato-Sandrucci *et al.* (1962a, b, c), De Graeff and Leijnse (1964), Houlihan and Eversole (1964), and Moses (1965).

It should be pointed out that the most diverse substances will modify the aqueous and electrolyte compartments. One can cite nicotine (Aizawa *et al.* 1960) and the adreno- and cholinolytics (Yusunov and Makhumudov, 1964). Thus atropine increases the volumes of total and extracellular water, and reduces the ion content of the blood and urine.

An important practical application of the measurement of ionic and fluid compartments arises in the study of radioprotectors. These substances can to some extent prevent the hydroelectrolyte disorders which accompany the gastrointestinal troubles of the irradiation syndrome, and which can cause death (Zsebok and Petranyi, 1964).

The study of calcium transport has made it possible to analyze the action of various substances on the mechanisms of muscular contraction and bone calcium renewal.

In the muscular field we shall leave aside the question of cardiotonic substances since their mode of action has been studied at the cellular level by Lamb in the present work. With reference to the effects of "tetracemate" (EDTA) on the heart (Valette *et al.*, 1964), where the pharmacological effect of a perfusion of disodium tetracemate has been related to a modification of the calcium content of the extracellular fluid, it has been found that since the cellular calcium concentration is not altered, chemical estimates of total calcium in the heart are not significantly altered by the treatment either; but the kinetic study of ^{45}Ca discloses an appreciable decrease of extracellular calcium in the organism. The rapidity of exchange of calcium in the myocardium explains the particular sensitivity of this tissue to the chelation of calcium (Stoclet, 1958).

In the same field we have proposed a simplified method for studying the effect of drugs on the movements of calcium in striated muscle at rest and during contraction (Stoclet, 1964b, 1966). The complete kinetic study, presented above, of the distribution of ^{45}Ca in the rat organism has shown that the calcium content of striated muscle can be divided into two fractions. The first fraction, which is very rapidly renewed, is probably confined to the extracellular medium in the muscle at rest, but increases relatively more than the extracellular volume when the muscle engages in activity. The other fraction, which is renewed much more slowly, undoubtedly corresponds to the cellular calcium. The exchanges of calcium in this case are not accelerated during contraction. The renewal of these two fractions takes place at rates so different that 5 min after injection of the tracers (^{45}Ca and ^{82}Br) the specific radioactivity of extracellular calcium can be considered to be identical to that of plasma calcium, and the specific radioactivity of cellular calcium can be considered to be zero. Under these conditions the ratio of the radioactivity per gram of muscle to the specific plasma radioactivity is, after 5 min, a measure of the so-called "rapidly exchangeable" calcium that is localized in the extracellular medium of the muscle at rest and which mediates the contraction. The simplified method consists in simultaneously measuring the "rapidly exchangeable" calcium and the extracellular volume in the two gastro-cnemius muscles of the rat (Cohen and Stoclet, 1967): one is at rest and serves as control, the other is stimulated in a suitable rhythm via the sciatic nerve. In these conditions it was found that the potentiation of the contractions by veratrine is accompanied by a marked increase of the mass of rapidly exchangeable calcium of the muscle in activity, whereas the same substance has no effect at all on the muscle at rest. This method is of interest in allowing experiments on living animals, the muscles of which show physiological hyperemia in functioning.

With reference to bone calcium, compartmental analysis is prospectively of interest to the pharmacologist not only in studying the action of factors which normally influence osteogenesis and osteolysis such as the thyroid or parathyroid hormones (Aubert *et al.*, 1964; Aubert, 1965), or vitamine D (Milhaud *et al.*, 1960a), but also in studying the pharmacological effect of cortisone (Milhaud *et al.*, 1960b) and of its derivatives (Garrett *et al.*, 1962, 1963). It is known that the administration of these hormones in therapeutic doses leads to a syndrome reminiscent of osteoporosis. In particular, there is a distinct increase of calcium excretion accompanied by reduced osteogenesis and increased osteolysis. Conversely, the administration of an anabolic androgen (nor-testosterone) increases retention of ^{45}Ca by the organism without at the same time abolishing the effect of cortisone (Bohr and Dawids, 1964). This research shows that among the synthetic steroids the pharmacologist now has a means of selecting the substances which have the least side-effects on the skeleton, or, alternatively, those having an anabolic effect there. The use of a radioisotope of calcium in conjunction with an analog or digital computer enables investigations of this kind to be carried out on a large scale.

The study of the effect of drugs on body compartments is not restricted to the hydro-mineral compartments. In this respect no great difficulty arises unless metabolism of organic matter complicates the study. In certain cases compartmental analysis is simple and provides irreplaceable data. Sufficient proof of this is forthcoming from the interest aroused by the action of anti-uricemic or "uricosuric" substances on the kinetics of uric acid labeled with ^{14}C. After intravenous injection of a single dose of tracer, the exchangeable pool and the renewal rate are determined from the decrease of specific plasma radioactivity over a period of 4 days, the decrease here being represented by a straight line on semi-logarithmic coordinates (except during the first hours). In this way Sörensen (1960) showed that the urinary elimination of uric acid cannot be taken as an index of urate production because some of the uric acid is not excreted in the urine. The simultaneous study of urinary excretion and of the kinetics of uric acid ^{14}C in the blood only enables the action of a drug on the production and elimination of uric acid in man to be known.

It seems possible to conclude that the field of application for measurements of the size and renewal rate of body compartments under the influence of drugs is immense, but only partially exploited up to the present time. As a result, in order to use the method, the pharmacologist has to draw upon relevant physiological data which have often only recently been obtained. There is no doubt that this method is full of promise in pharmacology.

4. COMPARTMENTAL ANALYSIS OF DRUG DISTRIBUTION

The use of labeled drugs has made possible great advances in the general problem of the fate of drugs in the organism. In the present volumes this problem has been approached at the cellular level by Lamb in Chapter 13, and from the metabolic point of view by Glasson in Chapter 17 (see also Glasson, 1965). We will confine ourselves to some particular kinetic aspects of the problem.

A theoretical study of the circumstances of the distribution of therapeutic substances was made by Teorell (1937), but his equations for the concentration of these substances as a function of time in various parts of the body and in relation to extra- or intra-vascular modes of administration, were formulated before the labeled molecules necessary for the experiments were available.

In connection with compartmental analysis of the distribution of drugs in the organism, the reader's attention is drawn to some recent reviews: Segre (1965), Wang and Willis (1965), and Rescigno and Segre (1966). We shall restrict ourselves to mentioning some special features of the methods which can be used.

The labeled medicament may be a molecule occurring naturally in the organism, or it may be a foreign molecule.

With natural molecules, the use of the tracer is the same in pharmacology as in physiology; the applicable methods have already been considered above. The principal studies of this kind have been concerned with hormones and biogenic amines. As we have seen already, a kinetic study of transition to isotopic equilibrium can be made in respect of aldosterone (Peterson, 1965), or a study at equilibrium by perfusion of L-nor-adrenaline-^{14}C at a constant rate for several hours (Kopin and Gordon, 1963).

The study of biogenic amines raises special problems, which have been examined by Kopin (1965) and Beaven (1965). As regards the catecholamines, use has mostly been made of racemic tracers, whilst the natural forms belong to the L-series. The L and D isomers penetrate the tissues in different circumstances (Iversen, 1963) and they are not metabolized at the same rate; after some hours, however, only the L-isomer still remains in the tissues and it can be assumed that, once there, it follows the same fate as the endogenous catecholamine. But labeled histamine, which enters mast cells anything but slowly, can for this reason be used to study nonmastocyte histamine.

Tracers foreign to the organism are more specifically a pharmacological question. The theoretical aspects have been treated by Robertson in Chapter 10. It has already been seen that certain foreign substances are used as indicators to measure particular fluid spaces (antipyrine for instance). Labeled drugs are studied in the same way.

In cases of apparent equilibrium after injection of a single dose of indicator, a dilution space can be determined and compared with the volume of an aqueous portion of the organism which has been determined simultaneously. Thus Watkins *et al.* (1964) studied simultaneously the tissue distribution of alloxan-^{14}C and D-mannitol-^{3}H in conditions where the alloxan was only slowly destroyed. The results support a hypothesis according to which alloxan would not penetrate cells but would remain in the extracellular fluid with its site of action on the cell membrane.

More often, however, distribution is more complex in a system with several compartments. Note, for example, the compartmental analysis after injection of a single dose of digoxin-^{3}H (Harrisson *et al.*, 1964) or of psychofuranine (Garrett *et al.*, 1960). The latter study was carried out using an analog computer. The authors set forth the advantages of a method which enables them to study the mechanisms and rates of gastrointestinal absorption, diffusion in the tissues and urinary elimination of a drug, but the use of an electron microscope, together with an analog computer, would possibly enable the intracellular compartments to be localized as well (Chance, 1963); although this goes beyond the scope of the present contribution.

One very specifically pharmacological application of kinetic studies using labeled drugs, concerns the absorption of drugs when administered in different ways and the influence of excipients. The cutaneous, intestinal and other permeabilities are the subject of other chapters in this volume, so we shall not stress this application. The theoretical side is treated by Teorell (1937a, b). Interpreting the results is greatly assisted by using an analog computer, as observed by Borzelleca *et al.* (1966) in a study on drug absorption per rectum.

The services rendered to pharmacology by medicaments labeled with a radioisotope are very numerous (see the book edited by Roth, 1965). Any list of the drugs which have been the subject of special monographs in the various sections of this volume would be tiresome and of little use. The reader is therefore recommended to a recent review by Buyske (1965) in which some examples of the utility of labeled drugs are to be found in reference to the discovery and evaluation of pharmacological activities.

CONCLUSION

The methods of compartmental analysis using nuclear indicators enable body composition and its modifications under the influence of drugs or the distribution of the drug to be analyzed. Drug distribution is only one aspect of the more general problem of studying the fate of the drug in the organism, which also includes the study of metabolism. Labeled molecules also make it possible to study the metabolism, distribution, absorption, and excretion of the drug simultaneously.

The methods of analysis are very diverse, since they range from simple determination of one dilution space to kinetic study of the distribution of the tracer in a system comprising numerous compartments. Generally speaking, the technical and theoretical difficulties are greater for a larger number of compartments, but in any case the results cannot be interpreted without a schematic representation of the organism in the form of a model with one or more compartments. This model is necessarily a simplification of reality, and one has to ask whether it may not be an oversimplification.

The objections which are raised to the methods of compartmental analysis are discussed in Chapter 10. The greatest caution is required in physiological interpretation of the parameters measured, for even the term "compartment" cannot be defined precisely. A close analogy is no proof in itself, although agreement between experimental results and values calculated from the model is always a favorable presumption in such reasoning.

We have deliberately set aside one factor which may be involved in interpreting the results, i.e. the circulation, studied in this volume by Winbury (Chapter 12). The rate of entry of a tracer into the tissues clearly can be deduced from its rate of disappearance from the blood only if the flow of blood is the factor limiting the phenomenon rather than the rate of passage through the capillaries.

In spite of the theoretical and practical difficulties that arise in giving effect to the methods of compartmental analysis, these methods render great service to the pharmacologist, in research in general and in measuring the pharmacological activity of new molecules, as well as in analyzing the mode of action of drugs. In fact, it is sometimes possible to adopt simplified methods in the light of earlier experience.

The interpretation of the results of these studies is always more dependable when support is provided by other experiments. In this regard, methods which use several tracers simultaneously are particularly valuable.

Compartmental methods of analysis of the organism have the decisive advantage of being generally applicable to the living, entire animal under physiological conditions, since the experimenter often only has to administer the tracer, collect excreta, and take a few blood samples. Doubtless these methods are due for still greater development in the future owing to the constant improvement of apparatus for measuring radioactivity, enabling the concentration of several radioisotopes to be measured in the same sample, and of analog and even digital computers for data-processing.

REFERENCES

(A) BOOKS, REVIEWS AND MONOGRAPHS

BEAVEN, M. A. (1965) Use of tracers in the study of biogenic amine compartments, in *Advances in Methodology* Rotschild, S. (ed.). Plenum Press, New York, U.S.A., pp. 243–52.

BERNARD, C. (1866) *Leçons sur les propriétés des tissus vivants*. Baillière, Paris, France.

CHEVALLIER, F. (1963) La méthode d'équilibre isotopique, in *L'emploi des radioisotopes en sciences nutritionnelles et des rayonnements ionisants en technologie alimentaire*. C.N.R.S., Paris, France.

COSTA, E., BOULLIN, D. J., HAMMER, W., VOGEL, W. and BRODIE, B. B. (1966) Interactions of drugs with adrenergic neurons. *Pharmacol. Rev.*, **18**:577–97.

DE GRAEFF, J. and LEIJNSE, B. (1964) *Water and Electrolyte Metabolism*. Elsevier, New York, U.S.A.

ELKINTON, J. R. and DANOWSKI, T. S. (1955) *The Body Fluids.* Williams & Wilkins, Baltimore, Mass., U.S.A.

GLASSON, B. (1965) Le problème de la localisation des substances médicamenteuses et de leurs métabolites dans l'organisme. *Therapie,* **20**:222–40.

HAXHE, J. J. (1964) Mesure des compartiments corporels. Méthodes et résultats. *J. Physiol., Paris,* **58**:7–109.

MANERY, J. F. (1954) Water and electrolyte metabolism. *Physiol. Rev.,* **34**:334–417.

MOORE, F. D., OLESEN, K. H., McMURREY, J. D., PARKER, H. V., BALL, M. R. and BOYDEN, C. M. (1963) *The Body Cell Mass and its Supporting Environment. Body Composition in Health and Disease,* Saunders, Philadelphia, Penn., U.S.A.

RESCIGNO, A. and SEGRE, G. (1966) *Drug and Tracer Kinetics.* Blaisdell Pub. Co., Waltham, Mass., U.S.A.

ROBERTSON, J. S. (1957) Theory and use of tracers in determining transfer rates in biological systems. *Physiol. Rev.,* **37**:133–54.

ROBERTSON, J. S. (1962) Mathematical treatment of uptake and release of indicator substances in relation to flow analysis in tissues and organs, in *Handbook of Physiology,* Section 2, Circulation I., pp. 617–44. Amer. Physiol. Soc., Washington, D.C., U.S.A.

ROTH, L. J. (ed.) (1965) *Isotopes in Experimental Pharmacology.* University of Chicago Press, Chicago, Ill., U.S.A.

SEGRE, G. (1965) Compartmental analysis of labeled drug kinetics, in *Isotopes in Experimental Pharmacology.* Roth, L. J. (ed.). University of Chicago Press, Chicago, Ill., U.S.A.

SHEPPARD, C. W. (1962) *Basic Principles of the Tracer Method.* John Wiley, New York, U.S.A., pp. 157–67.

SOLOMON, A. K. (1953) Kinetics of biological processes. Special problems connected with the use of tracers. *Advanc. Biol. Med. Phys.,* **3**:65–97.

SOLOMON, A. K. (1960) Compartmental methods of kinetic analysis, in *Mineral Metabolism. An Advanced Treatise,* pp. 119–67. Vol. 1, Part A. Academic Press, New York, U.S.A.

TEORELL, T. (1937a) Kinetics of substances administered to the body. I: Extravascular modes of administration. *Arch. Int. Pharmacodyn.,* **57**:205–25.

TEORELL, T. (1937b) Kinetics of substances administered to the body. II: Intravascular modes of administration. *Arch. Int. Pharmacodyn.,* **57**:226–40.

WANG, C. H. and WILLIS, D. L. (1965) *Radiotracer Methodology in Biological Science.* Prentice-Hall, Englewood Cliffs, N.J., U.S.A.

ZIERLER, K. L. (1962) Circulation times and the theory of indicator-dilution methods for determining blood flow and volume, in *Handbook of Physiology,* Section 2, Circulation I. pp. 585–615. Amer. Physiol. Soc., Washington, D.C., U.S.A.

ZILVERSMIT, D. B., ENTEMAN, C. and FISHLER, M. C. (1943) On the calculation of "turnover time" and "turnover rate" from experiments involving the use of labelling agents. *J. Gen. Physiol.,* **26**:325.

(B) ORIGINAL PAPERS

AIZAWA, K., KOMORIYAMA, K. and OHNO, S. (1960) Influence of nicotine on serum protein and the amounts of circulatory blood and extracellular fluid, *Excerpta Med.,* Section 2, 16, Abstr. n-7251.

ANBAR, M. and LEWITUS, Z. (1958) Rate of body water distribution studied with triple labelled water. *Nature, Lond.,* **181**:344.

AUBERT, J. P. (1965) Quantitation of calcium metabolism by multicompartmental analysis, in *Isotopes in Experimental Pharmacology,* pp. 169–75. Roth, L. J. (ed.). University of Chicago Press, Chicago, Ill., U.S.A.

AUBERT, J. P., BRONNER, F. and RICHELLE, L. (1963) Quantitation of calcium metabolism theory. *J. Clin. Invest.*, **42**:885–97.

AUBERT, J. P., CHERIAN, A. G., MOUKHTAR, M. S. and MILHAUD, G. (1964) Étude du métabolisme du calcium chez le Rat à l'aide de calcium 45. V: La thyroparathyroïd-ectomie et l'effet de la thyroxine et de la parathormone. *Biochem. Pharmacol.*, **13**:31–44.

AUBERT, J. P. and MILHAUD, G. (1960) Méthode de mesure des principales voies du métabolisme calcique. *Biochim. Biophys. Acta*, **39**:122–39.

AUBERT, J. P., MILHAUD, G., MONOUSSOS, G. and DORMARD, Y. (1958) Mesure de l'échange chimique et du renouvellement physiologique du calcium osseux chez l'Homme et chez le Rat. *C.R. Acad. Sci. Paris*, **246**:2817–20.

AUBERT, J. P., MOUKHTAR, M. S. and MILHAUD, G. (1961) Étude du métabolisme du calcium chez le Rat à l'aide de calcium 45. III: Les relations entre les divers processus chez le rat normal. *Rev. Franc. Etud. Clin. Biol.*, **6**:1034–43.

BAKER, C. H. (1963a) Cr^{51} labeled red cell, I^{131} fibrinogen, and T-1824 dilution spaces. *Amer. J. Physiol.*, **204**:176–80.

BAKER, C. H. (1963b) Fibrinogen I^{131}, T-1824 and red cell–Cr^{51} spaces following hemorrage. *Amer. J. Physiol.*, **205**:527–32.

BAUER, G. C. H., CARLSSON, A. and LINDQUIST (1955a) A comparative study on the metabolism of Sr^{90} and Ca^{45}. *Acta Physiol. Scand.*, **35**:36–66.

BAUER, G. C. H., CARLSSON, A. and LINDQUIST, B. (1955b). Some properties of the exchangeable bone calcium. *Acta Physiol. Scand.*, **35**:67–72.

BELCHER, D. H., FRASER, T. R., JOPLIN, G. F., SLATE, J. D. H. and TAYLOR, R. G. S. (1960) Simultaneous determinations of total body water, extracellular fluid volume, total exchangeable sodium and total exchangeable potassium in man. A simplified technique and some clinical results. *Strahlentherapie*, **45**:195–202.

BOHR, H. H. and DAWIDS, S. G. (1964) The effect of cortiosne and anabolic steroids on the retention of radioactive calcium and strontium in rats. *Acta Endocr. Copenhagen*, **47**:223–30.

BONET-MAURY, P., DEYSINE, A. and PATTI, F. (1954) Enregistrement continu sur la souris vivante de la concentration sanguine en ^{14}C. *C.R. Soc. Biol. Paris*, **148**:798–800.

BONFILS, S., MAJOIS, J. and PELLETIER, C. (1963) Étude de contenu sanguin (volume total et hématocrite) des organes du rat, par double marquage isotopique. *C.R. Soc. Biol. Paris*, **157**:21–4.

BORZELLECA, J. F. and LOWENTHAL, W. (1966) Drug absorption from the rectum. II: Rates of absorption and elimination from the blood for various suppository bases. *J. Pharm. Sci.*, **55**:151–4.

BOZLER, E. (1963) Distribution and exchange in connective tissue and smooth muscle. *Amer. J. Physiol.*, **205**:686–92.

BRODIE, B. B. and BEAVEN, M. A. (1963) Neurochemical transducer systems, *Med. Exp.*, **8**:320–51.

BRODIE, B. B., BRAND, E. and LESHIN, S. (1939) The use of bromide as measure of extra-cellular fluid. *J. Biol. Chem.*, **130**:555–63.

BRONNER, F. (1958) Disposition of intraperitoneally injected calcium 45 in suckling rats. *J. Gen. Physiol.*, **41**:767–82.

BROOKS, S. A., DAVIES, J. W. L., GRABER, I. G. and RICKETTS, C. R. (1960) Labelling of inulin with radioactive iodine, *Nature, Lond.* **188**:675–6.

BUCHANAN, D. L. (1961) Analysis of continuous dosage isotopes experiments. *Arch. Biochem. Biophys.*, **94**:489–99.

BUYSKE, D. A. (1965) Isotopically labelled agents in the discovery of evaluation of pharmacological activities, in *Isotopes in Experimental Pharmacology*, Roth, L. J. (ed.). University of Chicago Press, Chicago, Ill., U.S.A., pp. 275–94.

CACHERA, R. and BARBIER, P. (1941) L'épreuve au rhodonate de sodium, méthode de mesure du volume des liquides interstitiels. *C.R. Soc. Biol. Paris*, **135**:1175–9.

CHANCE, B. (1963) Localization of intracellular and intramitochondrial compartments. *Ann. N.Y. Acad. Sci.*, **108**:322–30.

CHAPLIN, H., Jr. and MOLLISON, P. (1952) Correction for plasma trapped in the red cell column of the hematocrit. *Blood*, **7**:1227–38.

CHEEK, D. B. (1961) Extracellular volume its structure and measurement and the influence of age and disease. *J. Pediat.*, **58**:103–25.

CHEVALLIER, F., BRIERE, M., SERRELL, F. and CORNU, M. (1962) Mesure en continu de la radioactivité spécifique du gaz carbonique expiratoire d'un animal après administration de composés marqués au carbone 14. Recherches d'équilibres isotopiques. *J. Physiol. Paris*, **54**:701–10.

CHIVOT, C. (1967) *Les colloïdes radioactifs dans l'exploration fonctionnelle du système reticulo-endothélial*. Rapport CEA R3240. Saclay, France.

COHEN, Y. and DELASSUE, H. (1959) Étude comparative du métabolisme du ^{35}S chez la souris après administration par voie orale ou sous-cutanée de radiosulfate et de radiosulfure de sodium. *C. R. Soc. Biol. Paris*, **153**:999–1003.

COHEN, Y. and INGRAND, J. (1960) Étude et contrôle du marquage des globules rouges au chrome 51. *Rev. Hemat.*, **15**:217–32.

COHEN, Y. and STOCLET, J. C. (1960) Application au Rat de la mesure du volume sanguin circulant et du volume sanguin des organes par les hématies marquées au ^{51}Cr. *C. R. Soc. Biol. Paris*, **154**:2023–5.

COHEN, Y. and STOCLET, J. C. (1967) Mesure du volume des liquides extracellulaires. Application en pharmacodynamie. *Ann. Phys. Biol. Med.*, **1**:63–70.

COSMOS, E. and VAN KIEN, L. K. (1961) Autoradiography of calcium 45 in frog skeletal muscle using ashed tissue sections. *Int. J. Appl. Radiat. Isotopes*, **12**:118–21.

COTLOVE, E. (1954) Mechanism and extent of distribution of inulin and sucrose in chloride space of tissues. *Amer. J. Physiol.*, **176**:396–410.

COTLOVE, E. and HOGBEN, C. A. M. (1962) Chloride, in *Mineral Metabolism*, 2 B (Comar, C. L. and Bronner, F. (eds.)). Academic Press, New York and London, pp. 109–73.

CRISPELL, K. R., PORTER, B. and NIESET, R. T. (1950) Studies of plasma volume using human serum albumin tagged with radioactive iodine[131]. *J. Clin. Invest.*, **29**:513–16.

DALTON, R. G. (1964) Measurement of body water in calves with urea. *Brit. Vet. J.*, **120**:378–84.

DAVIDSON, D., McINTYRE, I., RAPOPORT, A. and BRADLEY, J. E. S. (1956) Determination of total fat *in vivo* with ^{85}Kr. *Biochem. J.*, **62**:34P.

DAWSON, A. B., EVANS, H. M. and WHIPPLE, G. H. (1920) Blood volume studies. III: Behaviour of large series of dyes introduced into the circulating blood. *Amer. J. Physiol.*, **51**:232–56.

EDELMAN, I. S., JAMES, A. H., BROOKS, L. and MOORE, F. D. (1954a) Body sodium and potassium. IV: The normal total exchangeable sodium: its measurement and magnitude. *Metabolism*, **3**:530–8.

EDELMAN, I. S., JAMES, A. H., BADEN, H. and MOORE, F. D. (1954b) Electrolyte composition of bone and the penetration of radiosodium and deuterium oxide into dog and human bone. *J. Clin. Invest.*, **33**:122–31.

EDELMAN, I. S., OLNEY, J. M., JAMES, A. H., BROOKS, L. and MOORE, F. D. (1952) Body composition: Studies in the human being by the dilution principle. *Science*, **115**:447–54.

EVERETT, N. B., SIMMONS, B. and LASHER, E. P. (1956) Distribution of blood (Fe^{59}) and plasma (I^{131}) volume of rats determined by liquid nitrogen freezing. *Circulation Res.* **4**:419–24.

FALLER, I. L., PETTY, D., LAST, J. H., PASCALE, L. R. and BOND, E. E. (1955) A comparison of the deuterium oxide and antipyrine dilution method for measuring total body water in normal and hydropic human subjects. *J. Lab. Clin. Med.*, **45**:748–58.
FERNANDEZ, L. A., RETTORI, O. and MEJIA, R. H. (1966) Correlation between body fluid volumes and body weight in the rat. *Amer. J. Physiol.*, **210**:877–9.
FINE, J. and SELIGMAN, A. M. (1944) Traumatic shock. VII: A study of the problem of "lost plasma" in hemorrhagic tourniquet and burn shock by the use of radioactive iodo-plasma proteins. *J. Clin. Invest.*, **23**:720–30.
FLORA, J. H., PHILLIPS, D. F., ARCIDIACONO, F. and SAPIRSTEIN, L. A. (1962) Distribution of 4-iodo-antipyrine after intravenous injection in the rat. *Circulation Res.*, **11**: 252–6.
FORBES, G. B. and HURSH, J. B. (1961) Estimation of total body fat from potassium-40 content. *Science*, **133**:1918.
GAEBLER, O. H. and CHOITZ, H. C. (1964) Studies of body water and water turnover determined with deuterium oxide added to food. *Clin. Chem.*, **10**:13–20.
GARRETT, E. R., JOHNSTON, R. L. and COLLINS, E. J. (1962) Kinetics of steroid effects on Ca^{47} dynamics in dogs with the analog computer, I. *J. Pharm. Sci.*, **51**:1050–7.
GARRETT, E. R., JOHNSTON, R. L. and COLLINS, E. J. (1963) Kinetics of steroid effects on Ca^{47} dynamics in dogs with the analog computer, II. *J. Pharmac. Sci.*, **52**:668–78.
GARRETT, E. R., THOMAS, R. C., WALLACH, D. P. and ALWAY, C. D. (1960) Psychofuranine: Kinetics and mechanisms *in vivo* with the application of the analog computer. *J. Pharmacol.*, **130**:106–18.
GAUDINO, M. and LEVITT, M. G. (1949) Inulin spaces a measure of extracellular fluid, *Amer. J. Physiol.*, **157**:387–93.
GILBERT, D. L. and FENN, W. C. (1957) Calcium equilibrium in muscle. *J. Gen. Physiol.* **40**:393–408.
GOMIRATO-SANDRUCCI, M., MUSSA, G. C., PAVESIO, D. and VISCONTI DI OLEGGIO, A. (1962a) Influence of varying doses of prednisone on the chloride space and chloride exchangeable pool. *Minerva Pediat.*, **14**:584–8.
GOMIRATO-SANDRUCCI, M., MUSSA, G. C., PAVESIO, D. and VISCONTI DI OLEGGIO, A. (1962b) Effects of prolonged administration of cortisone derivatives on the volume of extracellular water. *Minerva Pediat.*, **14**:589–93.
GOMIRATO-SANDRUCCI, M., MUSSA, G. C., PAVESIO, D. and VISCONTI DI OLEGGIO, A. (1962c) Behavior of sodium space and total exchangeable sodium during treatment with varying doses of prednisone. *Minerva Pediat.*, **14**:715–18.
GREHANT, N. and QUINQUAUD, E. (1882) Mesure du volume sanguin contenu dans l'organisme d'un mammifère vivant. *C. R. Acad. Sci. Paris*, **44**:1450–3.
HAHN, P. F., BALFOUR, W. M., ROSS, J. F., BALE, W. F. and WHIPPLE, G. H. (1941) Red cell volume circulating and total as determined by radio-iron. *Science*, **93**:87–8.
HAMMETT, F. S. (1925a) A biochemical study of bone growth. I: Changes in the ash, organic matter, and water during growth (*Mus norvegiens albinus*). *J. Biol. Chem.*, **64**:409–29.
HAMMETT, F. S. (1925b) A biochemical study of bone growth. II: Changes in the calcium, magnesium and phosphorus of bone during growth. *J. Biol. Chem.*, **64**:685–96.
HANSARD, S. L. (1964) Total body water in farm animals. *Amer. J. Physiol.*, **206**:1369–72.
HARRISON, C. E. JR., BRANDENBURG, R. O., ONGLEY, P. A., ORVIS, A. L. and OWEN, C. A. JR. (1964) A compartmental analysis of single intravenously administered doses of tritiated digoxin in dogs. *Ann. Intern. Med.*, **60**:709.
HAXHE, J. J. (1963) *La composition corporelle normale. Ses variations au cours de la sous-alimentation et de l'hyperthyroïdie.* Arscia, Bruxelles.
HEVESY, G. and HOFER, E. (1934) Die Verweilzeit des Wassers im menschlichen Korper, untersucht mit Hilfe von "scheweren" Wasser als Indicator. *Klin. Wschr.*, **13**:1524–6.
HOULIHAN, R. T. and EVERSOLE, W. J. (1964) Effects of various adrenal steroids on water

and electrolyte shifts in the adrenalectomized force-fed rat. *Proc. Penn. Acad. Sci.*, **38**:13.

IVERSEN, L. L. (1963) The reuptake of noradrenaline by the isolated perfused rat heart. *Brit. J. Pharmacol.*, **21**:523–37.

KEITH, N. M., ROWNTREE, L. G. and GERAGHTY, J. T. (1915) A method for the determination of plasma and blood volume. *Arch. Int. Med.*, **16**:547–76.

KIMBEL, K. H. (1965) Continuous *in vivo* measurement of absorption, accumulation, distribution and excretion of radio-opaque media, in *Isotopes in Pharmacology*, Roth, L. J. (ed.). Univ. of Chicago Press, Chicago, pp. 249–58.

KOPIN, I. J. (1965) Origin, disposition and metabolic fate of catecholamines, in *Isotopes in Pharmacology*, Roth, L. J. (ed.).University of Chicago Press, Chicago, Ill., U.S.A., pp. 307–13.

KOPIN, I. J. and GORDON, E. K. (1963) Origin of norepinephrine in the heart. *Nature, Lond.*, **199**:1289.

KYLE, L. H., WERDEIN, J. J. and CANARY, J. J. (1963) Nitrogen balance and total body water in the measurement of change in body fat. *Ann. N.Y. Acad., Sci.*, **110**:55–61.

LANGHAM, W. H., EVERSOLE, W. S., HAYES, F. N. and TRUJILLO, T. T. (1956) Assay of tritium activity in body fluids, with use of a liquid scintillation system. *J. Lab. Clin. Med.*, **47**:819–25.

LEROY, G. V., OKITA, G. T., TOCUS, E. C. and CHARLESTON, D. (1960) Continuous measurement of specific activity of $C^{14}O_2$ in expired air. *Int. J. Appl. Radiat. Isotopes*, **7**:273–86.

LESSER, G. T., BLUMBERG, A. G. and STEELE, J. M. (1952) Measurement of total body fat in living rats by absorption of cyclopropane. *Amer. J. Physiol.*, **169**:545–53.

LESSER, G. T., PERL, W. and STEELE, J. M. (1960) Determination of total body fat by absorption of an inert gas: measurements and results in normal human subjects. *J. Clin. Invest.*, **39**:1791–806.

LESSER, G. T. and ZAK, G. (1963) Measurement of total body fat in man by the simultaneous absorption of two inert gases. *Ann. N.Y. Acad. Sci.*, **110**:40–54.

LIM, TH. P. K. (1963) Critical evaluation of the pneumatic method for determining body volume: Its history and technique. *Ann. N.Y. Acad. Sci.*, **110**:72–4.

LJUNGGREN, H., IKKOS, D. and LUFT, R. (1957a, b) Studies on body composition. I: Body fluid compartments and exchangeable potassium in normal males and females. II: Body fluid compartments and exchangeable potassium in obese females. *Acta Endocrinol.*, **25**:187–98, 199–208.

MANERY, J. F. (1961) Minerals in non-osseous connective tissue (including the blood-lens and cornea), in *Mineral Metabolism*, **1** B (Comar, C. L. and Bronner, F. (eds.)). Academic Press, New York, U.S.A., pp. 551–608.

MANERY, J. F. and HASTINGS, A. B. (1939) The distribution of electrolytes in mammalian tissues. *J. Biol. Chem.*, **127**:657–76.

McFARLANE, A. S. (1958) Efficient trace-labelling of proteins with iodine. *Nature, Lond.*, **182**:53.

MARSHALL, E. K. and DAVIS, E. M. (1914) Urea: Its distribution in and its elimination from the body. *J. Biol. Chem.*, **18**:53–80.

MILHAUD, G., REMAGEN, W., GOMES DE MATOS, A. and AUBERT, J. P. (1960a) Étude du métabolisme du calcium chez le Rat rachitique. I: Le rachitisme expérimental. *Rev. Franc. Étud. Clin. Biol.*, **5**:254–61.

MILHAUD, G., REMAGEN, W., GOMES DE MATOS, A. and AUBERT, J. P. (1960b) Étude du métabolisme du calcium chez le Rat à l'aide de calcium 45. II: Action de la cortisone. *Rev. Franc. Étud. Clin. Biol.*, **5**:354–8.

MILLER, I. and WEIL, W. B. (1963) Some problems in expressing and comparing body composition determined by direct analysis. *Ann. N.Y. Acad. Sci.*, **110**:153–60.

MOLLISON, P. L. and VEAL, N. (1955) The use of the isotope ^{51}Cr as a label for red cells. *Brit. J. Haematol.*, **1**:62–74.
MONTANARI, R., COSTA, E., BEAVEN, M. A., and BRODIE, B. B. (1963) Turnover rates of norepinephrine in hearts of intact mice, rats, and guinea pigs using tritiated norepinephrine. *Life Sci.*, **2**:232–40.
MOORE, F. D. (1946) Determination of total body water and solids with isotopes. *Science*, **104**:157–60.
MOORE, F. D. and BOYDEN, C. M. (1963) Body cell mass and limits of hydration of the fat-free body: their relation to estimated skeletal weight. *Ann. N.Y. Acad. Sci.*, **110**:62–71.
MOORE, F. D., McMURREY, J. D., PARKER, H. V. and MAGNUS, I. C. (1956) Body composition: Total body water and electrolytes: Intravascular and extravascular phase volumes. *Metabolism*, **5**:447–67.
MOREL, F. (1950) Techniques de la mesure des échanges capillaires à l'aide des indicateurs radioactifs. *Helv. Physiol. Pharmacol. Acta*, **8**:52–73.
MOSES, A. M. (1965) Influence of adrenal cortex on body water distribution in rats. *Amer. J. Physiol.*, **208**:662–5.
NEUMAN, W. F. and NEUMAN, M. W. (1953) The nature of the mineral phase of bone. *Chem. Rev.*, **53**:1–45.
NEUMAN, W. F. and NEUMAN, M. W. (1958) *The Chemical Dynamics of Bone Mineral.* University of Chicago Press, Chicago, Ill., U.S.A.
NICHOLSON, J. P. and ZILVA, J. F. (1957) A 6 hours method for determining the extracellular fluid volume in human subjects. *Clin. Chim. Acta*, **2**:340–4.
NOBLE, R. P. and GREGERSEN, M. I. (1946) Blood volume in clinical shock. I: Mixing time and disappearance rate of T-1824 in normal subjects and in patients in shock; determination of plasma volume in man from 10-minutes sample. *J. Clin. Invest.*, **25**:158–71.
OKITA, G. T. (1965) *In vivo* oxidation of C^{14} labelled intermediates and of drugs as measured by a continuous C^{14}O$_2$ monitor, in *Isotopes in Experimental Pharmacology* (Roth, L. J. (ed.)). University of Chicago Press, Chicago, Ill., U.S.A., pp. 191–203.
PACE, N., KLINE, L., SCHACHMAN, H. K. and HARFENIST, M. (1947) Studies on the body composition. IV: Use of radioactive hydrogen for measurement *in vivo* of total body water. *J. Biol. Chem.*, **168**:459–69.
PACE, N. and RATHBON, E. N. (1945) Studies on body composition. III: The body water and chemically combined nitrogen content in relation to fat content. *J. Biol. Chem.*, **158**:685–91.
PEARLMAN, W. H. (1957) 16-^{3}H-progesterone metabolism in advanced pregnancy and in oophorectomized hysterectomized women. *Biochem. J.*, **67**:1–5.
PERRAULT, G., BAZIN, J. P., and PAGES, J. P. (1967) Influence de la décroissance physique d'un traceur radioactif dans la résolution d'un système de compartiments. *Int. J. Appl. Radiat. Isotopes*, **18**:7–10.
PETERSON, R. E. (1965) Studies of radioactive aldosterone in man, in *Radioisotopes in Pharmacology* (Roth, L. L. (ed.)). University of Chicago Press, Chicago, Ill., U.S.A., pp. 177–90.
POLOSA, C. and HAMILTON, W. F. (1962) The relation between cells and plasma within the renal vasculature. *Arch. Int. Pharmacodyn.*, **140**:294–307.
PRENTICE, T. C., SIRI, W., BERLIN, N. I., HYDE, G. M., PARSONS, R. J., JOINER, E. E. and LAWRENCE, J. H. (1952) Studies of total body water with tritium. *J. Clin. Invest.*, **31**:412–8.
PRITCHARD, W. H., MOIR, TH. W. and MACINTYRE, W. J. (1955) Measurement of the early disappearance of iodinated (I^{131}) serum albumin from circulating blood by a continuous recording method. *Circulation Res.*, **3**:18–23.
RAWSON, R. A., CHIEN, S., PENG, M. T. and DENNENBACK, R. J. (1959) Determination

of residual blood volume required for survival in rapidly hemorrhaged splenecto-mized dog. *Amer. J. Physiol.*, **196**:179–83.

REEVE, E. B. and VEALL, N. (1949) A simplified method for determination of circulating red-cell volume with radioactive phosphorus. *J. Physiol. Lond.*, **108**:12–23.

SAVOIE, J. C. and JUNGERS, P. (1965) Mesure de l'espace extra-cellulaire chez l'homme à l'aide du radio-sulfate S^{35}. *Rev. Franc. Étud. Clin. Biol.*, **10**, 99–106.

SCHLOERB, P. R., FRISS-HANSEN, B. J., EDELMAN, I. S., SOLOMON, A. K. and MOORE, F. D. (1950) The measurement of total body water in the human subject by deuterium oxide dilution, with a consideration of the dynamics of deuterium distribution. *J. Clin. Invest.*, **29**:1296–1310.

SCHWARTZ, I. L., SCHACHTER, D. and FREINKEL, N. (1949) The measurement of extra-cellular fluid in man by means of a constant infusion technique. *J. Clin. Invest.*, **28**:1117–28.

SEITCHIK, J., ALPER, C. and SZUTA, A. (1963) Changes in body composition during pregnancy. *Ann. N.Y. Acad. Sci.*, **110**:821–9.

SHEPPARD, C. W., OVERMAN, R. R., WILDE, W. S. and SANGREN, W. C. (1953) The disappearance of K^{42} from the non-uniformly mixed circulation pool in dogs. *Circulation Res.*, **1**:284–97.

SOLOMON, A. K., EDELMAN, I. S. and SOLOWAY, S. (1950) The use of the mass spectro-meter to measure deuterium in body fluids. *J. Clin. Invest.*, **29**:1311–19.

SÖRENSEN, L. D. (1960) The elimination of uric acid in man. *Scand. J. Clin. Lab. Invest.*, **12**, suppl. 54, 1–214.

STERLING, K. and GRAY, S. J. (1950) Determination of circulating red cell volume in man by radioactive chromium. *J. Clin. Invest.*, **29**:1614–19.

STOCLET, J. C. (1958) Étude à l'aide de ^{45}Ca des échanges de calcium entre le plasma sanguin et différents organes chez le Rat. *C.R. Acad. Sci. Paris*, **247**:974–6.

STOCLET, J. C. (1959) Étude comparative de la répartition de ^{45}Ca et ^{24}Na entre le plasma sanguin et différents organes du Rat. *C.R. Acad. Sci. Paris*, **248**: 3229–31.

STOCLET, J. C. (1960a) Les échanges calciques rapides analysés par le calcium 45 chez le Rat. *C.R. Acad. Sci. Paris*, **251**:1834–6.

STOCLET, J. C. (1960b) Les échanges calciques entre le plasma sanguin et divers organes étudiés chez le Rat mâle et femelle à l'aide de ^{45}Ca. *C.R. Acad. Sci. Paris*, **251**: 1934–6.

STOCLET, J. C. (1964a) Étude des mouvements du calcium dans l'organisme de Rat. *C.R. Soc. Biol. Paris*, **158**:1208–11.

STOCLET, J. C. (1964b) Mouvements du calcium dans le muscle strié au repos et en fonctionnement, étudiés chez le Rat *in vivo*. *C.R. Soc. Biol. Paris*, **158**:1277–80.

STOCLET, J. C. (1966) Mouvements du calcium dans le muscle au repos et en activité chez le Rat *in vivo*. *J. Physiol. Paris*, **58**, suppl. 4, 1–131.

STOCLET, J. C. and COHEN, Y. (1963) L'élution plasmatique de ^{45}Ca injecté au Rat, analysée en fonction du sexe et de l'âge. *Ann. Nutr. Paris*, **17**:B193–B205.

SWANN, R. C., MADISSO, M. and PITTS, R. F. (1954) Measurement of extracellular fluid volume in nephrectomized dogs. *J. Clin. Invest.*, **33**:1447–53.

TALA, P., LIETO, J. V. and KYLLÖNEN, K. E. J. (1956) Practical blood volume measure-ments with radioactive chromic chloride and iodinated human serum albumin. *Ann. Med. Exp. Fenn.*, **34**:226–34.

TALSO, P. J., LAHR, TH. N., STAFFORD, N., FERENZI, G. and JACKSON, H. R. O. (1955) A comparison of the volume of distribution of antipyrine, N-acetyl-4-amino-anti-pyrine and I^{131} labelled 4-iodo-antipyrine in human beings. *J. Lab. Clin. Med.*, **46**: 619–23.

TALSO, P. J., MILLER, CH. E., CARBALLO, A. J. and VASQUEZ, I. (1960) Exchangeable potassium as a parameter of body composition. *Metabolism*, **9**:456–71.

VALETTE, G., COHEN, Y. and STOCLET, J. C. (1964) Interprétation des effets de l'E.D.T.A. sur le coeur au moyen des échanges de ^{45}Ca. *J. Physiol. Paris*, **56**:454–5.

WALKER, W. C. and WILDE, W. S. (1952) Kinetics of radiopotassium in the circulation, *Amer. J. Physiol.*, **170**:401–13.

WALSER, M., SELDIN, D. W. and GROLLMAN, A. (1953) An evaluation of the radiosulfate for the determination of the volume of extra-cellular fluid in man and dogs. *J. Clin. Invest.*, **32**:299–308.

WATKINS, D. COOPERSTEIN, S. J. and LAZAROW, A. (1964) Alloxan distribution (*in vitro*) between cells and extracellular fluid. *Amer. J. Physiol.*, **207**:431–5.

YALOW, R. S. and BERSON, S. A. (1951) The use of K^{42}-tagged erythrocytes in blood volume determinations. *Science*, **114**:14–15.

YUSUNOV, A. Y. and MAKHUMUDON, E. S. (1964) Effect of adreno and cholinolytic agents on water and mineral metabolism (in dogs) under conditions of high temperature and solar radiation. *Med. Zh. Uzbekistana*, **30**:4.

ZSEBOK, Z. and PETRANYI, G. (1964) The protective action of AET against the destruction of sodium and liquid metabolism in gastrointestinal radiation syndrome. *Strahlentherapie*, **125**:449–55.

CHAPTER 12

USE OF RADIOISOTOPIC TRACERS IN THE STUDY OF NUTRITIONAL CIRCULATION

Martin M. Winbury

Department of Pharmacology, Warner-Lambert Research Institute, Morris Plains, New Jersey

1. INTRODUCTION

1.1. DEFINITION OF REGIONAL MICROCIRCULATION AND NUTRITIONAL CIRCULATION

The primary function of the circulation is to provide materials for tissue nutrition such as oxygen and substrates and the removal of products of tissue metabolism. The rate of blood flow to any region or organ is usually in balance with the requirements of the tissues of that organ or region. In addition to providing for tissue nutrition, the circulation is involved in maintenance of heat balance of the organism. This necessitates a large volume of blood flow through regions with low metabolic demands such as the skin.

Exchange of materials between the blood and tissues can only occur in functional capillary beds. The larger vessels which lead to and from these capillary beds serve merely as mixing chambers and avenues of transport (Robertson, 1962). This tissue exchange function requires circulation to the capillary beds, and capillaries of sufficient length and adequate diffusion capacity (Kitchin, 1963; Goresky, 1965; Renkin, 1965). Capillaries that are not open do not contribute to the exchange between blood and tissues.

Capillaries are a part of the regional microcirculation, and it is in that segment of the system that exchange can occur to support tissue nutrition. Therefore the term "nutritional circulation", originated by Kety (1949) and by Hyman (Hyman, 1957; Hyman *et al.*, 1959), has been used by many others to describe the function of this area.

The purpose of this chapter is to demonstrate how radioactive tracers can be used to study the transport function of the capillary circulation which is, in reality, the nutritional circulation of any specific region or organ. The theoretical basis for the use of these techniques will be considered in some detail together with a general description of the various methodological approaches. Finally, there will be a brief description of specific techniques employed for various organ systems and the effect of pharmacological agents thereon.

1.2. TOTAL REGIONAL CIRCULATION VERSUS NUTRITIONAL CIRCULATION

The total blood flow to an area can be estimated by various types of blood flow meters, direct observation of microcirculatory beds (Grant, 1964), plethysmographic techniques (Braithwaite *et al.*, 1959; Coffman, 1963), thermal conductivity methods (Barlow *et al.*, 1961), heat elimination methods (Elkin and Cooper, 1951), angiographic techniques (Lehan *et al.*, 1966), and indicator-dilution methods based on the Fick principle using diffusible or nondiffusible indicators (Kety, 1951; Goodale and Hackel,

TABLE 1. DICHOTOMY OF RESPONSE OF ARTERIOLAR RESISTANCE (AR) AND NUTRITIONAL CIRCULATION (E ^{86}Rb)

	AR	E ^{86}Rb	Drug
		Hind limb	
Constriction	↑	↑	Epinephrine
	↑	↑	Norepinephrine
	↑	↑	Serotonin I[a]
Dilatation	↓	↑	Histamine
	↓	↑	Isoproterenol
	↓	↑	Nitroglycerin
	↓	↑	Pentaerythritol Tetranitrate (PETN)
	↓	↑	Serotonin II[a]
	↓	↓	Acetylcholine
	↓	↓	Serotonin III[a]
	↓	↓	Histamine-Skeletal Muscle[b]
		Heart	
Dilatation	↓	↑	Nitroglycerin
	↓	↑	Pentaerythritol Tetranitrate
	↓	↓	Norepinephrine
	↓	↓	Isoproterenol

[a] Serotonin produced different effects in different animals.
[b] Histamine in isolated gastrocnemius muscle.

1953; Munck and Lassen, 1957; Fox, 1962; Robertson, 1962). The total circulation does not indicate what fraction of the regional blood flow is available for nutritional purposes (Kety, 1951; Hirvonen and Sonnenschein, 1962). A portion of the regional flow may pass through areas of the microcirculation through which exchange does not occur and be "nonnutritional" (Walder, 1955; Gemmell and Veall, 1956; Hyman, 1957; Barlow *et al.*, 1961; Friedman, 1965; Schroeder, 1966). From the functional viewpoint, the nonnutritional flow can be considered a shunt between the arteries and veins since there is no exchange between the blood and tissues (Elkin and Cooper, 1951; Hyman, 1957; Hyman *et al.*, 1959; Kety, 1960a). An example of this is the diversion of blood flow from muscle to skin, where metabolic needs are low (Elkin and Cooper, 1951; Gabel *et al.*, 1964). A similar diversion of blood flow can occur within a tissue, and will be discussed in detail at a later point.

There can be a dichotomy between the response of the nutritional circulation and the total circulation after the administration of drugs and stimulation of various nerves (Table 1). This has been amply demonstrated in skeletal muscle (Walder, 1953; Hyman *et al.*, 1959; Coffman, 1963; Gabel *et al.*, 1964; Winbury *et al.*, 1965a), and in heart muscle (Winbury *et al.*, 1963). Since the arterioles regulate the total blood flow to the region, while the precapillary sphincters regulate the distribution of blood flow to the capillary beds (Kitchin, 1963; Renkin, 1965; Gosselin and Audino, 1966; Mellander, 1966), it may be inferred that there can be different effects on the arterioles and precapillary sphincters.

Diffusible tracers can be used for investigation of the transport function or nutritional circulation. The first practical application was that of Kety (1949), who studied the clearance of ^{24}Na from skeletal muscle in humans. The movement of these substances, like oxygen and substrates, depends upon capillary permeability and cell membrane permeability (Miller and Wilson, 1951; Robertson, 1962; Landis and Pappenheimer, 1963). Some indicators enter the extracellular fluid, while others enter the cells. Regardless of this, as long as the transport between the blood and tissues (or vice versa) is a flow-limited process, these indicators can be used to measure the nutritional circulation.

2. FUNCTIONAL ORGANIZATION OF REGIONAL MICROCIRCULATION

The regional microcirculation is that section of the circulatory system intimately involved with the regulation of blood flow to the tissue requirements. It is important to review the morphologic and functional organization of the microcirculation in order to better understand the concept of nutritional circulation and how diffusible tracers can be used for study of this function.

2.1. ANATOMIC ORGANIZATION

Although it is convenient to consider the terminal vascular bed as a system in series between the arterioles and venules, the actual pattern is much more complex. Furthermore the terminal vascular beds differ

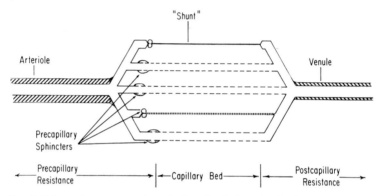

FIG. 1. Schematic representation of microcirculation. Capillaries are represented by $=====$ open or $------$ closed. The "shunt" could be anatomic or physiologic. A short capillary or one with poor diffusion capacity (low PS/Q) would act as a physiological shunt. This diagram represents the heart which has a capillary reserve at rest of 25% of the total.

markedly in different regions (Lutz and Fulton, 1962; Burton, 1965). In general, arteries and arteriolar branches anastomose freely with each other, and together with the thoroughfare channels form a complex network of the capillaries in which blood flow may be intermittent and forward and backward (Zweifach, 1957; Lutz and Fulton, 1962; Burton, 1965).

Nonetheless, for functional purposes we can consider that the terminal vascular bed is composed of several sections in series (Kitchin, 1963; Mellander, 1965). First there are the arteriolar resistance vessels, and then precapillary sphincters. This is followed by the capillary, the post capillary resistance vessel, and, finally, the venular capacitance vessels (Fig. 1). We can add to this the possibility of shunts or nonnutritive capillaries (Schroeder, 1966). The presence of morphologic arteriovenous shunts has not been demonstrated in many tissues, but physiologic studies indicate the presence of shunting mechanisms.

Arteriovenous anastomosis has been found in the skin, liver, mesentery, and intestine (Lutz and Fulton, 1962; Burton, 1965). "Thoroughfare" or "preferential" channels is another type of morphologic shunt permitting blood to flow directly from the arterial to venous system (Zweifach, 1961; Lutz and Fulton, 1962; Burton, 1965). There is a question about the presence of large morphological shunts in skeletal muscle (Grant, 1964), and the general consensus based on direct observation or pellet injection studies is that shunts are absent (Schroeder, 1966).

Finally, there are capillaries through which exchange between blood and tissue does not occur, and these can act as a shunting mechanism, in the physiological sense at least (Walder, 1955; Landis and Pappenheimer, 1963; Burton, 1965).

"Physiological" or "functional" shunting has been inferred in those tissues lacking morphologic shunts, when the increase in total blood flow is out of proportion to the change in the nutritional circulation; in fact there are circumstances where the nutritional circulation shows no change in the face of a marked increase in blood flow (Hyman, 1957). Physiological shunting has been suggested in the case of skeletal muscle (Prentice *et al.*, 1955; Walder, 1955; Hyman, 1957; Renkin, 1965; Schroeder, 1966) and heart (Winbury and Pensinger, 1966). This will be discussed in more detail in Section 4.3.

Total regional blood flow measurements include the volume of blood passing between the major artery and vein of the region. Both nutritive and nonnutritive (shunt) blood flow are included in this value (Kety, 1965). On the other hand, the uptake or washout of a diffusible indicator measures only the capillary (nutritive) function (Dobson and Warner, 1957).

2.2. REGULATION OF MICROCIRCULATION

Functionally the microcirculation can be considered as a series-coupled system. The arterioles (resistance vessels) determine the blood flow to the region, and the precapillary sphincters determine the distribution of flow and the number of open capillaries (Kitchin, 1963; Renkin, 1965; Gosselin and Audino, 1966; Mellander, 1966). In addition, there are post-capillary resistance vessels and capacitance vessels (Kitchin, 1963; Mellander, 1965). The ratio of the pre- to the post-capillary resistance regulates the mean hydrostatic capillary pressure and transcapillary filtration. The capacitance vessels regulate the regional blood volume. Drugs and neurohumoral agents can have more or less specific and different effects on each of these variables (Mellander, 1966).

The tone of the arterioles is under the regulation of the autonomic nervous system (sympathetic), but it can be influenced by various circulating neurohumoral agents and by drugs. Since the main source of regional vascular resistance resides in the smaller arterioles, these vessels are of prime importance in the regulation of the total regional flow. There is local autonomy of the regional blood flow in certain organs (heart, skeletal muscle, kidney), which is known as autoregulation. This phenomenon can easily be demonstrated in the heart, and is the mechanism that permits the coronary blood flow to adjust to changing metabolic requirements by an intrinsic mechanism (Berne, 1967).

The precapillary sphincters determine the number of open capillaries and capillary surface area available for exchange (Kitchin, 1963; Mellander, 1965; Renkin, 1965; Gosselin and Audino, 1966). These sphincters do not appear to grade their tone; consequently the opening of capillaries is an all or none process (Hyman and Lenthall, 1962; Gosselin and Audino, 1966). Precapillary sphincters can respond in a different way to drugs than can resistance or capacitance vessels. In skeletal muscle, norepinephrine dilates the precapillary sphincters, but constricts the resistance and capacitance vessels (Mellander, 1966). At constant blood flow the overall effect is an increase in the nutritional circulation (Gabel *et al.*, 1964; Winbury *et al.*, 1965a). It is well to keep in mind that the determinants of nutritional circulation are the capillary surface area and the total volume of blood flow available for perfusion of capillaries. This involves the arteriolar resistance vessels, and the precapillary sphincters. Autoregulation may occur at the capillary level through precapillary sphincter control (Braithwaite *et al.*, 1959).

The arteriovenous shunts of the skin are intimately related to heat dissipation and are under neurohumoral control. It has been suggested that during reactive hyperemia of the skin there is a reciprocal relationship between the capillaries and shunts (Braithwaite *et al.*, 1959). The ischemia produces dilatation of the capillaries, which then close down as oxygenation becomes adequate. At the same time the shunts enlarge and divert the blood from the capillaries. Studies by Hyman *et al.* (1959) demonstrated that stimulation of the hypothalamic vasodilator center of the cat produced a large increase in blood flow of skeletal muscle but no change in nutritional circulation (^{24}Na clearance). Several workers concluded that the sympathetic cholinergic vasodilator nerves produce shunting of some type (Hyman *et al.*, 1959; Hirvonen and Sonnenschein, 1962; Schroeder, 1966).

Renkin (1965) has suggested that shunting in skeletal muscle assumes importance only when an excessive load results in the failure of local circulatory regulation.

2.3. FUNCTIONAL STUDIES

2.3.1. *Homogeneous or nonhomogeneous perfusion*

Skeletal muscle is considered to have two or more parallel components which represent regions of the tissue with different perfusion rates. Thus the circulation of the region is nonhomogeneous. An increase in the nutritional circulation (clearance of tracer) may be the result of improved circulation to the poorly perfused area, producing a more uniform circulation or increasing perfusion of an already well perfused area (Dobson and Warner, 1957; Renkin, 1959a, b). Washout curves of diffusible tracers from skeletal muscle show two or more exponential components in dog (Prentice *et al.*, 1955; Dobson and Warner, 1957; Tønnesen and Sejrsen, 1967) and man (Dobson and Warner, 1957; Freis *et al.*, 1957).

A comprehensive study by Barlow *et al.* (1961) demonstrated two parallel pathways in skeletal muscle. One has a rapid capillary circulation supplying the muscle fibers themselves, and the other has a slow capillary circulation supplying the intramuscular septum and tendons. Epinephrine had a different effect on the two components. Comparison of autoradiographs with the ^{24}Na washout curve demonstrated that ^{24}Na was evenly distributed throughout the muscle during the initial, fast clearance phase, but during the slow phase the ^{24}Na was found only in the intramuscular septa and tendons. These results support the concept of Renkin (1959a, b) that skeletal muscle has well perfused and poorly perfused areas.

The skin of the rabbit also has a dual capillary circulation based on areas of high and low metabolic rates (Thorburn *et al.*, 1966); the fast compartment is associated with the hair follicles and the slow compartment is associated with the remainder of the skin. There was a marked increase in the size of the fast compartment during the active phase of hair growth (anagen phase), but the flow rate per unit weight was the same. As a consequence, the mean or total cutaneous flow was increased.

^{85}Kr washout curves from the kidney are a series of exponentials associated with blood flow through localized regions of the kidney (Thorburn *et al.*, 1963). The outer cortex has the fastest rate, the outer medullary and inner cortical flow is about 28%, the outer cortical rate, and the inner medulla 4% of the cortical rate, respectively. Since the outer cortical compartment contains 80 % of the renal blood volume, this area represents the major portion of blood flow to the kidney.

Based on washout of ^{85}Kr or ^{133}Xe the normal myocardium has homogeneous perfusion (Ross *et al.*, 1964; Sullivan *et al.*, 1965). However, in the presence of coronary artery disease there is heterogeneity of myocardial flow (Sullivan *et al.*, 1965). An analysis of flow rate at various depths of the myocardium demonstrated that the flow rate in the endocardium was 25 % lower than the epicardium, indicating a nonhomogeneity associated with specific areas (Kirk and Honig, 1964).

Analysis of ^{133}Xe or ^{85}Kr clearance curves from the brain shows two distinct homogeneously perfused areas, which can respond differently to drugs (Lassen *et al.*, 1964a; Skinhoj *et al.*, 1964; Häggendal, 1966). The grey matter has a much higher flow rate than the white matter (Høedt-Rasmussen *et al.*, 1966; Obrist *et al.*, 1967).

2.3.2. *Independent response of arterioles and nutritional circulation*

The microcirculatory mechanisms that control the transcapillary exchange or nutritional circulation are the arteriolar resistance vessels, which control total blood flow through the vascular bed, and precapillary sphincters, which determine the number of open capillaries. The response of the arterioles and the precapillaries of both skeletal and heart muscle to drugs, neurohumoral agents, and nerve stimulation can be different.

Stimulation of the hypothalamic vasodilator center produced no change in ^{24}Na clearance from the skeletal muscle of the cat in spite of large increases in blood flow (Hyman *et al.*, 1959). The authors concluded that the sympathetic vasodilator fibers influence nonnutritional vessels (physiological shunts) principally. Nonetheless, these results demonstrate arteriolar dilatation in the absence of an increase in nutritional circulation. Using the capillary filtration coefficient as a measure of precapillary sphincter function, it was found that norepinephrine constricted resistance vessels (arterioles) but dilated precapillary sphincters (Mellander, 1966). This confirmed previously reported results demonstrating that epinephrine and norepinephrine increased skeletal muscle nutritional circulation (^{86}Rb clearance) in spite of increased arteriolar resistance, suggesting precapillary sphincter dilatation (Gabel *et al.*, 1964; Winbury *et al.*, 1965a). On the other hand, acetylcholine decreased arteriolar resistance and reduced ^{86}Rb clearance suggesting precapillary sphincter constriction (Gabel *et al.*, 1964; Winbury *et al.*, 1965a).

A similar dichotomy was observed in the canine heart. Norepinephrine decreased arteriolar resistance and reduced ^{86}Rb clearance (Winbury *et al.*,

1962; Winbury *et al.*, 1965a). A study in pigs showed that pentaerythritol tetranitrate can increase fractional ^{86}Rb uptake in the absence of a change in blood flow (Winbury and Pensinger, 1966).

Table 1 compares the response of arteriolar resistance and ^{86}Rb clearance for a number of agents in the heart and skeletal muscle.

2.3.3. *Nutritional and nonnutritional blood volume*

As previously discussed, skeletal muscle may have parallel flow channels. The capacity of these parallel systems was determined by means of a variation of the indicator dilution technique using ^{86}Rb and ^{131}I serum albumin. Approximately 75% of the total circulating blood volume of the hindlimb is in the nonnutritional channel, and about 25% in the nutritional channel. Since the nonnutritional network includes large and small arteries and veins as well as any shunt-like channels, it is difficult to draw any conclusion about the capacity of the shunts themselves.

3. TRACER TECHNIQUE FOR STUDY OF REGIONAL CIRCULATION

Radioactive tracers have been used to measure various aspects of regional blood flow. This includes the total volume of flow per unit time or nutritional flow alone. The development of equipment for detection of radioactivity in blood or tissues has contributed to the use of radioactive tracers and has made for ease in performing such studies.

The radioactive tracers used include large nondiffusible molecules (^{131}I albumin, ^{51}Cr red cells, ^{55}Fe siderophilin), which remain within the vascular system and have a small volume of distribution and diffusible substances (^{86}Rb, ^{84}Rb, ^{42}K, ^{24}Na, ^{131}I, ^{133}Xe, ^{85}Kr, etc.) which pass through capillary walls and equilibrate with the extravascular space and have a large volume of distribution (Ross and Friesinger, 1965). The nondiffusible tracers are used to measure total regional flow based on the indicator-dilution principle. On the other hand, the diffusible tracers can be used for determining total flow based on the Fick principle or for the determination of effective capillary flow (nutritional) based on the extraction or clearance principle.

Extraction is defined as the percentage of a substance extracted from the arterial blood in a single passage through a vascular bed $(A - V)/A$, where A and V represent concentration of the tracer in the arterial and venous blood respectively. Clearance is defined as the virtual volume of plasma or blood required to account for the tracer added to (uptake) or removed from the tissue (washout) in a unit time; it has the dimensions of ml/min:

$$\frac{\Delta \text{ amount in tissue in time } t}{\text{integrated arterial or venous concentration} \times \text{time } t}$$

or, if extraction E and blood flow Q are known, clearance $= Q \times E$.

3.1. INDICATOR DILUTION PRINCIPLE

The familiar indicator-dilution principle of Stewart for the estimation of cardiac output has been applied to the measurement of blood flow through various organs (Fox, 1962). If a nondiffusible indicator is injected into the arterial supply of an organ system, a venous dilution curve will be obtained which depends upon the amount of indicator injected and the volume of blood flow. The same principle can be applied by the determination of the time–concentration curve of a nondiffusible radioactive tracer in an organ by external counting techniques, since all the indicators will be confined to the vascular system. An application of this approach employed ^{32}P labeled red cells as the tracer (Grängsjö et al., 1966). The red cells were injected into the renal artery of the dog, and indicator dilution curves of beta activity were recorded from a needle detector in the renal medulla and an end detector on the renal surface.

Sevelius and Johnson (1959) developed a method which would theoretically estimate the total coronary flow as a fraction of the cardiac output after intravenous injection of ^{131}I-albumin. This approach is based on the assumption that the coronary circuit is the shortest circuit between the aorta and right ventricle. After the intravenous injection of the tracer, the initial indicator dilution curve of the right ventricle is an estimate of cardiac output, and it is assumed that the first curve due to recirculation is related to the coronary circulation (Conn, 1962). The validity of this method has been questioned because it is difficult to differentiate the primary cardiac output curve from the coronary recirculation curve (Rowe, 1962). More important is the fact that some of the blood from the systemic circuit returns to the right ventricle nearly simultaneously with the blood from the coronary sinus, resulting in unduly high values (Marchioro et al., 1961; Conn, 1962).

The volume of blood in an organ system may be determined using nondiffusible indicators (Pensinger et al., 1965; Friedman, 1966). The effect of various drugs has been studied in the foot (Geraud et al., 1960) and in the heart (Bloor and Roberts, 1965; Winbury and Pensinger, 1966).

3.2. KETY–SCHMIDT TECHNIQUE

The Kety–Schmidt technique, used extensively for measurement of *total* cerebral or myocardial flow with N_2O gas as an indicator, is a specialized application of the Fick principle. The Fick method has as its basis the principle of conservation of matter (Kety, 1951; Kety, 1960a). Thus the quantity of indicator accumulated or removed by a region per unit time is equal to the quantity brought to the region minus the quantity transported out (Kety, 1951, 1960a, b). The classical application of the Fick principle as used for determination of cardiac output requires representative arterial (C_a) and venous concentrations (C_v) of the indicator (O_2 or CO_2) as well as the rate of uptake or removal q/t, which results in the familiar equation for blood flow (f); $f = (q/t)/(C_a - C_v)$ (Kety, 1951; 1960a).

Blood flow can be measured on the basis of the quantity of a substance (N_2O, ^{85}Kr) which accumulates or leaves the region during the transition from one steady state to another (Kety, 1960a). An inert, freely diffusible tracer, abruptly injected into the arterial blood, will become equally distributed in the volume of the region, and the concentration or partial pressure there will be equal to that in the arterial blood. Thus $(dq/dt) = f(C_a - C_v)$. An application of this principle was applied for measurement of cerebral blood flow using ^{79}Kr. q was estimated by a scintillation detector, and C_a and C_v by direct sampling (Kety, 1960a; Fox, 1962; Robertson, 1962). This equation may be applied without determining q directly by permitting a sufficient time of exposure of the region to the gas, so that equilibration between the gas concentration in the brain or heart and in the venous blood draining the region has occurred, as in the Kety–Schmidt (1948) N_2O method. This is achieved by having the subject breathe 15% N_2O for 10 min or ^{85}Kr in air for 14 min (Lassen and Munck, 1955; Munck and Lassen, 1957). At equilibrium, the tissue concentration equals the venous concentration times the blood: tissue partition coefficient λ. The arteriovenous concentration difference is determined either during the period of N_2O saturation or during desaturation (Goodale and Hackel, 1953) after cessation of N_2O breathing. The integrated arteriovenous difference is divided into the equilibrium organ concentration ($C_v \times \lambda$) to derive blood flow in ml/min per 100 g:

$$f = \frac{C_v \times \lambda}{\int_0^{10} (C_a - C_v)\, dt}$$

(Kety, 1951; 1960a).

To apply this approach properly it is necessary to obtain mixed venous blood from the region with minimal contamination (coronary sinus, internal jugular vein), and the time for the tissue and venous blood to reach equilibrium must not be too long to be practical (Kety, 1951, 1960a). Areas that do not drain into the venous outflow from the region will not contribute to the flow measurement. Other diffusible indicators have been employed with the Kety–Schmidt procedure for *total* coronary or cerebral flow. These include ^{131}I-antipyrine (Sapirstein and Mellette, 1955; Krasnow *et al.*, 1963), [79]Kr, and [85]Kr (Lassen and Munck, 1955; Lewis *et al.*, 1955; Tybjaerg Hansen *et al.*, 1956; Munck and Lassen, 1957; Lassen and Høedt-Rasmussen, 1966). It is important to remember that this procedure is based on concentration of indicator in the venous blood from the region, and includes blood passing through capillary beds (nutritional) as well as blood passing directly from arterial to venous channels without permitting exchange (nonnutritional). Therefore *total* regional blood flow is measured (Kety, 1951, 1960a, 1960b).

3.3. DIFFUSIBLE TRACERS FOR NUTRITIONAL CIRCULATION

3.3.1. *Theory and principles*

The exchange between the tissues and blood can be studied with rapidly diffusible inert tracers (Kety, 1951; Landis and Pappenheimer, 1963). Since the diffusion of lipid-soluble (^{133}Xe, [85]Kr) molecules and small lipid-insoluble molecules ([24]Na, ^{131}I, ^{86}Rb, [42]K, etc.) between the capillary and most tissues is not limiting, blood-tissue exchange depends upon the distribution and rate of capillary blood flow (Kety, 1951, 1960a, b; Landis and Pappenheimer, 1963). On this basis the exchange of an inert, freely diffusible tracer between the blood and tissues can be used for the measurement of local nutrient flow (effective capillary transport function) (Renkin, 1959a; Robertson, 1962; Kety, 1965). It is assumed that the exchange of the tracer is similar to that of normal metabolites from the standpoint of diffusion and distribution (Hyman, 1960). Studies in isolated skeletal muscle have demonstrated parallel qualitative changes in the extraction of ^{86}Rb and O_2 after nerve stimulation or administration of vasoactive agents. This indicates that ^{86}Rb exchange is a measure of blood-tissue transport, as related to normal metabolites (Renkin and Rosell, 1962; Gabel *et al.*, 1964; Winbury *et al.*, 1965a), and justifies the term nutritional circulation.

The use of diffusible tracers for measurement of local nutritional circulation is an extension of the principles discussed in the previous section. Kety (1949) introduced the use of radioactive diffusible tracers for local tissue circulation with the depot clearance (washout) technique. [24]Na was injected into the gastrocnemius muscle, and the exponential washout was followed with a Geiger–Müller counter over the muscle. Under these circumstances, C_a is negligible, and the following equation describes this function: $C = C_0 e^{-kt}$, where C represents the concentration in the tissue under study at time t, C_0 represents the initial concentration of indicator, and k represents the effective blood and lymph flow per volume of extra-cellular water of the tissue under study (f/V) (Kety, 1949; 1960a). The tissue concentration of tracer should decrease as a single exponential function, and when plotted semilogarithmically will yield a straight line, the slope of which is the clearance constant k. This is the quantitative measure of the ability of the local capillary circulation to remove (or supply) freely diffusible substances. The dose injected is not critical provided the radioactivity is sufficiently high so that counts can be recorded over a reasonable period of time, since

$$k = \frac{\log C_1 - \log C_2}{0.4343\,(t_2 - t_1)}.$$

Uptake of indicators has also been used to study nutritional circulation, and the following equations are the theoretical basis of this approach When C_a is constant, $C(T) = \lambda\,C_a\,(1 - e^{-kT})$; when C_a is variable but zero at time zero, $C(T) = \lambda k e^{-kT} \int_0^T C_a e^{kt}dt$. It is important to bear in mind that these clearance approaches do not require the tracer concentration in venous blood, and are therefore related only to capillary flow (Kety, 1960a, b). For details on the derivation of the equations described in this section, one should check the original references of Kety (1949; 1951; 1960a, b).

3.3.2. *Blood-flow-limited exchange*

The factors that are involved in the exchange of substances between the blood and tissue are the rate of capillary blood flow, capillary surface area and the permeability of the capillary and cell membrane (Kety, 1949; Gemmell and Veall, 1956; Renkin, 1959a; Landis and Pappenheimer, 1963). When the blood-tissue permeability is great in comparison to blood flow, the exchange between the blood and tissues is essentially a flow-limited process, and can be used as an estimate of local nutrient circulation. Lipid-soluble molecules and small lipid-insoluble molecules have a rate of diffusion across capillary (and cell) membranes which is far in excess of the rate of supply or removal by the capillary blood (Renkin, 1959a; Conn, 1962; Landis and Pappenheimer, 1963; Love, 1964). This makes them suitable for the determination of the effective capillary (nutritional) blood flow. Assuming that permeability is not limiting and constant, the clearance of tracer is a function of the volume of capillary blood flow and the capillary surface area available for exchange (Renkin, 1959a). Both of these are involved in tissue nutrition.

3.3.3. *Properties of tracers*

Although all of the tracers can be used for the measurement of local tissue blood flow, the area and volume of distribution differ. ^{24}Na and ^{131}I are hydrophilic ions which do not readily cross cell membranes; therefore the distribution is in the extracellular fluid (Dobson and Warner, 1957; Lassen *et al.*, 1964b). Because these ions enter and leave the extracellular fluid rapidly, they are more useful for the tissue washout approach after intraarterial or depot injection (Kety, 1949; Dobson and Warner, 1957). In order to measure the extraction of ^{24}Na by the heart muscle after intraarterial injection, it was necessary to make rapid multiple determinations in the venous outflow, and extrapolate back to zero time (Yudilevich and Martin de Julian, 1965).

^{86}Rb and ^{42}K enter the cells, and have a larger volume of distribution. The K pool of the heart and skeletal muscle cells provide an almost infinite sink, since the ^{86}Rb and ^{42}K leaving the capillaries and efflux is slow (Renkin, 1959a; Robertson, 1962; Grupp, 1963). At normal blood flow rates the exchange between the interstitial fluid and intracellular fluid is much more rapid than between the plasma and interstitial fluid, eliminating cell membrane permeability as a limiting factor (Conn, 1962). These properties make these ions particularly suitable for the uptake approach (Love and Burch, 1957; Love, 1964). ^{42}K leaves the circulation at a rate 4–5 times that of ^{24}Na, making it a more accurate tracer at higher blood flow rates (Robertson, 1962).

^{133}Xe, ^{79}Kr, ^{85}Kr, ^{131}I-antipyrine and D_2O are lipophilic, and extremely permeable to cell membranes. This results in a more complete and even distribution throughout the tissue compared to the lipid-insoluble ions such as ^{24}Na, ^{131}I, ^{42}K, and ^{86}Rb (Landis and Pappenheimer, 1963; Lassen, 1964; Lassen *et al.*, 1964b). The gases (^{133}Xe and ^{85}Kr) have been used extensively for the measurement of total cerebral blood flow by the Kety–Schmidt technique previously discussed, and for local tissue flow by the Kety washout technique, after local intraarterial or depot injections (Herd *et al.*, 1962; Lassen, 1964; Lassen *et al.*, 1964b; 1965).

Although the exchange of most tracers is blood-flow-limited at low flow rates, the lipid-insoluble substances may become diffusion-limited at high flow rates, and do not faithfully predict local tissue flow (Prentice *et al.*,

1955; Landis and Pappenheimer, 1963). Lassen (1964) compared the clearance of ^{133}Xe and ^{24}Na from the skeletal muscle of man simultaneously under a variety of conditions. At rest, the clearance of ^{133}Xe and ^{24}Na were the same; however, during reactive hyperemia, clearance of ^{133}Xe greatly exceeded that of ^{24}Na (4–5 times), indicating a diffusional limitation for ^{24}Na at high flows. Others also demonstrated that the clearance of ^{24}Na tended to a plateau as the flow rate increased (Prentice *et al.*, 1955; Walder, 1955). It was concluded that the clearance of ^{24}Na at high flow rates is a measure of the capillary diffusion capacity or permeability-surface area product. ^{133}Xe clearance truly reflects capillary blood flow (Lassen, 1964; Lassen *et al.*, 1964b). A similar study by Reller *et al.* (1964) compared the clearance of ^{42}K and ^{131}I-antipyrine in the skeletal muscle of the dog, and demonstrated that the ^{42}K values fell off substantially, relative to ^{131}I-antipyrine, as tissue flow increased.

Finally, we must realize that permeability to tracers differs among regions (Crone, 1963). For example, pulmonary capillaries are impermeable to ^{24}Na but not to D_2O (Chinard *et al.*, 1962). Thus it is necessary to consider the permeability characteristics of the particular region in the selection of a tracer substance.

3.3.4. *Factors in tissue clearance approach*

The validity of the tissue clearance approach is based on the premise that the uptake or removal of a tracer is a blood-flow-dependent process. We have previously mentioned that membrane permeability to most tracers is not limiting, except at high flow rates, and that the nonhomogeneity of a region can influence the results. Now it is appropriate to discuss some of the other factors that might influence clearance.

One of the questions that arises is the direct effect of drugs or nerve stimulation on tissue permeability to the tracer. The work of Barlow *et al.* (1961) clearly demonstrated that the blood flow:^{24}Na-clearance ratio was not influenced by agents that might alter membrane permeability. For example, administration of serotonin, hydrocortisone, or calcium, or increasing blood pH, all of which are believed to decrease permeability or inhibit Na movement, did not alter the above ratio.

When using ^{42}K or ^{86}Rb, it is important to establish that a change in the K flux does not influence ^{42}K or ^{86}Rb uptake. It has been demonstrated that the net exchange of K by the heart or the plasma level of K did not influence ^{86}Rb extraction (Love and Burch, 1959; Love, 1964). Further efflux of ^{42}K and ^{86}Rb is very slow, and not markedly influenced by changes in blood flow rate (Renkin, 1959a; Grupp, 1963).

Diffusion of tracers is little influenced by net fluid movement (Landis and Pappenheimer, 1963). An elevation of venous pressure will increase outward fluid filtration owing to an increased hydrostatic pressure, but will decrease the transport of the tracer (Rapaport *et al.*, 1952). The comparison of the clearance of ^{24}Na or ^{131}I, when injected in a depot of hypertonic albumin or isotonic saline, indicated no significant effect of the diluent (Rapaport *et al.*, 1952). Since the hypertonic albumin produces outward filtration of fluid from the capillary, it can be concluded that diffusion of tracer and ultrafiltration of fluid are independent.

Another point to be considered in the use of tracers that accumulate in the tissues (such as ^{42}K or ^{86}Rb) is the effect of the gradual saturation which may occur with prolonged administration of the tracer. As the tissue levels of ^{42}K or ^{86}Rb increase or become significant, the percentage extraction from the arterial blood may decline and would influence the clearance value. Studies in the dog heart and hindlimb demonstrate that continuous exposure to ^{42}K, ^{86}Rb or ^{84}Rb, with a rise in tissue level, will result in a gradual decline in the percentage extraction with time (Love and Burch, 1959; Mack *et al.*, 1959; Renkin, 1959b; Bing *et al.*, 1964). This does not occur with "slug" injections or with short periods of exposure to the tracer.

Significant removal of tracer from a depot by the lymphatic system or diffusion along intramuscular planes from the range of the detection probe will produce falsely high capillary clearance values. Experiments in dogs established that no more than 1.1 % of the ^{24}Na injected into the gastrocnemius muscle could be accounted for in the thoracic duct lymph (Stone and Miller, 1949); there was a good correlation between the percentage mobilized from the depot and that actually recovered in the venous blood from the limb. Likewise, diffusion along local tissue planes has been eliminated (Miller and Wilson, 1951). This establishes that the mobilization of tracer from a depot is a function primarily of the capillary blood flow (Stone and Miller, 1949; Gosselin, 1966a).

When using the depot injection approach (washout), it is critical that the injection produces minimal disturbance of the tissue (Hyman, 1960). The volume of injection can influence the clearance—large volumes will decrease the apparent clearance (Hyman, 1960). The depth of injection is also important. For example, the endocardial layers of the heart have a slower clearance than the epicardial layers (Kirk and Honig, 1964). In addition, in skeletal muscle epinephrine has a different effect on ^{24}Na clearance from deep or superficial sites (Barlow *et al.*, 1961).

Another problem that may be encountered in depot injections is the loss through the needle track (Wisham and Yalow, 1952), and the failure to inject in the same region of the tissue. To obviate some of these difficulties, a very fine catheter was inserted into the muscle (through a hypodermic needle) and left *in situ* for many days, permitting repeat injections in the exact same site (Gosselin, 1966a). The difference between two consecutive clearances was much smaller by the catheter injection technique than by injections with a needle.

One must remember that clearance from a local depot may not always provide an estimate of the overall clearance rate of the region, particularly if there is inhomogeneity. Intraarterial administration of tracer results in a more uniform distribution of the tracer to the various components of a tissue, i.e. muscle fibers and connective tissue of skeletal muscle (Hyman *et al.*, 1959; Barlow *et al.*, 1961). Since various capillaries are opening and closing in the normal state, intraarterial labeling is more effective if the muscle is dilated when the tracer is injected (Hyman and Lenthall, 1962). If the muscle was labeled in the normal state, dilator agents such as bradykinin or ATP increased blood flow but not ^{131}I clearance; if the capillaries were maximally dilated during labeling, the drugs increased ^{131}I clearance (Hyman and Lenthall, 1962). Apparently the heart is more homogeneous than skeletal muscle since ^{85}Kr or ^{133}Xe clearance values by depot injection were similar to those by intraarterial injection (Linder, 1966).

The reserve capacity of the capillary bed differs in various tissues and will influence the response to drugs. The reserve is much greater in muscle than skin (Reller *et al.*, 1964), and is small in the heart. Under basal conditions, nitroglycerin could open additional capillaries; however, if capillary dilatation was maximal, nitroglycerin had no significant effect (Winbury *et al.*, 1965c; Renkin, 1966; Winbury, 1967).

4. PHYSIOLOGICAL ASPECT OF BLOOD-TISSUE EXCHANGE

Clearance of a tracer from the tissue (washout) or blood (uptake) is related to the capillary blood flow rate, the permeability of the capillary (and cell) membrane, and the capillary surface area (Kety, 1949; Gemmell and Veall, 1956; Renkin, 1959a, 1965; Gosselin and Audino, 1966). Therefore clearance is a measure of effective capillary blood flow when permeability is not a limiting factor. With lipophilic tracers such as ^{85}Kr and ^{133}Xe, this is the case over a wide range of blood flow because of the infinite capillary permeability to these substances. Diffusional equilibrium is achieved in a single passage through a capillary, resulting in complete extraction. Permeability to ionic (lipophobic) tracers is not as great, and extraction of the tracer is less than 100%, except at low flow rates. None-theless, these tracers are of value since tissue clearance is a function of nutritional capillary circulation except at high blood flow rates.

The theoretical relationship between blood flow Q, functional extraction E, clearance C, and permeability-surface area product PS has been reviewed by Renkin (1959a, 1965, 1966). These relationships will be considered only briefly, and the original references should be consulted for further details.

Extraction is the fractional extent to which diffusional equilibrium is attained in a single capillary passage (Renkin, 1965). It is influenced by the diffusional barrier of the capillary and the time spent by blood in the capillary (blood flow) (Yudilevich and Martín de Julián, 1965). In the passage through a single capillary there is an exponential decline in the concentration of tracer, which is related to the permeability–capillary surface area product PS and the capillary blood flow Q (Renkin, 1959a; Renkin, 1965). Thus $E = 1 - e^{-PS/Q}$: e is the base of natural logarithms. Clearance is considered the minimum volume of blood/unit time required to supply or remove the tracer. In terms of the previous equation, $C = QE = Q(1 - e^{-PS/Q})$. Finally, PS is considered the maximal clearance possible for a specific tracer; it represents the diffusional capacity of the capillary bed for that tracer. On the basis of extraction, $PS = -Q \ln(1 - E)$. The interrelationship between blood flow Q and the measures of capillary transport function E, C, and PS of ionic tracers will now be discussed.

4.1. RELATION OF BLOOD FLOW TO EXTRACTION AND CLEARANCE

When a tracer substance such as ^{42}K or ^{86}Rb in the capillary diffuses into an infinite sink, the concentration in the blood falls progressively as it proceeds from the arterial to the venous end owing to cumulative diffusional loss (Renkin, 1959a; Renkin, 1965). Because permeability to ionic tracers is not infinite, the extent of diffusional equilibrium attained is related to the time the blood spends in a capillary or, in other words, to the velocity of blood flow. The theoretical equation for this function (see above) states that extraction decreases with increasing blood flow at constant PS. How do the actual data fit theory?

In the majority of studies on the hindlimb, skeletal muscle, or heart, E had an inverse relationship with Q. This was true if Q was varied mechanically (altered perfusion rate) or by vasodilator drugs (reduction in arteriolar resistance). Several groups have demonstrated the inverse relationship between E and Q in skeletal muscle using ^{86}Rb as the tracer. Some determined fractional extraction by the steady state arteriovenous difference method (Renkin, 1959a, b, 1965; Friedman, 1965; Renkin *et al.*, 1966); others used the "slug" injection method (Laurence *et al.*, 1963). The inverse relationship between E and Q has been described as linear (Renkin, 1959a, b; Laurence *et al.*, 1963), or exponential (Friedman, 1965). Much depends

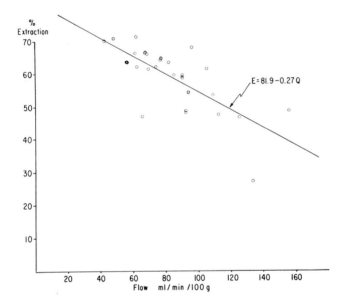

FIG. 2. Relationship of myocardial extraction of ^{86}Rb to coronary blood flow (dog). The equation represents the best linear fit to the data.

upon the range of flow studied and the assumptions made in the computations. If *PS* is assumed to be constant, then the relationship will be curvilinear, but if one determines the best fit to the data it could well be linear (Laurence *et al.*, 1963; Winbury *et al.*, 1965b). Certainly over a restricted range of blood flow values the E/Q relationship would appear to be linear.

The inverse relationship of fractional extraction to blood flow has been repeatedly demonstrated in the isolated or intact heart perfused with blood or saline at various flow rates. The isotopes [42]K, ^{86}Rb, and [84]Rb were administered by constant infusion or a "slug", and the species included rabbit and dog (Nolting *et al.*, 1958; Love and Burch, 1959; Mack *et al.*,

1959; Winbury *et al.*, 1965b; Moir, 1966). Figure 2 illustrates this relationship in the intact dog heart perfused with blood at various flow rates.
Likewise, when coronary blood flow was increased by graded doses of
nitroglycerin, E fell progressively, and all the control and drug Q and E
values fit an inverse linear relationship (Winbury *et al.*, 1965a; Winbury
and Gabel, 1967).

Others originally reported that fractional extraction by the heart of dog
and man was independent of blood flow (Bennish and Bing, 1962; Bing

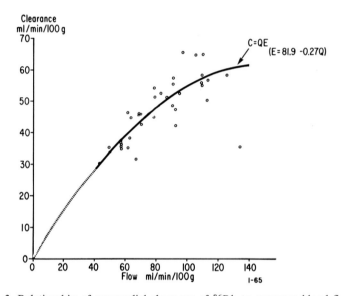

FIG. 3. Relationship of myocardial clearance of ^{86}Rb to coronary blood flow
(dog). The equation describing this function is based on the E versus Q function
of Fig. 1. Note that clearance becomes asymptotic at higher blood flow (Winbury,
1967).

et al., 1964; Martin and Yudilevich, 1964; Cohen *et al.*, 1965a; Yudilevich
and Martín de Julián, 1965). This may be due to the restricted range of
blood flow studied, and the fact that multiple values were not obtained in
the same heart. Recently one of these groups reinvestigated the E/Q
relationship over a wider range of Q and changed their opinions, reporting
that as Q increased E declined, and when Q decreased E rose (Cohen *et al.*,
1967).

It would appear that the majority of studies agree that E has an inverse
relationship with Q. It has been suggested that this is not a result of in-

complete equilibrium across the capillary wall but rather that extraction in the capillary is complete and the E/Q relationship expresses the ratio of blood passing through nutritional and nonnutritional paths (Friedman, 1965). As flow declines, a larger portion of the total flow goes to capillary (nutritional) paths. This concept has been questioned by Yudilevich and Martín de Julián (1965), since it would be necessary for 30% of the blood flow of the heart to pass through nonnutritional paths. Such a large shunt flow is unlikely.

Clearance of ^{86}Rb is highly correlated with Q in the heart and skeletal muscle, but increases less than proportionally (Renkin, 1965). In some studies C was determined directly on the basis of tissue concentration/arterial concentration (Love and O'Meallie, 1963; Love *et al.*, 1965b; Moir, 1966); in other studies C was derived from $E \times Q$ (Renkin, 1959a; Bennish and Bing, 1962; Laurence *et al.*, 1963; Winbury *et al.*, 1965b; Yudilevich and Martín de Julián, 1965).

At low flow rates, C and Q are similar, but as Q increases the difference between Q and C becomes greater, and C tends to become limited by PS. Over a restricted range of Q values, the interrelationship between C and Q in the heart and skeletal muscle may appear to be linear (Winbury *et al.*, 1965a). However, analysis over a more extensive blood flow range demonstrated that the C/Q relationship of the heart is curvilinear (Winbury *et al.*, 1965b; Winbury, 1967), and may be logarithmic (Love and O'Meallie, 1963) or parabolic (Love *et al.*, 1965b). In general C ^{86}Rb/Q relationship for the heart has a steep slope at Q values of < 70 ml/min per 100 g, but tends to flatten out and become asymptotic at $Q > 100$. Figure 3 from Winbury (1967) illustrates this relationship, which has the equation $C = Q (81.9 - 0.27Q)$.

4.2. PERMEABILITY–SURFACE AREA PRODUCT PS. RELATION TO BLOOD FLOW AND DRUGS

PS depends on the permeability per unit surface area of the capillary to the tracer P and on the effective capillary surface area S (Renkin, 1959a; 1965). It has the dimensions of ml/min per 100 g, and corresponds to the maximal clearance possible in a capillary bed of given permeability and surface area. At normal blood flow values, capillary or tissue permeability to most tracers is not limiting and constant; PS can therefore be considered as related to the capillary surface area available for the transport of nutritional substances (Landis and Pappenheimer, 1963). However, at excessive blood flow, diffusion of ionic tracers may be limiting, and PS is then a measure of the diffusion capacity of the capillary bed for the tracer (Renkin, 1959a; 1966).

At constant blood flow, a change in E or C is a result of a similar directional change in PS. This is evident on the basis of the theoretical equations relating these variables to PS (see above). The capillary surface area S is a function of the number of open capillaries, and at the maximal PS value for a specific substance, it is assumed that all functional capillaries are open (Walder, 1953; Kitchin, 1963; Renkin, 1966; Winbury, 1967).

PS is altered by many factors, including neurogenic and humoral agents, drugs, and by changes in the rate of blood flow. At constant blood flow, sympathetic stimulation or infusion of norepinephrine decreased PS for ^{86}Rb in skeletal muscle to about one fourth the resting level, while metabolic vasodilatation due to stimulation of the muscle or reactive hyperemia doubled the PS (Renkin, 1966; Renkin *et al.*, 1966). The total range of control is 8–10 fold from the lowest to highest value (Renkin, 1966). Nitroglycerin can increase PS in the heart and skeletal muscle perfused at constant flow (Winbury and Gabel, 1967).

Although PS is considered to be relatively constant in a basal metabolic state, it is related to the blood flow rate in skeletal muscle and heart (Renkin, 1959b; Winbury *et al.*, 1965b, c; Renkin, 1966; Winbury, 1967). When the coronary arteries of the intact dogs were perfused with blood at various rates above and below the basal values, it was found that the C ^{86}Rb/Q relationship did not conform to a single PS value (Winbury, 1967). At lower flows, PS was about 60 ml/min per 100 g, and at the highest flows it was about 80. The theoretical PS/Q curve was calculated on the basis of the C ^{86}Rb/Q relationship ($PS = -Q \ln [1 - (81.9 - 0.27Q)]$). PS increased rapidly at low flow values, but reached a plateau of 80 ml/min per 100 g at a total coronary blood flow rate of 100 ml/min per 100 g (Fig. 4). This is the point of maximal capillary surface area with all functional myocardial capillaries open. At the basal coronary blood flow rate of 60–80 ml/min per 100 g, PS had a value of about 60. Assuming that the plateau PS value of 80 represents maximal surface area with all myocardial capillaries open, it can be inferred that under basal conditions 75% (60/80) of the capillaries are open. The coronary capillary reserve, one quarter of the total, is smaller than the skeletal muscle capillary reserve, one half of the total (Renkin, 1966).

The importance of the myocardial capillary reserve was demonstrated by some studies with nitroglycerin and pentaerythritol tetranitrate. Coronary flow was constant, and the drugs were injected into the coronary circuit. With $PS > 80$ ml/min per 100 g the "nitrate" coronary dilator drugs produced no change, or a decrease in *PS*, while with *PS* values < 80 there was usually an increase (Winbury, 1967). These data confirm the concept that with *PS* equal to 80 ml/min per 100 g, the capillary surface area is maximal, and coronary reserve is exhausted.

A vasodilator drug may increase capillary clearance by increasing blood flow (arteriolar dilatation), and/or by opening more capillaries, thereby

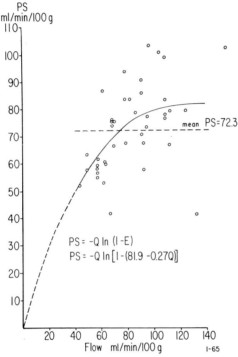

$$PS = -Q \ln (1 - E)$$
$$PS = -Q \ln [1 - (81.9 - 0.27Q)]$$

FIG. 4. Relationship of myocardial capillary surface area *PS* to coronary blood flow (dog). The theoretical curve is derived from the equations. Note that *PS* plateaus at a total coronary blood flow rate of about 100 ml/min per 100 g (Winbury, 1967).

increasing *PS* (precapillary sphincter dilatation). The influence of drug induced changes in *Q* on *PS* and *C* is illustrated (Fig. 5) by a comparison of the effects of intracoronary injection of nitroglycerin at constant blood flow and at constant pressure (Winbury, 1967; Winbury and Gabel, 1967). The increase in $C\,^{86}Rb$ was augmented considerably when the blood flow was permitted to increase, while *PS* was augmented slightly. It would appear that the enhanced effect on $C\,^{86}Rb$ results from the additive effect

of an increase in capillary surface area (*PS*) and blood flow. However, when
PS is maximal, the only mechanism for increasing clearance is a rise in
blood flow.

Since lipophilic tracers have almost infinite permeability it is difficult to
determine a *PS* value, because *P* is not limiting even at high blood flows.
PS can be computed for ionic tracers, because permeability becomes the
limiting factor at high flow rates. Studies comparing both types of tracers
have been considered previously in Section 3.3.

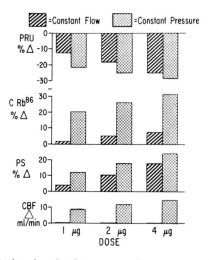

FIG. 5. Effect of nitroglycerin (intracoronary) at constant flow or constant
pressure. When blood flow increased (constant pressure) the changes in clearance
($C^{86}Rb$) were augmented. This demonstrates that clearance is influenced by
capillary surface area *PS* and blood flow *CBF* (Winbury and Gabel, 1967).

4.3. PHYSIOLOGICAL SHUNTING

The questions about the existence of anatomic shunts have already been
covered in Section 2. Opinions differ about such shunts; however, there is
evidence for physiological shunting. The best example is the marked increase in skeletal muscle blood flow with no change in $C^{24}Na$ produced by
stimulation of the medullary cholinergic vasodilator center (Hyman *et al.*,
1959). The mechanisms involved in physiological shunting will be considered in this section.

When shunting occurs there is competition between the functional capillary bed and the bypass circulation for the available blood. The bypass is

assumed to be a vessel or bed through which transport of solutes is limited, or cannot occur. This could be a true arteriovenous shunt or a capillary bed with poor diffusional capacity or small surface area (short capillaries) (Renkin *et al.*, 1966). These will have a low PS/Q ratio compared with normal functional capillaries. Another bypass mechanism would be nonuniform distribution of blood flow between regions of different metabolic function and rate (Barlow *et al.*, 1961; Landis and Pappenheimer, 1963).

4.3.1. *Skeletal muscle*

Total extraction of ^{86}Rb by skeletal muscle is always less than 100%, even at exceedingly low flows. On the assumption that extraction of ^{86}Rb is complete in true capillaries, Friedman (1965) concluded that there must be a bypass flow in skeletal muscle. Dilatation of precapillary sphincters produced a passive redistribution of blood flow from bypasses to capillaries as a result of a reduction in the distending pressure and the closure of bypasses. In the isolated hindlimb of the rabbit or cat it was noted that there was a critical blood flow rate below which there was no clearance of ^{24}Na from a depot. At higher rates, clearance was linearly related to flow. The critical flow was assumed to represent flow through arteriovenous capillaries or shunts (Walder, 1955).

Others do not agree with the reasoning that there must be a bypass circulation or arteriovenous shunting to explain some of these data (Freis *et al.*, 1957; Renkin, 1959a, b). The definition of a shunt in physiological terms might help to clarify matters. Any pathway between the artery and vein which has a smaller extraction ratio than the average for the vascular bed acts as a type of shunt; this means any capillary pathway in which the ratio PS/Q is less than that for the entire system of capillaries. There is nonuniformity of the capillary circulation, which can be altered under various circumstances and results in an alteration in PS. For example, during excessive skeletal muscle contraction at constant blood flow, PS reached a peak and then declined during the period of contraction, even though arteriolar dilatation persisted (Renkin, 1965; Renkin *et al.*, 1966). This secondary reduction in PS is probably associated with the nonuniform distribution of blood flow in relation to surface area, which has an effect similar to shunting. The following hypothesis proposed by Renkin *et al.* (1966) explains the secondary decline in PS, and may serve to explain the physiological shunting seen in other studies.

There are short capillary pathways (low PS/Q; low surface area) which are all completely closed at rest; in addition some of the long capillaries (high surface area and high PS/Q) are closed. In the microcirculation scheme (Fig. 1), the shunt could be considered as short capillaries. Moderate exercise opens up additional long capillaries and produces an increase in PS. However, during excessive exercise, all capillaries open and there is redistribution of available blood with an increase through short capillaries and a decrease through the long capillaries. This produces a reduction in the overall PS, and is, in effect a form of physiological shunting. This hypothesis is attractive in that it can explain the phenomenon of shunting in areas where the existence of anatomic shunts has been challenged. In this case the short capillaries, which have small surface area, act as a bypass mechanism. One prerequisite to this hypothesis is that the precapillary sphincters of the short capillary beds have a low sensitivity to the substance involved in autoregulation of capillary blood flow. Likewise, as there are differences in the response of arterioles and precapillary sphincters to drugs, there may be qualitative differences in the response of precapillary sphincters.

4.3.2. *Heart*

The response of the dog heart maintained at constant coronary flow to vasodilator agents is somewhat dependent upon the level of PS. When PS was below the maximal value, nitroglycerin produced an increase; however, when the control PS was equal to or above the maximum, nitroglycerin produced no change or a decrease in PS. Assuming that all capillaries are open at maximal PS, then the reduction in PS produced by nitroglycerin could be a result of shunting and diversion of blood from functional capillaries (Winbury *et al.*, 1965c; Winbury, 1967). Another possible explanation of these data is opening of capillaries with a low PS (short capillaries) leading to redistribution of blood and a fall in total PS. This is in accord with the hypothesis of Renkin *et al.* (1966) just discussed.

Other studies on the heart have been interpreted to indicate a shunt phenomenon. Comparison of the effects of pentaerythritol tetranitrate (PETN) with those of dipyridamole on fractional myocardial ^{86}Rb uptake and total coronary flow showed a different pattern of response (Winbury and Pensinger, 1966; Winbury, 1967). PETN increased ^{86}Rb uptake 40% in the absence of any change in blood flow. Dipyridamole also increased ^{86}Rb uptake 40%, but blood flow was increased more than 100%. Further, in some animals dipyridamole increased blood flow but produced no change in ^{86}Rb uptake. Presumably dipyridamole produced some form of shunting even though PS was not maximal. We can conclude that PS was not maximal because PETN increased ^{86}Rb uptake in the absence of any change in blood flow and the only mechanism for this effect would be enhancement of capillary surface area. Another group studying dipyrida-mole and the effect on E ^{86}Rb also concluded that when blood flow was elevated by this agent, the effect could be due to a shunting through non-nutritional vessels (Moir, 1966). On the other hand, when myocardial capillary function was assessed on the basis of transport of tritiated water, it was concluded that all of the blood flow increase due to dipyridamole is a result of an increase in capillary flow (Palmer *et al.*, 1966).

If we think in terms of the concept proposed by Renkin *et al.* (1966), the difference in the results with dipyridamole between the groups using ^{86}Rb and tritiated water can be explained. There is infinite permeability of the capillaries to tritiated water, which means that when short capillaries are open the overall clearance of the tritiated water would not decline. On the other hand, if there is excessive flow through shorter channels, clearance and *PS* measured by ^{86}Rb will fall owing to increasingly impaired distri-bution. The apparent shunting based on studies with ionic tracers is physiological in nature and would apply to other substances involved in tissue nutrition. If there were true anatomic shunts, this would be dis-tinguished with tritiated water as well as ^{86}Rb.

There is another type of shunting that is of importance from the meta-bolic standpoint but which may not be detected by the conventional approach to the study of regional nutritional blood flow. This involves the distribution of blood flow within a region to areas of high and low metabolic requirements (Barlow *et al.*, 1961). If a drug were to produce a plethora of blood flow to the area of low metabolic requirements at the expense of the blood flow to the area of high metabolic requirement, there would be regional ischemia, and a form of shunting. This may not be recognized if there is uniformity in the PS/Q ratio of the capillary beds throughout the region.

5. METHODS FOR STUDY OF NUTRITIONAL CIRCULATION WITH DIFFUSIBLE INDICATORS

There are two basic approaches to the study of capillary transport func-tion (nutritional circulation) (Dobson and Warner, 1957; Love, 1964; Ross and Friesinger, 1965; Winbury *et al.*, 1965a). One depends upon washout of the diffusible tracer from the region following direct injection into the tissue or administration through the arterial supply; the decline in the tissue level is determined by a Geiger–Müller tube or an external scintillation probe. The other basic approach is the measurement of the uptake of the diffusible tracer from the arterial blood. Uptake by the tissue can be measured directly by scintillation probe or indirectly by difference between the amount in arterial and venous blood. The clearance of particulate tracers from the blood by the liver and the clearance of labeled hippurate by the kidney are considered as special applications of the uptake method.

Different types of isotopes are best suited for each approach. Washout depends on the rapid movement of the tracer from the extracellular fluid (or tissue) to the capillary blood, whereas uptake depends on the tracer remaining in the tissue after the removal from the arterial blood. Various isotopes have been used for either approach, but it is easier to select the isotope on the basis of the approach and the property of the tracer. The general requirement is similar for both approaches, namely that clearance of the tracer from the tissue or blood is a flow-limited process. This means that the blood-tissue permeability should be great in relation to blood flow. As mentioned previously, this is satisfied by the lipophilic tracers over a very wide range of blood flow and by the lipophobic ionic tracers over the physiological blood flow range. In general, the tracer should have transport characteristics similar to normal metabolites but should be stable and not enter into metabolic processes (Hyman, 1960). The ionic tracers satisfy these requirements and they are therefore considered related to the nutritional effectiveness of the capillary circulation.

5.1. WASHOUT APPROACH

5.1.1. *Principle*

The rate of removal of a diffusible tracer introduced into a limited part of a tissue is a function of local tissue nutrient circulation. This is the basis of the original ^{24}Na tissue-clearance method described by Kety (1949). On the basis of the theoretical equations in Section 3.3.3, the tissue concentration should decrease exponentially. Of course, the validity of the approach depends upon a rapid equilibration of the tracer in the extracellular fluid with the capillary blood. Blood flowing through nonnutritional beds (shunting) does not contribute to the washout.

5.1.2. *Depot washout*

The procedure described by Kety (1949) has been used extensively by others in the original form or with various modifications. The common basis for all of the washout procedures is that clearance of a diffusible tracer from a local depot in the tissue is a reflection of functional capillary blood flow to that area, as described by the following equation:

$$C = C_0 e^{-kt}; \quad k = f/V.$$

^{24}NaCl in 0.5–1.0 ml of isotonic saline was injected into the gastrocnemius muscle of the human, and the radioactivity was determined with a shielded Geiger–Müller tube placed next to the calf. Counts were recorded at one-minute intervals and corrected for background radiation. The corrected values were plotted semilogarithmically against time, and a straight line of the slope k (clearance constant) drawn through the points. As previously shown (Section 3.3), the clearance constant

$$k = \frac{\log C_1 - \log C_2}{0.4343 \, (t_2 - t_1)};$$

C_1 and C_2 are cpm at time t_1 and t_2, respectively; $0.4343 = \log e$.

The clearance function satisfied the requirements of a simple exponential curve, suggesting that the disappearance of ^{24}Na is a flow-limited process, and that perfusion is homogeneous. The resting clearance constant of 5% per min was reduced to 0.2% per min by a tourniquet applied above the depot, and increased to 12% per min by reactive hyperemia, and to 11.3% per min by exercise. Addition of epinephrine to the depot injection reduced k to 1% per min. These original studies established the validity of the approach and developed the concept of nutritional circulation.

In the same year, Stone and Miller (1949) determined k in dogs on the basis of disappearance of ^{24}Na from a depot in the gastrocnemius muscle and the isotope appearing in the venous blood. There was a good agreement between the percentage of ^{24}Na mobilized and that recovered in the blood from the limb; little was removed by the lymphatic system, which indicates that the washout is related to capillary blood flow. Franke *et al.* (1950) failed to demonstrate an exponential function for the rate of removal of ^{24}Na from the hamstring muscles of the dog, particularly after the first 10 min. They suggested using the simpler calculation of percentage of activity remaining per unit time. For example, the average intramuscular clearance constant for 10 min in the dog was 0.0534 or 59.4% activity remaining.

Semple *et al.* (1951) modified the original Kety method by using "half dispersal time" instead of the clearance constant k. The "half dispersal time" represents the time required for the tissue depot concentration to decrease 50% ($t_{\frac{1}{2}}$); this was obtained from a semilog plot of cpm versus time. The longer the time the slower the clearance. McGirr (1952) observed variation in the counting rate for the first few minutes after injection of the depot, but there was an exponential decrease in count rate if the first 5 min were ignored. Results were also expressed as "half time" from which the clearance constant can be calculated since

$$k = \frac{\ln 2}{t_{\frac{1}{2}}} = \frac{0.693}{t_{\frac{1}{2}}}.$$

Others (Rapaport *et al.*, 1952; Coffman, 1963) also found it necessary to discard the data from the first few minutes after injection of ^{24}Na or ^{131}I; this was followed by a straight line of constant slope.

Wisham and Yalow (1952) were able to reconcile the difference between the results of Kety (1949) and Franke *et al.* (1950). Clearance was determined in skin, subcutaneous tissue and muscle, and the raw data indicated that muscle had a curve consisting of two components while the other tissues had a single component. It was suggested that the second component of the muscle clearance curve was from ^{24}Na deposited in the subcutaneous tissue when the needle was withdrawn. The second component, which is a straight line based on the final 8–10 points, was subtracted stepwise from the original raw data to yield the net activity from the muscle alone. This net activity is a single exponential of much shorter "half time" than the second component. The average percentage of the total activity due to the second component (subcutaneous) at the initial time of recording was 44%.

The same basic depot "washout" approach has been applied to other tissues including uterus (McClure Browne and Veall, 1953; Munck *et al.*, 1964), testis (Setchell *et al.*, 1966), heart (Madoff and Hollander, 1961; Salisbury *et al.*, 1962; Kirk and Honig, 1964; Linder, 1966), liver (Sigel and Que, 1965), etc. All have demonstrated an exponential "washout" rate.

With ionic tracers such as ^{24}Na or ^{131}I, these methods have been used to determine the clearance constant, which is a function of blood flow, since the basic equation can be expressed as $C = C_0 e^{-(f/V)t}$, where f represents blood flow and V the volume in which the tracer is distributed, i.e. extracellular fluid volume for ^{24}Na (Kety, 1949; McClure Browne and Veall, 1953). It follows then that

$$f = k \times V = \frac{0.693}{t_{\frac{1}{2}}} V.$$

Using these equations, Kirk and Honig (1964) have estimated coronary capillary flow with ^{131}I on the assumption that the tracer was distributed in the same compartment as ^{24}Na.

Estimation of capillary blood flow in terms of milliliters per unit weight per unit time is easily accomplished with gases such as ^{133}Xe and ^{85}Kr, because the blood-tissue partition coefficient has been or can be determined experimentally. The applicable equation follows:

$$f \text{ (ml per 100 g/min)} = \frac{k\,\lambda\,\times\,100}{\rho},$$

where λ is the blood-tissue partition coefficient and ρ the specific gravity of the tissue (Herd *et al.*, 1962; Tønnesen, 1964; Regan *et al.*, 1966; Setchell *et al.*, 1966). Because ρ is very close to 1, it is frequently omitted in the computations. Lassen *et al.* (1964b, 1965) have recently described modifications of the depot clearance method which permits calculation of blood flow at any time during the ^{133}Xe clearance curve from muscle. The output of the ratemeter (coupled to a scintillation probe) was recorded on a logarithmic potentiometer writing on linear paper, and the clearance rate can be determined from the tangent of the curve.

5.1.3. *Washout after intraarterial injection*

The depot injection technique measures blood flow in a circumscribed small area, which may not reflect the flow rate in the entire region. This is especially true when there is heterogeneous perfusion of the region, and a drug may have a selective effect on the capillary flow of one component. Intraarterial administration of a tracer labels the entire region supplied by the vessel (Ross *et al.*, 1964), and washout studies then permit a qualitative and quantitative measure of the regional circulation. It is thus possible to determine, simultaneously, tissue perfusion as well as the relative homogeneity or heterogeneity of the region, and the relative volume of the compartments (Dobson and Warner, 1957).

Methods have been developed for the determination of the clearance, on the basis of washout after intraarterial administration of the tracer to various regions. These include skeletal muscle (Prentice *et al.*, 1955; Dobson and Warner, 1957; Hyman *et al.*, 1959; Dobson and Warner, 1960; Hyman and Lenthall, 1962; Paldino *et al.*, 1962), skin (Rubinstein *et al.*, 1964; Thorburn *et al.*, 1966), heart (Herd *et al.*, 1962; Johansson *et al.*, 1964; Ross *et al.*, 1964; Klein *et al.*, 1965; Rees and Redding, 1966; Rees *et al.*, 1966), brain (Ingvar and Lassen, 1962; Lassen *et al.*, 1964a; Skinhoj *et al.*, 1964; Høedt-Rasmussen *et al.*, 1966; Lassen and Høedt-Rasmussen, 1966), kidney (Thorburn *et al.*, 1963; Ladefoged *et al.*, 1965), liver (Rees *et al.*, 1964), and testis (Setchell *et al.*, 1966). The disappearance of tracer (^{24}Na, ^{131}I, ^{85}Kr, or ^{133}Xe) was followed in the usual manner by an external probe. In some of the procedures developed for the heart, the tracer was injected into the left ventricular cavity (Cohen *et al.*, 1964), the ascending aorta close to the coronary ostia (Holmberg *et al.*, 1967), or into the coronary venous system (Harman *et al.*, 1966). Analysis of the washout curves after intraarterial injection is the same as previously described for the depot clearance method.

5.1.4. *Analysis of multi exponential washout curves*

Dobson and Warner (1957) observed that the ^{24}Na washout from the hindlimb of man after rapid intraarterial injection was a multiexponential function, and developed an approach to the analysis of data from a multi-compartmental vascular system, and estimation of regional blood flow. A similar approach to the study of cerebral circulation was developed by Lassen *et al.* (1964a) and by Høedt-Rasmussen *et al.* (1966), and for skeletal muscle circulation by Tønnesen and Sejrsen (1967).

In a one-component system (homogeneous perfusion), washout from the tissue after intraarterial injection of isotope follows the familiar mono-exponential clearance function: $A = A_0 e^{-kt}$, where A represents the counting rate at time t and A_0 the rate at zero time. The clearance constant k is determined in the usual manner from a semilog plot of activity relative to time. When there are several compartments in parallel (differing per-fusion rate and/or volumes of distribution), the washout curve is a series of exponentials corresponding to the number of compartments. The general equation describing this function is

$$A = A_{o1} \times e^{-k_1 t} + A_{o2} \times e^{-k_2 t} + A_{o3} \times e^{-k_3 t} + \ldots A_{on} \times e^{-k_n t},$$

where n denotes the number of compartments.

This type of function can be analyzed graphically by plotting the recorded decrease in total radioactivity as a function of time on a semi-logarithmic basis. Sequential "curve striping" will yield a series of mono-exponential curves corresponding to the number of individual compart-ments. Extrapolation of each curve back to zero time will yield the initial concentration A_0. Thus one obtains the A_0 (zero intercept) and k (clearance constant) for each compartment. Nutrient blood flow for each compart-ment can be computed in the conventional manner: $f = k\lambda/\rho$.

Since the isotope injection was of short duration the concentration in each compartment at the onset of desaturation C_0 is not equal, the faster perfused tissue dominates the washout curve and results in too high a per-fusion value and volume of distribution. Therefore it is necessary to correct for the unequal saturation by determination of the relative and fractional volumes of each compartment and then compute the weighted flow. From the *relative volume* of each compartment (A_{o1}/k_1) the *fractional volume* of each can be obtained by

$$(\text{fractional}) \ V_1 = \frac{A_{o1}}{k_1} \bigg/ \frac{A_{o1}}{k_1} + \frac{A_{o2}}{k_2} + \frac{A_{o3}}{k_3} + \ldots + \frac{A_{on}}{k_n}.$$

This equation has been simplified by Tønnesen and Sejrsen (1967) by direct use of the individual $t_{\frac{1}{2}}$ values as follows:

$$(\text{fractional}) \ V_1 =$$

$$\frac{A_{o1} \times t_{\frac{1}{2},1}}{(A_{o1} \times t_{\frac{1}{2},1}) + (A_{o2} \times t_{\frac{1}{2},2}) + (A_{o3} \times t_{\frac{1}{2},3}) + (A_{on} \times t_{\frac{1}{2},n})}$$

The sum of the V values is unity. The *weighted* flow (or k) of each compartment can be obtained by the product of the fractional volume times the flow (or k) of the respective compartment: weighted f_1 (or k_1) $= V_1 \times f_1$ (or k_1). The mean flow is the sum of the weighted flows.

By means of this method of analysis it has been possible to determine the nutritive blood flow and the relative weight of the gray and white matter in the brain (Skinhoj *et al.*, 1964; Høedt-Rasmussen *et al.*, 1966; Obrist *et al.*, 1967) of various compartments in skeletal muscle (Dobson and Warner, 1957; Tønnesen and Sejrsen, 1957) and skin (Thorburn *et al.*, 1966) of the cortex and the medulla in the kidney (Thorburn *et al.*, 1963; Carriere *et al.*, 1966), and of normal and ischemic area of the heart (Johansson *et al.*, 1964; Johansson *et al.*, 1965).

Ingvar and Lassen (1962) avoided the necessity of these corrections for unequal saturation by producing the same C_0 in all compartments. This was accomplished by using a stepwise procedure for intraarterial administration of ^{85}Kr over a few minutes. The initial slope of the curve of log tissue concentration versus time is obtained by drawing the tangent at zero time. This line represents a single exponential function from which the *average* blood flow can be determined from $t_{\frac{1}{2}}$ and the average λ.

Recently Høedt-Rasmussen *et al.* (1966) and Tønnesen and Sejrsen (1967) have applied the stochastic theory to the measurement of *mean* cerebral and skeletal muscle blood flow. ^{133}Xe or ^{85}Kr was injected rapidly into the artery supplying the region, and the buildup and subsequent clearance of isotope was recorded with a scintillation detector. It is necessary to determine the maximum height and total area of the radioactivity curve. Average flow is derived from the following equation:

$$f = \lambda \left(\frac{\text{height}}{\text{area}} \right) \text{ ml/g per min.}$$

In this case λ is the average value for the compartments of the tissue and should be determined experimentally. There was good agreement between blood-flow values derived from the stochastic method and multicompartment method of analysis. However, by the stochastic method the relative weight and perfusion of the compartments cannot be determined.

5.2. UPTAKE APPROACH

5.2.1. *Principle*

Clearance of a tracer from the arterial blood passing through a region is a measure of the local nutritional circulation. Extraction by the tissues is a flow-limited process, because the blood-tissue permeability is great in comparison with the blood flow. ^{42}K and ^{86}Rb have been used for the uptake approach because: (1) there is rapid exchange between the capillary blood and the tissues; (2) the K content within cells is great, and therefore provides an almost infinite sink for the ^{42}K or ^{86}Rb that leaves the capillary, and (3) the efflux of ^{42}K or ^{86}Rb is very slow and does not appear to influence uptake (Love and Burch, 1957b; Renkin, 1959a; Renkin and Rosell, 1962; Love, 1964). Therefore the accumulation of ^{42}K or ^{86}Rb by a tissue is an approach to the measurement of nutritional circulation. Accumulation within the tissue is an important advantage for the uptake method but not a requisite. However, uptake studies with tracers that do not accumulate (^{24}Na, ^{131}I) are more difficult, and require corrections for washout in order to determine extraction at zero time (Martin and Yudilevich, 1964; Yudilevich and Martín de Julián, 1965).

The uptake approach has been used by measurement of extraction using a single or double isotope procedure or by direct determination of blood clearance by the tissues. In order to use the first procedure, arterial and venous samples are required; for the second procedure, a measure of tissue concentration and arterial concentration are required.

The determination of renal blood flow or glomerular filtration rate using a single intravenous injection of ^{131}I (or ^{125}I) Hippuran and/or ^{131}I Hypaque, respectively, is an uptake approach. These substances are removed only by the kidney, being ultimately excreted in the urine. Therefore the tracer removed from the blood accumulates in an infinite sink—the urine. Since the purpose of these newer tracer methods is to eliminate collection of urine, the clearance is based on the decline in blood level (Gott *et al.*, 1962; Stokes and Ter-Pogossian, 1964; Pritchard *et al.*, 1965; Dabaj *et al.*, 1966).

The hepatic circulation can be studied by means of uptake of colloidal substances such as ^{32}P-labeled colloidal chromic phosphate or colloidal ^{198}Au. This is based on the fact that the reticuloendothelial system of the liver (and spleen) is highly effective in removing these colloidal substances in a single passage (Dobson and Jones, 1952; Vetter *et al.*, 1954). Here again we have a type of infinite sink, and the liver blood flow can be estimated on the basis of the disappearance rate of colloid from the blood stream or accumulation in the liver (Dobson and Jones, 1952; Vetter *et al.*, 1954; Iio *et al.*, 1960; Restrepo *et al.*, 1960; Stroun *et al.*, 1962).

5.2.2. *Extraction*

Extraction of a tracer such as ^{42}K or ^{86}Rb is determined on the basis of the concentration or amount of tracer in the arterial and venous blood: $E = (A - V)/A$, where E is the extraction ratio and A and V the concentration or amount of tracer in the arterial and venous blood, respectively. If blood flow Q is known, clearance C and permeability-surface area coefficient, PS, can be calculated from E; $C = Q \times E$; $PS = -Q \ln (1 - E)$. At constant blood flow, changes in E are directly related to changes in C and PS, and predict direct effects on capillary surface area via the precapillary sphincters. However, when Q can vary, it is difficult to make predictions directly from E. It was previously shown (Section 4) that E varies inversely with Q, when varied by alteration of perfusion rate or a vasodilator agent such as nitroglycerin. Under these circumstances, it is difficult to determine whether changes in E are a result of changes in Q or a direct action on the nutritional circulation.

With nonconstant flow it is necessary to compare the E/Q relationship in the absence and presence of the drug and to determine whether there is a significant difference of the slope (Winbury *et al.*, 1965a; Renkin *et al.*, 1966). Friedman (1965) demonstrated that papaverine, muscle contraction, or arterial occlusion reduced the $E\,^{86}$Rb$/Q$ slope of skeletal muscle but did not alter the zero intercept indicating that the capillary surface area was increased. Renkin *et al.* (1966) noted that the rise in skeletal muscle blood flow produced by stimulation of the muscle was accompanied by a slight increase in $E\,^{86}$Rb, and an increase in C and PS that was proportional to the increased blood flow. When the muscle was at rest, a like increase in blood flow reduced E, and the change in C and PS were much less than proportional to Q, which demonstrates that metabolic vasodilatation produced a direct relaxation of precapillary sphincters.

(*a*) *Single isotope methods for extraction*

Constant arterial level. It is possible to determine E continuously by perfusion of the region at a constant rate with blood containing ^{86}Rb or ^{42}K, and constant recording of venous radioactivity. Renkin *et al.* (Renkin, 1959a; Renkin and Rosell, 1962; Renkin *et al.*, 1966) have developed such a procedure for studies on skeletal muscle, and the same fundamental method can be applied to most any region.

Basically, the procedure requires isolation of the muscle (gracilis in dog or gastrocnemius-plantaris in cat) from the remainder of the circulation. Blood containing ^{86}Rb or ^{42}K was perfused at a constant rate by a special pump from a reservoir into the arterial supply to the muscle. The venous outflow from the isolated muscle was passed through a coil of tubing in a well counter coupled with a ratemeter and a direct writing recorder. Any change in venous radioactivity indicates a change in E ^{86}Rb that is directly related to like changes in C and PS, since the blood flow is constant. Corrections for ^{86}Rb taken up by red cells amount to about 5%. After prolonged perfusion runs it is also necessary to make a correction for ^{86}Rb accumulated by the tissue. If this is not done, the small amount of ^{86}Rb diffusing back into the capillary blood will produce an apparent reduction in E. Back-diffusion is measured by perfusing the tissue with ^{86}Rb free blood and by estimation of tissue level, C_T, by $C_T = C_v/E$, where C_v is the venous radioactivity. It is also possible to determine E on the basis of the outflow of ^{86}Rb in venous blood. After 1–2 hr of perfusion, C_T was about 10–20% of the arterial level (Renkin and Rosell, 1962).

Extraction was determined in the isolated rabbit heart by perfusion with blood containing ^{86}Rb for a period of 20 min (Mack *et al.*, 1959). The outflow was collected and the concentration of ^{86}Rb determined. The average extraction over the 20-min period was calculated in the usual fashion.

"Slug" injection. Gabel *et al.* (1964) developed a single "slug" isotope method which avoided continuous perfusion of ^{86}Rb and the buildup of tissue levels. The hindlimb or gastrocnemius muscle (Winbury *et al.*, 1965a) of the dog was isolated from the systemic circulation. Arterial blood from the systemic circulation was pumped into the arterial supply of the region at a constant rate. The total venous outflow from the limb was passed through a well counter for the determination of the venous radioactivity, and back to the systemic circulation. ^{86}Rb was rapidly injected (as a slug) into the arterial supply, and the radioactivity in the venous blood was recorded continuously as a time–concentration curve. The area under the curve represents the unextracted ^{86}Rb. Extraction was calculated as follows:

$$E = \frac{{}^{86}\text{Rb injected} - {}^{86}\text{Rb in venous blood}}{{}^{86}\text{Rb injected}}.$$

The ^{86}Rb not extracted by the region is diluted by the systemic circulation and extracted by other tissues. Thus recirculation of ^{86}Rb is insignificant. Since the tissue is exposed to ^{86}Rb for only short periods, there is minimal buildup of tissue level, and correction is not required.

The flow rate through the well counter must be constant throughout the entire experiment because the area under the curve for a given amount of radioactivity varies inversely with the flow rate through the well counter (Winbury *et al.*, 1965a). An improved procedure for calibration, which permits variation of flow rate through the counter, was subsequently developed (Laurence *et al.*, 1963; Winbury *et al.*, 1965a).

(*b*) *Double isotope methods.* The double isotope procedure using a diffusible and nondiffusible tracer has more universal application since it can be applied to regions where circulatory isolation is not possible and/or where total venous outflow cannot be collected (heart *in situ*).

The principle of the approach developed by Winbury *et al.* (1962; 1965a) for the heart and hindlimb involves simultaneous slug injection of ^{86}Rb as the diffusible tracer and ^{131}I-albumin as the nondiffusible tracer. The nondiffusible tracer remains within the vascular compartment, and the diffusible tracer is taken up by the tissues. Extraction of ^{86}Rb is based on the ratio of ^{86}Rb:^{131}I-albumin injected to that in a sample of venous blood as

$$E\,^{86}\text{Rb} = \frac{\left(\dfrac{^{86}\text{Rb}}{^{131}\text{I}-\text{alb}}\text{ injected}\right) - \left(\dfrac{^{86}\text{Rb}}{^{131}\text{I}-\text{alb}}\text{ venous blood}\right)}{\left(\dfrac{^{86}\text{Rb}}{^{131}\text{I}-\text{alb}}\text{ injected}\right)}.$$

The basic procedure requires timed collection of aliquots of venous blood from the region for the determination of the venous ^{86}Rb:^{131}I-albumin ratio after the injection of tracers into the arterial supply. A sample of arterial blood is required to correct for ^{131}I-recirculation and of venous blood to correct for efflux of ^{86}Rb.

The left coronary artery of the heart was perfused at a constant rate with blood from the systemic circulation. Venous blood (coronary sinus) was drawn at constant rate by a pump through a mixing chamber and well counter, and returned to the venous circulation. ^{86}Rb and ^{131}I-albumin were injected simultaneously into the arterial inflow close to the organ, and an aliquot of coronary sinus blood was collected from the mixing chamber at a constant rate for 2.5 min starting at the time the isotopes are expected to traverse the dead space of the system and the coronary circuit. Since there is recirculation of the ^{131}I-albumin a sample of arterial blood was also taken, and corrections were applied to the venous sample. Likewise, before the isotope run an aliquot of coronary sinus blood was collected to correct for efflux. Corrections are as follows: corrected ^{86}Rb = (venous ^{86}Rb after injection — venous ^{86}Rb efflux); corrected ^{131}I-albumin = (venous ^{131}I after injection — arterial ^{131}I after injection). It was found that the mixing chamber was required to eliminate stratification of isotopes in the flow stream. The 2.5-min collection of coronary sinus was required to achieve a constant ratio of ^{86}Rb:^{131}I-albumin (Winbury *et al.*, 1965a).

Copp and Shim (1965) described a similar double-isotope method for determination of extraction by bone (tibia) in the dog. Evans blue (T-1824) as the reference nondiffusible tracer, and ^{85}Sr as the diffusible tracer, were injected over a minute into the nutrient artery. The percentage of T-1824 and ^{85}Sr was determined in the femoral vein blood collected for 5 min.

Martin and Yudilevich (1964) developed a theory for the quantification of transcapillary exchange in the isolated dog heart based on first dilution curves of two tracers—one that crosses the capillary barrier and the other that remains in the plasma. By appropriate computations it is possible to obtain extraction E, fractional turnover rate k, and extracellular compartment size. The procedure was further studied by Yudilevich and Martín de Julián (1965), using ^{86}Rb, ^{42}K, ^{22}Na and ^{131}I as the diffusible tracers, and ^{131}I-albumin and ^{59}Fe-siderophilin as the reference nondiffusible tracer. A slug injection of mixtures of tracers was administered to the Langendorff isolated dog heart preparation perfused with blood, and the venous outflow was collected in 40–60 samples over 3–10 min. The ratio of the percentage of the administered dose of test substance (diffusible) ($c(t)$) to that of the reference substance (nondiffusible) ($C(t)$), was calculated for each venous sample from the time of peak activity. With ^{86}Rb and ^{42}K, this ratio was constant for about 2 min, thus allowing a direct determination of E on the basis of

$$E = 1 - \left[\frac{c(t)}{C(t)} \right].$$

However, with ^{22}Na and ^{131}I, E decreased with time after the peak radioactivity. The apparent decrease in E for ^{22}Na or ^{131}I is due to the backflux of the tracer into the blood. In order to determine the true E of substances that are not sequestered in the cells it is necessary to apply the following equation:

$$k \frac{\int_0^t [C(t) - c(t)]\, dt}{C(t)} - \frac{c(t)}{C(t)} + (1 - E) = 0.$$

This is done graphically by plotting

$$\left[\frac{\int_0^t [C(t) - c(t)]\, dt}{C(t)} \right] \text{ versus } \left[\frac{c(t)}{C(t)} \right].$$

The integral is estimated by summation after a smoothing procedure of the experimental points (Yudilevich and Martín de Julián, 1965). At a zero intercept

$$E = 1 - \left[\frac{c(t)}{C(t)} \right]$$

and the reciprocal of k is equal to the slope.

Dobson and Warner (1960) analyzed washout curves for ^{24}Na and ^{131}I-albumin injected intraarterially into the dog hindlimb. They suggested that comparison of simultaneous washout curves for diffusible and nondiffusible tracers can be used for the determination of the regional blood flow as well as the transcapillary exchange rate and the intracellular penetration rates.

5.2.3. *Direct determination of clearance*

Tissue clearance of a tracer from the arterial blood is another approach to the study of nutritional circulation. The requisites for the determination of clearance on the basis of uptake are a measure of arterial concentration of the tracer and a relatively complete retention in the tissue (Love and Burch, 1957a; Bacaner and Beck, 1964). Thus, for ^{86}Rb,

$$\text{mean } C\,(\text{ml/min per g}) = \frac{\text{tissue } {}^{86}\text{Rb (cpm/g)}}{\text{mean arterial } {}^{86}\text{Rb (cpm/ml)} \times \text{duration (min)}}.$$

The same principles and equations for the determination of clearance on the basis of tissue washout apply here as well (Sections 3.3 and 5.1). With a constant arterial level of tracer, a clearance constant k can be determined on the basis of $C = C_\infty (1 - e^{-kt})$ when C is the ^{86}Rb concentration in the tissue at time t; C_∞ is the tissue concentration at infinity, which is assumed to be the same as the plasma concentration. The fractional turn-over rate k can be determined graphically on the basis of $t_{\frac{1}{2}}$ of the tissue ^{86}Rb concentration, estimated by a scintillation probe (Love, 1964).

Love and Burch (1957a) investigated a procedure for the estimation of the rate of myocardial ^{86}Rb uptake in dogs, which might be useful in man.

^{86}Rb was infused intravenously for 30 min at a declining rate in order to maintain a constant arterial level. The rise in the myocardial ^{86}Rb concentration was obtained with a ratemeter connected to a scintillation probe over the precordium. It was assumed that the initial rate of increase of myocardial radioactivity is related to the initial rate of clearance of ^{86}Rb from the plasma by the heart, and that the final level of radioactivity achieved at the end of the ^{86}Rb infusion is related to the average clearance during the infusion.

The initial clearance of ^{86}Rb is considered the clearance at a time before ^{86}Rb begins to return from the myocardium to the plasma. The following equation applies:

$$\text{initial } C \ ^{86}\text{Rb (ml/g per min)} = k \ \frac{\text{mean myocardial } ^{86}\text{Rb conc.}}{\text{mean plasma } ^{86}\text{Rb conc.}}.$$

The turnover constant k is obtained graphically by determining $t_{\frac{1}{2}}$ from a semilogarithmic plot of the myocardial radioactivity versus time. The average myocardial $C \ ^{86}$Rb can be derived from

$$\text{mean } C \ ^{86}\text{Rb (ml/g per min)} = \frac{\text{final myocardial } ^{86}\text{Rb conc.}}{\text{plasma } ^{86}\text{Rb} \times \text{duration}}.$$

The greater the degree of equilibrium of the heart with the plasma, the poorer is the average clearance a reflection of initial clearance. It was found that the mean $C \ ^{86}$Rb reflects the true uptake rate when there is less than 40% equilibrium. There was a good correlation between ^{86}Rb clearance values (initial and mean) obtained by scintillation probe compared with those from direct myocardial ^{86}Rb concentration at the end of the experiment. Changes in clearance produced by drugs (vasopressin or norepinephrine) could be reliably predicted from the *initial* $C \ ^{86}$Rb, but not from the *mean* $C \ ^{86}$Rb. Vasopressin infusion reduced the initial $C \ ^{86}$Rb, while norepinephrine produced an increase (Love and Burch, 1957b). Further investigations (Love and Burch, 1959) suggest that this method can be used to estimate coronary blood flow in man without cardiac catheterization provided the myocardial radioactivity can be measured accurately with an external probe.

In later studies in dogs ^{86}Rb was infused for 10 min after which the heart was removed and the mean clearance determined on the basis of the final myocardial concentration and of the mean arterial level over the same time period. This method was used to study the relationship between the coronary blood flow and $C \ ^{86}$Rb (Love and O'Meallie, 1963), and the effect of norepinephrine, angiotension, dipyridamole, digitoxin (Love *et al.*, 1965a, 1965b), hypoxemia and hypercapnia (Love and Tyler, 1965) on C ^{86}Rb and coronary blood flow.

One of the difficulties in the measurement of myocardial uptake by precordial counting after the intravenous injection or infusion of a tracer is the problem of the isolation of the myocardial component of activity from the chest wall, lungs, and heart chambers by any form of simple collimation (Ross and Friesinger, 1965). Another problem is the estimation of the absolute flow, which is difficult to determine by precordial techniques because the variability in the depth and size of the heart prevents an absolute estimate of cardiac uptake of the isotope. These problems have been approached by Donato *et al.* (1964, 1966) by a comparison of precordial curve of ^{131}I-albumin with that of ^{86}Rb, and by Bing *et al.* (1964) and Cohen *et al.* (1965a) with ^{84}Rb and coincidence counting. Each of these techniques will be described.

Donato *et al.* (1964, 1966) based their method of the determination of myocardial clearance of ^{86}Rb on the premise that the average extraction of the indicator by the myocardium during the first minutes after intravenous injection of a slug of ^{86}Rb does not differ from the average total body extraction, and that myocardial radioactivity is constant after the primary arterial curve. This appears to be the case for rats, dogs, and man (Donato *et al.*, 1964; Sapirstein, 1965; Donato *et al.*, 1966). Thus the fraction of injected tracer taken up by the myocardium is equal to the fraction of the cardiac output perfusing the myocardium, which is the basis of the fractional distribution technique of Sapirstein (1958).

The method of Donato *et al.* used in humans requires successive intravenous injection of a slug of ^{131}I-albumin, and 2–3 min later ^{86}Rb, to determine the intravascular and intravascular $+$ myocardial precordial activity respectively. Arterial blood was drawn at a constant rate for 1 min starting 30 sec after the injection of each isotope for the arterial dilution curves. The precordial count rate between 30 and 90 sec after the injection of the isotope was used for computations. The original procedure described in 1964 (Donato *et al.*, 1964) employed a single scintillation probe; in 1966 (Donato *et al.*, 1966) a twin counter system was used. The purpose of the later system is to reduce the dependence of the counting values on geometry.

The precordial counting rate for ^{131}I-albumin (R_B) equals the arterial concentration ($\bar{c}B$) times the effective intravascular volume (W_B); or $W_B = R_B/\bar{c}B$. After the injection of ^{86}Rb, the precordial activity (R_{Rb}) is equal to the intravascular (R_B) plus the extravascular (R_E) components:

$R_{Rb} = R_B + R_E$. The extravascular component (R_E) is composed of myocardial activity (R_m) and the striated muscles of the chest wall. Fortunately, after a single injection of ^{86}Rb, the myocardial activity is 15–30 times that of the anterior chest wall, so that the contribution of nonmyocardial tissue to the precordial count rate is small. Thus with proper shielding the R_m shortly after the injection of ^{86}Rb is assumed to be equal to R_E. The amount of ^{86}Rb taken up by the myocardium in the first 30 seconds (R_m) can be estimated by subtracting from the precordial counting rate between 30–90 sec (R_{Rb}) the contribution due to intravascular radioactivity: ^{86}Rb content $(R_m) = R_{Rb} - W_B \times$ ^{86}Rb concentration in the arterial blood. This value is equal to the average myocardial ^{86}Rb concentration times the effective volume of the myocardium. Since neither concentration nor volume are known, clearance must be determined indirectly.

The area under the ^{86}Rb radiocardiographic curve (RCG) is measured after semilogarithmic extrapolation of the downslope of the apparent recirculation. This value equals the integral of the primary arterial concentration curve times the effective volume of the heart chambers, and any other vessels contributing to the curve. Myocardial C ^{86}Rb (ml/g per min) is equal to the ratio of the myocardial ^{86}Rb content (R_m) to the area of RCG. This is equivalent to the myocardial ^{86}Rb concentration (cpm/g)/area of primary arterial concentration curve (cpm)/ml blood $\times$ duration of curve.

$$C(\text{ml/g min}) \text{ per} = \frac{R_m}{\text{area RCG}}$$

$$= \frac{\text{myocardial conc. (cpm/g)}}{\text{area of primary arterial conc. curve (cpm/ml} \times \text{duration)}}.$$

Two successive measurements of C ^{86}Rb performed in a series of patients showed an average difference of about 7% of the mean values. There was excellent agreement between coronary blood flow values obtained by the N_2O saturation method and C ^{86}Rb (Donato et al., 1966). Nitroglycerin increased C ^{86}Rb significantly in normal subjects (Donato et al., 1964).

This method measures the average nutritional flow of the entire myocardial mass. Thus under-perfused areas which do not contribute to the Fick (N_2O) values contribute to the clearance value by the Donato method.

Bing et al. (1964) and Cohen et al. (1965a) developed the coincidence counting technique with ^{84}Rb to circumvent the principle disadvantage of methods using ^{86}Rb—namely, the problem of determination of the specific activity of the heart muscle as distinct from the other tissues. [84]Rb, which is a positron emitter, results in the production of two gamma photons of 0.51 MeV, 180° apart. By means of a pair of scintillation detectors 180° apart, it is possible to record the activity of [84]Rb with a minimum of background radiation, and easily to calibrate the equipment in absolute terms.

Two pairs of coincidence detectors are required for use in man. One pair is positioned over the precordial area (above and below left side of chest); the other pair is placed over the right side of the chest (*B*). The difference between precordial activity (*H*) and *B*, (*H* − *B*), expresses the uptake of [84]Rb by the heart muscle alone. [84]Rb was infused intravenously at a constant rate for 30 min. Simultaneously, arterial blood was withdrawn at a constant rate, and passed through a well counter. *H*, *B*, and the arterial radioactivity were recorded continuously. A calibration coefficient (cal) takes into account the various factors such as geometry of the heart and detectors, etc., and permits the determination of the clearance in absolute units (ml/min) (Cohen *et al.*, 1965a). The clearance is calculated from the following equations:

$$\text{clearance (ml/min)} = \frac{dC/dt}{C_a} = \left(\frac{d(H-B)/dt}{Aw}\right) \times \text{cal},$$

with *Aw* representing arterial radioactivity (disintegrations/min) in the well counter, d(*H* − *B*)/d*t* is the first derivative of the myocardial uptake of [84]Rb and cal the correction factor. Clearance is calculated from values at 8-sec intervals using a digital computer by dividing the first derivative of the myocardial uptake by the arterial activity. The ratio is then multiplied by the correction factor. The initial 5 min of recording was not used. After this the clearance declined exponentially with time. The values were therefore plotted semilogarithmically against time to obtain a straight line which was extrapolated back to zero time. The clearance at zero time is assumed to be the same as the coronary blood flow on the premise that the extraction of [84]Rb is 100 % at this point (Cohen *et al.*, 1965a). At zero time there should be no [84]Rb in the coronary sinus blood resulting in an extraction ratio of 1. In the initial studies of this group (Bing *et al.*, 1964; Cohen *et al.*, 1965a) the extraction ratio of the isolated dog heart was reported to be independent of blood flow rate, but a later study (Cohen *et al.*, 1967) demonstrated that extraction was inversely related to flow. Theoretically, this does not alter the validity of the clearance values since extraction and clearance are extrapolated back to zero time. Comparison of the observed and derived flow in the isolated dog heart indicates an average difference of 7 % (Cohen *et al.*, 1965a). In normal man, nitroglycerin increased the myocardial clearance value. This method, like that of Love and of Donato, measures nutritional flow rather than total flow (Cohen *et al.*, 1967).

Bacaner and Beck (1964) described a method for the determination of intestinal blood flow in dogs which has been applied to man. ^{32}P (as $Na_2H^{32}PO_4$), administered as an intravenous slug, is completely removed in a single pass through the intestine and retained for 12–15 sec, a time well past the peak of the arterial curve. Intestinal radioactivity was obtained with a critically shielded gut detector in the lumen, and the arterial dilution curve is determined by continuous withdrawal of arterial blood at a constant rate through a coil around a Geiger–Müller tube. Methods are described for calculating the coefficients which permit relating the counting rates to concentrations in the arterial blood and tissue. The clearance is calculated from the derivative form of the clearance equation

$$f = \frac{(\mathrm{d}C/\mathrm{d}t)\, t - t_0}{C_a\,(t_0)},$$

where C is the concentration in the tissue and C_a the concentration in the arterial blood. A graph is constructed of the regional concentration curve versus time, on which is superimposed the arterial concentration, with the peak arterial concentration coinciding with the inflection point of the regional curve. The values computed in the interval of constant ratio of $(\mathrm{d}C/\mathrm{d}t)/C_a$ is considered the clearance (ml/min per 100 g). There was good agreement between the venous outflow and the calculated flow. In human use, the method requires only an arterial puncture and the passage of a detector into the intestine via the mouth or rectum.

In the previously described methods, tissue uptake has been estimated by a probe; this permits multiple determinations in the same subject or animal with no damage to the region. In animals, tissue uptake has been determined by the removal of the tissue and direct reading of the radioactivity. These methods are easy to use, and the clearance can be expressed directly in ml/min per unit weight (or volume). For studies on the heart, ^{86}Rb was infused at a constant rate intravenously (Levy *et al.*, 1961; Levy and Chansky, 1965), or directly into the coronary circulation (Moir, 1966) for 1 or 2 min, and the heart was fibrillated and removed at the end of the infusion. Arterial blood samples were taken at 10- or 20-sec intervals, and the clearance calculated from the tissue concentration (cpm/g) divided by the mean arterial concentration (cpm/g × min). A similar method for the determination of the clearance of various portions of the gastrointestinal tract has been described (Delaney and Grim, 1964a). ^{42}K was injected intravenously as a slug, and the arterial concentration was measured continuously by a well counter. The animal was sacrificed at 30 sec, and the clearance calculated from the ^{42}K content of tissue divided by the area under primary arterial dilution curve. Derived flows correlated well with directly measured flow.

Bone clearance and extraction can be studied with ^{45}Ca, ^{47}Ca, and ^{85}Sr. Bone acts as an infinite sink for these isotopes, and uptake is a flow-limited process which makes them suitable for the study of nutritional circulation. The tracer was administered intravenously (Frederickson *et al.*, 1955; Weinman *et al.*, 1963; Lehan *et al.*, 1966) and arterial samples were taken continuously or at frequent intervals. Animals were sacrificed 5–10 min after the injection and the clearance calculated in the conventional manner. In some studies the tracer was injected directly into the nutrient artery of the tibia of the dog, permitting the simultaneous determination of the clearance and extraction (Weinman *et al.*, 1963; Copp and Shim, 1965).

5.2.4. *Fractional distributional approach*

The fractional distribution method with ^{86}Rb or ^{42}K as the tracer has been used extensively for the simultaneous determination of blood flow in several organs and the distribution of blood flow within an organ. We are indebted to Sapirstein (1958) for the concept and principle of the fractional distribution of indicators. Delaney *et al.* (Delaney and Grim, 1964a, 1965; Delaney and Custer, 1965; Delaney and Grim, 1966) confirmed the validity of the concept in a series of investigations.

(a) *Principle.* The fractional distribution of ^{42}K or ^{86}Rb in various regions corresponds to the fractional distribution of the cardiac output. This principle is valid if the extraction ratio of indicator by the organ under study is the same as the overall extraction ratio of the body. Tracers such as ^{86}Rb and ^{42}K are particularly useful for fractional distribution studies because these isotopes enter the organ K pool which acts as an infinite sink for the tracer. Since the tissue uptake of ^{86}Rb and ^{42}K from the arterial blood is a flow-limited process, the fractional distribution method measures the ratio of the organ nutritional circulation to the total body nutritional circulation.

Uptake of ^{86}Rb by a region is a function of the product of the capillary blood flow, Q, times the integrated arterial concentration ($\int_0^T C_a \, dt$) times the extraction ratio, E, of ^{86}Rb by the organ. Likewise, the uptake by the entire body is the cardiac output, CO, times the integrated arterial concentration times the extraction ratio of ^{86}Rb for the body:

$$\text{Regional } ^{86}\text{Rb uptake} = Q \left(\int_0^T C_a \, dt \right) E \, ^{86}\text{Rb regional;}$$
$$\text{Body } ^{86}\text{Rb uptake} = CO \left(\int_0^T C_a \, dt \right) E \, ^{86}\text{Rb body.}$$

The indicator is injected intravenously and mixes with the blood in the heart resulting in a uniform C_a to all areas of the body. When E for the region is the same as E for the entire body, Q/CO is equal to organ uptake divided by the body uptake. Thus the latter ratio describes the fraction of the cardiac output received by the region. Because physiological or anatomical shunts do not participate in ^{86}Rb uptake, the cardiac output in this case represents the total body nutritional circulation, and the ratio is the fraction of the total nutritional circulation received by the organ. The total body uptake is equivalent to the amount of indicator injected leading to the equations: flow fraction = regional ^{86}Rb content divided by ^{86}Rb injected, and regional blood flow = flow fraction $\times$ CO.

If all organs of the body extracted 100% of the arterial ^{86}Rb or ^{42}K and retained the indicator for a finite time, the arterial level would be zero after the first circulation, there would be no recirculation of tracer, and the uptake of each organ would represent its blood flow (Sapirstein, 1958; Delaney and Grim, 1964a). Extraction of ^{86}Rb and ^{42}K is less than 100%, which results in the recirculation of the tracer. However, as Sapirstein (1958) indicated, when the organ tracer content remains stable for a finite time after the initial delivery by the arterial blood, the extraction ratio of the organ is the same as that of the entire body. With the exception of the brain, the ^{86}Rb or ^{42}K organ content was constant from 9 to 64 sec in rats, and to 120 sec in dogs (Sapirstein, 1958). The brain takes up the isotope for the first 6 sec, but loses it rapidly thereafter, indicating an extraction ratio much lower than the rest of the body. Thus ^{86}Rb or ^{42}K is suitable for the estimation of regional nutritional circulation for most areas other than the brain.

Delaney *et al.* (Delaney and Grim, 1964a; Delaney and Custer, 1965; Delaney and Grim, 1966) were concerned about the amount of ^{86}Rb that remains in the blood at the time of sacrifice. Approximately 25% of the injected dose was found in the blood stream of the dog 30–35 sec after the injection of the indicator. This suggests that the calculated organ blood flow could be in error by as much as 25%, even though the extraction ratios were identical. However, they found that the venous loss of ^{86}Rb or ^{42}K was almost exactly balanced by the uptake of recirculating isotope, which means, in fact, that each organ contained an amount of tracer equivalent to 100% of its share of the cardiac output, providing further justification for the use of ^{86}Rb and ^{42}K as tracers for the fractional distributional approach.

Takács *et al.* (1964) also investigated the content of isotope in the circulating blood at the time of sacrifice, and reported much lower values than

Delaney. At 50–80 sec after intravenous injection, the entire circulating blood of the normal rat contained 7% of the ^{42}K and 5% of the ^{86}Rb injected. Disappearance was slower in the dog, and at 60 sec there was 14% of the ^{86}Rb injected, but by 120 sec this amount was reduced to 7%.

(b) *Method.* The fractional distribution procedure was originally developed by Sapirstein in 1958. The tracer was injected intravenously as a slug, and the animals were killed at various intervals thereafter. The isotope uptake was determined in one group of rats, and the cardiac output in another group of rats of the same strain, on the basis of the primary arterial indicator dilution curve for the tracer. In dogs, the cardiac output and the fractional ^{86}Rb distribution were determined in the same animal. The organ content and arterial blood concentration were measured by direct counting procedures. Three indicator substances, ^{42}K, ^{86}Rb, and ^{131}I-antipyrine, were studied in this first investigation to determine the characteristic pattern for various organs and indicators. This included brain, heart, kidneys, liver, gut, spleen, skin, and carcass for the rat; and heart, kidneys, skin, gut, stomach, pancreas, spleen, liver, tongue, lungs, and carcass for the dog. The organ content of ^{86}Rb and ^{42}K was constant, except for the brain, from 9 to 64 sec in the rat, and from 20 to 120 sec in the dog. The content of ^{131}I-antipyrine was stable only in the brain, skin, and carcass of the rat.

A later study by Sapirstein and Goldman (1959) showed that ^{86}Rb and ^{131}I-antipyrine are satisfactory indicators of adrenal blood flow in the rat. Both isotopes were retained at a constant level during the first 30 sec after injection, and, when administered together, the ratio of ^{131}I to ^{86}Rb in the adrenal gland was 0.99. Blood flow values obtained by direct catheterization of the adrenal vein were almost identical to those calculated from ^{86}Rb uptake.

A modification by Goldman (1961) permitted the use of unanesthetized, unrestrained rats. Three days prior to the experiment catheters were implanted in the right femoral vein for the injection of ^{86}Rb, and in the left femoral artery for the withdrawal of blood samples. For the study, the animals were placed in a small box which allowed manipulation of the catheters without restraint. After filling the venous catheter with ^{86}Rb, it was rapidly flushed in, and blood was collected from the arterial catheter on a circular sample collector. At 30 sec after the injection the animals were killed with an intravenous injection of saturated KCl solution, and the organs removed, weighed, and radioactivity determined. This method has been used to determine the flow fraction and regional flow of several organs simultaneously in the same animal by the determination of the

[86]Rb content of the appropriate organ, and the cardiac output from the indicator dilution curve (Goldman, 1963; Goldman, 1965/1966; Goldman, 1966). The organ blood flow can be expressed as ml/min per organ, or as ml/min per g by dividing organ blood flow by organ weight.

The flow values obtained by the fractional uptake approach are really clearance values. In fact, Delaney and Grim (1964a, 1965) calculated the clearance of various parts of the gastrointestinal tract of the dog directly, by dividing the organ content of ^{86}Rb or [42]K by the primary arterial dilution curve, the downslope of which was extrapolated exponentially. The basis of this calculation is as follows: fractional distribution $= (Ir/I)$; regional flow $= (Ir/I) \times CO$; $CO = I/(\int_0^T C_a \, dt)$, where Ir is the indicator content of region and I the amount of indicator injected. I cancels out when the equations for fractional distribution and cardiac output are combined, leaving the clearance $= Ir/\int_0^T C_a \, dt$. The simultaneous determination of [42]K clearance and total gastric venous outflow shows good correlation with a mean difference of 5.4%.

Rathmacher *et al.* (1965) found that the fractional ^{86}Rb uptake method could be applied to swine. There were no significant changes in tracer content from 30 to 180 sec in skeletal muscle, testicle, ovary, spleen, liver, adrenal, or heart. The lung and uterus decreased and the kidney increased with time. Winbury and Pensinger (1966) and Pensinger *et al.* (1965) employed the fractional distribution approach to the study of myocardial nutritional circulation of swine and determined the blood content simultaneously with ^{131}I-albumin. The animals were sacrificed 10 min after the simultaneous injection of both tracers. Levy and Martins de Oliveira (1961) have used this technique for the determination of the regional distribution of canine myocardial blood flow. Likewise, King and associates (1966) evaluated the effect of epicardiectomy on canine myocardial nutrient flow in normal and chronic ischemic areas with this method. Actual coronary blood flow was compared with calculated values in 32 dogs by perfusing the coronary arteries with blood taken from the left atrium by a pump. There was a good correlation of calculated flow with actual flow above 16 ml/min per 100 g. When the pump flow was zero, the calculated flow was 16 ml/min per 100 g, which probably represents coronary nutrition from the chambers of the heart.

Blood flow in the testis and epididymis of the rat and ram was determined by fractional uptake of ^{131}I-antipyrine (Setchell *et al.*, 1964). Concentration of the tracer was constant for 10–60 sec in the rat and for 90–120 sec in the ram.

One of the major advantages of the fractional distribution approach for the study of drugs is the ability to determine the flow fraction of cardiac output of several organs simultaneously. This permits the evaluation of selective effects of drugs on the nutritional circulation of specific regions, or the redistribution of blood flow independently of effect on clearance. For example, pentaerythritol tetranitrate and dipyridamole increased the fractional ^{86}Rb uptake of the heart without a similar increase in skeletal muscle (Winbury and Pensinger, 1966). In comparing the effects of various catecholamines on the circulation, it was found that epinephrine altered fractional uptake of many organs whereas norepinephrine altered only a few (Goldman, 1966).

5.2.5. *Renal blood flow*

The renal blood flow can be estimated by the measurement of the disappearance from the blood of a tracer solely removed by the kidney. This is really a specialized application of the direct determination of clearance based on uptake. The tracer cleared by the kidney is excreted into an infinite sink, the urine. Gott *et al.* (1962) indicated the basic requirements for a material to be suitable are: (1) that it be cleared from the blood by the kidneys only, (2) that it reach its volume of distribution rapidly, and (3) that the changes in the blood concentration observed reflect the change in the entire apparent volume of distribution of the tracer. Orthoiodohippurate ([131]-I-Hippuran) satisfied these requirements and is suitable to measure the effective renal blood flow.

[131]I-Hippuran was injected as a single intravenous dose into patients or dogs, and the blood concentration determined at intervals over a period of 30 or more minutes (Gott *et al.*, 1962; Pritchard *et al.*, 1965; Dabaj *et al.*, 1966). Blood disappearance curves, plotted semilogarithmically versus time, disclosed three phases. There was an initial rapid fall in concentration for the first 9 min which probably represents establishment of equilibrium. The second slower exponential phase started at 10 min and ended at 20–25 min after the injection. This represents the renal clearance of Hippuran, and the slope k can be determined in the conventional manner. By extrapolation of the slope of this phase back to zero time the volume of distribution V can be calculated from the injected dose/blood concentration at zero time. Clearance equals kV, which for Hippuran is the effective renal blood flow. There was good agreement between the values derived from the single injection blood disappearance method and the conventional constant infusion urine collection method (man and dog), or direct renal vein outflow (dog) (Gott *et al.*, 1962; Pritchard *et al.*, 1965; Dabaj *et al.*, 1966).

A method for the simultaneous determination of the glomerular filtration rate and the effective renal blood flow was developed by Stokes and
Ter-Pogossian (1964). The ^{131}I-Hypaque clearance from the blood
measured the glomerular filtration rate, and the ^{125}I-Hippuran clearance
measured the renal blood flow. Both tracers were administered in the same
intravenous injection into dogs or man, and serial blood samples were
taken at frequent intervals. The radioactivity was determined in a well
counter for ^{131}I and ^{125}I, by the appropriate selection of the energy windows
and correction for the overlap of spectra. The relationship log of the blood
concentration versus time was plotted for each isotope for 60 min. The
^{125}I-Hippuran curve showed an early mixing slope (rapid) which was
followed by the slope (slower) due to renal clearance (ERBF). The ^{131}I-
Hypaque curve also has two components; the second component represents
glomerular filtration. There was good correlation between the values for
the filtration rate and renal plasma flow calculated by this method and the
conventional clearance approach with urine collection.

These procedures have the advantage of not requiring a constant
intravenous infusion and urine collection. Glomerular filtration and renal
blood flow can be determined after a single intravenous injection of a
suitable tracer. Clearance is based on the slope of the exponential decline
in blood concentration and the apparent volume of distribution.

5.2.6. *Hepatic blood flow*

Dobson and Jones (1952) established that the liver blood flow can be
measured by the rate of disappearance of intravenously injected particulate
matter from the blood stream. This is based on the ability of the reticulo-
endothelial system of the liver and spleen to remove colloidal particulate
matter from the blood passing through the liver. The spleen is in series with
the liver and drains into the portal system, making it an integral part of the
portal circulation. These organs together can account for 90–95% of the
removal of particulate matter of a certain size from the blood stream
(Restrepo *et al.*, 1960). The uptake of colloidal tracer by the liver is flow-
limited, and it should be possible to calculate the liver blood flow from the
disappearance rate constant as the fraction of blood volume perfusing the
liver per unit time (Vetter *et al.*, 1954). Thus the liver blood flow is determined by an uptake procedure measured either as blood disappearance of
a colloidal tracer or liver accumulation of the tracer, and the method of
computation is similar to that for clearance constants k for washout or
uptake of diffusible tracers.

Using colloidal chromic phosphate (^{32}P), Dobson and Jones in 1952 demonstrated that the disappearance curve of ^{32}P from the blood is exponential, and the liver blood flow can be calculated from the rate constant k. This was determined from a semilogarithmic plot of blood concentration versus time, the slope of this function being k. When the extraction of the tracer by the liver and spleen is complete, k will be an estimate of the circulating blood volume which passes through the liver in a unit time. Actually, extraction in rabbit, dog, and mouse was 80–90%, so that k represents minimal liver perfusion.

When blood concentration was monitored over a period of 30 min, the blood disappearance curve could be resolved into three exponential components by curve stripping. The fastest component was considered to be dependent upon liver blood flow. A probe over the liver showed that radioactivity rose logarithmically to a constant maximum; an uptake constant could be calculated from the curve of liver accumulation.

Vetter and coworkers (1954) introduced the use of colloidal radioactive gold (^{198}Au) as the tracer. This is labeled with a γ-emitting isotope and is suitable for external counting techniques—an advantage over chromic phosphate. Another advantage of colloidal ^{198}Au is the uniformity of particle size around an average of about 250 Å. The tracer was injected intravenously and the decline in blood ^{198}Au was measured with a counter placed between the calves of the subject. The semilogarithmic plot of the disappearance curve shows that it is a composite of a series of simple exponentials. The first (fastest) component was separated from the others, and used for the determination of the disappearance constant k. The constant k obtained by external counting was compared with that obtained from serial arterial blood samples. The mean difference was only 2.7%, indicating that external measurement of the blood disappearance rate was a valid method. When k was determined twice at a 1-hr interval in several subjects, there was excellent agreement of the two values. The apparent liver blood flow can be calculated from k, and the blood volume determined with Evans blue, but there are reservations to this because the liver does not clear the blood completely in one passage (90%).

Several groups have determined the blood clearance and liver uptake of colloidal ^{198}Au simultaneously in man and dogs with scintillation probes over the liver and other areas that permit measurement of peripheral activity (i.e. thigh, neck, heart, or head). Restrepo *et al.* (1960) found that the liver uptake and blood disappearance constants did not differ significantly in dog, but the uptake constants had a tendency to be higher and had a wider range than disappearance constants. Iio *et al.* (1960) determined the liver, heart, and periphery (thigh) constants simultaneously in humans, and observed that they were equal in those patients without heart failure or splenomegalic liver cirrhosis. Likewise, Stroun *et al.* (1962) determined k from liver and a number of other areas simultaneously in addition to direct determination of blood disappearance. The k values derived from blood, liver, and the parietal region of the brain (peripheral) were almost identical. Agreement of blood with finger or thigh was not as good. All three groups of investigators reported that the blood and peripheral disappearance curve was of more than one component, and used the initial (fast) component for calculation of the constant k. Ueda *et al.* (1961) have described the application of electronic digital computers to the analysis of the ^{198}Au colloid uptake by the liver.

The size of the colloidal particles is of importance. The optimal size is 150–300 Å (Taplin, 1965). Particles that are too large will be trapped in the lung, and those too small will be cleared with very low efficiency and at a much slower rate. This explains the two main components of the blood disappearance curve; the first is the fast component reflecting the clearance of the major fraction of the injected dose by the liver. The second slower component reflects the small fraction of the dose comprised of very small particles that are cleared with poor efficiency. It is necessary to subtract this component from the original curve to arrive at a correct k for the fast component.

Another factor that may affect the accuracy of the results is the quantity of particulate matter injected (Vetter *et al.*, 1954). Patients initially received 250 mcg of colloidal ^{198}Au. When the experiment was repeated in 1 hr using six times that amount, the disappearance constant was reduced. However, when twice the amount was given the second constant was the same as the first. Presumably with the largest dose the reticuloendothelial system of the liver is unable to remove all of the particles passing through the liver in a given time.

5.3. COMPARISON OF CLEARANCE WITH TOTAL BLOOD FLOW

The clearance of an inert diffusible tracer is a measure of nutritional blood flow and may or may not agree with total flow. The extent of agreement depends upon the tissue studied, the tracer used, the method of alteration of blood flow, and the range of blood flow studied.

Previously it was stressed that the lipophilic tracers, such as ^{85}Kr and ^{133}Xe, have minimal diffusional barriers, and when used appropriately are good indicators of true capillary flow. If all of the blood supply to a tissue passes through functional capillary beds (nutritional), one would expect good agreement between clearance of such tracers and total blood flow.

5.3.1. *Heart*

The clearance of ^{85}Kr or ^{133}Xe determined with a counter over the heart compared well with the total coronary blood flow determined by a rota-meter (Herd *et al.*, 1962; Ross *et al.*, 1964; Rees and Redding, 1966) or the Kety–Schmidt technique using N_2O or ^{131}I-antipyrine (Cohen *et al.*, 1964). Another investigator found good agreement of ^{86}Rb clearance and blood flow when the canine heart was perfused over a broad range (King *et al.*, 1966). Likewise, using ^{84}Rb it was found that clearance agreed with total perfusion rate in isolated dog heart using a coincidence counting technique (Lübs *et al.*, 1965). On the other hand, pentaerythritol tetranitrate increased fractional ^{86}Rb uptake of the swine heart without any change in total flow measured by an electromagnetic flow meter; dipyridamole increased both blood flow and fractional ^{86}Rb uptake (Winbury and Pensinger, 1966).

An ingenious approach was the measurement of the transit time of tritiated water, which was compared with total coronary flow based on the Fick (O_2) principle. Dogs treated with dipyridamole showed an increased flow of about 1.5 times as calculated by both methods (Palmer *et al.*, 1966).

Using angiographic techniques, the diameter of the large coronary arteries was compared with ^{85}Kr clearance (intracoronary). Nitroglycerin produced a prolonged increase in the diameter of the arteries, but only a short increase in ^{85}Kr clearance; dipyridamole produced no change in arterial diameter, but a prolonged increase in ^{85}Kr clearance (Lehan *et al.*, 1966). It can be concluded that in the majority of studies there is good agreement of blood flow and tissue clearance in the heart particularly when ^{85}Kr or ^{133}Xe is used as the tracer.

5.3.2. *Kidney*

Effective renal blood flow, determined in man by a blood clearance method based on measurement of the decrease in blood level of ^{131}I-Hippuran after a single intravenous injection, compared well with values obtained by the conventional para-aminohippuric acid infusion method. One group found an average difference between the two methods of 2.9% (Dabaj *et al.*, 1966), and another group 6.9% (Gott *et al.*, 1962). Using two isotopes of iodine it was possible to determine the glomerular filtration rate (^{131}I-Hypaque) and renal blood flow (^{125}I-Hippuran) simultaneously after a single intravenous injection of both tracers (Stokes and Ter-Pogossian,

1964). These values agreed with simultaneously determined conventional clearances of inulin or creatinine and para-aminohippurate.

5.3.3. *Gastric*

Studies in the dog compared venous outflow from the stomach with ^{42}K clearance (uptake) over a wide range of flow values which were altered by epinephrine, norepinephrine, or histamine. The two methods showed a good correlation, with an average difference of 5.4% (Delaney and Grim, 1964a).

5.3.4. *Cerebral*

Studies in man compared the cerebral clearance of ^{85}Kr by a scintillation detector following intraarterial administration with the ^{85}Kr modification of the Kety–Schmidt (washout) method. There was a significant correlation between the two techniques with no systematic difference (Lassen and Høedt-Rasmussen, 1966).

5.3.5. *Skeletal muscle*

There are as many reports showing agreement of the clearance of the tracer with the blood flow in skeletal muscle as those showing disagreement of the two values. Some of this inconsistency may be related to the tracer used or the method of alteration of blood flow.

When the blood flow to the biceps of the dog was varied mechanically by a pump, there was a linear relationship of the flow with ^{24}Na clearance from a depot; however, the variation for any single point was considerable (Prentice *et al.*, 1955). A similar linear agreement between the perfusion rate and the ^{24}Na clearance from a depot was observed in cat and rabbit except at high flows when clearance plateaued (Walder, 1955). Bradykinin infusion into the cat or rabbit produced a similar increase in ^{131}I clearance (intraarterial) and venous outflow from skeletal muscle (Paldino *et al.*, 1962).

In a careful study in the cat on the validity of the clearance approach, Barlow *et al.* (1961) determined the blood flow by the Hensel needle, direct microscopic observation, and venous outflow in comparison with clearance of ^{24}Na, ^{42}K, or ^{131}I after intraarterial or depot injection. Infusion of epinephrine produced changes in blood flow that were not paralleled by the clearance of the ions. Likewise, Hyman *et al.* (1959) using cats showed that stimulation of the hypothalamic vasodilator center in the medulla increased the venous outflow from the muscle but produced no change in the

[24]Na clearance (depot). Sympathetic stimulation produced a greater reduction in muscle blood flow than [24]Na clearance (Hyman *et al.*, 1959).

In humans, muscle blood flow was determined by the venous occlusion plethysmographic method, which provides a reasonable estimate of total arterial inflow. Epinephrine was found to produce a similar increase in the ^{131}I clearance (depot) and the blood flow, up to a plateau value for clearance by one group of workers (Coffman, 1963). Others reported that epinephrine produced no change in [24]Na clearance (Walder, 1953) or an increase in [24]Na clearance considerably less than that of blood flow (Dobson and Warner, 1957). Exercise resulted in a parallel increase in muscle blood flow and [24]Na clearance (Walder, 1955). Priscolene had different effects on skeletal muscle blood flow and clearance in humans. Blood flow and skin temperature were increased, but [24]Na clearance was decreased (Murphy *et al.*, 1950; Elkin and Cooper, 1951). Shunting to skin and subcutaneous tissue was suggested as the mechanism of action (Murphy *et al.*, 1950).

Comparison of ^{133}Xe clearance and muscle blood flow in humans demonstrated higher values for blood flow at rest (Lassen *et al.*, 1965). This difference was greater during reactive hyperemia, for blood flow almost doubled while ^{133}Xe clearance increased only slightly. It was suggested that most of the increased flow was in the skin.

5.3.6. *Cutaneous*

Cutaneous blood flow was based on heat elimination techniques and compared with [24]Na clearance from a cutaneous depot. The cutaneous blood flow was altered by reflex heating or cooling; these procedures produced little change in [24]Na clearance (Miller and Wilson, 1951).

5.4. SPECIFIC USE OF SPECIAL PROPERTIES OF TRACERS

It has already been mentioned that specific properties of tracers can be used to advantage in particular approaches. The purpose of this section is to summarize that aspect of tracer techniques.

Nondiffusible tracers are confined to the vascular system and have a small volume of distribution. They have been used to measure *total* regional flow and regional blood volume (Geraud *et al.*, 1960). Further, nondiffusible tracers can be used as reference substances in conjunction with diffusible tracers (Freis *et al.*, 1953; Dobson and Warner, 1957; Freis *et al.*, 1957; Chinard *et al.*, 1962; Crone, 1963; Copp and Shim, 1965). This has the advantage of allowing a direct comparison of the two types of tracers and eliminates the necessity of complete circulatory isolation (Martín and Yudilevich, 1964; Winbury *et al.*, 1965a; Yudilevich and Martjn de Julián, 1965). Nondiffusible tracers also permit correction for blood content of diffusible tracers (Donato *et al.*, 1964; Bloor and Roberts, 1965; Donato *et al.*, 1966).

Tracers that are selectively accumulated or removed by a region can be used to measure blood flow in that area. The kidney clears the blood of para-aminohippuric acid and ^{125}I- or ^{131}I-Hippuran clearance from the blood is used as a measure of the effective renal blood flow (Gott *et al.*, 1962; Stokes and Ter-Pogossian, 1964; Pritchard *et al.*, 1965; Dabaj *et al.*, 1966). Glomerular filtration rate has been estimated by clearance of ^{131}I-Hypaque from the blood (Stokes and Ter-Pogossian, 1964).

The unique property of the liver to clear the blood of particulate matter has been used to determine liver blood flow (Taplin, 1965). The tracers include colloidal chromic phosphate (^{32}P) (Dobson and Jones, 1952) and colloidal ^{198}Au (Vetter *et al.*, 1954; Iio *et al.*, 1960; Restrepo *et al.*, 1960; Stroun *et al.*, 1962).

Bone selectively accumulates ^{45}Ca, ^{47}Ca, and ^{85}Sr, which is diluted in the large pool of bone Ca. Thus the clearance of these isotopes from the blood is a measure of bone blood flow (Frederickson *et al.*, 1955; Weinman *et al.*, 1963; Copp and Shim, 1965).

^{84}Rb has an advantage over ^{86}Rb for precordial counting, because of the geometric properties of the emissions (Bing *et al.*, 1964; Cohen *et al.*, 1967). The isotope decays by positron emissions 19% of the time. These ultimately yield a pair of gamma photons 180 degrees apart. With coincidence counters 180 degrees apart, above and below the organ (heart), it is possible to detect activity specifically from the organ with a minimum of background and stray counts.

Table 2 lists the organs studied with the approach and isotopes used.

6. ALTERATIONS IN NUTRITIONAL CIRCULATION PRODUCED BY PHARMACOLOGICAL AGENTS

In this section the changes in nutritional circulation produced by drugs, neurohumoral agents, and other procedures will be described as well as the changes due to disease states such as arterial occlusion. In many cases there was a dichotomy between the response of the arteriolar resistance vessels

TABLE 2. METHODS FOR NUTRITIONAL CIRCULATION IN VARIOUS ORGANS

Organ	Method[a] and route	Isotope	Radioactivity measurement[b]	References
Skeletal muscle	Washout—depot	^{24}Na	Indirect—tissue	Barlow et al., 1961; Elkin and Cooper, 1951; Franke et al., 1950; Kety, 1949; McGirr, 1952; Miller and Wilson, 1951; Moulton et al., 1958; Murphy et al., 1950; Prentice et al., 1955; Rapaport et al., 1952; Semple et al., 1951; Stone and Miller, 1949; Tønnesen, 1963; Walder, 1953, 1955; Wisham and Yalow, 1952
	Washout—depot	^{131}I	Indirect—tissue	Coffman, 1963; Gosselin, 1966a, 1966b; Hyman et al., 1959; Pabst, 1958; Rapaport et al., 1952
	Washout—depot	^{133}Xe	Indirect—tissue	Alpert et al., 1966; Lassen et al., 1964b, 1965; Lassen and Kampp, 1965; Lindbjerg et al., 1964; Lindbjerg, 1965; Tønnesen, 1964, 1965
	Washout—depot	^{133}Xe + ^{24}Na	Indirect—tissue	Lassen, 1964
	Washout—depot	^{133}Xe + ^{131}I	Indirect—tissue	Gosselin and Audino, 1966
	Washout, i.a.	^{24}Na	Indirect—tissue	Barlow et al., 1961; Bacaner and Beck, 1964
	Washout, i.a.	^{131}I	Indirect—tissue	Hyman et al., 1959; Hyman and Lenthall, 1962; Paldino et al., 1962
	Washout, i.a.	^{24}Na + ^{131}I-alb.	Indirect—tissue	Dobson and Warner, 1960
	Washout, i.a.	^{133}Xe	Indirect—tissue	Tønnesen and Sejrsen, 1967
	Uptake (E), i.a.	^{42}K	Direct—venous	Renkin, 1959a; 1959b
		^{86}Rb	Direct—venous	Friedman, 1965; Renkin and Rosell, 1962; Renkin et al., 1966; Sheehan and Renkin, 1965; Winbury and Gabel, 1967
		^{86}Rb + ^{131}I-alb.	Direct—venous	Winbury et al., 1965a

[a] In uptake method E = extraction, C = clearance and F = fractional. i.a. = intra-arterial; i.v. = intravenous.
[b] Indirect measurement refers to external counting. Direct measurement refers to direct counting of tissue or blood samples.

TABLE 2—cont.

Organ	Method[a] and route	Isotope	Radioactivity measurement[b]	References
Heart	Washout—depot	^{133}Xe	Indirect—tissue	Harley et al., 1966
(collateral)	Washout—depot	^{133}Xe or Kr^{85}	Indirect—tissue	Linder, 1966
	Washout—depot	^{131}I	Indirect—tissue	Hollander et al., 1963; Kirk and Honig, 1964; Madoff and Hollander, 1961
	Washout—depot	^{24}Na	Indirect—tissue	Salisbury et al., 1962
	Washout, i.a.	^{133}Xe	Indirect—tissue	Bernstein et al., 1965; Lichtlen et al., 1966; Rees and Redding, 1966; Rees et al., 1966
	Washout, i.a.	^{133}Xe	Autoradiography	Shaw et al., 1966
(collateral)	Washout, i.a.	^{133}Xe or ^{85}Kr	Indirect—tissue	Linder, 1966
	Washout, i.a.	^{85}Kr	Indirect—tissue	Herd et al., 1962; Lehan et al., 1966
(collateral)	Washout, i.a.	^{85}Kr	Indirect—tissue	Johansson et al., 1964, 1965, 1966
	Washout, i. aorta	^{133}Xe	Direct—venous	Holmberg et al., 1967
	Washout, i.a. + cor. v.	^{85}Kr	Indirect—tissue	Harman et al., 1966
	Washout, left ventricle	^{85}Kr	Direct—venous	Cohen et al., 1964, 1966; Elliott and Gorlin, 1966
	Washout, left ventricle	^{85}Kr	Indirect—tissue + Direct—venous	Klein et al., 1965
	Uptake (E), i.a.	^{84}Rb	Indirect coincidence—tissue	Bennish and Bing, 1962
	Uptake (E), i.a.	^{86}Rb	Direct—arterial + venous	Mack et al., 1959
	Uptake (E), i.a.	^{86}Rb + ^{131}I-alb.	Direct—venous	Winbury et al., 1962, 1963, 1965a, b, c; Winbury and Gabel, 1967; Winbury, 1967
	Uptake (E), i.a.	^{22}Na + ^{59}Fe-siderophilin	Direct—venous	Martin and Yudilevich, 1964
	Uptake (E), i.a.	^{131}I, ^{22}Na, ^{42}K, ^{86}Rb ^{131}I-alb., ^{59}Fe-siderophilin	Direct—venous	Yudilevich and Martin de Julián, 1965

	Uptake (E), i.v.	^{86}Rb	Direct—arterial + venous	Love and Burch, 1959
	Uptake (C), i.v.	^{84}Rb	Indirect coincidence—tissue + Direct—arterial	Bing et al., 1964; Cohen et al., 1965a, b; Lübs et al., 1965, 1966
	Uptake (C), i.v.	^{86}Rb	Indirect—tissue + Direct—tissue + arterial	Love and Burch, 1957a, b
	Uptake (C), i.v.	^{86}Rb	Direct—tissue + arterial	Love and O'Meallie, 1963; Love et al., 1965a, b; Love and Tyler, 1965
(collateral)	Uptake (C), i.v.	^{86}Rb	Direct—tissue + arterial	Levy et al., 1961; Levy and Chanksy, 1965
	Uptake (C), i.v.	^{86}Rb + ^{131}I-alb.	Indirect—tissue + Direct—arterial	Donato et al., 1964, 1966
(collateral)	Uptake (C), i.v.	^{3}H$_2$O	Direct—tissue + arterial	Bloor and Roberts, 1965
	Uptake (C), i.a.	^{86}Rb	Direct—tissue + arterial	Moir, 1966
	Uptake (F), i.v.	^{86}Rb	Direct—tissue	Galysh and Salazar, 1966; King et al., 1966; Levy and Martins de Oliveira, 1961; Pensinger et al., 1965; Winbury and Pensinger, 1966
Skin, subcutaneous and adipose	Washout—depot	^{133}Xe	Indirect—tissue	Larsen et al., 1966
	Washout—depot	^{24}Na	Indirect—tissue	Braithwaite et al., 1959; McGirr, 1952; Miller and Wilson, 1951; Wisham and Yalow, 1952
	Washout—depot	^{24}Na or ^{22}Na	Indirect—tissue	Gemmell and Veall, 1956
	Washout—depot	^{24}Na or ^{131}I	Indirect—tissue	Barany, 1955
	Washout—depot	^{125}I	Indirect—tissue	Dern and Leaverton, 1966
	Washout, i.a.	^{85}Kr	Indirect—tissue	Rubinstein et al., 1964; Thorburn et al., 1966
Hand	Uptake (F), i.v.	^{42}K	Indirect—tissue	Sapirstein and Goodwin, 1958
Synovia	Washout—depot	^{24}Na	Indirect—tissue	Wisham and Dworecka, 1966

TABLE 2—*cont.*

Organ	Method[a] and route	Isotope	Radioactivity measurement[b]	References
Bone	Uptake (E + C), i.a. + i.v.	^{85}Sr	Direct—tissue + arterial + venous	Copp and Shim, 1965
	Uptake (C), i.v.	^{45}Ca	Direct—tissue + arterial	Frederickson et al., 1955
	Uptake (C), i.a. or i.v.	^{47}Ca + ^{85}Sr	Direct—tissue + arterial	Weinman et al., 1963
Brain	Washout, i.a.	^{85}Kr	Indirect—tissue	Häggendal, 1966; Ingvar and Lassen, 1962; Lassen et al., 1964a; Skinhøj et al., 1964
	Washout, i.a.	^{85}Kr or ^{133}Xe	Indirect—tissue	Høedt-Rasmussen et al., 1966
	Washout, i.a. or inhalation	^{85}Kr	Indirect—tissue	Lassen and Høedt-Rasmussen, 1966
	Washout, inhalation	^{133}Xe	Indirect—tissue	Obrist et al., 1967
	Uptake (C), i.v.	CF_3 ^{131}I, ^{131}I-antipyrine, ^{14}C-pentobarbital, ^{14}C-antipyrine	Direct—arterial + autoradiograph	Kety, 1960b; Kety, 1965
Gastrointestinal	Uptake (C), i.v.	^{42}K	Direct—tissue + arterial	Delaney and Grim, 1964a, 1965
	Uptake (C), i.v.	^{86}Rb	Direct—tissue + arterial	Delaney and Custer, 1965
	Uptake (C), i.v.	$Na_2H^{32}PO_4$	Indirect—tissue + Direct—arterial	Bacaner and Beck, 1964
	Uptake (F), i.v.	^{86}Rb	Direct—tissue	Steiner and Mueller, 1961

Organ	Method	Tracer	Type	References
Pancreas	Uptake (F), i.v.	^{42}K	Direct—tissue	Delaney and Grim, 1964b
	Uptake (F), i.v.	^{42}K or ^{86}Rb	Direct—tissue	Delaney and Grim, 1966
	Uptake (F), i.v.	^{86}Rb	Direct—tissue	Papp et al., 1965
Kidney	Washout, i.a.	^{133}Xe	Indirect—tissue	Ladefoged et al., 1965; Carriere et al., 1966; Sparks et al., 1965; Thorburn et al., 1963
	Washout, i.a.	^{85}Kr	Indirect—tissue	
	Uptake (C), i.v.	^{131}I-Hippuran	Direct—venous	Dabaj et al., 1966; Gott et al., 1962; Pritchard et al., 1965
	Uptake (C), i.v.	^{131}I-Hippuran + ^{131}I-Hypaque	Direct—venous	Stokes and Ter-Pogossian, 1964
	Uptake (F), i.v.	^{86}Rb	Direct—tissue	Deutsch and Dreichlinger, 1963
Liver	Washout—depot	^{22}Na	Indirect—tissue	Sigel and Que, 1965
	Washout, i.a.	^{133}Xe	Indirect—tissue	Rees et al., 1964
	Uptake (C), i.v.	$Cr^{32}PO_4$ (colloid)	Direct—venous	Dobson and Jones, 1952
	Uptake (C), i.v.	^{198}Au (colloid)	Indirect—tissue (liver)	Ueda et al., 1961
	Uptake (C), i.v.	^{198}Au (colloid)	Indirect—tissue (liver + peripheral)	Iio et al., 1960; Restrepo et al., 1960; Stroun et al., 1962; Vetter et al., 1954
	Uptake (C), i.v.	^{198}Au (colloid)	Indirect—tissue (peripheral)	

TABLE 2—*cont.*

Organ	Method[a] and route	Isotope	Radioactivity measurement[b]	References
Endocrines				
Placenta	Washout—depot	^{24}Na	Indirect—tissue	McClure Browne and Veall, 1953
Pituitary	Uptake (F), i.v.	^{86}Rb	Direct—tissue	Goldman and Sapirstein, 1958
Adrenal	Uptake (F), i.v.	^{86}Rb + ^{131}I-antipyrine	Direct—tissue	Sapirstein and Goldman, 1959
Various	Uptake (F), i.v.	^{86}Rb	Direct—tissue	Goldman, 1961, 1963
Uterus	Washout—depot	^{133}Xe	Indirect—tissue	Lysgaard and Lefévre, 1965; Munck *et al.*, 1964, 1965
Testis	Washout—depot + i.a.	^{85}Kr	Indirect—tissue	Setchell *et al.*, 1966
	Uptake (F), i.v.	^{131}I-antipyrine	Direct—tissue	Setchell *et al.*, 1964
Various organs	Uptake (F), i.v.	^{86}Rb	Direct—tissue	Goldman, 1966; 1965/1966; Rathmacher *et al.*, 1965; Takács, 1965; Takács and Albert, 1965
	Uptake (F), i.v.	^{86}Rb or ^{42}K	Direct—tissue	Sapirstein, 1958; Takács *et al.*, 1964

and the nutritional circulation. These have been mentioned previously and some illustrative results are tabulated in Table 1. Any reference made to blood flow in the section refers to *nutritional* blood flow rather than *total* flow unless otherwise specified. The methods employed in the various regions are summarized in Table 2.

Nutritional circulation is measured by the clearance of a diffusible tracer from the blood or tissue. It is important to remember that the clearance of a tracer is related to the capillary blood flow rate, Q, and the capillary surface area available for transport of the tracer. Therefore, when *total* blood flow can vary, a change in nutritional circulation may be the result of a change in Q and/or PS. However, when the *total* blood flow is constant any change in the nutritional circulation will be the result of a like change in the capillary surface area.

6.1. SKELETAL MUSCLE (TABLE 3)

Reactive hyperemia following the interruption of the arterial supply (Kety, 1949; McGirr, 1952; Lassen *et al.*, 1964b) or during perfusion with venous blood (Gabel *et al.*, 1964; Winbury *et al.*, 1965a) increased nutritional circulation in animals or man. The increase in man was more than fivefold (Rapaport *et al.*, 1952; Pabst, 1958) and exceeded that due to exercise (Elkin and Cooper, 1951; Tønnesen, 1964). Exercise alone increased nutritional flow in skeletal muscle in animals or man (Kety, 1949; Walder, 1953; Pabst, 1958; Hyman *et al.*, 1959; Fox, 1962; Lassen and Kampp, 1965; Renkin *et al.*, 1966), but the response was smaller in patients with occlusive arterial disease (Tønnesen, 1965).

Vasodilator agents that normally increase *total* peripheral blood flow did not have the same effect on skeletal muscle nutritional flow after intravenous injection in man. Nicotinic acid, papaverine, and priscoline *decreased* nutritional flow in man (Murphy *et al.*, 1950; Elkin and Cooper, 1951), although intraarterial administration in the dog produced an increase. Since the patients did show a reactive hyperemia response, the blood flow reserve was not exhausted; this raises a question about the value of "peripheral dilators" for the treatment of occlusive arterial disease.

Comparison of ^{133}Xe clearance in normal patients with those having occlusive arterial disease demonstrated no difference at rest. However, with an impaired skeletal muscle circulation there was a diminished response to exercise, alone (Lassen and Kampp, 1965; Alpert *et al.*, 1966), or exercise during arterial occlusion (Lassen, 1964; Lassen *et al.*, 1964b; Lindbjerg

TABLE 3. ALTERATIONS IN NUTRITIONAL CIRCULATION

Organ	Drug	Species	Route[a]	Response	Comment	References
Skeletal muscle	Norepinephrine	Man	depot	→	Inhibited by alpha-blocker	Moulton et al., 1958
		Dog	i.a.	→		Sheehan and Renkin, 1965
		Dog	i.a.	↑		Gabel et al., 1964; Winbury et al., 1965a
		Cat	depot	→		Gosselin, 1966a
		Rabbit	depot	→		Pabst, 1958
	Epinephrine	Man	i.a. or i.v.	↑		Coffman, 1963
		Man	s.c.	↑		Dobson and Warner, 1957
		Man	i.v.	no change		Walder, 1953
		Man	depot			Kety, 1949; McGirr, 1952; Walder, 1953
		Dog	i.a.	↓ then ↑	Biphasic Increase-low conc. Decrease-high conc.	Gabel et al., 1964
		Dog	i.a.	↑ or ↓		Sheehan and Renkin, 1965
		Cat	depot			Gosselin, 1966a
	Isoproterenol	Dog	i.a.	↑	Inhibited by beta-blocker	Sheehan and Renkin, 1965
		Cat	depot	↑	Inhibited by beta-blocker	Gosselin, 1966a, 1966b
	Histamine	Man	depot	↑		Lindbjerg, 1965; McGirr, 1952; Walder, 1953
		Dog	i.a.	→	Hindlimb	Winbury et al., 1965a
		Dog	i.a.	↑		Gabel et al., 1964
	Acetylcholine or Mecholyl	Dog	i.a.	→		Gabel et al., 1964; Winbury et al., 1965a
		Cat	i.a.	↑		Hyman et al., 1959

[a] i.a. = intra-arterial; i.v. = intravenous; s.c. = subcutaneous; s.l. = sublingual; p.o. = oral; i.m. = intramuscular; i.p. = intraperitoneal.

	Animal	Route	Change		References
Bradykinin	Cat and Rabbit	i.a.	↑		Hyman and Lenthal, 1962; Paldino et al., 1962
Nitroglycerin	Dog	i.a.	↑		Gabel et al., 1964; Winbury and Gabel, 1967
PETN	Dog	i.a.	↑		Gabel et al., 1964; Winbury and Gabel, 1967
Vasopressin	Dog	i.a.	→		Gabel et al., 1964
Priscoline	Man	i.v.	→		Elkin and Cooper, 1951; Murphy et al., 1950
Nicotinic Acid	Man	i.v.	→		Elkin and Cooper, 1951; Murphy et al., 1950
Papaverine	Man	i.v.	→		Elkin and Cooper, 1951; Murphy et al., 1950; Friedman, 1965
	Dog	i.a.	←		
ATP	Cat and Rabbit	i.a.	←		Hyman and Lenthal, 1962
48/80	Cat	i.a.	←		Hyman et al., 1959
Sympathetic stimulation	Dog		→		Renkin and Rosell, 1962
	Cat		→		Hyman et al., 1959
Hyperemia	Man		←		Kety, 1949; Lassen et al., 1964b; McGirr, 1952
	Man		←	> 5-fold	Pabst, 1958; Rapaport et al., 1952
	Man		←	> exercise	Elkin and Cooper, 1951; Tønnesen, 1964

TABLE 3—*cont.*

Organ	Drug	Species	Route[a]	Response	Comment	References
Skeletal muscle —*cont.*	Hyperemia —*cont.*	Dog		↑	Venous blood	Gabel et al., 1964; Winbury et al., 1965a
		Dog		↑		Friedman, 1965
	Exercise	Man		↑		Alpert et al., 1966; Elkin and Cooper, 1951; Lassen et al., 1964b, 1965; Lassen and Kampp, 1965; McGirr, 1952; Pabst, 1958; Kety, 1949; Tønnesen, 1964; Walder, 1953
		Man		Inconsistent		Tønnesen, 1965
		Man		↑	Greater in normal	Semple et al., 1951
		Dog		↑		Friedman, 1965; Renkin et al., 1966
		Cat		↑	Nerve stimulation	Hyman et al., 1959
	Shock	Dog		↓		Gabel et al., 1964
Heart	Norepinephrine	Man	i.v.	↑		Cohen et al., 1964
		Dog	i.v.	↑		Lehan et al., 1966; Love and Burch, 1957a, b; Love et al., 1965a
		Dog	i.a.	↓	Constant flow	Winbury et al., 1962
	Epinephrine	Dog	i.a.	↑		Regan et al., 1966
	Isoproterenol	Man	i.v.	↑	Normal and anginal	Cohen et al., 1964, 1966; Elliott and Gorlin, 1966

Drug	Species	Route	Effect		References
Vasopressin	Dog	i.v.	↓	Constant flow	Love and Burch, 1957a, b
	Dog	i.a.	↓		Winbury et al., 1962
Nitroglycerin	Man	s.l.	↑—Normal ↓—Anginal		Bing et al., 1964; Cohen et al., 1965a, b, 1967; Donato et al., 1964; Lübs et al., 1966
	Man	s.l.	↑—Normal		Lübs et al., 1965
	Man	s.l.	No change—Anginal Variable—Normal		Ross et al., 1964
	Man	s.l.	↓—Anginal	Normal and anginal	Bernstein et al., 1965; Lichtlen et al., 1966
	Man	s.l.	No change	Anginal	Hollander et al., 1963
	Man	i.a.	↑	Greater in normal	Bernstein et al., 1965; Lichtlen et al., 1966
	Dog	i.v.	↓		Bernstein et al., 1965
	Dog	i.a.	←		Bernstein et al., 1965; Lehan et al., 1966; Rees and Redding, 1966; Rees et al., 1966; Winbury and Gabel, 1967
	Dog	i.a.	↑ Variable	Constant flow	Winbury et al., 1962, 1963
	Dog	i.a.		Depends on state of capillary circulation	Winbury et al., 1965c
Angiotensin	Dog	i.v.	No change	Increase blood pressure	Frank et al., 1965
	Dog	i.v.	No change	Total flow increase	Love et al., 1965a
PETN	Dog	i.v.	←		Rees and Redding, 1966
	Dog	i.a.	←	Variable flow or constant flow	Winbury and Gabel, 1967

TABLE 3—*cont.*

Organ	Drug	Species	Route[a]	Response	Comment	References
Heart —cont.	PETN—*cont.*	Dog	i.a.	↑	Constant flow	Winbury et al., 1962, 1963
		Dog	i.a.	Variable	Depends on state of capillary circulation	Winbury et al., 1965c
		Pig	p.o.	↑	Chronic	Winbury and Pensinger, 1966
	Dipyridamole	Dog	i.v.	↑		Lehan et al., 1966; Love et al., 1965a; Palmer et al., 1966; Rees and Redding, 1966 Moir, 1966
		Dog	i.a.	↑↑	Constant flow	Winbury et al., 1963
		Dog	i.a.	↑	Chronic	Winbury and Pensinger, 1966
		Pig	p.o.	↑		
	Isoptin	Man	i.v.	↑ / ←—Normal	Normal	Cohen et al., 1965b
		Man	i.v.	↓—Anginal		Lübs et al., 1966
	Intensain	Man	i.v.	Inconsistent / ←—Normal		Cohen et al., 1965b
		Man	i.v.	↓—Anginal		Lübs et al., 1966
	Papaverine	Man	i.v.	No change	Normal	Cohen et al., 1965b
		Man	i.v.	No change	Normal and anginal	Lübs et al., 1966
	Digitoxin	Dog	i.m.	↓	Chronic effect	Love et al., 1965a
	Reserpine	Dog	i.m.	↓	Chronic effect	Love et al., 1965a

		Species	p.o.		Chronic	Reference
Heart	Thyroxine	Rat		↑		Galysh and Salazar, 1966
	Hyperemia	Dog		↑		Hollander et al., 1963; Johansson et al., 1964; Madoff and Hollander, 1961
		Dog		↑	Systemic hypoxia	Lehan et al., 1966; Love and Tyler, 1965
	Exercise	Man		↑	Normal and anginal	Cohen et al., 1966; Hollander et al., 1963
		Man		↑	Greater in normal	Holmberg et al., 1967
Skin	Norepinephrine	Man	depot	→		Barany, 1955
	Epinephrine	Man	depot	→		Barany, 1955; McGirr, 1952
	Histamine	Man	depot	↑		Gemmell and Veall, 1956; McGirr 1952
	Angiotensin	Man	depot	→	Greater in hypertensive	Dern and Leaverton, 1966
	Veritol	Man	depot	↑	Greater in normal than diabetic	Barany, 1955
	Hyaluronidase	Man	depot	No change		Gemmell and Veall, 1956
	Hyperemia	Man		↑		Braithwaite et al., 1959; Sapirstein and Goodwin, 1958
	Nerve block	Man		↑		Barany, 1955

Table 3—*cont.*

Organ	Drug	Species	Route[a]	Response	Comment	References
Brain	Norepinephrine	Dog	i.v.	→	Gray matter	Häggendal, 1966
	Aramine	Dog	i.v.	→	Gray matter	Häggendal, 1966
	Papaverine	Dog	i.v.	↑	Gray matter	Häggendal, 1966
	Metrazol	Dog	i.v.	↑	Cortex	Ingvar and Lassen, 1962
	Pentobarbital	Rat	i.p.	No change	Anesthesia	Sapirstein, 1965
Adrenal	ACTH	Rat	i.v.	↑		Sapirstein and Goldman, 1959
Testis	Norepinephrine	Ram	i.a.	→		Setchell *et al.*, 1966
	Epinephrine	Ram	i.a.	→	Inhibited by alpha-blocking agent	Setchell *et al.*, 1966
	Isoproterenol	Ram	i.a.	↑		Setchell *et al.*, 1966
	Acetylcholine	Ram	i.a.	No change		Setchell *et al.*, 1966
Gastric	Norepinephrine	Dog	i.v.	→		Delaney and Grim, 1965
	Epinephrine	Dog	i.v.	↑		Delaney and Grim, 1964a, 1965
	Histamine	Dog	i.v. or i.m.	↑		Delaney and Grim, 1964a, 1965

Organ	Agent	Species	Route	Effect	Reference
Pancreas	Secretin	Dog	i.v.	No change	Delaney and Grim, 1965
	Norepinephrine	Dog	i.v.	No change	Delaney and Grim, 1964b, 1966
	Epinephrine	Dog	i.v.	→	Delaney and Grim, 1964b, 1966
		Rat	i.v.	No change	Papp et al., 1965
	Histamine	Dog	i.v.	No change	Delaney and Grim, 1964b
		Dog	i.v.	→	Delaney and Grim, 1966
		Rat	i.v.	↑	Papp et al., 1965
	Vasopressin	Dog	i.v.	→	Delaney and Grim, 1966
	Dibenzyline	Dog	i.v.	No change	Delaney and Grim, 1966
	Secretin	Dog	i.v.	↑	Delaney and Grim, 1964b, 1966
	Pancreozymin	Dog	i.v.	No change	Delaney and Grim, 1966
	Decholin	Rat	i.v.	↑	Papp et al., 1965
	Cortisone	Dog	i.v.	↑	Delaney and Grim, 1966
Liver	Norepinephrine	Man	i.v.	↑	Iio et al., 1960
	Epinephrine	Mouse	i.v.	→	Dobson and Jones, 1952
		Man	i.v.	↑	Iio et al., 1960
	Decholin	Man	i.v.	↑	Iio et al., 1960
	Aminophylline	Man	i.v.	↑	Iio et al., 1960

et al., 1964; Lassen *et al.*, 1965; Tønnesen, 1965). Likewise histamine administered in the depot of ^{133}Xe produced a smaller increase in clearance in diseased patients compared with normals (Lindbjerg, 1965). These procedures are of value in the diagnosis of peripheral vascular disease. The clearance of ^{24}Na from a depot in skeletal muscle was similar in normotensive and hypertensive patients, but when norepinephrine was added to the depot, the reduction in clearance in the hypertensives was twice that of normals (Moulton *et al.*, 1958).

Among the catecholamines, isoproterenol produced an increase in the nutritional circulation, which could be blocked by beta-adrenergic blocking agents (Sheehan and Renkin, 1965; Gosselin, 1966a; 1966b). Norepinephrine usually decreased the nutritional circulation (Moulton *et al.*, 1958; Pabst, 1958; Sheehan and Renkin, 1965; Gosselin, 1966a), but one laboratory reported an increase in skeletal muscle and the hindlimb of the dog in the face of arteriolar constriction (Gabel *et al.*, 1964; Winbury *et al.*, 1965a). This difference could be due to the mode of administration of norepinephrine. The increase in nutritional circulation occurred with abrupt intraarterial injection; the decreases were observed with norepinephrine, in a depot or administered as an intraarterial infusion. The reduction in clearance could be blocked by an alpha-adrenergic blocking agent (Sheehan and Renkin, 1965). Epinephrine has been reported to produce an increase (Dobson and Warner, 1957; Coffman, 1963; Gabel *et al.*, 1964), decrease (Kety, 1949; Walder, 1953; King *et al.*, 1966), biphasic response (decrease then increase) (Sheehan and Renkin, 1965), or no change in the skeletal muscle nutritional circulation of animals and man. Again, these differences could be due to the mode or route of administration as well as dosage. For example, a low concentration in a depot increased flow but a high concentration decreased local flow (Gosselin, 1966a).

Stimulation of the sympathetic outflow reduced the clearance of ^{24}Na or ^{86}Rb (Hyman *et al.*, 1959; Renkin and Rosell, 1962), but stimulation of the medullary cholinergic vasodilator center did not change the ^{24}Na clearance in spite of a marked augmentation of *total* skeletal muscle blood flow.

Elevation of nutritional flow was also observed with histamine (McGirr, 1952; Walder, 1953; Gabel *et al.*, 1964), bradykinin (Hyman and Lenthall, 1962; Paldino *et al.*, 1962), mecholyl (Hyman *et al.*, 1959), ATP (Hyman and Lenthall, 1962), the nitrates, nitroglycerin, and pentaerythritol tetranitrate (Winbury and Gabel, 1967), and the histamine releaser, 48/80 (Hyman and Lenthall, 1962). Nutritional flow was reduced by shock and by vasopressin (Gabel *et al.*, 1964).

6.2. HEART (TABLE 3)

A number of groups have investigated the effect of nitroglycerin on myocardial nutritional circulation in man. A qualitative difference in the response of the normal (increase) and coronary disease patient (decrease or no change) was observed on sublingual treatment (Hollander *et al.*, 1963; Bing *et al.*, 1964; Donato *et al.*, 1964; Ross *et al.*, 1964; Cohen *et al.*, 1965a, 1965b; Lübs *et al.*, 1965; Lübs *et al.*, 1966; Cohen *et al.*, 1967). Others found a decrease in both types of patients after sublingual dosage, but an increase when the nitroglycerin was given directly into the coronary artery (Bernstein *et al.*, 1965; Lichtlen *et al.*, 1966).

A similar pattern was observed in the dog administered nitroglycerin by the intracoronary (increase) or intravenous (decrease) route (Bernstein *et al.*, 1965). Other animal studies indicated that nitroglycerin by the intravenous (Lehan *et al.*, 1966; Rees and Redding, 1966; Rees *et al.*, 1966) or intracoronary route augmented myocardial nutritional flow (Winbury *et al.*, 1962; 1963; Winbury and Gabel, 1967). The response can be dependent upon the myocardial nutritional flow reserve, for when coronary flow was constant and all of the myocardial capillaries open there was either no change or a decrease in flow (Winbury *et al.*, 1965c). This may be similar to the condition in the patient with coronary heart disease, and could be the reason for the decrease in the nutritional flow that has been reported.

Another nitrate, PETN, was studied in the dog and pig. When administered by intracoronary injection, nutritional circulation was elevated if total coronary inflow was held constant or permitted to increase (Winbury and Gabel, 1967). Chronic oral treatment of pigs for 7 days elevated the fractional ^{86}Rb uptake, but did not change the *total* coronary flow; this is in contrast to dipyridamole, which increased ^{86}Rb uptake and *total* blood flow (Fig. 6) (Winbury and Pensinger, 1966). It was suggested that PETN has a specific effect on precapillary sphincters, while dipyridamole acts directly on arteriolar resistance vessels.

A number of other coronary dilators have been studied in animals and man. Isoptin and Intensain increased nutritional flow in normal humans but decreased the flow in coronary patients; papaverine caused no change in either type of patient (Cohen *et al.*, 1965b; Lübs *et al.*, 1966). Dipyridamole augmented the nutritional circulation after intravenous (Love *et al.*, 1965a; Lehan *et al.*, 1966; Palmer *et al.*, 1966; Rees and Redding, 1966), oral (Winbury and Pensinger, 1966), or intracoronary (Winbury *et al.*, 1963) administration in dogs. The response to exercise or intravenous injection of isoproterenol has been used for the diagnosis of coronary heart disease. Although both increase myocardial tracer clearance, the normal individual had a greater response (Hollander *et al.*, 1963; Cohen *et al.*, 1964, 1966; Harman *et al.*, 1966; Holmberg *et al.*, 1967).

Chronic treatment of dogs with digitoxin or reserpine reduced nutritional circulation (Love *et al.*, 1965a), but chronic treatment of rats with

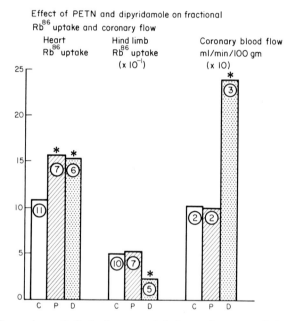

FIG. 6. Comparison of effect of pentaerythritol tetranitrate *P* and dipyridamole *D* on coronary blood flow and fractional uptake of ^{86}Rb in swine heart. The control group is represented by *C*. Both drugs significantly (*) increased ^{86}Rb uptake but only dipyridamole increased blood flow. Animals received drugs *per os* for 7 days at a dose of 40 mg/kg per day.

thyroxine elevated flow (Galysh and Salazar, 1966). Acute injection of angiotensin did not alter tracer clearance in dogs even though *total* coronary flow was enhanced (Frank *et al.*, 1965; Love *et al.*, 1965a). On the other hand, vasopressin lowered the myocardial nutritional blood flow. In the majority of studies norepinephrine and epinephrine enhanced nutritional flow. The same effect was observed during reactive hyperemia (Madoff and Hollander, 1961; Hollander *et al.*, 1963; Johansson *et al.*, 1964; Love and Tyler, 1965; Lehan *et al.*, 1966).

6.3. SKIN (TABLE 3)

The vasoconstrictor agents, norepinephrine, epinephrine, and angiotensin, reduced nutritional circulation in the skin (McGirr, 1952; Barany, 1955; Dern and Leaverton, 1966). The vasodilator, histamine, increased dermal nutritional circulation (McGirr, 1952; Gemmell and Veall, 1956), and hyaluronidase produced no change (Gemmell and Veall, 1956). The agents were administered as a depot with the tracer, so that these are local effects.

Patients with hypertension or diabetes showed an abnormal response of the local dermal nutritional circulation. The hypertensive patient had an increased response to angiotensin (Dern and Leaverton, 1966). In the diabetic, ^{131}I clearance was lower before and after nerve block, and veritol produced an attenuated response compared to normal man (Barany, 1955).

Indirect heating or cooling caused large alterations in *total* cutaneous blood flow, not always accompanied by similar changes in nutritional circulation (Miller and Wilson, 1951). During reflex vasodilatation clearance of [24]Na from a skin depot was not changed, but there was a decrease during reflex vaso-constriction. The failure of clearance to increase during reflex vasodilatation may be due to blood passing through the arteriovenous shunts present in the skin (Miller and Wilson, 1951). Local cooling of the skin led to reduced clearance and local heating to an increased clearance (McGirr, 1952; Rubinstein *et al.*, 1964).

[85]Kr washout from the skin of the rat indicated the presence of two components with markedly different perfusion rates (Thorburn *et al.*, 1966). The fast component (30 ml/min per 100 g) was associated with the hair follicles and the slow component (4.5 ml/min per 100 g) with the remainder of the skin. During the resting phase of hair growth (telogen), the fast component comprised 21% of the tissue mass, but during rapid hair growth (anagen) it increased to 67% of the tissue mass but the basic nutritional perfusion rate of each compartment was not altered.

As in skeletal muscle and heart, there was increased nutritional circulation of the skin during reactive hyperemia (Sapirstein and Goodwin, 1958; Braithwaite *et al.*, 1959).

6.4. BRAIN (TABLE 3)

By use of washout of diffusible tracers ([85]Kr and ^{133}Xe) it was found that the white and gray matter have different perfusion rates (Lassen *et al.*, 1964a; Skinhoj *et al.*, 1964; Høedt-Rasmussen *et al.*, 1966; Obrist *et al.*,

1967). The washout curve has two exponentials, with the fast component corresponding to the gray matter and the slower component corresponding to the white matter. These two compartments are considered to be in parallel.

The gray matter appeared to be more sensitive to drugs and contributed more to the overall changes in brain blood flow produced by drug than did the white matter. Specific measurements of nutritional circulation in the gray matter demonstrated a reduction with norepinephrine and aramine and an increase with papaverine (Häggendal, 1966). Metrazol increased average brain clearance of tracer (Ingvar and Lassen, 1962) while pentobarbital did not alter fractional uptake of ^{131}I-antipyrine (Sapirstein, 1965).

Average nutritional flow (gray and white) was reduced in cerebrovascular disease (Lassen *et al.*, 1964a).

6.5. GASTROINTESTINAL TRACT, LIVER, AND PANCREAS (TABLE 3)

The fractional distribution of blood flow to various portions of the gastrointestinal tract was estimated by uptake of ^{86}Rb or [42]K. In the rat the nutritional circulation of the stomach was less than one half that of the duodenum; there was a progressive decline down the small intestine (Steiner and Mueller, 1961). A more extensive regional analysis has been made in the dog. The ^{86}Rb clearance for various portions follows: esophagus, 21 ml/min per 100 g; stomach, 51; duodenum, 70; remainder of intestine, 72; and colon, 82 (Delaney and Custer, 1965). Further analysis of gastric nutritional flow revealed that the corpus of the stomach received eight times as much circulation as the antrum but weighs only four times as much (Delaney and Grim, 1965). The mucosal layer receives 70% of the flow to the corpus, with the remainder equally divided between the submucosa and muscularis (Delaney and Grim, 1965).

Drugs not only alter total gastric nutritional circulation, but the distribution as well (Delaney and Grim, 1964a; 1965). Histamine increased gastric blood flow and did not alter the ratio of antrum to corpus perfusion. In contrast, epinephrine, which also increased overall gastric perfusion, had a greater effect on the antrum, thereby increasing the antrum:corpus ratio. Norepinephrine decreased the gastric nutritional flow primarily at the expense of the corpus. Thus there was a rise in the antrum:corpus ratio. Finally, secretin produced a selective increase in the antrum which was not adequate to result in a significant elevation of overall gastric blood flow.

The catecholamines, epinephrine and norepinephrine, had variable effects on pancreatic nutritional blood flow; the same was true for histamine (Delaney and Grim, 1964b; Papp *et al.*, 1965; Delaney and Grim, 1966). Blood flow was increased by secretin, cortisone, and decholin, and decreased by vasopressin (Delaney and Grim, 1964b; Papp *et al.*, 1965; Delaney and Grim, 1966). Pancreozymin and dibenzyline were without effect.

In man, hepatic circulation was enhanced by the intravenous injection of epinephrine, norepinephrine, decholin, and aminophylline (Iio *et al.*, 1960). In the mouse, epinephrine had the opposite effect (Dobson and Jones, 1952).

6.6. EPIDIDYMIS, TESTIS AND KIDNEY (TABLE 3)

The regional distribution of nutritional blood flow in the testis and epididymis of the rat and ram was determined by fractional uptake of ^{131}I-antipyrine (Setchell *et al.*, 1964). Perfusion of the testis was one and one half that of the average rate of the epididymis in the rat. However, in the ram the nutritional flow was the same in the testis and epididymis. There was stratification of flow rate in the epididymis with the head having the highest rate in the rat, whereas in the ram it is lowest in the first portion of the head but increased farther down. Changes in nutritional circulation of the testis were measured by [85]Kr washout (Setchell *et al.*, 1966). Epinephrine and norepinephrine produced a reduction in flow that was blocked by an alpha-adrenergic blocking agent. Isoproterenol improved testicular nutritional flow but acetylcholine had no effect.

The perfusion rates of different regions of the dog kidney were affected by hemorrhagic hypotension (Carriere *et al.*, 1966). A marked decrease in average renal clearance of [85]Kr was observed; this due to a reduction in the fast phase of cortical perfusion accompanied by a marked redistribution of available circulation between the cortex and medulla.

6.7. VARIOUS ORGANS—FRACTIONAL DISTRIBUTION

Several investigators have used the fractional distribution approach to determine the effect of pharmacological agents on a number of organs simultaneously. Changes in the fraction of the cardiac output received by an organ will indicate a specific effect on the nutritional circulation of that organ in relation to the total nutritional circulation. Changes in clearance of the tracer (flow fraction × cardiac output) in an organ may be non-specific via an increase in cardiac output.

Epinephrine and norepinephrine, given intravenously, had different effects on the regional distribution of nutritional blood flow in the rat (Takács, 1965; Goldman, 1966). Epinephrine altered the flow fraction to many organs whereas norepinephrine altered only a few (Goldman, 1966). For example, an infusion of epinephrine at the rate of 0.5 mcg/kg per min reduced the fractional distribution of ^{86}Rb to the adrenal, thyroid, spleen, and skin, and caused an increase to the kidney. A like dose of norepinephrine increased adrenal, thyroid, and gut fractional distribution. At higher doses of either agent other organs or regions such as skin, gut, kidney, pineal, heart, and skeletal muscle were affected. Distribution to the heart was increased by the higher doses of both agents. Vasopressin infusion in rats increased flow fraction to posterior pituitary, pineal, liver, and lung and decreased the fraction to the skin and skeletal muscle (Goldman, 1965/1966). Bradykinin had little effect on fractional distribution throughout the various organs (Takács and Albert, 1965).

7. SUMMARY AND CONCLUSION

Diffusible tracers have been employed for the study of the nutritional circulation or capillary transport function. This dimension of the regional microcirculation is possibly more important than the *total* regional blood flow since the exchange between the blood and tissues can occur only in functional capillary beds. Pharmacologic agents have produced changes in nutritional circulation independent of those on regional *total* blood flow or vascular resistance, suggesting that these variables are under independent control. *Total* blood flow or vascular resistance is controlled by the arteriolar resistance vessels and the nutritional circulation by the pre-capillary sphincters.

The diffusible tracers are well suited for the measurement of nutritional blood flow because the exchange between the blood and tissues is limited by capillary blood flow rate and not by the permeability of the capillary or cell membrane. Therefore clearance of a tracer is related to the rate of capillary blood flow and to the capillary surface area available for transport of the tracer. The latter is a function of the number of open capillaries regulated by the precapillary sphincters.

Lipid soluble tracers such as ^{85}Kr or ^{133}Xe have almost infinite permeability even at high blood flow rate; thus extraction is complete and clearance of the tracer is a measure of capillary blood flow even at high flow rates. On the other hand, with lipid insoluble tracers such as ^{42}K, ^{86}Rb, ^{84}Rb, ^{24}Na, ^{131}I, etc., permeability is not as great and extraction varies inversely with the rate of capillary blood flow. Clearance of these tracers follows blood flow but is not proportional, and at high flow rates permeability may become limiting. At that point clearance is a measure of the diffusion capacity of the tissue for the particular tracer.

The two basic approaches for the study of nutritional circulation with diffusible tracers are the *washout* principle and the *uptake* principle. Washout depends upon the removal of a diffusible tracer from the tissue by the effective capillary blood flow in the region. The tracer may be placed in the tissue as a local depot or by addition to the tissue via the arterial supply. The rate of washout from the tissue is exponential; therefore the clearance constant is a measure of the function of the nutritional circulation.

The uptake approach depends upon removal of the tracer from the arterial blood by the tissue. The principal methods are the measurement of extraction from the arterial blood, the direct determination of clearance of arterial blood, and the fractional distribution of cardiac output.

Clearance may or may not agree with the *total* blood flow depending on the tracer used and whether or not there is physiological shunting of the particular tracer in the tissue.

The use of diffusible tracers for the study of various tissues has been described. Perfusion is not homogeneous in skeletal muscle, brain, kidney, and skin. It is possible to analyze the perfusion rate and the size of each of the compartments in these areas by the appropriate use of diffusible tracers. In addition, by the proper experimental design it is possible to determine the effect of a drug on the arteriolar resistance vessels and on the precapillary sphincters at the same time. Further, lipid insoluble tracers permit the measurement of the effect of pharmacological agents on the capillary surface area.

REFERENCES

(A) BOOKS, REVIEWS AND MONOGRAPHS

BARANY, F. R. (1955) Abnormal vascular reactions in diabetes mellitus. *Acta Medica Scand.*, **152**:1–129.

BERNE, R. M. (1967) Autoregulation of coronary blood flow: Possible role of adenosine, in *Problems in Laboratory Evaluation of Antianginal Agents*, Winbury, M. M. (ed.). North-Holland Publishing C., Amsterdam, pp. 8–16.

BURTON, A. C. (1965) *Physiology and Biophysics of the Circulation.* Year Book Medical Publishers Inc., Chicago, Ill., U.S.A.

DOBSON, E. L. and JONES, H. B. (1952) The behavior of intravenously injected particulate material: Its rate of disappearance from the blood stream as a measure of liver blood flow. *Acta Medica Scand.* **144**:273–344.

DOBSON, E. L. and WARNER, G. F. (1960) Clearance rates following intra-arterial injections in the study of peripheral vascular beds, in *Methods in Medical Research*, Vol. 8, Bruner, H. D. (ed.). Year Book Publishers, Inc., Chicago, Ill., U.S.A., pp. 242–8.

HYMAN, C. (1960) Peripheral blood flow measurements: Tissue clearance, in *Methods in Medical Research*, Vol. 8, Bruner, H. D. (ed.). Year Book Publishers Inc., Chicago, Ill., U.S.A., pp. 236–42.

KETY, S. S. (1951) The theory and applications of the exchange of inert gas at the lungs and tissues. *Pharmacol. Rev.*, **3**:1–41.

KETY, S. S. (1960a) Theory of blood-tissue exchange and its application to measurement of blood flow, in *Methods in Medical Research*, Vol. 8. Bruner, H. D. (ed.). Year Book Publishers Inc., Chicago, Ill., U.S.A., pp. 223–7.

KETY, S. S. (1960b) Measurement of local blood flow by the exchange of an inert, diffusible substance, in *Methods in Medical Research*, Vol. 8, Bruner, H. D. (ed.). Year Book Publishers Inc., Chicago, Ill., U.S.A., pp. 228–36.

KETY, S. S. (1965) Measurement of regional circulation in the brain and other organs by isotopic techniques, in *Isotopes in Experimental Pharmacology*, Roth, L. J. (ed.). University of Chicago Press, Chicago and London, pp. 211–18.

KITCHIN, A. H. (1963) Peripheral blood flow and capillary filtration rates. *Brit. Med. Bull.*, **19**:155–60.

LANDIS, E. M. and PAPPENHEIMER, J. R. (1963) Exchange of substances through the capillary walls, in *Handbook of physiology*, Section 2, Circulation, Vol. 2, Hamilton, W. F. and Dow, P. (eds.). American Physiological Society, Washington, D.C., U.S.A., pp. 961–1034.

LUTZ, B. R. and FULTON, G. P. (1962) Structural basis of the microcirculation, in *Blood Vessels and Lymphatics* Abramson, D. I. (ed.). Academic Press, New York and London, pp. 137–45.

RENKIN, E. M. (1967) Blood flow and transcapillary exchange in skeletal and cardiac muscle, in *Coronary Circulation and Energetics of the Myocardium*. Karger, Basel, pp. 18–30.

ROBERTSON, J. S. (1962) Mathematical treatment of uptake and release of indicator substances in relation to flow analysis in tissues and organs, in *Handbook of Physiology*, Section 2: Circulation, Vol. 1, Hamilton, W. F. and Dow, P. (eds.). American Physiological Society, Washington, D.C., U.S.A., pp. 617–44.

TAPLIN, G. V. (1965) Liver blood flow, in *Radioisotopes and Circulation*, Sevelius, G. (ed.). Little Brown & Co., Boston, Mass., U.S.A., pp. 205–25.

WINBURY, M. M. (1967) Role of myocardial nutritional circulation in evaluation of antianginal agents, in *Problems in Laboratory Evaluation of Antianginal Agents*, Winbury, M. M. (ed.). North-Holland Publishing Co., Amsterdam, pp. 26–40.

WINBURY, M. M., KISSIL, D. and LOSADA, M. (1965a) Approaches to the study of nutritional blood flow—extraction of Rb^{86} by the heart and hind limb, in *Isotopes in Experimental Pharmacology*, Roth, L. J. (ed.). University of Chicago Press, Chicago and London, pp. 229–48.

ZWEIFACH, B. W. (1961) *Functional Behavior of the Microcirculation* (American Lecture Series). Charles C. Thomas, Springfield.

(B) ORIGINAL PAPERS

ALPERT, J., GARCIA DEL RIO, H. and LASSEN, N. A. (1966) Diagnostic use of radioactive xenon clearance and a standardized walking test in obliterative arterial disease of the legs. *Circulation*, **34**:849–55.

BACANER, M. B. and BECK, J. S. (1964) Regional blood flow measurement *in vivo* for a definable geometry. *Amer. J. Physiol.*, **206**:962–6.

BARLOW, T. E., HAIGH, A. L. and WALDER, D. N. (1961) Evidence for two vascular pathways in skeletal muscle. *Clin. Sci.*, **20**:367–85.

BENNISH, A. and BING, R. J. (1962) Determination of nutrient coronary microcirculation by external coincidence counting with the use of rubidium-84. *Clin. Med.*, **60**:859.

BERNSTEIN, L., FRIESINGER, G. C., LICHTLEN, P. R. and ROSS, R. S. (1965) The effect of nitroglycerin on the systemic and coronary circulation in man and dogs. *Circulation*, **33**:107–16.

BING, R. J., BENNISH, A., BLUEMCHEN, G., COHEN, A., GALLAGHER, J. P. and ZALESKI, E. J. (1964) The determination of coronary flow equivalent with coincidence counting technic. *Circulation*, **29**:833–46.

BLOOR, C. M. and ROBERTS, L. E. (1965) Effect of intravascular isotope content on the isotopic determination of coronary collateral blood flow. *Circulation Res.*, **16**:537–44.

BRAITHWAITE, F., FARMER, F. T., EDWARDS, J. R. G. and INKSTER, J. S. (1959) Simultaneous measurements of blood flow and sodium-24 clearance in the skin. *Brit. J. Plast. Surgery*, **12**:189–99.

CARRIERE, S., THORBURN, G. D., O'MORCHOE, C. C. C. and BARGER, A. C. (1966) Intrarenal distribution of blood flow in dogs during hemorrhagic hypotension. *Circulation Res.*, **19**:167–79.

CHINARD, F. P., ENNS, T. and NOLAN, M. F. (1962) Indicator-dilution studies with "diffusible" indicators. *Circulation Res.*, **10**:473–90.

COFFMAN, J. D. (1963) Effects of intra-arterial and intravenous epinephrine on disappearance of NaI[131] from calf muscle and on calf blood flow. *Circulation Res.*, **13**:56–63.

COHEN, A., GALLAGHER, J. P., LUEBS, E.-D., VARGA, Z., YAMANAKA, J., ZALESKI, E. J., BLUEMCHEN, G. and BING, R. J. (1965a) The quantitative determination of coronary flow with a positron emitter (rubidium-84). *Circulation*, **32**:636–49.

COHEN, A., ZALESKI, E., LUEBS, E.-D. and BING, R. J. (1965b) The use of positron emitter in the determination of coronary blood flow in man. *The Physiologist*, **8**:137.

COHEN, A., ZALESKI, E. J., BALEIRON, H., STOCK, T. B., CHIBA, C. and BING, R. J. (1967) Measurement of coronary blood flow using rubidium[84] and the coincidence counting method—A critical analysis. *Amer. J. Cardiol.*, **19**:556–62.

COHEN, L. S., ELLIOTT, W. C. and GORLIN, R. (1964) Measurement of myocardial blood flow using krypton-85. *Amer. J. Physiol.*, **206**:997–9.

COHEN, L. S., ELLIOTT, W. C., KLEIN, M. D. and GORLIN, R. (1966) Coronary heart disease—Clinical, cinearteriographic and metabolic correlations. *Amer. J. Cardiol.*, **17**:153–68.

CONN, H. L., JR. (1962) Use of external counting technics in studies of the circulation. *Circulation Res.*, **10**:505–17.

COPP, D. H. and SHIM, S. S. (1965) Extraction ratio and bone clearance of Sr^{85} as a measure of effective bone blood flow. *Circulation Res.*, **16**:461–7.

CRONE, C. (1963) The permeability of capillaries in various organs as determined by use of the "indicator diffusion" method. *Acta Physiol. Scand.*, **58**:292–305.

DABAJ, E., MENGES, H., JR., and PRITCHARD, W. H. (1966) Determination of renal blood flow by single injection of Hippuran-I[131] in man—a comparison with the standard clearance technique. *Amer. Heart J.*, **71**:79–83.

DELANEY, J. P. and CUSTER, J. (1965) Gastrointestinal blood flow in the dog. *Circulation Res.*, **17**:394–402.

DELANEY, J. P. and GRIM, E. (1964a) Canine gastric blood flow and its distribution. *Amer. J. Physiol.*, **207**:1195–1202.

DELANEY, J. P. and GRIM, E. (1964b) Drug influences on pancreatic blood flow. *Fed. Proc.*, **23**:252.

DELANEY, J. P. and GRIM, E. (1965) Experimentally induced variations in canine gastric blood flow and its distribution. *Amer. J. Physiol.*, 208:353–8.

DELANEY, J. P. and GRIM, E. (1966) Influence of hormones and drugs on canine pancreatic blood flow. *Amer. J. Physiol.*, 211:1398–1402.

DERN, P. L. and LEAVERTON, P. (1966) The effect of angiotensin-II on the "clearance" of radioiodine from the skin in hypertension. *J. Lab. Clin. Med.*, 67:265–72.

DEUTSCH, G. and DREICHLINGER, O. (1963) Differential determination of blood flow in kidney functional areas with Rb^{86}. *Studii. Cerc. Stint. Med.*, 10:59–67.

DOBSON, E. L. and WARNER, G. F. (1957) Measurement of regional sodium turnover rates and their application to the estimation of regional blood flow. *Amer. J. Physiol.*, 189:269–76.

DONATO, L., BARTOLOMEI, G., FEDERIGHI, G. and TORREGGIANI, G. (1966) Measurement of coronary blood flow by external counting with radioactive rubidium—Critical appraisal and validation of the method. *Circulation*, 33:708–18.

DONATO, L., BARTOLOMEI, G. and GIORDANI, R. (1964) Evaluation of myocardial blood perfusion in man with radioactive potassium or rubidium and precordial counting. *Circulation*, 29:195–203.

ELKIN, D. C. and COOPER, F. W., JR. (1951) The effect of vasodilator drugs on the circulation of the extremities. *Surgery*, 29:323–33.

ELLIOTT, W. C. and GORLIN, R. (1966) Isoproterenol in treatment of heart disease—Hemodynamic effects in circulatory failure. *J. Amer. Med. Ass.*, 197:315–20.

FOX, I. J. (1962) Indicators and detectors for circulatory dilution studies and their application to organ or regional blood-flow determination. *Circulation Res.*, 10:447–71.

FRANK, M. J., NADIMI, M., CASANEGRA, P. and STEIN, P. (1965) The effect of angiotensin on myocardial function. *Clin. Res.*, 13:525.

FRANKE, F. R., BOATMAN, J. B., GEORGE, R. S. and MOSES, C. (1950) Effect of physical factors on radiosodium clearance from subcutaneous and intramuscular sites in animals. *Proc. Soc. Exp. Biol. Med.*, 74:417–21.

FREDERICKSON, J. M., HONOUR, A. J. and COPP, D. H. (1955) Measurement of initial bone clearance of Ca^{45} from blood in the rat. *Fed. Proc.*, 14:49.

FREIS, E. D., HIGGINS, T. F. and MOROWITZ, H. J. (1953) Transcapillary exchange rates of deuterium oxide and thiocyanate in the forearm of man. *J. Appl. Physiol.*, 5:526–32.

FREIS, E. D., SCHNAPER, H. W. and LILIENFIELD, L. S. (1957) Rapid and slow components of the circulation in the human forearm. *J. Clin. Invest.*, 36:245–53.

FRIEDMAN, J. J. (1965) Microvascular flow distribution and rubidium extraction. *Fed. Proc.*, 24:1099–1103.

FRIEDMAN, J. J. (1966) Total, non-nutritional, and nutritional blood volume in isolated dog hindlimb. *Amer. J. Physiol.*, 210:151–6.

GABEL, L. P., WINBURY, M. M., ROWE, H. and GRANDY, R. P. (1964) The effect of several pharmacological agents upon Rb^{86} uptake by the perfused dog hindlimb. *J. Pharmacol.*, 146:117–22.

GALYSH, F. T. and SALAZAR, M. A. (1966) Cardiac output and functional myocardial blood flow in rats treated with sodium D- or L-thyrozine (D-T_4 or L-T_4). *Pharmacologist*, 8:213.

GEMMELL, W. and VEALL, N. (1956) The factors influencing the tissue clearance of radioactive sodium. *Strahlentherapie Sonderbaende*, 36:120–7.

GERAUD, J., BRU, A. and BES, A. (1960) Méthode de mesure des variations de la capacité vasculaire périphérique par l'utilisation de sérumalbumine humaine marquée par ^{131}I. *Compte Rendus*, 154:1647–51.

GOLDMAN, H. (1961) Endocrine gland blood flow in the unanesthetized, unrestrained rat. *J. Appl. Physiol.*, 16:762–4.

GOLDMAN, H. (1963) Effect of acute stress on the pituitary gland: Endocrine gland blood flow. *Endocrinology*, **72**:588–91.

GOLDMAN, H. (1965/1966) Vasopressin modulation of the distribution of blood flow in the unanesthetized rat. *Neuroendocrinology*, **1**:23–30.

GOLDMAN, H. (1966) Catecholamine-induced redistribution of blood flow in the unanesthetized rat. *Amer. J. Physiol.*, **210**:1419–23.

GOLDMAN, H. and SAPIRSTEIN, L. A. (1958) Determination of blood flow to the rat pituitary gland. *Amer. J. Physiol.*, **194**:433–5.

GOODALE, W. T. and HACKEL, D. B. (1953) Measurement of coronary blood flow in dogs and man from rate of myocardial nitrous oxide desaturation. *Circulation Res* **1**:502–8.

GORESKY, C. A. (1965) The nature of transcapillary exchange in the liver. *Canad. Me Ass. J.*, **92**:517–22.

GOSSELIN, R. E. (1966a) Local effects of catecholamines on radioiodide clearance in skeletal muscle. *Amer. J. Physiol.*, **210**:885–92.

GOSSELIN, R. E. (1966b) Mechanism of isoproterenol-induced vasodilatation in muscle. *Pharmacologist*, **8**:174.

GOSSELIN, R. E. and AUDINO, L. F. (1966) Dual control of the microcirculation in muscle. *Fed. Proc.*, **25**:594.

GOTT, F. S., PRITCHARD, W. H., YOUNG, W. R., and MACINTYRE, W. J. (1962) Renal blood flow measurement from the disappearance of intravenously injected Hippuran I^{131}. *J. Nucl. Med.*, **3**:480–5.

GRÄNGSJÖ, G., ULFENDAHL, H. R. and WOLGAST, M. (1966) Determination of regional blood flow by means of small semiconductor detectors and red cells tagged with phosphorus-32. *Nature*, **211**:1411–12.

GRANT, R. T. (1964) Direct observation of skeletal muscle blood vessels (rat cremaster). *J. Physiol.*, **172**:123–37.

GRUPP, G. (1963) Potassium exchange in the dog heart *in situ*. *Circulation Res.*, **13**:279–89.

HÄGGENDAL, E. (1966) Effects of some vasoactive drugs on the vessels of the cerebral grey matter in the dog. *Acta Physiol. Scand.*, **66**:55–79.

HARLEY, A., HARPER, J. R. and ESTES, E. H. (1966) Distribution of blood flow in the myocardium measured by clearance of xenon^{133}. *Circulation*, **34**:122.

HARMAN, M. A., MARKOV, A., LEHAN, P. H., OLDEWURTEL, H. W. and REGAN, T. J. (1966) Coronary blood flow measurements in the presence of arterial obstruction. *Circulation Res*, **19**:632–7.

HERD, J. A., HOLLENBERG, M., THORBURN, G. D., KOPALD, H. H. and BARGER, A. C. (1962) Myocardial blood flow determined with krypton-85 in unanesthetized dogs. *Amer. J. Physiol.*, **203**:122 4.

HIRVONEN, L. and SONNENSCHEIN, R. R. (1962) Relation between blood flow and contraction force in active skeletal muscle. *Circulation Res.*, **10**:94–104.

HØEDT-RASMUSSEN, K., SVEINSDOTTIR, E. and LASSEN, N. A. (1966) Regional cerebral blood flow in man determined by intra-arterial injection of radioactive inert gas. *Circulation Res.*, **18**:237–47.

HOLLANDER, W., MADOFF, I. M., and CHOBANIAN, A. V. (1963) Local myocardial blood flow as indicated by the disappearance of NaI^{131} from the heart muscle: Studies at rest, during exercise and following nitrite administration. *J. Pharmacol.*, **139**:53–9.

HOLMBERG, S., PAULIN, S., PŘEROVSKÝ, I. and VARNAUSKAS, E. (1967) Coronary blood flow in man and its relation to the coronary arteriogram. *Amer. J. Cardiol.*, **19**:486–91.

HYMAN, C. (1957) Physiological implications of dual circulation in muscle. *Angiologie*, **9**:25–7.

HYMAN, C. and LENTHALL, J. (1962) Analysis of clearance of intra-arterially administered labels from skeletal muscle. *Amer. J. Physiol.*, **203**:1173–8.

HYMAN, C., ROSELL, S., ROSEN, A., SONNENSCHEIN, R. R. and UVNÄS, B. (1959) Effects of alterations of total muscular blood flow on local tissue clearance of radio-iodide in the cat. *Acta Physiol. Scand.*, **46**:358–74.

Iio, M., KAMEDA, H. and UEDA, H. (1960) The study on hepatic blood flow determination by Au^{198} colloid using deviced recording method. *Jap. Heart J.*, **1**:17–36.

INGVAR, D. H. and LASSEN, N. A. (1962) Regional blood flow of the cerebral cortex determined by krypton[85]. *Acta Physiol. Scand.*, **54**:325–38.

JOHANSSON, B., LINDER, E. and SEEMAN, T. (1964) Collateral blood flow in the myocardium of dogs measured with krypton[85]. *Acta Physiol. Scand.*, **62**:263–70.

JOHANSSON, B., LINDER, E. and SEEMAN, T. (1965) Coronary collateral blood flow in relation to the mass of ischemic myocardium, studied with krypton. *Acta Physiol. Scand.*, **63**:495–504.

JOHANSSON, B., LINDER, E. and SEEMAN, T. (1966) Effects of heart rate and arterial blood pressure on coronary collateral blood flow in dogs. *Acta Physiol. Scand.*, **68**:33–46.

KETY, S. S. (1949) Measurement of regional circulation by the local clearance of radioactive sodium. *Amer. Heart J.*, **38**:321–8.

KETY, S. S. and SCHMIDT, C. F. (1948) The nitrous oxide method for the quantitative determination of cerebral blood flow in man: Theory, procedure and normal values. *J. Clin. Invest.*, **27**:476–83.

KING, R. D., STEINER, S. H. and HEIMBURGER, I. L. (1966) Effect of epicardiectomy on myocardial blood flow. *J. Thoracic Card. Surg.*, **51**:660–6.

KIRK, E. S. and HONIG, C. R. (1964) Nonuniform distribution of blood flow and gradients of oxygen tension within the heart. *Amer. J. Physiol.*, **207**:661–8.

KLEIN, M. D., COHEN, L. S. and GORLIN, R. (1965) Krypton-85 myocardial blood flow: Precordial scintillation versus coronary sinus sampling. *Amer. J. Physiol.*, **209**:705–10.

KRASNOW, N., LEVINE, H. J., WAGMAN, R. J. and GORLIN, R. (1963) Coronary blood flow measured by I^{131} Iodo-antipyrine. *Circulation Res.*, **12**:58–62.

LADEFOGED, J., PEDERSEN, F., DOUTHEIL, U., DEETJEN, P. and SELKURT, E. E. (1965) Renal blood flow measured with Xenon-133 wash-out technique and with an electromagnetic flow meter. *Pflügers. Arch. ges. Physiol.*, **284**:195–200.

LARSEN, O. A., LASSEN, N. A. and QUAADE, F. (1966) Blood flow through human adipose tissue determined with radioactive xenon. *Acta Physiol. Scand.*, **66**:337–45.

LASSEN, N. A. (1964) Muscle blood flow in normal man and in patients with intermittent claudication evaluated by simultaneous Xe^{133} and Na^{24} clearances. *J. Clin. Invest.* **43**:1805–12.

LASSEN, N. A. and HØEDT-RASMUSSEN, K. (1966) Human cerebral blood flow measured by two inert gas techniques. *Circulation Res.*, **19**:681–8.

LASSEN, N. A. and KAMPP, M. (1965) Calf muscle blood flow during walking studied by the Xe^{133} method in normals and in patients with intermittent claudication. *Scand. J. Clin. Lab. Invest.*, **17**:447–53.

LASSEN, N. A. and MUNK, O. (1955) The cerebral blood flow in man determined by the use of radioactive krypton. *Acta Physiol. Scand.*, **33**:30–49.

LASSEN, N. A., HØEDT-RASMUSSEN, K., SØRENSEN, S. C., SKINHØJ, E., CRONQUIST, S., BODFORSS, B. and INGVAR, D. H. (1964a) Regional cerebral blood flow in man determined by krypton[85]. *Neurology*, **13**:719–27.

LASSEN, N. A., LINDBJERG, I. F., and MUNCK, O. (1964b) Measurement of blood-flow through skeletal muscle by intramuscular injection of xenon-133. *Lancet*, **i**:686–9.

LASSEN, N. A., LINDBJERG, I. F. and DAHN, I. (1965) Validity of the xenon[133] method for measurement of muscle blood flow evaluated by simultaneous venous occlusion plethysmography: Observations in the calf of normal man and in patients with occlusive vascular disease. *Circulation Res.*, 16:287:93.

LAURENCE, R., GRANDY, R. P., WARREN, P. and WINBURY, M. M. (1963) Studies on Rb[86] uptake by the dog hind limb. *Pharmacologist*, 5:274.

LEHAN, P. H., OLDEWURTEL, H. A., WEISSE, A. B., ELLIOTT, M. S. and REGAN, T. J. (1966) Relationship of angiographic coronary artery diameter to blood flow. *Circulation*, 34:154.

LEVY, M. N. and CHANSKY, M. (1965) Collateral circulation after coronary artery constriction. *Amer. J. Physiol.*, 208:144–8.

LEVY, M. N. and MARTINS DE OLIVEIRA, J. (1961) Regional distribution of myocardial blood flow in the dog as determined by Rb[86]. *Circulation Res.*, 9:96–8.

LEVY, M. N., IMPERIAL, E. S. and ZIESKE, H., JR. (1961) Collateral blood flow to the myocardium as determined by the clearance of rubidium[86] chloride. *Circulation Res.*, 9:1035–43.

LEWIS, B. M., SOKOLOFF, L., WENTZ, W. B., WECHSLER, R. L., and KETY, S. S. (1955) Determination of cerebral blood flow using radioactive krypton. *Fed. Proc.*, 14:92.

LICHTLEN, P., ROSS, R. S., FRIESINGER, G. C. and BERNSTEIN, L. (1966) Die Wirkung von Nitroglyzerin auf die Koronardurchblutung am Menschen, Unter Berücksichtigung der selektiven Koronarangiographie und Messung der Koronardurchblutung mit Xenon 133. *Cardiologia*, 48:371–3.

LINDBJERG, I. F. (1965) Measurement of muscle blood-flow with ^{133}Xe after histamine injection as a diagnostic method in peripheral arterial disease. *Scand. J. Clin. Lab. Invest.*, 17:371–80.

LINDBJERG, I. F., LASSEN, N. A. and MUNCK, O. (1964) Musklernes Blodgennemstrømning ved Claudicatio Intermittens Bestemt med [133]xenon. *Nord. Med.*, 72:1013–19.

LINDER, E. (1966) Measurements of normal and collateral coronary blood flow by close arterial and intramyocardial injection of krypton-85 and xenon-133. *Acta Physiol. Scand.*, 68:5–31.

LOVE, W. D. (1964) Isotope clearance and myocardial blood flow. *Amer. Heart J.*, 67:579–82.

LOVE, W. D. and BURCH, G. E. (1957a) A study in dogs of methods suitable for estimating the rate of myocardial uptake of Rb[86] in man, and the effect of L-norepinephrine and Pitressin® on Rb[86] uptake. *J. Clin. Invest.*, 36:468–78.

LOVE, W. D. and BURCH, G. E. (1957b) Differences in the rate of Rb[86] uptake by several regions of the myocardium of control dogs and dogs receiving L-norepinephrine or Pitressin®. *J. Clin. Invest.*, 36:479–84.

LOVE, W. D. and BURCH, G. E. (1959) Influence of the rate of coronary plasma flow on the extraction of Rb[86] from coronary blood, *Circulation Res.*, 7:24–30.

LOVE, W. D. and O'MEALLIE, L. P. (1963) Relationship of blood flow and myocardial Rb[86] clearance in right and left ventricles. *Amer. J. Physiol.*, 205:382–4.

LOVE, W. D. and TYLER, M. D. (1965) Effect of hypoxemia and hypercapnia on regional distribution of myocardial blood flow. *Amer. J. Physiol.*, 208:1211–16.

LOVE, W. D., MUNFORD, R. S. and ABRAHAM, R. E. (1965a) Comparison of the effects of L-norepinephrine, angiotensin, dipyridamole, digitoxin, and reserpine on the regional distribution of coronary blood flow. *J. Lab. Clin. Med.*, 66:423–32.

LOVE, W. D., TYLER, M. D., ABRAHAM, R. E. and MUNFORD, R. S. (1965b) Effects of O_2, CO_2, and drugs on estimating coronary blood flow from Rb[86] clearance. *Amer. J. Physiol.*, 208:1206–10.

LÜBS, E. D., COHEN, A., ZALESKI, E., ZÜHLKE, V. and BING, R. J. (1965) Die Bestimmung der Koronardurchflussmenge beim Menschen mit dem Isotop Rubidium-84 und einem koinzidenzmess System und ihre diagnosticheAuswertung. *Z. Kreislaufforsch.* 54:1217–28.

LÜBS, E. D., COHEN, A., ZALESKI, E. J. and BING, R. J. (1966) Effect of nitroglycerin, Intensain, Isoptin, and papaverine on coronary blood flow in man—measured by the coincidence counting technic and rubidium[84]. *Amer. J. Cardiol.*, **17**:535–41.

LYSGAARD, H. and LEFÈVRE, H. (1965) Myometrial blood flow in pregnancy measured with xenon[133]. *Acta Obst. Gynec. Scand.*, **44**:401–7.

MACK, R. E., NOLTING, D. D., HOGANCAMP, C. E. and BING, R. J. (1959) Myocardial extraction of Rb[86] in the rabbit. *Amer. J. Physiol.* **197**:1175–7.

MADOFF, I. M. and HOLLANDER, W. (1961) Experiences with NaI[131] injected into the myocardium as an estimate of coronary blood flow. *J. thoracic card. Surg.*, **42**: 755–63.

MARCHIORO, T., FELDMAN, A., OWENS, J. C. and SWAN, H. (1961) Measurement of myocardial blood flow: Indicator-dilution technique. *Circulation Res.*, **9**:541–6.

MARTÍN, P. and YUDILEVICH, D. (1964) A theory for the quantification of transcapillary exchange by tracer-dilution curves. *Amer. J. Physiol.*, **207**:162–8.

McCLURE BROWNE, J. C. and VEALL, N. (1953) The maternal placental blood flow in normotensive and hypertensive women. *J. Obstet. Gynaec. Brit. Empire*, **60**:141–7.

McGIRR, E. M. (1952) The rate of removal of radioactive sodium following its injection into muscle and skin. *Clin. Sci.* **11**:91–9.

MELLANDER, S. (1964) Skeletal muscle circulation. *Nord. Med.*, **72**:1311–16.

MELLANDER, S. (1966) Comparative effects of acetylcholine, butyl-norsynephrine (Vasculat), noradrenaline. and ethyl-adrianol (Effontil) on resistance, capacitance, and precapillary sphincter vessels and capillary filtration in cat skeletal muscle. *Angiologica*, **3**:77–99.

MILLER, H. and WILSON, G. M. (1951) The measurement of blood flow by the local clearance of radioactive sodium. *Brit. Heart J.*, **13**:227–33.

MOIR, T. W. (1966) Measurement of coronary blood flow in dogs with normal and abnormal myocardial oxygenation and function—Comparison of flow measured by a rotameter and by Rb[86] clearance. *Circulation Res.*, **19**:695–9.

MOULTON, R., SPENCER, A. G. and WILLOUGHBY, D. A. (1958) Noradrenaline sensitivity in hypertension measured with a radioactive sodium technique. *Brit. Heart J.*, **20**: 224–8.

MUNCK, O. and LASSEN, N. A. (1957) Bilateral cerebral blood flow and oxygen consumption in man by use of krypton[85]. *Circulation Res.*, **5**:163–8.

MUNCK, O., LYSGAARD, H., PONTONNIER, G., LEFÈVRE, H. and LASSEN, N. A. (1964) Measurement of blood-flow through uterine muscle by local injection of [133]Xenon. *Lancet*, **i**:1421.

MUNCK, O., PONTONNIER, G., LYSGAARD, H., LEFÈVRE, H., and LASSEN, N. A. (1965) Détermination du débit du muscle utérin par injection locale de xénon 133. *Rev. Franc. Étud. Clin. Biol.*, **9**:750–3.

MURPHY, R. A., JR., McCLURE, J. N., JR., COOPER, F. W., JR. and CROWLEY, L. G. (1950) The effect of priscoline, papaverine, and nicotinic acid on blood flow in the lower extremity of man—A comparative study. *Surgery*, **27**:655–63.

NOLTING, D., MACK, R., LUTHY, E., KIRSCH, M. and HOGANCAMP, C. (1958) Measurement of coronary blood flow and myocardial rubidium uptake with Rb[86]. *J. Clin. Invest.*, **37**:921.

OBRIST, W. D., THOMPSON, H. K., JR., KING, C. H. and WANG, H. S. (1967) Determination of regional cerebral blood flow by inhalation of 133-xenon. *Circulation Res.*, **20**:124–35.

PABST, H. W. (1958) Isotopenstudien uber die Regulation der Muskeldurchblutung. *Strahlentherapie Sonderbaende*, **38**:313–22.

PALDINO, R. L., HYMAN, C. and LENTHALL, J. (1962) Bradykinin-induced increase in total and effective blood flow in skeletal muscle. *Circulation Res.*, **11**:847–52.

PALMER, W. H., FAM, W. M. and McGREGOR, M. (1966) The effect of coronary vasodilatation (dipyridamole-induced) on the myocardial distribution of tritiated water. *Canad. J. Physiol. Pharmacol.*, **44**:777–82.

PAPP, M., ÁCS, Z. and VARGA, B. (1965) The effect of agents influencing circulation on pancreatic blood flow. *Acta Physiol. Acad. Sci. Hung*, **26**:44–5.

PENSINGER, R. R., WINBURY, M. M., LOSADA, M. and KISSIL, D. (1965) Functional regional circulation in the myocardium of pig and dog determined by Rb^{86} uptake and I^{131}-albumin. *Circulation*, **32**:170.

PRENTICE, T. C., STAHL, R. R., DIAL, N. A. and PONTERIO, F. V. (1955) A study of the relationship between radioactive sodium clearance and directly measured blood flow in the biceps muscle of the dog. *J. Clin. Invest.*, **34**:545–58.

PRITCHARD, W. H., ECKSTEIN, R. W., MACINTYRE, W. J. and DABAJ, E. (1965) Correlation of renal blood flow determined by the single injection of hippuran-I^{131} with direct measurements of flow. *Amer. Heart J.*, **70**:789–96.

RAPAPORT, S. I., SAUL, A., HYMAN, C. and MORTON, M. E. (1952) Tissue clearance as a measure of nutritive blood flow and the effect of lumbar sympathetic block upon such measures in calf muscle. *Circulation*, **5**:594–604.

RATHMACHER, R. P., ANDERSON, L. L., and MELAMPY, R. M. (1965) Regional organ blood flow in the immature pig. *The Physiologist*, **8**:255.

REES, J. R. and REDDING, V. J. (1966) Myocardial blood flow measurement. *Proc. Roy. Soc. Med.*, **59**:30–4.

REES, J. R., REDDING, V. J. and ASHFIELD, R. (1964) Hepatic blood-flow measurement with Xenon-133; Evidence for separate hepatic-arterial and portal-venous pathways. *Lancet*, **ii**:562–3.

REES, J. R., REDDING, V. J., ASHFIELD, R., GIBSON, D. and GAVEY, C. J. (1966) Myocardial blood flow measurement with ^{133}xenon effect of glyceryl trinitrate in dogs. *Brit. Heart J.*, **28**:374–81.

REGAN, T. J., MOSCHOS, C. B., LEHAN, P. H., OLDEWURTEL, H. A. and HELLEMS, H. K. (1966) Lipid and carbohydrate metabolism of myocardium during the biphasic inotropic response to epinephrine. *Circulation Res.*, **19**:307–16.

RELLER, C. R., JR., SHERIDAN, J. D. and AUST, J. B. (1964) Tissue blood flow during varied perfusion conditions. *Amer. J. Physiol.*, **207**:1354–60.

RENKIN, E. M. (1959a) Transport of potassium-42 from blood to tissue in isolated mammalian skeletal muscles. *Amer. J. Physiol.*, **197**:1205–10.

RENKIN, E. M. (1959b) Exchangeability of tissue potassium in skeletal muscle. *Amer. J. Physiol.* **197**:1211–15.

RENKIN, E. M. (1965) Blood flow and transcapillary exchange in skeletal muscle. *Fed. Proc.*, **24**:1092–8.

RENKIN, E. M. and ROSELL, S. (1962) The influence of sympathetic adrenergic vasoconstrictor nerves on transport of diffusible solutes from blood to tissues in skeletal muscle. *Acta Physiol. Scand.*, **54**:223–40.

RENKIN, E. M., HUDLICKÁ, O., and SHEEHAN, R. M. (1966) Influence of metabolic vasodilatation on blood-tissue diffusion in skeletal muscle. *Amer. J. Physiol.*, **211**:87–98.

RESTREPO, J. E., WARREN, W. D., NOLAN, S. P. and MULLER, W. H., JR. (1960) Radioactive gold technique for the estimation of liver blood flow: Normal values and technical considerations. *Surgery*, **48**:748–57.

ROSS, R. S. and FRIESINGER, G. C. (1965) Anatomic and physiologic considerations in measurements of myocardial blood flow. *Circulation*, **32**:630–5.

ROSS, R. S., UEDA, K., LIGHTLEN, P. R. and REES, J. R. (1964) Measurement of myocardial blood flow in animals and man by selective injection of radioactive inert gas into the coronary arteries. *Circulation Res.*, **15**:28–41.

ROWE, G. G. (1962) The regulation of coronary blood flow in man in normal and abnormal conditions. *Med. Clin. N. Am.* **46**:1421–44.

RUBINSTEIN, H. M., DIETZ, A. A. and CZEBOTAR, V. (1964) Measurement of regional blood flow through the skin from the clearance of krypton-85. *Nature*, **202**:704–5.

SALISBURY, P. F., CROSS, C. E., OBLATH, R. W. and RIEBEN, P. A. (1962) Local circulation in heart muscle studied with Na^{24} clearance method. *J. Appl. Physiol.*, **17**:475–8.

SAPIRSTEIN, L. A. (1958) Regional blood flow by fractional distribution of indicators. *Amer. J. Physiol.*, **193**:161–8.

SAPIRSTEIN, L. A. (1965) Effect of anesthesia on the distribution of cerebral blood flow in the rat. *The Physiologist*, **8**:267.

SAPIRSTEIN, L. A. and GOLDMAN, H. (1959) Adrenal blood flow in the albino rat. *Amer. J. Physiol.*, **196**:159–62.

SAPIRSTEIN, L. A. and GOODWIN, R. S. (1958) Measurement of blood flow in the human hand with radioactive potassium. *J. Appl. Physiol.*, **13**:81–4.

SAPIRSTEIN, L. A. and MELLETTE, H. (1955) Use of antipyrine in regional blood flow measurements in the dog. *Fed. Proc.*, **14**:129.

SCHROEDER, W. (1966) Nutritive und nicht-nutritive Skelettmuskeldurchblutung. *Arch. Kreisl.-Forsch.*, **40**:36–49.

SEMPLE, R., McDONALD, L. and EKINS, R. P. (1951) Radioactive sodium (Na^{24}) in the measurement of local blood flow. *Amer. Heart J.*, **41**:803–9.

SETCHELL, B. P., WAITES, G. M. H. and THORBURN, G. D. (1966) Blood flow in the testis of the conscious ram measured with krypton^{85}: Effects of heat, catecholamines and acetylcholine. *Circulation Res.*, **18**:755–65.

SETCHELL, B. P., WAITES, G. M. H. and TILL, A. R. (1964) Variations in flow of blood within the epididymis and testis of the sheep and rat. *Nature*, **203**:317–18.

SEVELIUS, G. and JOHNSON, P. C. (1959) Myocardial blood flow determined by surface counting and ratio formula. *J. Lab. Clin. Med.*, **54**:669–79.

SHAW, D., FRIESINGER, G. C., PITT, A. and ROSS, R. S. (1966) Macro-autoradiography of Xe^{133} in the myocardium. *Fed. Proc.*, **25**:401.

SHEEHAN, R. M. and RENKIN, E. M. (1965) Influence of adrenergic drugs on blood-tissue diffusion. *Pharmacologist*, **7**:178.

SIGEL, B. and QUE, M. Y. (1965) Measurement of local hepatic circulation—A technique using tissue clearance of radioactive sodium (^{22}Na). *Arch. Surg.*, **90**:202–4.

SKINHOJ, E., LASSEN, N. A. and HØEDT-RASMUSSEN, K. (1964) Cerebellar blood flow in man. *Arch. Neurol.*, **10**: 464–7.

SPARKS, H. V., KOPALD, H. H., CARRIERE, S., CHIMOSKEY, J. E. and BARGER, A. C. (1965) Intrarenal distribution of blood flow in dogs with chronic congestive heart failure. *The Physiologist*, **8**:277.

STEINER, S. H. and MUELLER, G. C. E. (1961) Distribution of blood flow in the digestive tract of the rat. *Circulation Res.*, **9**:99–102.

STOKES, J. M. and TER-POGOSSIAN, M. M. (1964) Double isotope technique to measure renal functions—Single injection technique without urine collection. *J. Amer. Med. Ass.*, **187**:20–3.

STONE, P. W. and MILLER, W. B., JR. (1949) Mobilization of radioactive sodium from the gastrocnemius muscle of the dog. *Proc. Soc. Exp. Biol. Med.*, **71**:529–34.

STROUN, J., MEYKADEH, F. and WENGER, P. (1962) La mesure du débit sanguin hépatique chez l'adulte normal par la clearance kupfférienne de l'or colloidal radioactif. *Helv. Med. Acta*, **29**:597–606.

SULLIVAN, J. M., TAYLOR, W. J., ELLIOTT, W. C. and GORLIN, R. (1965) Clearance of intramyocardial radiokrypton as an index of regional myocardial blood flow. *Circulation*, **32**:204.

TAKÁCS, L. (1965) Effects of adrenalin and noradrenalin on cardiac output and regional blood flow in the rat. *Acta Physiol. Acad. Sci. Hung.*, **27**:205–12.

TAKÁCS, L. and ALBERT, K. (1965) Action of bradykinin on cardiac output and blood distribution of rats. *Arch. Int. Pharmacodyn.*, **155**:117–21.

TAKÁCS, L., KÁLLAY, K. and KARIA, A. (1964) Methodological remarks on Sapirstein's isotope indicator fractionation technique. *Acta Physiol. Hung.*, **25**:389–98.

THORBURN, G. D., CASEY, B. H. and MOLYNEUX, G. S. (1966) Distribution of blood flow within the skin of the rabbit with particular reference to hair growth. *Circulation Res.*, **18**:650–9.

THORBURN, G. D., KOPALD, H. H., HERD, J. A., HOLLENBERG, M., O'MORCHOE, C. C. and BARGER, A. C. (1963) Intrarenal distribution of nutrient blood flow determined with krypton[85] in the unanesthetized dog. *Circulation Res.*, **13**:290–307.

TØNNESEN, K. H. (1963) Clinical application of Na[24]-clearance during standard exercise in chronic arterial thrombosis. *Scand. J. Clin. Lab. Invest.*, **15**:64–5.

TØNNESEN, K. H. (1964) Blood-flow through muscle during rhythmic contraction measured by [133]xenon. *Scand. J. Clin. Lab. Invest.*, **16**:646–54.

TØNNESEN, K. H. (1965) The blood-flow through the calf muscle during rhythmic contraction and in rest by patients with occlusive arterial disease measured by Xe[133]. *Scand. J. Clin. Lab. Invest.*, **17**:433–46.

TØNNESEN, K. H. and SEJRSEN, P. (1967) Inert gas diffusion method for measurement of blood flow—Comparison of bolus injection to directly measured blood flow in the isolated gastrocnemius muscle. *Circulation Res.*, **20**:552–64.

TYBJAERG HANSEN, A., HAXHOLDT, B. F., HUSFELDT, E., LASSEN, N. A., MUNCK, O., RAHBEK SØRENSEN, H. and WINKLER, K. (1956) Measurement of coronary blood flow and cardiac efficiency in hypothermia by use of radioactive krypton 85. *Scand. J. Clin. Lab. Invest.*, **8**:182–8.

UEDA, H., IIO, M., KAMEDA, H. and MIGITA, T. (1961) Analysis of radioactive colloidal gold uptake rate in the liver by electronic digital computer—New analytical method for the determination of liver blood flow. *Jap. Heart J.*, **2**:460–72.

VETTER, H., FALKNER, R. and NEUMAYR, A. (1954) The disappearance rate of colloidal radiogold from the circulation and its application to the estimation of liver blood flow in normal and cirrhotic subjects. *J. Clin. Invest.*, **33**:1594–1602.

WALDER, D. N. (1953) The local clearance of radioactive sodium from muscle in normal subjects and those with peripheral vascular disease. *Clin. Sci.*, **12**:153–67.

WALDER, D. N. (1955) The relationship between blood flow, capillary surface area and sodium clearance in muscle. *Clin. Sci.*, **14**:303–15.

WEINMAN D. T., KELLY, P. J., OWEN, C. A., JR. and ORVIS, A. L. (1963) Skeletal clearance of Ca[47] and Sr[85] and skeletal blood flow in dogs. *Proc. Mayo Clin.*, **38**:559–70.

WINBURY, M. M. and GABEL, L. P. (1967) Effect of nitrates on nutritional circulation of heart and hindlimb. *Amer. J. Physiol.*, **212**:1062–6.

WINBURY, M. M., GABEL, L. and GRANDY, R. P. (1962) Effect of vasoactive agents on myocardial Rb[86]-uptake in the dog using a double-isotope technique. *Pharmacologist*, **4**:180.

WINBURY, M., GABEL, L. and GRANDY, R. P. (1963) Effect of vasoactive agents on nutritional blood flow and O$_2$ uptake in the myocardium of the dog, in *Abstracts*; *Second International Pharmacological Meeting, Prague, August 20–23, 1963*. p. 75. Hava, M., Palecek, F. and Volicer, L. (eds.). Pergamon Press, London, New York.

WINBURY, M. M., KISSIL, D. and LOSADA, M. (1965b) Influence of blood flow on myocardial extraction and clearance of Rb[86]. *Fed. Proc.*, **24**:235.

WINBURY, M. M., KISSIL, D. and LOSADA, M. (1965c) Functional organization of myocardial circulation: Effect of nitrites. *Circulation*, **32**:220.

WINBURY, M. M. and PENSINGER, R. R. (1966) Effect of pentaerythritol tetranitrate (PETN) and dipyridamole on the myocardial fractional Rb[86] uptake and coronary blood flow in pigs. *Pharmacologist*, **8**:222.

WISHAM, L. H. and DWORECKA, F. F. (1966) The effect of sympathectomy on radiosodium clearance from the knee joints of dogs. *J. Cardiovasc. Surg.*, **7**:66–8.

WISHAM, L. H. and YALOW, R. S. (1952) Some factors affecting the clearance of Na²⁴ from human muscle. *Amer. Heart J.*, **43**:67–76.

YUDILEVICH, D. and MARTÍN DE JULIÁN, P. (1965) Potassium sodium and iodide trans-capillary exchange in the dog heart. *Amer. J. Physiol.*, **208**:959–67.

ZWEIFACH, B. W. (1957) General principles governing the behavior of the microcirculation. *Amer. J. Med.*, **23**:684–96.

CHAPTER 13

RADIOISOTOPES COMPARTMENTAL ANALYSIS IN CELLULAR EXCHANGES

J. F. Lamb

*Department of Physiology, Bute Medical Buildings, St. Andrews,
Fife, Scotland*

1. INTRODUCTION

THE main object in writing this chapter has been to present a fairly complete account of the way in which exchanges of substances (mainly ions) across cell membranes may be measured, including the corrections which must be applied to them. The way in which the subject has been developed and the difficulties introduced is based on experience gained in teaching this subject to (medical) honours students over the last few years. The approach adopted is simple, perhaps oversimple. One justification for this is that there are numerous papers in the literature in which incorrect techniques or equations have been used or corrections omitted with a consequent uncertainty about the meaning of the results obtained. A second object has been to give some guidance as to the best kind of equipment to use. A third object is to provide some guidance on the interpretation of the results of these experiments once they are obtained. The literature in this field is very large. The choice of papers quoted is therefore somewhat arbitrary. I have tended to quote those papers that I have found useful and been most influenced by, and must apologize for omissions. In general it is hoped that this chapter will enable workers not familiar with the field to make meaningful measurements of exchanges across cell membranes without consulting the large number of separate papers on the subject. To this end, suggestions for improvements would be greatly welcomed.

Cells are continually exchanging materials between themselves and their environment. The rates of these exchanges may vary very widely from the rapid exchanges of water to the slow exchanges of ions. These exchanges will be called the fluxes of the substances across the cell membranes, either an influx or an efflux. In the past some confusion has arisen over the nomenclature of such measurements. In order to avoid this it is now customary to express the results of flux measurements in the absolute terms of an amount of a substance crossing unit area of cell membrane in unit time (see Keynes, 1951). Convenient units are pmole/cm² sec. Having measured the fluxes it is often desired to estimate the permeability of the cell membrane to a particular substance. Such a permeability is a property of the cell membrane. It is related to the flux of the substance by the following equation:

$$\text{Driving force} = (\text{flux})\,(\text{permeability}) \tag{1}$$

For uncharged substances the driving force is the concentration difference. For charged substances the driving force must incorporate the potential across the membrane as well as the concentration difference. Therefore the electrochemical potential must be used in Eq. (1) for ions. It cannot be assumed that the permeability as defined in Eq. (1) will remain constant with changes in the driving force. This point will be discussed later. For a general outline of this subject Dainty (1960) should be consulted.

The equations used to describe these fluxes will first be derived for the simplest experimental situation. Later the complications which arise in more complex situations will be considered. It will become apparent that the flux equations so derived are similar in many ways to those describing the gain and loss of heat by an object (Newton), or the charge and discharge of a condenser and so on. The present equations differ, however, in that they are suitable for nonsteady state conditions (i.e. where influx $\neq$ efflux), in that influx and efflux are measured separately.

2. THEORETICAL TIME COURSE OF EXCHANGE IN A SINGLE CELL

The model usually chosen for the derivation of these equations is that of a single cell suspended in a large volume of fluid. This fluid is kept well stirred to minimize any unstirred layer of fluid near the cell membrane, and it is assumed that diffusion is adequate to keep the contents of the cell mixed. It is further supposed that exchanges between the cell contents and the bathing fluid are limited only by the resistance of the cell membrane. This corresponds to one limiting case for the kinetics of transfer of substances across membranes discussed by Collander and Barlund (1933). Equations derived in this way are given by Levi and Ussing (1948), Harris and Burn (1949), Keynes and Lewis (1951), and Keynes (1951).

The equations can best be understood by considering the situation in a simple way first and then deriving them more formally. The lower part of Fig. 1 shows a situation in which a single large cell is moved from a solution containing an inactive substance S to one also containing a proportion of the radioactive substance S^* and then back to the inactive solution. In the upper part of Fig. 1 is plotted the change in the radioactivity in the cell

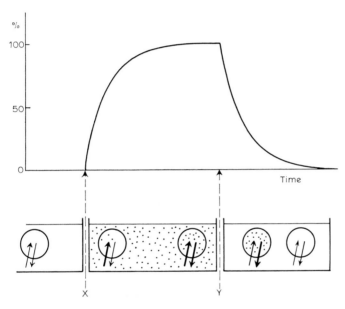

FIG. 1. Gain and loss of activity by a single "cell". Lower part—at x single cell moved from inert solution to solution containing some radioactive molecules (S_0^*); at y replaced in inert solution. Thick arrows represent flux of radioactivity, thin arrows flux of inactive molecules. Upper part—accumulation and loss of radioactivity in the cell; abscissa, time; ordinate specific activity in the cell/ specific activity in the solution, plotted on a linear scale.

contents. This is expressed such that at 100% the ratio of S^*/S in the cell equals that in the bathing solution (i.e. the specific activities are equal).

During the loading and unloading of the cell two processes may be distinguished—a constant influx of labeled ions into the cell driven by the fixed concentration of labeled ions outside and a varying efflux of labeled ions from the cell driven by the changing concentration of labeled ions in the cell. The actual net transfer of labeled ions at any time will be the algebraic sum of these processes.

On first putting the cell into labeled fluid (at X) the influx of labeled ions is large but the efflux is small, for the concentration of labeled ions in the cell is small. As the cell becomes loaded up the efflux of labeled ions increases until eventually, at equilibrium, it equals the influx. On replacing the cell in an inactive fluid (at Y) the influx drops to a low value, as the activity in the bathing fluid is low; initially the efflux is high, but it decreases as the internal concentration of labeled ions falls.

From Fig. 1 it is apparent that by suitable choice of conditions both the unidirectional influx and efflux may be measured separately. Thus, during the initial soaking of the cell in the radioactive solution, the radioactive efflux is negligible compared to the influx, and it may be neglected. The rate of gain of radioactivity by the cells under these conditions therefore measures the influx. During the washing out of activity the influx may be ignored and the rate of decrease of activity in the cells then gives a measure of the efflux.

With cells of similar shape, large cells have a greater volume per unit surface area than small cells. It is clear, therefore, that if the membrane permeability is similar for a large and a small cell then the large cell will take longer to fill and empty than the small one. The times of filling and emptying will be proportional to the ratio of volume/surface area of the cells (V/A). For cylindrical cells this may be simplified to $\pi r^2 l / 2\pi r l$ by omitting the ends of the cylinders, where l is the length of the cell and r the radius. This becomes $r/2$. In spherical cells V/A is $r/3$.

A simple analog may readily be made to demonstrate this to students. Arrange to fill a large burette from a constant flow bottle or tap. The burette represents the cell with a certain volume and a "surface area" for loss of fluid controlled by opening or closing the tap at the bottom. Such a burette empties exponentially (e.g. see Baylis, 1959, p. 24; in practice it is difficult to get it to do so exactly, probably due to turbulence at the emptying orifice), and in this case is filled at a constant flow rate. Start with the burette empty. Turn on the constant flow device. The fluid rises exponentially in the burette to a steady level where the gain and loss of water by the burette is the same. Then stop the inflow and observe the exponential emptying of the burette. Inflow and outflow may be calculated by timing the rise and fall of fluid in the burette and compared with the known flow rate from the constant flow device. A more sophisticated experiment very suitable for students is to produce large "cells" from dialysis tubing (Visking Tubing). These exchange ^{42}K with a $T_{\frac{1}{2}}^*$ of between 10–60* min, depending on the diameter.

* $T_{\frac{1}{2}}$: the time taken for the activity in the cell to fall to half its initial value.

These equations may be derived more formally as follows: let such a cell of area A cm^2 and volume V cm^3 and with an internal concentration of S_1 moles/cm^3 be suspended in a solution containing the same ion at a concentration S_0 moles/cm^3. Some of the external ions are then replaced by labeled ions S_0^*; the specific activity of the bathing fluid is then S_0^*/S_0 (usually expressed as so many counts per second (or minute) per mole of total ion present). It is required to measure the unidirectional fluxes of this ion S. Let the influx be M_{in} moles/cm^2 sec and the efflux be M_{out} moles/cm^2 sec. The radioactive fluxes are then M_{in*} and M_{out*} moles/cm^2 sec.

In unit time the amount of radioactive ion in the cell changes by $M_{in*}A - M_{out*}A$. Therefore the concentration changes by $M_{in*}A/V - M_{out*}A/V$, i.e.

$$\frac{d(S^*)_1}{dt} = M_{in*}\,A/V - M_{out*}\,A/V. \tag{2}$$

By suitable adjustment of the conditions either $M_{in*}A/V$ or $M_{out*}A/V$ may be eliminated and so the efflux or influx measured separately.

Influx. When the cell is first immersed in radioactive solution, $M_{out*}A/V$ is very small, and may be neglected, therefore, from Eq. (2),

$$\frac{d(S^*)_1}{dt} = M_{in*}\,A/V; \tag{3}$$

rearranging,

$$M_{in*} = \frac{d(S^*)_1}{dt} \cdot V/A. \tag{4}$$

M_{in} is then obtained by multiplying M_{in*} by S_0/S_0^*.

In practice the cell is allowed to accumulate a certain radioactivity $d(S^*)_1$ for a short time dt and then this multiplied by V/A and S_0/S_0^*. It will be noticed that it is not necessary to know $(S)_1$ to measure the influx.

If the time dt is short compared to the exchange time (say about 10% of the $T_\frac{1}{2}$), then little error is introduced into the result by the radioactivity lost in the efflux. Sometimes, however, the cells must be loaded up fairly considerably in order to get enough radioactivity to measure. It is then necessary to apply a correction to obtain the true influx from the data. In a paper on experiments with frogs' toe muscles, Keynes (1954) gives such a correction. This is based on either of two assumptions; that the inward and outward fluxes are equal or that they are proportional to the external and internal concentrations. The correction is

$$\left[\frac{dS}{dt}\right]_{t=0} = \frac{S}{T}\frac{kT}{1 - \exp - kT}, \tag{5}$$

where S is the amount entered in time T, k is the efflux rate constant, and dS is the amount estimated to enter in the short time dt.

Efflux. If the cell is allowed to accumulate radioactive ions until an equilibrium state is reached and then washed in inactive fluid, the influx term $M_{in*}A/V$ in Eq. (2) becomes very small, and the equation becomes

$$\frac{d(S^*)_1}{dt} = - M_{out*}\, A/V \qquad (6)$$

or

$$M_{out*} = - \frac{d(S^*)_1}{dt} \cdot V/A. \qquad (7)$$

If it is assumed that the efflux is proportional to the internal concentration of the radioactive ion, then Eq. (6) may be integrated to give

$$(S^*)_1 \underset{t=t}{} = (S^*)_1 \underset{t=0}{} e^{-kt}, \qquad (8)$$

where $(S^*)_1\underset{t=t}{}$ is the activity in the cell after time t and $(S^*)_1\underset{t=0}{}$ that at $t = 0$; k is a rate constant, i.e. the reciprocal of a time constant, and so is in units of $1/\text{time}$, e.g. $\min^{-1}$, $\sec^{-1}$, etc. If $\ln (S^*)^1$ is plotted against t, the graph will be a straight line of intercept $(S_1^*)\underset{t=0}{}$ and a slope of k.

Equation (8) is simply that for an exponential. For any particular situation, k must therefore contain the information unique to that situation. In this case this consists of the cell size (measured as V/A) and a term for the "leakiness" of the membrane. This "leakiness" from Eq. (1) is measured as

$$\frac{\text{flux}}{(S^*)_1}, \text{ i.e., } \frac{M_{out}}{(S^*)_1}.$$

Therefore

$$k \propto \frac{1}{V/A} \frac{M_{out}}{(S^*)_1}$$

or by adjustment of the units

$$k = \frac{-1}{V/A} \cdot \frac{M_{out*}}{(S^*)_1}. \qquad (9)$$

Rearranging, $$M_{out*} = k\,(V/A)\,(S^*)_1. \qquad (10)$$

M_{out} is then obtained by multiplying M_{out*} by the specific activity of the soak medium (S_0/S_0^*).

To obtain k directly, counts need to be plotted as $\log_e$. Usually counts are plotted on $\log_{10}$ graph paper; k may then be obtained by calculation. More simply, the $T_{\frac{1}{2}}$ may be measured directly. It can readily be shown that $k = 0.693/T_{\frac{1}{2}}$, and so the efflux can be calculated from

$$M_{\text{out}} = \frac{0.693}{T_{\frac{1}{2}}} (S)_1 \cdot V/A. \tag{11}$$

If $T_{\frac{1}{2}}$ is in seconds, S_1 in moles/cm^3, and V/A in cm, then the flux is moles/cm^2 sec.

In practice the cells do not need to be loaded completely with radioactivity, for k may be obtained from washout curves of partially loaded cells. It is, however, necessary to know $(S)_1$ at equilibrium.

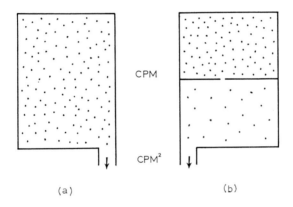

(a)   (b)

Fig. 2. Loss of radioactivity from (a) a homogeneous compartment, and (b) 2 compartments in series with a slow exchange between them. In *a* the radioactivity in the effluent (expressed as cpm^2) declines at the same rate as that in the cell (expressed as cpm). In *b* the effluent radioactivity declines at a faster rate than that in the cell.

In the type of experiment so far described, the content of radioactivity in the cell at any time is measured. The result is expressed as so many counts per minute or per second (cpm or cps), and later converted to an amount of the substance concerned. A more direct way of examining efflux, however, is to collect the total radioactivity leaving a cell in unit time and measure this. Thus 100 cpm may leave a cell in the first minute, 80 cpm may leave in the second minute, etc. It is conventional to express these results as 100 cpm per min or 100 cpm^2. This method appears to have first been used by Levi and Ussing (1949). It is a method particularly suitable for examination of changes in efflux, for it measures the change directly rather than a consequence of it.

Figure 2 illustrates another use which has been made of these two ways of expressing results. In Fig. 2a a cell is behaving as a single-compartment system in which the internal radioactive substance S^* is homogeneously distributed, and the total efflux of S^* (M_0^*) is directly proportional to the total internal concentration. The rate constant for the decrease of (S^*) is then equal to that for the decline of efflux S^*. Hodgkin and Keynes (1956)

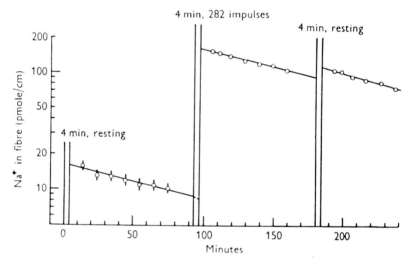

FIG. 3a. Exchanges of ^{24}Na in a single muscle fibre. *Abscissa*: time; *ordinate*: quantity of labeled Na per unit length of fiber, log scale. The vertical lines define the 4 min periods during which the fiber was exposed to ^{24}Na, in between it was washed in inactive Ringer. Stimulation greatly increased the ^{24}Na influx. Note the exponential loss of ^{24}Na.

used this kind of argument to show that squid axon did behave as a single-compartment system, at least over short periods of time. In Fig. 2b is shown a cell with two series compartments, one exchanging at a fast rate to the outside and the other at a slow rate with the faster compartment. In such a system the efflux largely reflects changes in the faster compartment, and therefore the rate constant for the decline of the efflux is faster than that for the decline of the contents. Most tissues lose radioactivity in this way. Unfortunately, two compartments in series is not a unique explanation for this phenomenon. Keynes and Swan (1959) found that frog muscle in lithium loses Na* in a complex way, which they ascribed to a carrier with several sites on it. Reference to this paper and to papers by Persoff (1960) and Dick and Lea (1964) should be made for an extensive discussion on this subject.

Figure 3a shows an example of an actual experiment measuring the Na* exchanges in a single muscle fiber (from Hodgkin and Horowicz, 1959). The Na* content is plotted on a log scale against time. The vertical lines

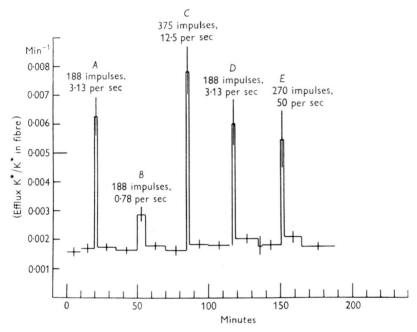

FIG. 3b. Effect of stimulation on K efflux. *Abscissa*: time; *ordinate*: fraction of labeled K lost per minute. Note (a) that the resting values of fractional loss is constant, indicating an exponential loss; and (b) the large effect of stimulation on the K loss. (Both from Hodgkin and Horowicz, *J. Physiol.*, 1959, with permission.)

indicate 4 min periods of influx in Na* Ringer, the rest are periods of efflux in inactive Ringer. The periods of influx of 4 min were short compared to the exchange time ($T_{\frac{1}{2}}$ of about 30 min), and therefore only a small quantity of Na* was lost during the influx. A correction for this was, however, applied, by extending the efflux curve during the 4 min influx with a slope appropriate to the stimulated or resting condition. Influx was then calculated from the end of this extended line. Note that the Na* is lost exponentially during the efflux.

Figure 3b shows another method of expressing results taken from the same paper. In this experiment the amounts of radioactivity leaving the fiber were collected and the activity left in the fiber at the end was measured. The ratio of efflux K* per min/K* in the fiber at the same time could then be calculated. As the loss follows an exponential law, this ratio did not vary with time. On stimulation the ratio rises greatly due to an increased K* loss. This method of expressing the results is very useful as it gives results which can be plotted on linear paper, which suits most people.

3. THEORETICAL EXCHANGES IN TISSUES

It is very seldom that the simple analysis described above can be applied. This may be because single cells are surrounded by layers of connective tissue which interfere to some extent with diffusion (e.g. squid axon (Caldwell and Keynes, 1960), or Purkinje tissues (Carmeliet, 1961)), or because the tissue being studied consists of a population of cells of various sizes. These and other changes introduce complications into the simple situation and will now be discussed.

3.1. EXTRACELLULAR SPACE

Most cells studied are not in direct contact with the bathing fluid but are surrounded by an extracellular space which then communicates with the bathing solution. The first consequence of this is that the system is now a two-compartment one, with intracellular and extracellular spaces as well as the bathing fluid. This type of situation is still capable of study, especially if the rate of exchange between the bathing fluid and the extracellular space is fast compared to the exchange between the extracellular space and the cell itself. This means that when the tissue is first immersed in the radioactive solution the extracellular space will fill up quickly but the intracellular space will fill more slowly. Similarly, on washing with nonradioactive fluid, the extracellular space will empty quickly followed by the slower emptying of the cell. This problem has been discussed by Defares and Sneddon (1961) in a slightly different context. The following account is from this book, with permission (pp. 582–5).

"We shall study the semi-logarithmic graph of a second order equation and the inverse problem, i.e. the question: how are we to know that an experimental curve plotted on semi-log paper may be represented by an equation of the type

$$y = C_1 e^{-k_1 t} + C_2 e^{-k_2 t}. \tag{12}$$

We have seen that a first order equation $y = Ae^{-\gamma t}$, when plotted on semi-log paper, yields a straight line, since $\log y = -\gamma t = \log A$. It is easily seen that the semi-log plot of (12) will not yield a straight line.

"Let us study an (experimental) curve $y = f(t)$, which when plotted on a semi-log paper yields a curve of the type shown in Fig. 4 (continuous curve). The ordinate of this continuous curve is obviously $\log_{10} y$.

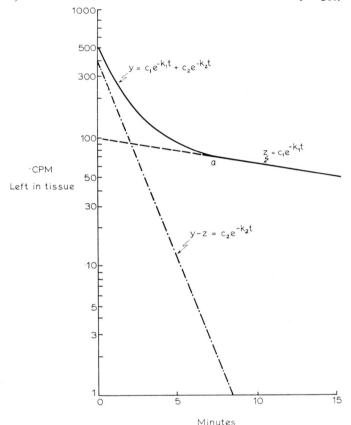

Fig. 4. The analysis of a typical washout curve of radioactivity from a tissue. *Abscissa*: time; *ordinate*: activity left in tissue on log scale. Continuous line indicates the usual experimentally obtained result of such an experiment. The (almost) straight part to the right of point a is extended to cut the ordinate. This line represents the loss of activity from the cells ($Z = C_1 e^{-k_i t}$). By graphical subtraction from the original curve the steep straight line is obtained. This represents the extracellular loss of activity ($y - z = C_1 e^{-k_2 t}$). Therefore the original curve is the sum of these lines ($y = C_2 e^{-k_2 t} + C_2 e^{-k_1 t}$). For simplicity the first component is shown as an exponential, in fact about the first 30% is lost faster than shown. (For example, see Fig. 2, Keynes, 1954.)

"We observe that the part of the non-linear curve to the right of the point *a* is (practically) a straight line.

"If now we extend this linear part to the left of *a* (broken line), we obtain a straight line starting at $t = 0$. Since this is a straight line on semi-log paper, we know that this straight line represents the function

$$\log_{10} z = -0.4343\, k_1 t = \log_{10} C_1, \tag{13}$$

$$\log z = -k_1 t = \log C_1. \tag{14}$$

Dropping logarithms this yields

$$z = C_1\, e^{-k_1 t}. \tag{15}$$

Let us now direct our attention to what happens to the left of the point *a*. Let us choose a value of *y* and a value of *z* at, say, the point $t = 2$. We then find $y = 190$, $z = 90$. Let us now form their difference, to find $y - z = 190 - 90 = 100$.

"If we plot this difference on (the same) semi-log paper, this means that we plot $\log_{10}(y - z)$ as the ordinate. If we repeat this process for a number of *y* and *z* values on the left of the point *a*, we notice from Fig. 4, that in this particular case, another straight line (steeper than the first) is obtained. What does this imply? It means that $\log_{10}(y - z)$ is some linear function of time, say

$$\log_{10}(y - z) = -0.4343\, k_2 t + \log_{10} C_2, \tag{16}$$

and where the modul 0.4343 is introduced for the sake of elegance, since this enables us to write (16) as

$$\log(y - z) = k_2 t + \log C_2. \tag{17}$$

Or, dropping logarithms,

$$y - z = C_2\, e^{-k_2 t}. \tag{18}$$

Combining (4) and (7), we thus find

$$y = C_1\, e^{-k_1 t} + C_2\, e^{-k_2 t}, \tag{12}$$

which is clearly a very interesting result with important implications.

"It means that by the method just explained we can test whether a given experimental curve may be represented by the second order equation (12). The following points should be noted:

"(1) Supposing that we are really dealing with a curve representing equation (12) on semi-log paper, then that part of the curve to the right of a is theoretically never a straight line, since the second exponential term is never zero. But in practice, we may find a straight line (to the right of a point a) which means that the second exponential has become negligibly small.

"It must be clearly realised that we are using semi-log paper. It should become very clear that if at, say, $t = 2$, the value of z (90 units) is subtracted from the value of y (190 units), and this difference (100 units) is plotted on semi-log paper, then we really have the effect of $\log(y - z)$ plotted against time on normal paper. This fact forms the key to a full understanding of the method.

"We shall now formulate the steps required for testing whether an experimental curve corresponds to the formula

$$y = C_1 e^{-k_1 t} + C_2 e^{-k_2 t}$$

(1) Plot the experimental values on semi-log paper.
(2) If the "latter" part of the curve is approximately a straight line, then extend this linear part to the left until it touches the y-axis.
(3) Take the differences of the values of the original curve and the extrapolated part of the linear curve. Plot these differences (with the symbols used above: $y - z$) on (the same) semi-log paper.
(4) If a straight line is thus obtained, this means that the curve may indeed be represented by equation (12)."

The presence of the extracellular space usually slows the diffusion of substances to and from the cell membrane. This affects both the intercept value discussed above and the apparent flux calculated from the rate constant of the exponential part of the curve.

A correction for the intercept value has been given by Huxley (1960) as follows: It is required to calculate the true value of C_1 (i.e. the intracellular concentration) in a situation which can be described by Eq. (12) and Fig. 4. The apparent values of the intercepts of the two exponential processes are C_1^1 and C_2^1, and these have rate constants of k_1 and k_2 respectively. The true value is then given by

$$C_1 = \frac{C_1^1 \times C_2^1 \times (k_2 - k_1)^2}{[C_1^1 \times k_1^2] + [C_2^1 \times k_2^2]}.$$

(19)

This correction should not be ignored, for it may sometimes be very large.

The following account of the correction which needs to be applied to the apparent flux is from Keynes (1954). After the initial 30% of the extracellular activity is lost, the remainder is lost exponentially (the steep line on

Fig. 4 representing Eq. (17), i.e. $y - z = C_2 e^{-k_2 t}$. From this the effective diffusion co-efficient for the ion in the extracellular space (D^1) can be calculated as follows:

For a cylindrical tissue of radius r,

$$D^1 = \frac{0.118r^2}{T_{\frac{1}{2}}}, \tag{20}$$

and for a plane sheet of thickness b washed on one side,

$$D^1 = \frac{0.28b^2}{T_{\frac{1}{2}}}. \tag{21}$$

(If the muscle is washed on both sides, use $2b$.)

At this stage the true flux M is guessed and then λ calculated as follows:

$$\lambda^2 = \frac{\epsilon}{1 - \epsilon} \frac{D^1 V C_0}{MA}, \tag{22}$$

where ϵ is the fraction (by volume) occupied by the extracellular space, V/A the volume/area ratio, and C_0 the ionic concentration in the extra-cellular space. λ has the units of length and is best calculated in μ.

The ratio of M_1 (the measured flux) to M (the true flux) for a cylindrical piece of tissue, is then given by

$$\frac{M^1}{M} = \frac{2\lambda}{a} \frac{I_1 (a/\lambda)}{I_0 (a/\lambda)}, \tag{23}$$

where a is the radius of the tissue. The ratio of $I_1(a/\lambda)/I_0(a/\lambda)$ are modified Bessel functions. It may be obtained from a set of tables, e.g. Watson (1922), p. 698, table II, columns $e^{-x}I_1(x)/e^{-x}I_0(x)$.

The equation for a plane sheet of muscle, thickness b, exposed to the medium on one side only, is

$$\frac{M^1}{M} = \frac{\lambda}{b} \tanh \frac{b}{\lambda}. \tag{24}$$

These equations are calculated for the influx condition, but they apparently can also be applied to efflux experiments. They are for tissues in a steady state. Similar equations have recently been worked out by Rennie, working in Professor Dainty's laboratory (to be published in *J. Theor. Biol.*). These equations do not require tables for working, and also apply a correction for slowness of diffusion to D^1.

In using this correction, M is guessed and a value of λ calculated. This is then substituted in Eqs. (23) or (24). If M was guessed correctly, then both sides of Eqs. (23) or (24) are approximately equal; if not, the process is repeated. The example Keynes gives is as follows: average $M^1 = 4.5$ pmole/cm^2 sec, $a = 260\,\mu$. $\epsilon = 0.27$, $V/A = 10.3\,\mu$. If $M = 5.0$ pmole/cm^2 sec, then $\lambda = 293\,\mu$. Therefore $a/\lambda = 0.89$. From Watson the value of $I_1(0.89)/I_0(0.89)$ is 0.405, therefore:

$$\frac{M^1}{M} = \frac{4.5^1}{50} = \frac{2 \times 0.405}{0.89} = 0.91.$$

Creese (1960) checked the predictions of these calculations and those of Harris and Burn (1949) experimentally on rat diaphragm. He found that the calculations slightly overestimated the correction required to allow for diffusion.

It has recently been shown that extracellular labeling substances leave skeletal muscle (Harris, 1965) and frog ventricle (Lindsay, 1966; Keenan and Niedergerke, 1967; Hannan and Lamb, unpublished observations) very slowly. This may mean that the substance being studied may cross the cell membrane more readily than it leaves the tissue. The interpretation of such experiments is therefore very difficult.

3.2. MULTICELLULAR TISSUE

Most tissues studied consist of many cells of a range of sizes. Thus in muscle the largest cell may have a diameter of 10 times that of the smallest (Creese *et al.*, 1956; Niedergerke, 1963; Lamb, unpublished observations). Two extreme views might be taken when considering exchanges in these tissues. It might be considered that the properties of all the cell membranes, expressed as per unit surface area, are similar irrespective of the cell size in the tissue. Alternatively, it might be considered that the properties of each cell membrane were such that all cells in a tissue exchanged substances at the same or similar rates. The first hypothesis means that cells would fill up and empty in times inversely proportional to their volume/surface area, which for cylindrical cells is $\frac{1}{2} \times$ radius. The second hypothesis means that in a tissue the membranes of large cells would have a higher permeability than the membranes of small cells.

The first hypothesis discussed above (i.e. that cells exchange in proportion to their volume/surface area) is generally held to apply to tissues. The evidence on which this is based is that cells of widely different sizes from different tissues have similar ionic fluxes (e.g. see Table 4 in Burrows and Lamb, 1962). Also, in single cells dissected from frog muscle, Hodgkin and Horowicz (1959) found some correlation between fibre size and rate constant of exchange of Na and K although it was not very marked. In a whole tissue each cell is presumed to exchange exponentially with its environment. The overall exchange of the tissue is therefore the sum of all these individual exponential exchanges. The time it takes each cell to fill or empty will depend on the size of the cell. Therefore, in general, the loading and washing out of the substance will not be exponential.

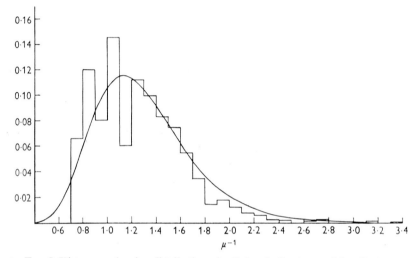

Fig. 5. Histogram showing distribution of cell sizes in frog's ventricle. *Abscissa*: the ratio of perimeter/area of the cells as an index of the ratio A/V; *ordinate*: relative area occupied by the cell cross-sections in any one class. Continuous curve, log-normal curve with geometric mean of 1.14 and S.D. of 0.3. (From Niedergerke, *J. Physiol.*, 1963, with permission.)

Various authors have studied this problem (e.g. see Creese *et al.*, 1956; Niedergerke, 1963) by computing the form of the efflux curves from the known population of cell sizes found in the tissue. To do this, histological sections need to be measured to determine the relative volumes occupied by cells of different sizes. Figure 5 shows a convenient way of expressing such data for frog's ventricle, from Niedergerke (1963). It can be seen that the cells are distributed in a log-normal way with a geometric mean of A/V of 1.14 μ^{-1}. From this data, curves of content, efflux, and ratio of efflux/content have been calculated (Fig. 6). For this the two assumptions that (1) all the cells have been loaded up to the same concentration, and (2) the permeabilities of all the cell membranes are the same, have been made.

From Fig. 6 it can be seen (1) that neither the efflux nor content curves deviate much from an exponential, (2) that they are almost parallel, (3) that the exponential of the geometric mean of the A/V distribution is a close fit to the content curve calculated from the whole distribution, and (4) the ratio of efflux activity/content activity changes slowly as the cells empty.

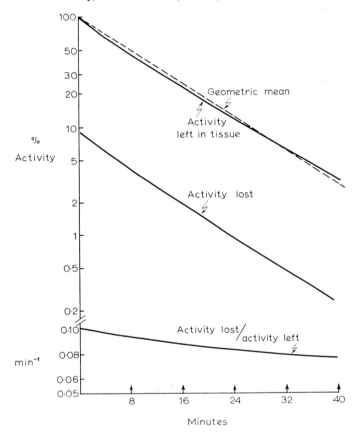

FIG. 6. Computed curves of outward movement of K* from previously loaded frog ventricle. *Abscissa*: time in minutes (arrows indicate elapse of each $T_{\frac{1}{2}}$); *ordinate*: upper—percentage radioactivity on log scale; lower—fractional radioactive loss per minute. Curves calculated from cell size distribution of Fig. 5 with assumptions that (1) all cells start with equal concentrations, and (2) the membranes of all cells have the same permeability. The upper continuous curve shows the activity remaining in the ventricle (cpm), the centre curve the activity lost per minute (i.e. cpm²), the lower curve shows the ratio of activity lost per minute/ activity remaining. The discontinuous curve shows the exponential calculated for the geometric mean value of A/V of 1.14 μ^{-1}.

Thus at 1, 2, 3, 4, and 5 halftimes it is 95, 90, 85, 82, and 79% of the starting value. From this it can be seen that over short times the content and efflux curves are parallel and exponential, and that the (geometric) mean value of A/V provides a reasonable fit to these curves.

Experimental results usually deviate more than would be expected from such theoretical considerations (Creese *et al.*, 1956; Niedergerke, 1963; Lamb, unpublished observations). The reason for this is not clear. It has been suggested that there may be a variation of permeability throughout the tissue, that cells may contain several compartments or perhaps that activity leaving small cells may then enter large cells and so be delayed in leaving the tissue. It should be noted that although whole frog sartorii lose K in a nonexponential way (Harris, 1957), single fibres lose K exponentially (Hodgkin and Horowicz, 1959). For a rigorous mathematical treatment of this subject reference should be made to Creese *et al.* (1956) and Niedergerke (1963).

3.3. MECHANICAL ARTEFACTS

In addition to measuring resting exchanges of ions and other substances, it is frequently desirable to measure these exchanges during electrical activity in the tissue. In nerve this raises no further problems; in muscle it may do so. This is because electrical activity in muscle is usually associated with alteration in the mechanical activity, and this mechanical activity in itself may cause interference with the normal exchanges across the membrane. This effect is likely to be minimal in those tissues which show very little mechanical activity (e.g. Purkinje fibers in the heart) or which can be isolated as single cells (single frog muscle cells; Hodgkin and Horowicz, 1959). In more complex tissues it may almost invalidate some kinds of measurements.

In the last few years we have examined this problem in frog's ventricle, and the following account is based on this (Lamb & McGuigan, 1968). A simple type of artefact which arises in this tissue is that if the heart is being used to perfuse itself, then alterations in rate of beating or force of contraction alters the perfusion rate. Consequently this alters the rates of loss or gain of substances simply by changing the rates of removal or presentation of the substance at the cell membranes. This may be overcome relatively simply by controlling the fluid flow through the heart by means of a constant flow system. The more intractable problem is as follows. In these tissues the cells exchange with the extracellular space, which then exchanges with the bathing solutions. Changes occurring in the characteristics of the extracellular space may affect the rates of diffusion of substances to and from the excitable membrane.

An experimental arrangement was made such that the fluid flow and pressure in the heart changed by $< 10\%$ during contraction. The efflux of various substances from the ventricle was collected over 30–40 action

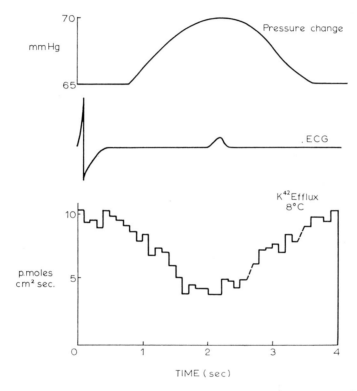

Fig. 7a (*above*) and b (*overleaf*). The loss of K* and SO_4* from frog's ventricle during one cardiac cycle. In each figure the upper trace represents intracellular pressure, the middle one the ECG and the lower one the isotope lost per 100 msec. In a is shown the K* loss, in b the SO_4* loss.

potentials. The results for a typical intracellular ion (K*) and extracellular ion (SO_4*) are shown in Figs. 7a and 7b together with the mean ECG and pressure wave. It can be seen that the loss of the extracellular ion is increased during the start of the twitch whereas the loss of the intracellular ion is decreased throughout the twitch. Similar results were obtained for Na, Ca, and sorbitol as extracellular substances. Altering the size of the

twitch by changing the calcium level in the Ringer altered these effects,
With no calcium present the twitch was abolished but the ECG unchanged
and there were then no alterations in the rates of loss of these substances.
   A probable explanation of these results is that contraction distorts and

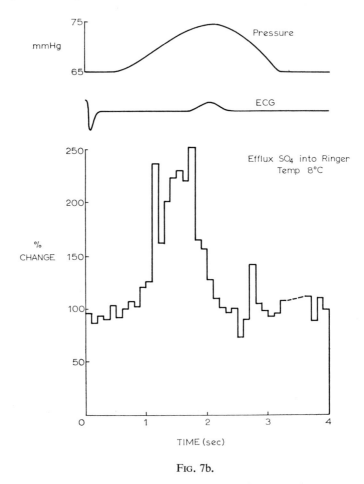

Fig. 7b.

diminishes the extracellular space. This has the effect of squeezing out
extracellular ions held in this space, the maximum effect being coincident
with the maximum rate of change of pressure in the tissue. It also decreases
the ease of diffusion of intracellular substances across the space during the
whole contraction period.

4. EXPERIMENTAL TECHNIQUES

There are basically two ways in which radioactive experiments may be done. Either the radioactivity in the tissue is measured directly, or the amount of radioactivity recovered from the tissue on washing with inert salt solution is measured. The first measures the content of the tissue directly (and hence gives an answer in so many counts per minute (cpm)); the second measures the effluent directly (and therefore has the units of cpm per time of collection). If the total radioactivity leaving the tissue is collected and counted, then it is clear that the total activity in the tissue at any given time can be obtained by summation of the activity lost. Therefore the second method described above (i.e. collecting and measuring the effluent) has the advantage that both efflux and content for any time may be obtained. It may be noted at this point that the content of radioactivity in the tissue, measured by summation of the radioactivity leaving the tissue, may not always be comparable with the content of radioactivity measured directly. This is because direct measurement of radioactivity is likely only to sample the activity in the part of the tissue nearest the detecting device, whereas collection of effluent radioactivity samples the whole tissue. Persoff (1960) examined this point (amongst others) in rabbit atria and in fact found no difference between the two methods.

4.1. DETECTORS

These may be either Geiger–Mueller (GM) tubes of various kinds or scintillation counters. At any particular level of sophistication (and hence the price) the background count of the GM tube is appreciably lower than that of the scintillation counter, e.g. the common thin end window GM tube (M6) has a background of about 12 cpm, a comparably priced scintillation counter has a background of 2–300 cpm; a low background gas flow GM counter may have a background count of 1 cpm whereas a comparably priced scintillation system may have a background count of 20–30 cpm. In general, isotope experiments across cell membranes are usually characterized by a low activity recovered from or measured in the tissue. For the common isotopes used to measure fluxes (^{22}Na, or ^{24}Na, ^{42}K, ^{86}Rb, ^{36}Cl, ^{45}Ca, ^{131}I, ^{82}Br) it can readily be calculated that if the sample activity is low, it takes a shorter time to count samples to a certain error level on a GM system than on a scintillation system. If money is scarce, a GM system should therefore have first preference.

If a large piece of tissue can be used (say 100 mg wet wt), then K and Na exchanges can readily be measured using simple GM tubes. For small tissues or compounds with low specific activities (e.g. ^{36}Cl) access to a low background gas flow counter is almost essential.

4.2. ČERENKOV COUNTING

A relatively new method of counting high energy beta emitters has recently been introduced (Garrahan and Glynn, 1966; Tothill, 1966; De Volpi and Porges, 1965). This Čerenkov emission of light takes place when a beta particle travels through a transparent medium at a speed greater than the speed of light in that medium. In certain circumstances this method has great advantages. These are where high energy beta emitters (e.g. ^{24}Na or ^{42}K) are being counted at low activities in large (20 ml) volumes. To use this method the sample is counted in a liquid scintillation system but without the liquid scintillator, i.e. the sample is simply poured into the glass counting vials. The counting is less efficient than that obtained with the liquid scintillator present (26% for ^{24}Na, 62% for ^{42}K; Garrahan and Glynn, 1966), but the volumes used are much higher (10–20 ml compared to 1 ml in a liquid scintillator). In our own experience we have obtained the following comparative data: 5 ml of sample counted on a Tracerlab Omni-guard low background counter 66 cpm; 20 ml of sample counted on a Packard Series 3000 liquid scintillation counter 564 cpm; backgrounds 2.0 cpm and 11 cpm. The ratio of (sample count rate)^2/background is therefore 2178 for the low background system and 28918 for the Čerenkov counting, an improvement of $\times$ 13 for the Čerenkov system. Quenching does occur, however.

4.3. EXAMPLES OF TECHNIQUES USED

(1) *Direct tissue counting.* Figure 8 shows an example of direct counting of the activity in a frog's muscle using a thin end window GM tube (Keynes, 1954). The bottom of the muscle bath is very thin to minimize absorption of radiation. A brass plate is interposed between the bath and the tube to limit the radiation reaching the tube to that from the centre of the muscle. In this kind of technique great care is necessary to ensure that the muscle remains in exactly the same position with respect to the tube if repeated measurements are made. Thus it is common to remove the muscle to another bath for exposure to the radioactive solution, reserving the counting bath for inactive solutions only. In this case some automatic system is desirable to replace the muscle in a standard position. The

apparatus may be calibrated by using an agar rod containing activity instead of the muscle.

If plenty of radioactivity is available from the preparation an easy way of doing these experiments is to use a wax plate (dental impression wax) on top of the brass plate. The muscle may then be pinned on to the plate with entomological pins. As the wax does not take up radioactivity, radio-active fluids may be applied directly (see Lamb and McGuigan, 1965). The wax halves the count obtained with ^{42}K.

An ingenious arrangement for counting the activity in single oocytes was devised by Dick and Lea (1964). This consisted of a plastic phosphor with a small tunnel in it into which the oocyte was put for counting. The

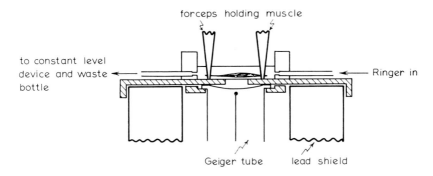

Fig. 8. Method of mounting a small muscle for direct counting of its radioactivity. The muscle is mounted in flowing Ringer, above a thin mica window covering a hole in the brass plate. The Geiger tube is mounted below the brass plate. The forceps are mounted on a Palmer screw stand. (From Keynes, *Proc. Roy. Soc.* 1954, with permission.)

rest of the phosphor was machined to a size calculated to give the optimum sample/background ratio for the isotope used.

(2) *Measurement of efflux.* Having loaded a muscle with radioactivity, the muscle may then be passed through a series of test tubes containing inactive salt solution. Finally, the muscle is weighed and dissolved in acid. The activity remaining in the muscle and in each tube can then be counted.

For the collection of the small amounts of activity from the frog's heart described earlier, a collecting device was devised (Fig. 9) which may be useful in other contexts. This consisted of a commercial gramophone turntable with a perspex top carrying 40 tubes around its edge. The effluent from the ventricle was directed into the tubes. The turntable rotated once every 4 sec and so each tube collected fluid for 100 msec. On each rotation a pair of contacts stimulated the ventricle, so each action potential occurred at a constant time with respect to the tubes. Some 40 action potentials were superimposed to give enough fluid to count.

4.4. EXPERIMENTS USING TWO ISOTOPES

Much experimental time may sometimes be saved by measuring two isotopes in the same experiment. The isotopes may be separately counted

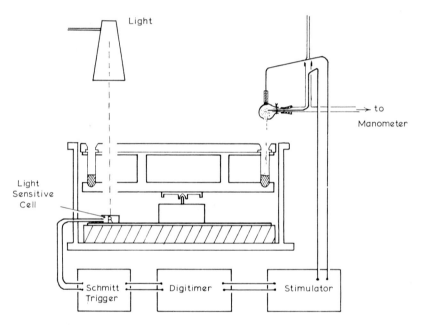

FIG. 9. Diagram of apparatus for collecting efflux during the cardiac cycle. A plastic turntable holding 40 test tubes is mounted on a commercial turntable. The ventricle is mounted on a cannula and positioned so that the efflux fluid falls into the test-tubes as they pass. The ventricle is stimulated once per cycle by the trigger arrangement shown. The pressure changes and ECG during each cycle were also monitored.

electronically or by using suitable counters. It is often possible, however, to do it more simply by suitable choice of the isotopes. Thus if ^{42}K and ^{36}Cl are used together, then an immediate count gives (^{42}K + ^{36}Cl). The count repeated one week later gives ^{36}Cl only, for the ^{42}K will have decayed by then. Working out such experiments tends to be very tedious and time-consuming. We have recently been using a small programme on the University KDF9 computer to do this, with much saving of time.

5. CORRECTIONS TO BE MADE TO THE OBSERVED COUNT RATES

Once obtained, the observed counts must be corrected before being used further. The corrections which need to be applied are as follows:

(1) *Background subtraction.* This must always be done unless the sample counts are very high compared to the background.

(2) *Correction for radioactive decay.* Usually all counts are corrected back to the start of the experiment. This may be done for the common ions ^{24}Na, ^{42}K, and ^{47}Ca by using the factors given in Table A 2 (p. 535). For example; to use with a sample of ^{24}Na 6 hr from the start of the experiment, multiply the observed counting rate by 1.319.

For ^{36}Cl, ^{14}C, ^{35}S, ^{45}Ca used in short-term experiments no correction is required.

(3) *Correction for self-absorption* of soft radiation within the thickness of the sample itself. This may be dealt with:

(a)   by elimination, in which equal weights of material are present in all samples (including the standards) counted;
(b)   by the use of a correction curve, best constructed by oneself;
(c)   by using an infinitely thick sample.

A common error is to count the effluent in Ringer or other salt solution, but dilute the standard solution with water only. Therefore more self-absorption occurs in the sample than in the standard.

(4) *Correction for resolving time of the detector.* This is usually only required with Geiger counters. At rates of 3000 cpm the error is 1–2%, and so at rates below this it may be ignored.

(5) *Corrections for variations in sensitivity of the counter during the experiment.* This may usually be ignored. It can be checked for by repeating a standard.

The error of the counts obtained must always be estimated or known. Basically this depends on the actual number of counts made, and to some extent on the background. If the sample counting rate exceeds 10 times the background, then the error = (total sample counts)$^{\frac{1}{2}}$. If the sample counting rate is less than 10 times the background rate, then it is necessary to include the background rate in the calculation of the counting error. By far the most convenient way of so doing is to refer to the nomogram given by

Loevinger and Berman (1951). A copy of this is reproduced as Fig. A.1 (p. 523). By reference to this the shortest time of counting to obtain a certain error may be obtained very easily.

6. INTERPRETATION OF THE FLUX MEASUREMENTS
6.1. EXCHANGES OF IONS ACROSS MEMBRANES

Ussing (1949) proposed that exchanges across cell membranes could occur in one of three ways:

(1) By diffusion down an electrochemical gradient.
(2) By exchange diffusion of a substance on one side of the cell membrane with the same substance on the other side. This involved no net movement of the substance across the cell membrane, but would allow a cell to gain or lose the radioactive form of the substance.
(3) By active movement of the substance across the cell membrane, the best known example being the coupled Na–K movement in squid axons and other cells.

Later he added solvent drag to this (1960; this reference also contains an extensive review of previous work). A classification of this kind can be made to embrace most of the exchanges found in cells under various conditions.

(1) *Passive diffusion.* By this is implied the movement of ions across a membrane due to thermal agitation driven by a concentration gradient or electrical potential. The net movement which occurs is always from a region of higher electrochemical potential. Probably all ions are continually crossing animal cells by this process. In discussing this it is convenient to consider these exchanges as occurring through passive permeability "channels". In general it is supposed that ions moving in one direction in these "channels" do not interact with ions moving in the opposite direction (the independence principle)—but there is at least one spectacular exception to this (K in squid axon; Hodgkin and Keynes, 1955). Enlargement of these "channels" leads to increased movement of the ion in question across the membrane, so that if the ion is not in electrochemical equilibrium, then an increased net movement of the ion will occur. As a consequence, the potential across the membrane may change. (To a smaller extent, usually, the ionic concentrations will also change.) Thus by changing the permeability to an ion which is not in equilibrium the membrane potential may be changed. This occurs during the action potential in squid axons and

probably in other tissues (see Hodgkin, 1958), when firstly the sodium permeability increases and then the potassium permeability increases. It also occurs during the end plate potential production (e.g. see Chapter XVI, Davson, 1964) and during various drug actions.

(2) *Active transport.* Certain net movements of ions occur in cells which cannot be explained by the operation of physical forces; this is active transport. Metabolic energy and chemical reactions clearly must be required for this to occur. Perhaps the most familiar example is the Na–K–ATPase system studied in red cells, see Whittam (1964) for references; squid axons, see Hodgkin (1964), and a few other tissues. In this, Na is moved into the cell, coupled with a K extrusion, and ATP is hydrolyzed. It is useful to consider briefly some of the uses to which active transport is put by cells. In all animal cells studied, active transport of Na and probably K, creates large ionic gradients across the resting cell, and in so doing controls the osmotic pressure of the cell interior and hence the volume of the cell (see, e.g., Hoffmann, 1964). In some cells large potentials are also set up, which then allow action potentials to occur. The resulting disturbance in Na and K distribution is corrected by active transport of Na and K. Many cells also use active transport to move substances across themselves from one medium to another. Thus, in the kidney and in frog's skin, active Na movement takes place across the cell. This probably occurs due to one side of the cell being "leaky" to Na, whereas the other side actively transports Na outwards (e.g. see Leaf, 1960; Ussing, 1960). Therefore, by orientation of the Na pumping, net transport across a layer of cells can be achieved. Many other substances are transported at many other sites.

Generally in the past the Na pump has been considered to be neutral, i.e. no charge was transferred across the membrane directly (Hodgkin, 1958). Recently, however, there has been evidence that the Na pump may produce a potential directly, by moving Na out of the cell uncoupled with K. This is the electrogenic action of the pump. Usually this is best shown during reaccumulation of Na after depletion (Kernan, 1962; Keynes and Rybová, 1963; Hashimoto, 1964; Cross *et al.*, 1965; Mullins and Awad, 1965; Frumento, 1965). Recent experiments by Adrian and Slayman (1966) using Rb as well as K also support this interpretation.

(3) *Exchange diffusion.* By this term is meant the exchange of a molecule on one side of the membrane with another molecule of the same kind on the other side with no energy expenditure. It is envisaged as occurring via a carrier molecule in the membrane. It owes its importance to the fact that radioactive ions can enter or leave cells by this route and thus confuse

measurements intended to reveal processes (1) and (2) above. There is some evidence that the amount of exchange diffusion occurring can be affected by ouabain (Glynn, 1956), and the presence of other ions, so that it is not necessarily a simple or unchanging process.

(4) Solvent drag. If large net flows of water are occurring, then ions may be swept through the membrane with the solvent. Usually, in fairly steady state conditions, this effect is ignored.

After measuring an ion flux it may be desired to try and apportion it into one or more of the above ways of movement across the membrane. Schatzmann (1953) showed that ouabain, a cardiac glycosicle, inhibited the active movement of Na across red cell membranes. This is widely used to characterize active transport of Na and K in various cells (e.g. see review by Glynn, 1964). Although this is generally true there is some recent evidence that there may be a Na–K coupled pump insensitive to ouabain in some cells (Lamb and McKinnon, 1967). Active ion transport is also energy dependent (Frazeri and Keynes, 1959) and therefore removal of energy supplies inhibits active transport and may also be used to identify an ion movement. In large cells both these methods may readily be used, in small cells inhibition of active movement of ions soon leads to changes in the internal environment of the cells and this may produce effects in itself.

If the active transport of an ion is blocked, the passive fluxes of the ion may then be measured. Comparison of the influx and efflux with the known electrochemical gradient will then produce one of the following situations —the flux against the electrochemical gradient is either (1) greater than expected, (2) less than expected, or (3) the same as expected. These will now be considered.

(1) This is the situation which arises when there is an appreciable exchange diffusion occurring. An example will illustrate this. Keynes and Swan (1959) found that a large sodium efflux from frog's sartorius still occurred after blocking the energy supply. This was against the electro-chemical gradient. On removal of the external sodium this efflux was greatly decreased. It was therefore concluded that there was a large sodium exchange diffusion occurring in these experiments.

(2) If the "uphill" flux is less than expected, then a "single-file effect" may be occurring. This was first described by Hodgkin and Keynes (1955) for K ions in squid axon. Their results could be explained by the supposi-tion that several sites were occupied in series as the ion crossed the mem-brane. In the presence of net losses of the ion (as occurs if pumping is blocked) labeled ions moving with the stream had a better chance of

crossing than those moving against the stream. This led to an apparently greater flux downhill.

(3) With a simple situation this is the expected result. A fuller treatment of this subject is given by Dainty (1962) and Briggs, *et al.* (1961) among others.

6.2. CALCULATION OF PERMEABILITY CHANGES

Once the flux measurements have been made, it is often desired to use these to calculate changes in permeability of the cells to the substance in question. This is generally much more complex than it seems at first sight. It is proposed only to outline some of the difficulties here.

For non-ionic substances the calculation of permeabilities is easier than for ions. The reason for this is that variation of the membrane potential across cells affects both the driving force on the ion and the "permeability" as usually defined. From Eq. (1):

$$\text{Flux} = \text{"permeability"} \times \text{driving force.}$$

As already stated the permeability so defined is not a constant. Goldman in 1943 developed an equation (the constant field or Goldman equation) which is widely used to describe ionic flux changes across cells. He defined the permeability Px in terms of the partition coefficient of the ion between the membrane and the solution, the mobility of the ion in the membrane and the membrane thickness. This way of defining permeability has the advantage that it remains constant with alterations in the driving force. He also assumed that the membrane potential was dropped uniformly across the membrane. The Goldman equation has the general form of

Flux $= (Px \times$ membrane potential factor$) \times$ electrochemical potential; for K, the fluxes can be calculated from

$$M_{\text{in}} = [PK \ VF/RT] \times \left(\frac{(K)_0}{(1 - \exp - VF/RT)} \right) \qquad (25)$$

and

$$M_{\text{out}} = [PK \ VF/RT] \times \left(\frac{(K)_1 \exp - VF/RT}{1 - \exp - VF/RT} \right), \qquad (26)$$

where M_{in} and M_{out} are the unidirectional fluxes, $(K)_0$ and $(K)_1$ are the external and internal concentrations of K respectively, RT and F are the gas constant, temperature, and Faraday, and V is the membrane potential. P_K is the potassium permeability as defined by Goldman. Net movements of K may be calculated by combining these two expressions. (See Katz, 1966).

It will be apparent from the above that flux measurements do not immediately lead to statements about permeabilities except under certain circumstances. The simplest such circumstance is when the effect being investigated is associated with no change in the membrane potential. This circumstance does not often arise naturally, but may be obtained by manipulation of the experimental conditions. Thus Jenkinson and Morton (1965, 1967) studied the effect of nor-adrenaline on the K fluxes in *taenia coli*, depolarized with high external KCl. Under these circumstances the adrenaline could be presumed to have no effect on the membrane potential. Therefore the observation that nor-adrenaline increased the K fluxes could be interpreted as an increase in permeability to potassium.

Generally speaking, drugs added to preparations do change the membrane potential, and it is then necessary to calculate the likely effects of such membrane changes on the flux being studied. Sometimes qualitative arguments are sufficient for this purpose. Thus Harris and Hutter (1956; also see Hutter, 1961) found that ACh added to frog's sinus venosis increased the K efflux by a factor of about 3. It was also known that ACh hyperpolarized the cells (Hutter and Trautwein, 1956). On the Goldman equation a hyperpolarization could be expected to decrease the K efflux. Harris and Hutter argued that they were probably therefore underestimating the true ACh effect because of the concomitant hyperpolarization. They proved this by depolarizing the cells with increased external K (and therefore stabilizing the membrane potential) and then found that ACh increased the K efflux by about 10 times.

This article has been concerned with the use of radioactive isotopes of ions for the measurement of unidirectional fluxes across cell membranes. We have seen that in principle the techniques used are very easy to use and understand. In practice reliable results are difficult to obtain in whole tissues, and difficult to interpret unless due consideration is given to other factors such as the membrane potential. In the past most information has been obtained from single squid axons, from single muscle cells, from red cells and in some cases from small skeletal muscles. From these few rather specialized tissues our present extensive knowledge of membrane passive properties and active transport has been derived. It is clear that there are still many more cell types and drugs to be investigated. These also should yield a great deal of information, if studied in ways which can give clear unequivocal answers.

REFERENCES

(A) BOOKS, REVIEWS AND MONOGRAPHS

BAYLIS, L. E. (1959) *Principles of General Physiology*, 1st ed., Longmans, London, p. 24·

BRIGGS, G. E., HOPE, A. B. and ROBERTSON, R. N. (1961) *Electrolytes and Plant Cells*, 1st ed., Blackwell, Oxford.

CARMELIET, E. E. (1961) Chloride and potassium permeability in cardiac Purkinje fibres, in *The Specialised Tissues of the Heart*. Elsevier Pub. Co., Amsterdam.

DAINTY, J. (1960) Electrical analogues in biology. *Symp. Soc. Exp. Biol.*, **14**.

DAINTY, J. (1962) Ion transport and electrical potentials in plant cells. *A. Rev. Pl. Physiol.*, **13**.

DAVSON, H. (1964) Transmission of the impulse, in *A Textbook of General Physiology*, chapter XVI. J. & A. Churchill, London.

DEFARES, J. G. and SNEDDON, I. N. (1960) *The Mathematics of Medicine and Biology*. North Holland Co., Amsterdam.

GLYNN, I. M. (1964) The action of cardiac glycosides on ion movements. *Pharmac. Rev.*, **16**:381–407.

HODGKIN, A. L. (1958) The Croonian Lecture—Ionic movements and electrical activity in giant nerve fibres. *Proc. Roy. Soc.*, B, **148**:1–37.

HODGKIN, A. L. (1964) *The Nervous Impulse*. Liverpool University Press.

HOFFMANN, J. F. (1964) *The Cellular Functions of Membrane Transport*. Prentice-Hall, N.J., U.S.A.

HUTTER, O. F. (1961) Ion movements during vagus inhibition of the heart, in *Nervous Inhibitions*. Proc. Int. Symp., Pergamon Press.

HUXLEY, A. F. (1960) Compartmental analysis, in *Mineral Metabolism*, Vol. 1. (Comar, C. L. and Bronner, F. (eds.)). Academic Press, London, England, pp. 163–6.

KATZ, B. (1966) *Nerve, muscle and synapse*. McGraw-Hill, London, pp. 59–64.

TOTHILL, P. (1966) *Measurement Techniques for the Clinical Application of Radioisotopes*. Radiochemical Centre, Amersham, England, p. 15.

USSING, H. H. (1960) The alkali metal ions in biology, in *Handb. Exper. Pharmakol.*, **13**:1–195. Springer-Verlag, Berlin.

USSING, H. H. (1949) Transport of ions across cellular membranes. *Phys. Rev.*, **29**:127–55.

WATSON, G. N. (1922) In *Theory of Bessel Functions*. Cambridge University Press, England, Table II, p. 698,

WHITTAM, R. (1964) *Transport and Diffusion in Red Blood Cells*, Monograph 13 of the Physiological Society, London. Edward Arnold.

(B) ORIGINAL PAPERS

ADRIAN, R. H. and SLAYMAN, C. L. (1966) Membrane potential and conductance during transport of sodium, potassium and rubidium in frog muscle. *J. Physiol.*, **184**:970–1014.

BURROWS, R. and LAMB, J. F. (1962) Sodium and potassium fluxes in cells cultured from chick embryo heart muscle. *J. Physiol.*, **162**:510–31.

CALDWELL, P. C. and KEYNES, R. D. (1960) The permeability of the squid giant axon to radioactive potassium and chloride ions. *J. Physiol.*, **154**:177–89.

COLLANDER, R. (1954) The permeability of Nitella cells to non-electrolytes. *Physiol. Plant*, **7**:420–45.

COLLANDER, R. and BARLUND, H. (1933) Permeabilitaütsstudien an Chara ceratophylla, II. *Acta. Bot. Fenn*, **11**:1–114.

CREESE, R. (1960) Potassium in different layers of isolated diaphragm. *J. Physiol.*, **154**:133–44.

CREESE, R., NEIL, M. W. and STEPHENSON, G. (1956) Effect of cell variation on potassium exchange in muscle. *Trans. Faraday Soc.*, **52**:1022–32.

CROSS, S. R., KEYNES, R. D. and RYBORÁ, RENATA (1965) The coupling of sodium efflux and potassium influx in frog muscles. *J. Physiol.*, **181**:865–80.

DE VOLPI, A. and PORGES, K. G. A. (1965) Čerenkov counting of aqueous solutions. *Int. J. Appl. Radiat. Isotopes*, **16**:8, 496–8.

DICK, D. A. T. and LEA, E. J. A. (1964) Na fluxes in single toad oocytes with special reference to the effect of external and internal Na concentration on Na efflux. *J. Physiol.*, **174**:55–90.

FRAZIER, H. S. and KEYNES, R. D. (1959) The effect of metabolic inhibitors on the sodium fluxes in sodium loaded frog sartorius muscle. *J. Physiol.*, **148**:362–78.

FRUMENTO, A. S. (1965) Sodium pump: Its electrical effects in skeletal muscle. *Science, N.Y.*, **147**:1442–3.

GARRAHAN, P. J. and GLYNN, I. M. (1966) Driving the sodium pump backwards to form adenosine triphosphate. *Nature, Lond.*, **211**:1414–15.

GLYNN, I. M. (1956) The action of cardiac glycosides on Na and K movements in human red cells. ('57) *J. Physiol.*, **136**:148–73.

HARRIS, E. J. (1957) Permeation and diffusion of K ions in frog muscle. *J. Gen. Physiol.*, **41**:169–95.

HARRIS, E. J. (1965) The dependence of efflux of sodium from frog muscle on internal sodium and external potassium. *J. Physiol.*, **177**:355–76.

HARRIS, E. J. and BURN, G. P. (1949) The transfer of sodium and potassium ions between muscle and the surrounding medium. *Trans. Faraday Soc.*, **45**:508–28.

HARRIS, E. J. and HUTTER, O. F. (1956) The action of acetylcholine on the movement of potassium ions in the sinus venosus of the heart. *J. Physiol., Lond.*, **133**:58–59P.

HASHIMOTO, Y. (1964) Resting potentials of Na-loaded sartorius muscle fibres of toads during recovery in high K Ringer. *Kumamoto Med. J.*, **18**:23–30.

HODGKIN, A. L. and HOROWICZ, P. (1959) Movements of Na and K in single muscle fibres. *J. Physiol.*, **145**:405–32.

HODGKIN, A. L. and KEYNES, R. D. (1955) The potassium permeability of a giant nerve fibre. *J. Physiol.*, **128**:61–88.

HODGKIN, A. L. and KEYNES, R. D. (1956) Experiments on the injection of substances into squid giant axons by means of a microsyringe. *J. Physiol.*, **131**:592–616.

HUTTER, O. F. and TRAUTWEIN, W. (1956) Vagal and sympathetic effects on the pace-maker fibres in the sinus venosus of the heart. *J. gen. Physiol.*, **39**:715–33.

JENKINSON, D. H. and MORTON, I. K. M. (1965) Effects of noradrenaline and isoprenaline on the permeability of depolarized intestinal smooth muscle to inorganic ions. *Nature, Lond.*, **205**:505–6.

JENKINSON, D. H. and MORTON, I. K. M. (1967) The role of α and β-adrenergic receptors in some actions of catecholamines on intestinal smooth muscle. *J. Physiol.*, **188**: 387–402.

KEENAN, MAY J. and NIEDERGERKE, R. (1967) Intracellular sodium concentration and resting sodium fluxes of the frog heart ventricle. *J. Physiol.*, **188**:235–60.

KERNAN, R. P. (1962) Membrane potential changes during sodium transport in frog sartorius muscle. *Nature, Lond.*, **193**:986–7.

KEYNES, R. D. (1951) The ionic movements during nervous activity. *J. Physiol.*, **114**: 119–50.

KEYNES, R. D. (1954) The ionic fluxes in frog muscle. *Proc. Roy. Soc.*, B, **142**:359–82.

KEYNES, R. D. and LEWIS, P. R. (1951) Potassium exchange in nerve. *J. Physiol.*, **113**: 73–98.

KEYNES, R. D. and RYBOVÁ, RENATA (1963) The coupling between sodium and potassium fluxes in frog sartorius muscle. *J. Physiol.*, **168**:58P.

KEYNES, R. D. and SWAN, R. C. (1959) The effect of external sodium concentration on the sodium fluxes in frog skeletal muscle. *J. Physiol.*, **147**:591–625.

LAMB, J. F. and McGUIGAN, J. A. S. (1965) Potassium fluxes in quiescent and beating frog ventricle. Nature, Lond. **205**, 1115–1116.

LAMB, J. F. and McGUIGAN, J. A. S. (1968) The efflux of potassium, sodium, chloride, calcium and sulphate ions and of sorbitol and glycerol during the cardiac cycle in frog's ventricle. *J. Physiol.*, **195**, 283–315.

LAMB, J. F. and McKINNON, M. G. A. (1967) Potassium influx in cultured cells in the presence of ouabaine. *J. Physiol.*, **191**, 33–34p.

LEAF, A. (1960) Some actions of neurohypophyseal hormones on a living membrane. *J. Gen. Physiol.*, **43**:suppl., 175–89.

LEVI, H. and USSING, H. (1948) The exchange of sodium and chloride ions across the fibre membrane of the isolated frog sartorius. *Acta Physiol., Scand.* **16**:232–49.

LOEVINGER, R. and BERMAN, M. (1951) Efficiency criteria in radioactivity counting. *Nucleonics*, **9**:26–39.

MULLINS, L. F and AWAD, M. Z. (1965) The control of the membrane potential of muscle fibres by the sodium pump. *J. Gen. Physiol.*, **48**:761–75.

NIEDERGERKE, R. (1963) Movements of Ca in beating ventricles of the frog heart. *J. Physiol.*, **167**:551–80.

PERSOFF, D. A. (1960) A comparison of methods for measuring efflux of labelled potassium from contracting rabbit atria. *J. Physiol.*, **152**:354–66.

SCHATZMAN, H. J. (1953) Herzglycoside als Hemmstoffe für den aktiven Kalcium und Natrium Transport durch die Erythro-cytenmembran. *Helv. physiol., Acta*, **11**:346–54.

USSING, H. H. (1960) The frog skin potential. *J. Gen. Physiol.*, **43**:suppl., 135–47.

APPENDIX

ISOTOPES USED IN PHARMACOLOGY AND NUCLEAR MEDICINE*

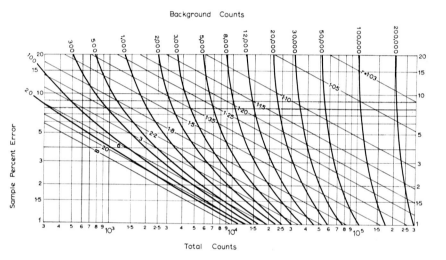

FIG. A1. Optimum Counts Chart. (1) If sample counting rate is > 10 times the background, then the error is √total count. Usually this is converted to the per cent error, e.g. a total count of 900 has an error of ± √900 = ± 30. So the percent is ± 3%. (2) If sample counting rate is < 10 times the background rate, use the graph to minimize the counting time to reach a certain error level

$$\text{Work out } r = \frac{\text{Total count rate}}{\text{Background rate}} \text{ roughly.}$$

Then enter the graph with the desired error and r and read off total counts and background counts required: e.g. if $r = 3$ and error is 3%, then total counts required are 4000 and background counts about 750. (From R. Loevinger and M. Berman, *Nucleonics*, **9** (1), 26–39 (1951) with permission.)

* Compiled by H. J. Glenn and J. F. Lamb.

TABLE 1

Data appearing in Table 1 were generated by consulting catalogs of commercial producers of isotopes and such standard sources of information as:

1. BEHRENS, C. F. and KING, E. R., *Atomic Medicine*, 4th ed., William and Wilkins, Baltimore, Maryland, U.S.A., 1964.
2. GOLDMAN, D. T., *Chart of the Nuclides*, 6th ed., distributed by Educational Relations Department, MWH, General Electric Company, Schenectady, N.Y., U.S.A., 1962.
3. LEDERER, C. M., HOLLANDER, J. M. and PERLMAN, I., *Table of Isotopes*, 6th ed., John Wiley, New York, U.S.A., 1968.
4. WAY, K. (ed.) *Journal of Nuclear Data* (Section B, Nuclear Data Sheets), Academic Press, New York, London.
5. WILSON, B. J. (ed.) *The Radiochemical Manual*, 2nd ed., the Radiochemical Centre, Amersham, England, 1966.

There may be some discrepancies in values from different sources. For more specific details, references (3) and (4) should be consulted.

The following abbreviations are used in Table 1:

d	day (half-life)
d	deuteron (production process)
EC	electron capture
f	fission
h	hour
IT	isomeric transition
m	minute
MeV	million electron volts. All particulate and radiation energies are given in MeV.
n	neutron
p	proton
t	triton
y	year
α	alpha particle
β^-	negative electron; beta particle
β^+	positive electron; positron
γ	gamma photon
%	percentage of the total number of transformations of the nuclide. Only radiation of greater than 1% is usually given.

ISOTOPES USED IN PHARMACOLOGY AND NUCLEAR MEDICINE

Isotope	Half-life	Type of decay and particle energies MeV		γ energies MeV	Production process
Arsenic-74	18 d	β^-	0.72–14.5% 1.36–17.7% 0.91–26.1%	0.635–14.5%	^{71}Ga (α,n) ^{74}As ^{74}Ge $(d,2n)$ ^{74}As
		β^+	1.51–3.6%	0.51 from β^+ 0.596–59.7%	
		EC	38.1%		
Arsenic-76	26.4 h	β^-	0.30–1.9% 1.20–6.6% 1.75–3.6% 2.41–30.6% 2.97–56.4%	0.56–44.6% 0.66–6.3% 1.21–6.2%	^{75}As (n,γ) ^{76}As
Barium-131	12.0 d	EC	100%	0.12–~31% 0.21–~23% 0.24–~5.6% 0.37–~17% 0.50–~56% 0.9 to 1.1–~2.8%	^{130}Ba (n,γ) ^{131}Ba
Bismuth-206	6.3 d	EC	100%	0.18–21% 0.34–25% 0.40–10% 0.50–15% 0.52–40% 0.54–31% 0.803–99%	^{206}Pb $(d,2n)$ ^{206}Bi

TABLE 1 (*cont.*)

Isotope	Half-life	Type of decay and particle energies MeV		γ energies MeV	Production process
Bismuth-206—*cont.*				0.88–68% 0.90–18% 1.02–8% 1.10–12% 1.60–5% 1.72–33%	
Bismuth-210 (Radium E)	5.0 d	α	$5 \times 10^{-5}\%$		^{209}Bi (n,γ) ^{210}Bi
		β^-	1.17–100%		
Bromine-82	35.5 h	β^-	0.46–100%	0.55–65% 0.61–42% 0.70–28% 0.78–83% 0.83–23% 1.04–29% 1.32–28% 1.48–17%	^{81}Br (n,γ) ^{82}Br
Cadmium-109	1.3 y	EC	100%	0.022 0.003 } Ag X-rays 0.088–4%	^{109}Ag (p,n) ^{109}Cd ^{109}Ag (d,2n) ^{109}Cd ^{108}Cd (n,γ) ^{109}Cd
Calcium-45	165 d	β^-	0.254–100%		^{44}Ca (n,γ) ^{45}Ca
Calcium-47	4.5 d	β^-	0.69–82% 2.00–18%	0.50–5.7% 0.81–5.7% 1.31–76.3%	^{46}Ca (n,γ) ^{47}Ca

Isotope	Half-life	Decay	β energy–%	γ energy–%	Production
Carbon-11	20 m	β^+	0.97–100%	0.51 from β^+	^{10}B (d,n) ^{11}C
Carbon-14	5760 y	β^-	0.155–100%		^{14}N (n,p) ^{14}C
Cesium-131	9.7 d	EC	100%	0.030 Xe X-rays 0.004	^{130}Ba (n,γ) ^{131}Ba $\xrightarrow[11.5\mathrm{d}]{\mathrm{EC}}$ ^{131}Cs
Cesium-137	30 y	β^-	0.51–92% 1.17–8%	0.662–86% via 2.6 m ^{137m}Ba	U (n,f) $\to$ ^{137}Cs
Chlorine-36	3×10^5 y	β^- EC	0.714–98.3% 1.7%		^{35}Cl (n,γ) ^{36}Cl
Chromium-51	27.8 d	EC	100%	0.32–~9% 0.005–V X-rays	^{50}Cr (n,γ) ^{51}Cr ^{51}V (d,2n) ^{51}Cr
Cobalt-57	270 d	EC	100%	0.014–8.2% 0.122–88.8% 0.136–8.8%	^{60}Ni (p,a)^{57}Co ^{58}Ni (p,pn) ^{57}Ni $\xrightarrow[37\mathrm{h}]{\mathrm{EC},\beta^-}$ ^{57}Co
Cobalt-58	71 d	β^+ EC	0.48–14.8% 85.2%	0.51 from β^+ 0.81–100%	^{58}Ni (n,p) ^{58}Co
Cobalt-60	5.24 y	β^-	0.31–100%	1.17–100% 1.33–100%	^{59}Co (n,γ) ^{60}Co
Copper-64	12.9 h	β^- β^+ EC	0.57–38% 0.66–19% 43%	0.51 from β^+	^{63}Cu (n,γ) ^{64}Cu ^{64}Ni (d,2n) ^{64}Cu ^{64}Ni (p,n) ^{64}Cu

R.I.P.—T★

TABLE 1 (*cont.*)

Isotope	Half life	Type of decay and particle energies MeV		γ energies MeV	Production process
Copper-67	61 h	β^-	0.40–45% 0.48–35% 0.58–20%	$\left.\begin{matrix}0.090\\0.092\end{matrix}\right\}24\%$ 0.182–44%	^{64}Ni $(\alpha,p)\,^{67}$Cu
Fluorine-18	110 m	β^+ EC	0.649–97% 3%	0.51 from β^+	^{16}O $(\alpha,np)\,^{18}$F ^{16}O $(t,n)\,^{18}$F
Gallium-68	68 m	β^+ EC	0.82–1% 1.89–86% 13%	0.51 from β^+ 1.08–4%	^{69}Ga $(p,2n)\,^{68}$Ge $\xrightarrow[280\text{d}]{\text{EC}}\,^{68}$Ga
Germanium-68	280 d	EC	100%	0.0092–Ga X-rays	^{69}Ga $(p,2n)\,^{68}$Ge
Gold-198	2.70 d	β^-	0.29–1.2% 0.96–98.8%	0.412–95.8% 0.68–1.0%	^{197}Au $(n,\gamma)\,^{198}$Au
Gold-199	3.15 d	β^-	0.25–23% 0.30–70% 0.46–7%	0.158–38.2% 0.208–9.4%	^{198}Pt $(n,\gamma)\,^{199}$Pt $\xrightarrow[30\text{m}]{\beta}\,^{199}$Au
Hydrogen-3 (Tritium)	12.26 y	β^-	0.018–100%		^{6}Li $(n,\alpha)\,^{3}$H
Indium-113m	1.7 h			0.39–67%	Daughter, ^{113}Sn
Iodine-123	13 h	EC	100%	0.16–84% 0.027–Te X-rays	^{121}Sb $(\alpha,2n)\,^{123}$I

Isotope	Half-life	Decay			Production
Iodine-125	60 d	EC	100%	0.035–7% 0.027–Te X-rays (138%)	^{124}Xe (n,γ) ^{125}Xe $\xrightarrow{\beta}$ ^{125}I 18h
Iodine-131	8.05 d	β⁻	0.25–2.8% 0.33–9.3% 0.61–87.2%	0.08–2.2% 0.28–6.3% 0.36–79% 0.64–9.3% 0.72–2.8%	^{130}Te (n,γ) ^{131}Te $\xrightarrow{\beta}$ ^{131}I 25m
Iodine-132	2.3 h	β⁻	0.80–21% 1.04–15% 1.22–12% 1.49–12% 1.61–21% 2.14–18%	0.38–4.8% 0.52–21.5% 0.62–5.2% 0.65–26.0% 0.67–100% 0.72–6.5% 0.78–84.0% 0.95–21.0% 1.14–5% 1.30–4% 1.39–8.5%	^{131}Te U (n,f) U (n,f) → ^{123}Te $\xrightarrow{\beta}$ ^{132}I 78h
Iridium-192	74 d	β⁻ EC	0.24–7.6% 0.54–41.8% 0.67–46.8% 4.6%	0.296–26% 0.308–29% 0.316–73% 0.468–47% 0.588–5% 0.605–9% 0.613–6%	^{191}Ir (n,γ) ^{192}Ir
Iron-52	8 h	β⁺ EC	0.80–~57% ~43%	0.51 from β⁺ 0.165–100%	^{52}Cr (α,4n) ^{52}Fe

TABLE 1 (*cont.*)

Isotope	Half life	Type of decay and particle energies MeV	γ energies MeV	Production process
Iron-55	2.9 y	EC 100%	0.0059–Mn X-rays	^{54}Fe (n,γ) ^{55}Fe ^{55}Mn (p,n) ^{55}Fe
Iron-59	45 d	β^- 0.13–1% 0.27–46% 0.46–53%	0.19–2.4% 1.10–57% 1.29–43%	^{58}Fe (n,γ) ^{59}Fe
Krypton-85	10.4 y	β^- 0.67–99.3%	0.54–0.7%	U (n,f) → ^{85}Kr
Lead-210 (Radium D)	22y	β^- 0.017–85% 0.063–15%	0.047–4.1% 0.010–Bi X-rays	Naturally occurring radioisotope
Manganese-54	314 d	EC 100%	0.84–100%	^{54}Fe (n,p) ^{54}Mn
Mercury-197	65 h	EC 100%	0.077–19.3% 0.069–Au X-rays (74.5%)	^{196}Hg (n,γ) ^{197}Hg
Mercury-203	47 d	β^- 0.21–100%	0.279–81.5%	^{202}Hg (n,γ) ^{203}Hg
Molybdenum-99	67 h	β^- 0.45–14% 1.23–85%	0.14–4.6% 0.18–4.5% 0.74–10.0% 0.78–4.0%	^{98}Mo (n,γ) ^{99}Mo U (n,f) → ^{99}Mo

	Half-life	Mode	β or α energies (MeV)-%	γ energies (MeV)-%	Production
Nitrogen-13	10 m	β^+	1.2-100%	0.51 from β^+	^{12}C (d,n) ^{13}N
Oxygen-15	2.0 m	β^+	1.7-100%	0.51 from β^+	^{14}N (d,n) ^{15}O
Palladium-103	17 d	EC	~100%	Rh X-rays	^{102}Pd (n,γ) ^{103}Pd ^{103}Rh (d,2n) ^{103}Pd
Phosphorus-32	14.3 d	β^-	1.71-100%		^{31}P (n,γ) ^{32}P ^{32}S (n,p) ^{32}P
Polonium-210 (Radium F)	138.4 d	α	5.30-~100%	0.8-0.0012%	^{209}Bi (n,γ) ^{210}Bi $\xrightarrow[5.01\text{d}]{\beta}$ ^{210}Po
Potassium-42	12.4 h	β^-	2.0-18% 3.6-82%	1.52-18%	^{41}K (n,γ) ^{42}K
Radium-226	1620 y	α	4.59-5.7% 4.78-94.3%	0.188-~4%	Naturally occurring radioisotope
Rhenium-186	88.9 h	β^- EC	0.93-95% 1.06-95% 5%	0.137-9% W, Os X-rays	^{185}Re (n,γ) ^{186}Re
Rhenium-188	17 h	β^-	low energy groups-~2% 1.96-20% 2.12-78%	0.155-10.5% and others Os X-rays	^{187}Re (n,γ) ^{188}Re
Rubidium-84	33 d	β^- β^+ EC	0.91-3.2% 0.8-10.9% 1.63-9.7% 76.3%	0.51 from β^+ 0.88-73.4%	^{81}Br (α,n) ^{84}Rb

TABLE 1 (*cont.*)

Isotope	Half life	Type of decay and particle energies MeV		γ energies MeV	Production process
Rubidium-86	18.7 d	β^-	0.68–8.5% 1.77–91.5%	1.08–8.5%	^{85}Rb (n,γ) ^{86}Rb
Scandium-46	84 d	β^-	0.36–99.5%	0.89–99.5% 1.12–100%	^{45}Sc (n,γ) ^{46}Sc
Selenium-75	120 d	EC	100%	0.096–3% 0.12–15% 0.14–54% 0.20–1.5% 0.27–56% 0.28–23% 0.31–1.4% 0.40–12.5%	^{74}Se (n,γ) ^{75}Se
Sodium-22	2.6 y	β^+ EC	0.54–90.5% 9.5%	0.51 from β^+ 1.28–100%	^{24}Mg (d,α) ^{22}Na
Sodium-24	15.0 h	β^-	1.39–100%	1.37–100% 2.75–100%	^{23}Na (n,γ) ^{24}Na
Strontium-85	64 d	EC	100%	0.51–100%	^{84}Sr (n,γ) ^{85}Sr ^{85}Rb (d,2n) ^{85}Sr

Nuclide	Half-life	Decay mode	%	Energy–%	Production
Strontium-87m	2.8 h	IT	99.35%	0.388–78%	$^{86}Sr\,(n,\gamma)\,^{87m}Sr$
		EC	0.65%		$^{85}Rb\,(\alpha,2n)\,^{87m}Y + {}^{87}Y \xrightarrow{EC} {}^{87m}Sr$ 80h
Strontium-90	28 y	β^-	0.54–100%		$U\,(n,f) \rightarrow {}^{90}Sr$
Sulfur-35	87.2 d	β^-	0.167–100%		$^{35}Cl\,(n,p)\,^{35}S$ $^{34}S\,(n,\gamma)\,^{35}S$
Technetium-99m	6 h	IT	100%	0.140–90.1%	$^{98}Mo\,(n,\gamma)\,^{99}Mo \xrightarrow{\beta} {}^{99m}Tc$ 67h
Tin-113	118 d	EC	100%	0.39–67% via 104 m ^{113m}In	$^{112}Sn\,(n,\gamma)\,^{113}Sn$
Xenon-133	5.3 d	β^-	0.34–~99%	0.081–35.5% 0.16–~0.5%	$U\,(n,f) \rightarrow {}^{133}Xe$
Yttrium-90	64.2 h	β^-	2.27–100%		$^{89}Y\,(n,\gamma)\,^{90}Y$ Daughter of ^{90}Sr
Zinc-65	245 d	β^+ EC	0.325–2% 98%	0.51 from β^+ 1.11–49%	$^{64}Zn\,(n,\gamma)\,^{65}Zn$ $^{65}Cu\,(p,n)\,^{65}Zn$ $^{65}Cu\,(d,2n)\,^{65}Zn$

TABLE A1. CHARACTERISTICS OF COMMONLY USED ISOTOPES*

Isotope	Half-life	Type of decay and particle energies MeV		γ energies MeV
Bromine-82	35.4 hr	β^-	0.44–100%	0.55–65% 0.62–42% 0.70–28% 0.78–83% 0.83–23% 1.04–29% 1.32–28% 1.48–17%
Calcium-45	165 days	β^-	0.254–100%	
Calcium-47	4.7 days	β^-	0.69–82% 2.00–18%	0.50–5.7% 0.81–5.7% 1.31–76.3%
Chlorine-36	3×10^5 years	β^- EC	0.714–98.3% 1.7%	
Iodine-131	8.04 days	β^-	0.25–2.8% 0.33–9.3% 0.61–87.2% 0.81–0.7%	0.08–2.2% 0.28–6.3% 0.36–79% 0.64–9.3% 0.72–2.8%
Potassium-42	12.4 hr	β^-	2.0–18% 3.6–82%	0.32–weak 1.52–18%
Rubidium-86	18.7 days	β^-	0.68–8.5% 1.77–91.5%	1.08–8.5%
Sodium-22	2.6 years	β^+ EC	0.54–90.5% 1.83–~0.06% 9.5%	0.51 from β^+ 1.28–100%
Sodium-24	15.0 hr	β^-	1.39–100%	1.37–100% 2.75–100%
Carbon-14	5760 years	β^-	0.159–100%	
Sulfur-35	87.2 days	β^-	0.167–100%	

* From *The Radiochemical Manual*, 2nd edition, 1966, the Radiochemical Centre Amersham, with permission.

TABLE A2. DECAY CORRECTIONS FOR Na-24, K-42 AND Ca-47 FOR 24 HOURS

t = elapsed time in hours (hr) or minutes (min). Correction factor is the ratio of amount of isotope initially to amount left not disintegrated after time t. To convert all counts back to the start of the experiment multiply each count by the factor appropriate to the elapsed time.

Na-24 and K-42 data reproduced from *Documenta Geigy, Scientific Tables*, 6th edition, by permission of J. R. Geigy, S.A., Basle, Switzerland.

| t | | Correction factor | | |
hr	min	Na-24	K-42	Ca-47
0	00	1.000	1.000	1.000
	10	1.007	1.009	
	20	1.015	1.018	
	30	1.023	1.028	
	40	1.031	1.037	
	50	1.039	1.047	
1	00	1.047	1.057	1.007
	10	1.055	1.066	
	20	1.063	1.076	
	30	1.071	1.086	
	40	1.080	1.096	
	50	1.088	1.107	
2	00	1.096	1.117	1.013
	10	1.105	1.127	
	20	1.113	1.138	
	30	1.122	1.148	
	40	1.131	1.159	
	50	1.139	1.170	
3	00	1.148	1.180	1.019
	10	1.157	1.191	
	20	1.166	1.203	
	30	1.175	1.214	

| t | | Correction factor | | |
hr	min	Na-24	K-42	Ca-47
8	00	1.447	1.558	1.051
	10	1.458	1.572	
	20	1.469	1.587	
	30	1.481	1.602	
	40	1.492	1.617	
	50	1.504	1.632	
9	00	1.515	1.647	1.057
	10	1.527	1.662	
	20	1.539	1.677	
	30	1.551	1.693	
	40	1.563	1.709	
	50	1.575	1.725	
10	00	1.587	1.741	1.064
	10	1.599	1.757	
	20	1.612	1.773	
	30	1.624	1.790	
	40	1.637	1.806	
	50	1.649	1.823	
11	00	1.662	1.840	1.070
	10	1.675	1.857	
	20	1.688	1.874	
	30	1.701	1.892	

| t | | Correction factor | | |
hr	min	Na-24	K-42	Ca-47
16	00	2.094	2.428	1.103
	10	2.110	2.450	
	20	2.127	2.473	
	30	2.143	2.496	
	40	2.160	2.519	
	50	2.176	2.543	
17	00	2.193	2.566	1.110
	10	2.210	2.590	
	20	2.227	2.614	
	30	2.244	2.639	
	40	2.262	2.663	
	50	2.279	2.688	
18	00	2.297	2.713	1.117
	10	2.315	2.738	
	20	2.333	2.763	
	30	2.351	2.789	
	40	2.369	2.815	
	50	2.387	2.841	
19	00	2.406	2.867	1.124
	10	2.424	2.894	
	20	2.443	2.921	
	30	2.462	2.948	

TABLE A2 (cont.)

t (hr)	t (min)	Na-24	K-42	Ca-47
3	40	1.184	1.225	
	50	1.193	1.236	
	00	1.203	1.248	
4	10	1.212	1.259	
	20	1.221	1.271	1.025
	30	1.231	1.283	
	40	1.240	1.295	
	50	1.250	1.307	
5	00	1.259	1.319	
	10	1.269	1.331	
	20	1.279	1.344	1.031
	30	1.289	1.356	
	40	1.299	1.369	
	50	1.309	1.381	
6	00	1.319	1.394	
	10	1.329	1.407	
	20	1.339	1.420	1.038
	30	1.350	1.433	
	40	1.360	1.447	
	50	1.371	1.460	
7	00	1.381	1.474	
	10	1.392	1.487	
	20	1.403	1.501	1.044
	30	1.414	1.515	
	40	1.425	1.529	
	50	1.436	1.543	

t (hr)	t (min)	Na-24	K-42	Ca-47
11	40	1.714	1.909	
	50	1.727	1.927	
12	00	1.741	1.945	
	10	1.754	1.963	
	20	1.768	1.981	1.076
	30	1.781	2.000	
	40	1.795	2.018	
	50	1.809	2.037	
13	00	1.823	2.056	
	10	1.837	2.075	
	20	1.851	2.094	1.083
	30	1.866	2.114	
	40	1.880	2.133	
	50	1.895	2.153	
14	00	1.909	2.173	
	10	1.924	2.193	
	20	1.939	2.214	1.090
	30	1.954	2.234	
	40	1.969	2.255	
	50	1.984	2.276	
15	00	2.000	2.297	
	10	2.015	2.318	
	20	2.031	2.340	1.096
	30	2.046	2.361	
	40	2.062	2.383	
	50	2.078	2.406	

t (hr)	t (min)	Na-24	K-42	Ca-47
19	40	2.481	2.975	
	50	2.500	3.003	
20	00	2.519	3.031	
	10	2.539	3.059	
	20	2.558	3.087	1.131
	30	2.578	3.116	
	40	2.598	3.145	
	50	2.618	3.174	
21	00	2.639	3.204	
	10	2.659	3.234	
	20	2.679	3.264	1.138
	30	2.700	3.294	
	40	2.721	3.324	
	50	2.742	3.355	
22	00	2.763	3.386	
	10	2.785	3.418	
	20	2.806	3.450	1.145
	30	2.828	3.482	
	40	2.850	3.514	
	50	2.872	3.547	
23	00	2.894	3.580	
	10	2.916	3.613	
	20	2.939	3.646	1.152
	30	2.962	3.680	
	40	2.985	3.714	
	50	3.008	3.749	
24	00	3.031	3.784	

AUTHOR INDEX

SUBJECT INDEX